AF147868

MEDICAL RADIOLOGY
Diagnostic Imaging

Editors:
A. L. Baert, Leuven
K. Sartor, Heidelberg

Springer-Verlag Berlin Heidelberg GmbH

J. N. Bruneton (Ed.)

In Collaboration with C. Raffaelli and O. Dassonville

Applications of Sonography in Head and Neck Pathology

With Contributions by

N. Amoretti · C. Arens · J. N. Bruneton · P. Brunner · B. Carlotti · P. Chevallier
O. Dassonville · C. Garel · A. Geoffray · N. Lassau · R. Lecesne · L. Leenhardt
T. Livraghi · P.-Y. Marcy · D. Matter · F. Meloni · M.-Y. Mourou · B. Padovani
G. Poissonnet · C. Raffaelli · J. Tramalloni · C. Tran · F. Tranquart · J. Viateau-Poncin

Translated from French into English by Nancy Reed-Rameau

Preface by
F. Weill

Foreword by
A. L. Baert

With 391 Figures in 716 Separate Illustrations, 272 in Color

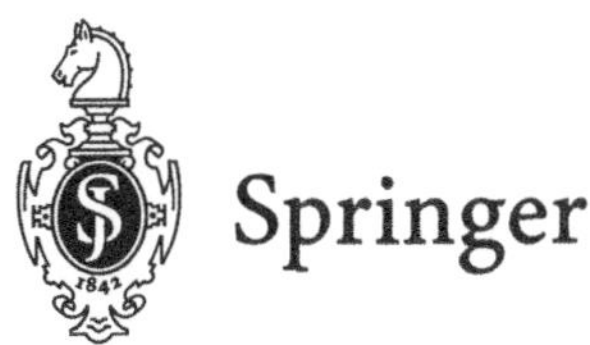

Springer

Jean Noël Bruneton, MD
Professor, Centre Régional de Lutte contre le Cancer
Centre Antoine-Lacassagne
Service de Radiodiagnostic
33, avenue de Valombrose
06189 Nice Cedex 2
France

Collaborators:

Charles P. Raffaelli, MD
Service de Radiodiagnostic
Hôpital Pasteur
30, avenue Voie Romaine, BP 69
06002 Nice Cedex 1
France

Olivier Dassonville, MD
Départment d'ORL
Centre Antoine-Lacassagne
33 avenue de Valombrose
06189 Nice Cedex 2
France

Translator:

Nancy Reed-Rameau
Villa Patricia
10 avenue Thérèse
06000 Nice
France

Medical Radiology · Diagnostic Imaging and Radiation Oncology
Continuation of
Handbuch der medizinischen Radiologie
Encyclopedia of Medical Radiology

ISBN 978-3-540-65498-8

Library of Congress Cataloging-in-Publication Data
Applications of sonography in head and neck pathology / J.N. Bruneton (ed.), in collaboration with C. Raffaelli and O. Dassonville ; with contributions by N. Amoretti ... [et al.] ; translated from French into English by Nancy Reed-Rameau ; preface by F. Weill ; foreword by A. L. Baert.
p. ; cm. -- (Medical radiology)
Includes bibliographical references and index.
ISBN 978-3-540-65498-8 ISBN 978-3-642-56213-6 (eBook)
DOI 10.1007/978-3-642-56213-6
1. Neck--Ultrasonic imaging. 2. Head--Ultrasonic imaging. I. Bruneton, J. N. II. Raffaelli, C. (Charles) III. Dassonville, O. (Oliver) IV. Series.
[DNLM: 1. Head--pathology. 2. Head--ultrasonography. 3. Neck--pathology. 4. Neck--ultrasonography. 5. Ultrasonography--methods. WE 705 A6527 2002a]
RC936 .A65 2002
617.5'107543--dc21 2001034200

http//www.springer.de

Originally published by Springer-Verlag Berlin Heidelberg New York in 2002

Cover-Design and Typesetting: Verlagsservice Teichmann, 69256 Mauer

SPIN: 107 099 57 21/3130 – 5 4 3 2 1 0 – Printed on acid-free paper

Foreword

Sonography, by virtue of its noninvasive nature, is used more and more in modern medicine as the first imaging modality for adults and children presenting with unexplained cervical mass lesions as well as for the study of the carotid arteries and jugular veins.

Remarkable advances have been achieved in ultrasound technology during the past 10 years, including color Doppler, power Doppler and the clinical use of new specific contrast agents . This technical progress has opened new and highly interesting diagnostic pathways for the study of a great variety of mass lesions affecting the various organs and anatomic areas of the head and neck region.

This book intends to provided the latest, much-needed update of our knowledge on the diagnostic potential of sonography in the cervical region and constitutes a very welcome addition to our series "Medical Radiology", which aims to cover all important clinical imaging fields of modern diagnostic radiology. It will be of great interest for general and specialized radiologists, for pediatricians, and for vascular and head and neck surgeons.

Professor J. N. Bruneton and his team in Nice are very well known experts in the field and they have, over the years, accumulated unique experience and a wealth of information on head and neck pathology as visualized with sonography. I would like to congratulate the editor and all contributors to this volume most sincerely for their outstanding work; the content is comprehensive, the illustrations superb.

I would be pleased to receive any constructive criticism or comments that readers may like to express.

Leuven ALBERT L. BAERT

Preface

Almost 25 years ago, I had the pleasure of showing Jean-Noel Bruneton, then an enthusiastic student, the first detailed pictures of thyroid nodules which had become available thanks to a new generation of gray-scale machines with high-frequency, handheld transducers. Today, Prof. Bruneton, a well-known workaholic, has become one of the most distinguished specialists in this field. After 8 years of retirement, far away from ultrasound screens, I can measure the extent of the technical and clinical progress achieved in recent years. Immense changes have occurred since we first visualized thyroid nodules 25 years ago. This book by Prof. Bruneton and his associates should be considered a milestone in thyroid, parathyroid, and components of the neck, including vessels, and associated pathologies. The authors employ all of the new technical modalities now available: high-definition gray scale, enhanced color Doppler, and ultrasound contrast agents. In the nine chapters the reader will find detailed morphological descriptions of numerous pathological processes, followed by thorough discussions of differential diagnosis. When appropriate, the rationale for selection of the best complementary procedures is proposed: fine-needle aspiration for thyroid nodules, for instance, thallium MIBI for parathyroid lesions, MRI for salivary gland disease, etc. The last chapter is devoted to cervical sonography in pediatrics. Cervical ultrasound has become a wide diagnostic field requiring, if not dedicated specialization, at least thorough postgraduate education: this is precisely what this comprehensive book permits. Readers will be grateful to its authors.

Francis Weill, MD
Professor Emeritus of Radiology
Former President of the WFUMB

Contents

1 Thyroid Gland

Jean Noël Bruneton, Tito Livraghi, Jocelyne Viateau-Poncin, Laurence Leenhardt, Jean Tramalloni

CONTENTS

J.N. Bruneton, MD
Service de Radiologie, Hôpital de l'Archet, 151, route de St.-Antoine Ginestière, B.P. 3079, F-06202 Nice Cedex 3, France
T. Livraghi, MD
Unita Raiologia, Ospedale Civile, Via C. Battisti, 23, I-20059 Vimercate (MI), Italy
J. Viateau-Poncin, MD
Clinique d'Aulnay, 28-36 avenue du 14 Juillet, F-93604 Aulnay-sous-Bois Cedex, France
L. Leenhardt, MD
Service Central de Médecine Nucléaire, Hôpital La Pitié-Salpêtrière, 83 Boulevard de l'Hôpital, F-75013 Paris, France
J. Tramalloni, MD
Cabinet de Radiologie, 25 rue du Docteur Paul Bruel, F-95350 Louvres, France

Evaluation of the thyroid gland is required in a number of clinical situations (Freitas and Freitas 1994): clinically solitary thyroid nodule, superior mediastinal mass, hyperthyroidism, diagnosis and postoperative follow-up of thyroid carcinoma, neonatal hypo-thyroidism, and anomalous thyroid development. For Gharib (1997), the main indications for ultrasound (US) in thyroid disease are determination of goiter size, evaluation of acute thyroiditis, difficulty in thyroid palpation, US-guided aspiration biopsy, US-guided percutaneous ethanol injection (PEI), diagnosis of thyroglossal duct cysts, and postoperative surveillance of thyroid carcinoma.

As the imaging modality of choice for assessment of thyroid morphology, sonography can generally determine the number and location of thyroid lesions and rule out nonthyroid pathologies. US facilitates the follow-up of treated patients and is less expensive than other imaging techniques. The technique also plays an essential role in nodular thyroid disease, in particular in the guidance of fine-needle aspiration (FNA) and surveillance of thyroid nodules not treated surgically (Barraclough and Barraclough 2000; Mirk et al. 1999; Sakaguchi et al. 2000).

1.1 Ultrasound Techniques for Thyroid Examination

For clinicians worldwide, US has become the first-line imaging modality for the thyroid (Massol et al. 1993). In addition to detection and accurate localization of thyroid nodules, US is highly effective in the guidance of FNA and in post-therapy follow-up (Bruneton et al. 1996; Reading and Gorman 1993).

Currently available US units equipped with high-frequency transducers (7.5–13 MHz) provide images of remarkable clarity. However, this increase in transducer frequency does not always allow examination of the entire gland in patients with a large goiter. In contrast, high resolution permits detailed analysis of thyroid nodules and visualization of normal laterocervical lymph nodes (Bruneton et al. 1994a). The data provided by US have not changed significantly over the past decade (Bruneton et al. 1996), but state-of-the art equipment allows identification of previously unrecognized anatomic structures, such as the laryngeal nerve (Solbiati et al. 1995).

1.1.1 Anatomy and Gray-Scale Imaging

1.1.1.1 Thyroid Gland

The thyroid is an endocrine gland located in the infrahyoid region of the anterior neck; its concave posterior surface lies against the anterolateral surfaces of the larynx and the first tracheal rings. The thyroid gland consists of paired lateral lobes connected by a midline bridge of tissue, the isthmus, at the junction of the lower and middle thirds of the gland.

The lateral lobes are shaped like triangular pyramids with their summit directed upward; they present three surfaces (anterior, medial, posterior), three borders (anterior, posterolateral, posteromedial), and two extremities (a narrow apex cephalad and a thicker base caudad).

Ultrasound allows volumetric analysis of the thyroid lobes. Each lobe can be considered a spheroid whose volume (v) is given by:

$$V = pi/6 + height + width + depth$$

Thyroid volume and gland diameters vary considerably. In normal adults, the height ranges from 4 to 6 cm and the width from 1 to 2 cm. The anteroposterior dimension is a particularly interesting parameter because it is relatively constant from one individual to another. An anteroposterior diameter greater than 2 cm suggests an underlying pathology not visible by US. Anteroposterior diameters greater than 2.5 cm are frankly abnormal, regardless of the results of morphological analysis of the gland. Thyroid volume can be determined from contiguous scans (mean, 10±4 ml) (Yokoyama et al. 1988; Jarlov et al. 1991).

Jarlov et al. (1993) underscored the problem of interobserver variation in interpretation of sonographically determined volumetric data (the kappa value for interobserver agreement ranges between 0.5 and 0.6). Interobserver agreement for measurement of nodules appears satisfactory, as variation did not exceed 6% for Bennedbaek et al. (1998). Berghout et al. (1987) and Hegedus et al. (1986) reported a similar concordance for measurement of thyroid volume, with variation ranging from 8% to 10%. For Wesche et al. (1998), measurement of thyroid volume using transverse scans at 5-mm intervals and measurement of the planimetric surface is more accurate than calculation of thyroid lobe volume by the ellipsoid formula (height + width + depth + pi/6), which underestimates thyroid size because the lobes tend to be elongated rather than spherical or oval (YEH et al. 1996). When a lobe appears triangular or rectangular on transverse scans, pi/6 must be replaced by 1. Thyroid enlargement may be suggested by bulging of the anterior aspect of the thyroid and thickening of the isthmus. This feature should be sought using sagittal scans, because the anterior border of the thyroid gland is normally concave or rectilinear.

The essential problem is not measurement of thyroid gland volume but rather determination of normal range limits. The mean volume in cubic centimeters (which generally corresponds to the weight in grams) varies as a function of the geographic area. In iodine-replete populations, for example, the mean weight of the normal thyroid is 10 g, with a maximum of 20 g. These values contrast with the normal volumes reported in the past century (20–25 g, with a maximum of 30 g) (LANGER 1999).

The base of each thyroid lobe is directed inferiorly to within 1 or 2 cm of the sternum, but this position varies from one individual to another. The base of one or both lobes may be located even lower, at the level of the cervicothoracic junction; this renders examination more difficult and requires considerable hyperextension of the neck for proper exploration. In other individuals, the base of one or both lobes lies higher up in the neck, 4–5 cm above the sternum; this is relatively frequent in young women.

Finally, the thyroid lobes are often slightly asymmetrical, with the right lobe tending to be larger than the left. Moreover, lobes are not always both located at the same level in the neck, and this can create a false impression of asymmetry on transverse scans. The isthmus varies from 1 to 2 cm in height. The pyramidal lobe (Lalouette's pyramid) is an inconstant conical structure projecting upward from the isthmus, either along the midline or off to one side, anterior to the thyroid cartilage.

Transverse, longitudinal, and in certain cases coronal scans allow assessment of the thyroid gland.

Thyroid tissue has a highly uniform, solid US pattern consisting of a dense agglomerate of very fine small echoes of equal size (Fig. 1.1). High-frequency transducers can sometimes demonstrate intrathyroid vessels as small rounded structures on scans perpendicular to the axis of the vessel or as small linear structures on scans parallel to the axis of the vessel. The isthmus is always well-visualized by US, especially when a high-frequency transducer or water bath is used. By contrast, the normal pyramidal lobe is rarely seen, owing to its small anteroposterior diameter (Fig. 1.2).

A decrease in thyroid volume is common in the elderly, as are modifications in the echotexture, which becomes discretely homogeneous, combining variable proportions of anechoic colloid zones and small areas of fibrosis. These modifications do not signify a pathological condition (GONCZI et al. 1994).

SZABOLCS et al. (1997) share this opinion, and confirmed that a hypoechoic pattern is not predictive of thyroid dysfunction in the elderly. ANDERSEN-RANBERG et al. (1999) reported US demonstration of a small thyroid gland in individuals aged 100 years (median volume 8.3 ml), but only 26% of the subjects in their unselected population had morphological alterations at US.

In children, the thyroid increases in volume between the ages of 7 and 16 years, then stabilizes, with the mean volume rising from 4.34±1.55 ml to 13.6±6.2 ml at puberty. Thyroid volume is greater in girls than in boys (MULLER-LEISSE et al. 1988). During pregnancy, the thyroid increases in size starting in the first trimester, and continues to enlarge until the end of pregnancy. This increase in volume does not exceed 50% for SMYTH et al. (1997). A pathological factor may accelerate the morphological phenomena of aging at the level of the thyroid: Chronic alcoholism, for example, is associated with both a decrease in thyroid volume and an increase in fibrosis (HEGEDUS 1990).

1.1.1.2
Anterior and Posteromedial Relations

The anterior relations of the thyroid lobe are common to the lateral lobes, the isthmus, and the parathyroid glands.

The superficial covering consists of skin, the platysma, and subcutaneous tissue. Sonographically, this covering corresponds to a thin, highly echogenic band averaging 2 mm in thickness; exact thickness depends on the person's weight. A stratified appearance is fairly common in obese individuals.

The investing layer of the deep cervical fascia forms a sheath encasing the sternocleidomastoid muscles laterally. These muscles are always well-visualized by US; although variable in thickness, they can be recognized by their elongated shape anterior to the lateral aspect of the thyroid lobes. The anteroinferior extremity of these muscles is located to one side of the midline. This investing layer of the cervical fascia contains the anterior jugular veins. Regardless of their thickness, the sternocleidomastoid mus-

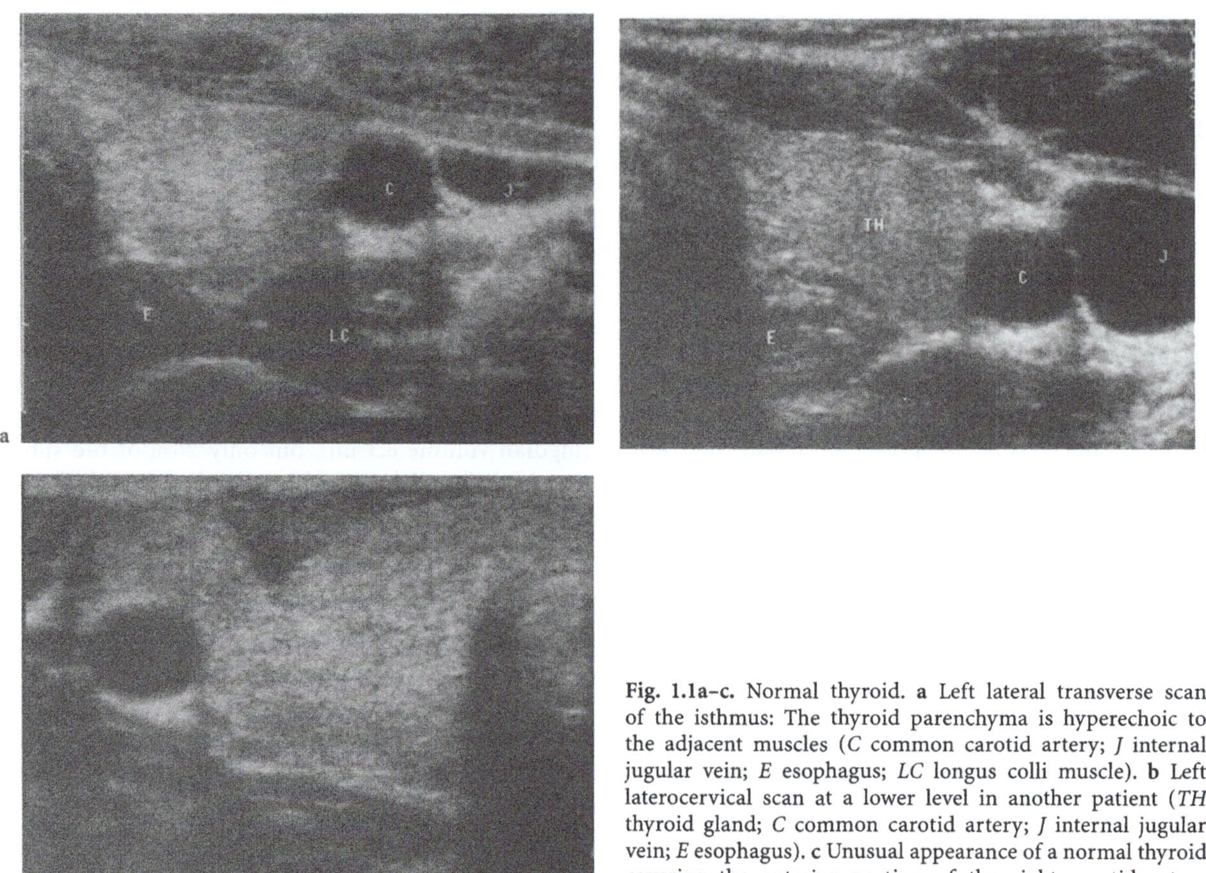

Fig. 1.1a–c. Normal thyroid. **a** Left lateral transverse scan of the isthmus: The thyroid parenchyma is hyperechoic to the adjacent muscles (*C* common carotid artery; *J* internal jugular vein; *E* esophagus; *LC* longus colli muscle). **b** Left laterocervical scan at a lower level in another patient (*TH* thyroid gland; *C* common carotid artery; *J* internal jugular vein; *E* esophagus). **c** Unusual appearance of a normal thyroid covering the anterior portion of the right carotid artery (transverse scan)

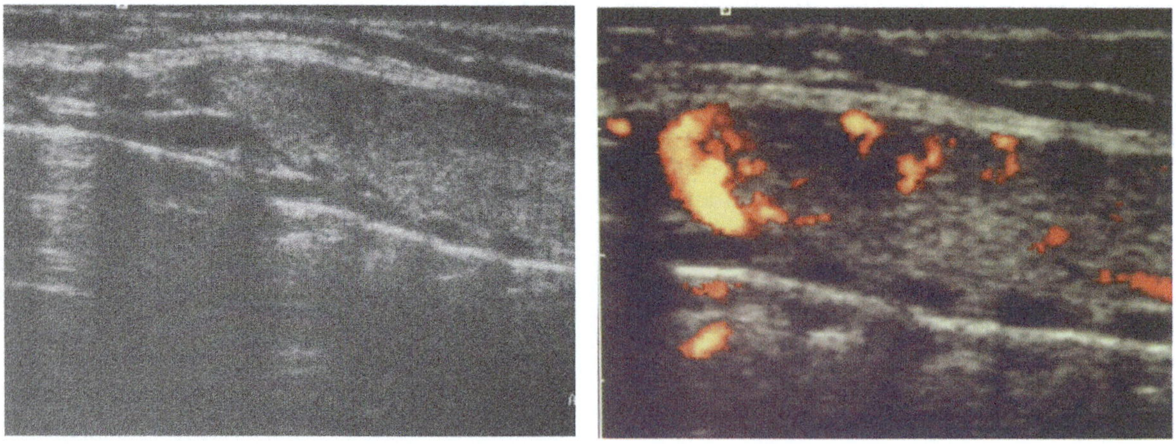

a b

Fig. 1.2a,b. Pyramidal lobe of the thyroid. **a** Sagittal scan. **b** Power Doppler (sagittal scan)

cles have a solid US pattern that is markedly less echogenic than the normal thyroid gland. This difference is of practical use for comparative analysis of the thyroid gland, in particular in cases of diffuse thyroid hypoechogenicity such as occur with thyroiditis.

Ying et al. (1998) compared the echogenicity of the thyroid gland with that of the sternocleidomastoid muscle using a transmission densitometer. The healthy thyroid was hyperechoic to the sternocleidomastoid muscle in all normal individuals, but the gland was relatively hyperechoic in only 70% of patients with thyrotoxicosis and 47% with thyroiditis. Despite the significant difference in relative echogenicity between the normal and the pathological thyroid, the hypoechogenicity observed in thyrotoxicosis and thyroiditis is not significantly different. An image density difference of less than 0.1 can be considered abnormal, while a value of more than 0.83 can be considered normal.

In addition to enclosing the sternocleidomastoid muscles, this investing fascial layer surrounds the trapezius muscle and forms the roof of the posterior cervical triangle, enclosing the omohyoid muscle; it also covers the infrahyoid muscles, forming the roof of the anterior triangle. This muscular layer is particularly well-visualized in patients with a muscular neck. The US image, similar to that of the sternocleidomastoid muscles, corresponds to a hypoechogenic band anterior and lateral to the thyroid lobes.

The posteromedial relations of the thyroid gland involve the thyroid lobes, the gastrointestinal tract, and the major neurovascular bundle.

The medial surface of the thyroid lobes is related, from front to back, to the upper airway (larynx and trachea) and to the pharynx and esophagus. These anatomic structures can be identified on sonograms as a very dense echogenic line, corresponding to the anterior wall, next to an acoustic shadow representing the air-filled cavity.

The gastrointestinal tract is represented by the inferior constrictor muscle of the pharynx and the esophagus. The esophagus crosses over the trachea on the left side and can be seen at the posteromedial border of the left thyroid lobe. The esophagus is well-visualized sonographically as a semicircular bull's-eye with a hyperechogenic center and less echogenic contours; the hyperechogenic area corresponds to the esophageal lumen and the less echogenic peripheral structure to the esophageal wall. This image is inconstant and visible to varying degrees depending on the subject. Particular care must be taken not to mistake an esophageal deviation on the left side of the neck for a cervical mass, and in particular a parathyroid gland. The mobility of this structure can be examined in real-time by having the patient swallow during scanning.

The posterior surface of the thyroid lobes is related to the cervical vertebrae, the longus colli muscle, and the major neurovascular bundle. From front to back are visualized sonographically the dense interface of the anterior surface of the cervical vertebrae, then the transversally elongated longus colli muscle, that is only slightly echogenic. The longus colli muscle may be shaped either like a trapezoid, with its largest base directed outwards, or like a triangle with its apex directed medially. This muscle is bounded anteriorly by the interface formed by the deep layer of the cervical fascia. In contrast to those muscles related to the thyroid gland anteriorly, the longus colli muscle is an important anatomic landmark for cervical US, yet it may be difficult or impossible to visualize in individuals with muscular atrophy (elderly patients or those with a neurologic pathology).

The major neurovascular bundle comprises the common carotid artery (with the internal carotid artery and external carotid artery located cephalad), the internal jugular vein (lateral to the artery and more or less spontaneously visible), and the vagus nerve. The sheath enclosing the major neurovascular bundle cannot be seen sonographically, but the common carotid artery is always recognizable on transverse scans as an anechoic circle with a solid circumference. Transverse scans provide a sectional view of the internal jugular vein external to the carotid artery. As the internal jugular vein is not always visible spontaneously, a Valsalva maneuver must be performed systematically; the resultant venous dilatation allows satisfactory examination. The vagus nerve lies in the posterior angle of the common carotid artery and the internal jugular vein and can be visualized by US.

The posteromedial border of the thyroid lobes is intimately related to the recurrent laryngeal nerve and the inferior thyroid pedicle. The recurrent nerve can be demonstrated by US. The inferior thyroid pedicle crosses over the posterior surface of the thyroid lobe and divides at the junction of the lower and middle thirds of the lobe; on sonograms, it corresponds to a thin, hypoechogenic zone lying transversely at the level of the lower third of the posterior surface of the thyroid lobe.

1.1.1.3 Blood Supply and Lymphatics

The arterial supply is provided by the terminal branches of the thyroid arteries:

- The superior thyroid artery is the main vascular structure. This paired, symmetrical artery arises from the external carotid artery and divides at the superior pole of the thyroid gland into three branches (superficial, medial, posterior). The medial branch anastomoses with its homologue from the contralateral superior thyroid artery; the posterior branch anastomoses with its homologue from the inferior thyroid artery.
- The inferior thyroid artery is also paired and symmetrical. It arises from the subclavian artery and divides at the junction of the lower and middle thirds of the posterior border of the thyroid lobe into three branches (medial, inferior, and posterior). The inferior branch forms the subisthmic anastomosis; the posterior branch forms the longitudinal retrolobar anastomosis with the homolateral branch of the superior thyroid artery. In contrast to the superior thyroid artery, the inferior thyroid artery is absent on rare occasions.
- The lowest thyroid artery is an inconstant branch that runs upward from the aortic arch or brachiocephalic trunk to the isthmus.

The superior thyroid artery represents the major blood supply of the thyroid gland and is easily visualized (Fig. 1.3). The inferior thyroid artery, with the adjacent venous trunk, is a particularly helpful landmark for localizing a normally positioned inferior parathyroid gland (Fig. 1.4).

The venous drainage of the thyroid gland begins from a dense subcapsular plexus, then divides into three trunks on each side:

- The superior thyroid vein is paired and a satellite of the artery; it drains into the internal jugular vein (thyrolinguofacial trunk).
- The inferior thyroid veins form several trunks, anastomosed together, and drain into the left innominate vein.
- The middle thyroid vein is inconstant; transverse on a normal-sized lobe, this vein may lie in an anteroposterior direction against a hypertrophic gland and thus complicate surgical hemostasis.

Sonographically, the thyroid veins may be easier to visualize than the arteries, especially if the internal jugular vein is thrombosed. However, in rare instances, intrathyroid varices can be visualized in the absence of jugular vein thrombosis (Figs. 1.5, 1.6).

The lymphatic vessels located at the periphery of the thyroid vesicles (follicles) form a subcapsular network giving rise to both medial and lateral collecting trunks. These collecting trunks are generally satellites of the thyroid veins. The two major lymph node groups are:

- The lateral and anterior nodes of the internal jugular chain
- The pretracheal nodes and the recurrent laryngeal nerve nodes, which drain parallel to the brachiocephalic trunks and to the origin of the superior vena cava

The existence of direct connections, without any nodal relays, between the thyroid lymphatics and the

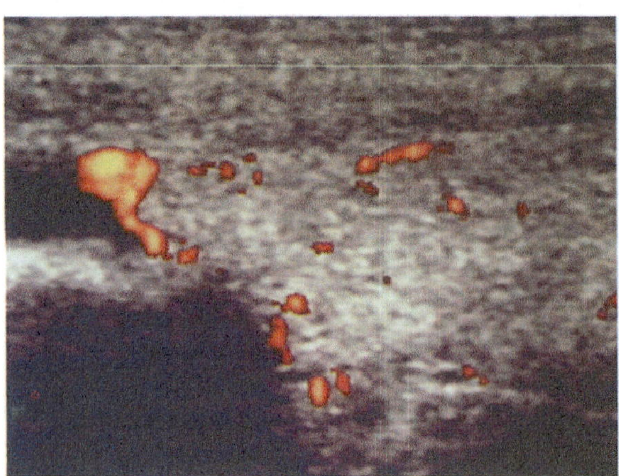

Fig. 1.3. Power Doppler analysis of the superior thyroid artery

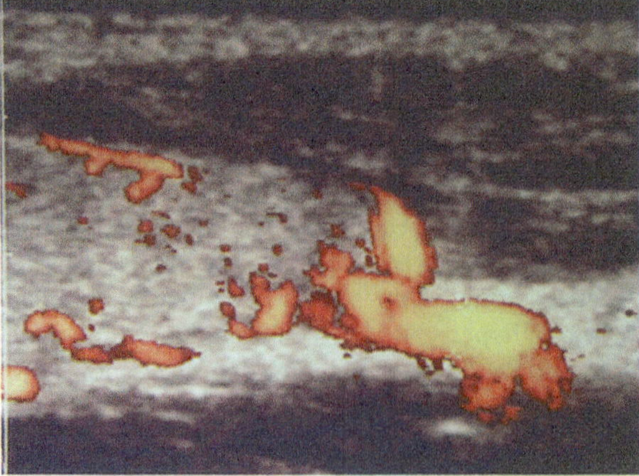

Fig. 1.4. Power Doppler analysis of the termination of the inferior thyroid artery

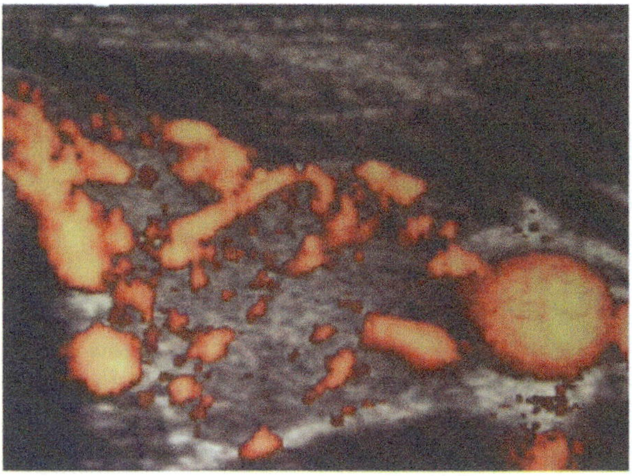

Fig. 1.5. Power Doppler analysis of the thyroid, permitting visualization of the perithyroid and intrathyroid veins

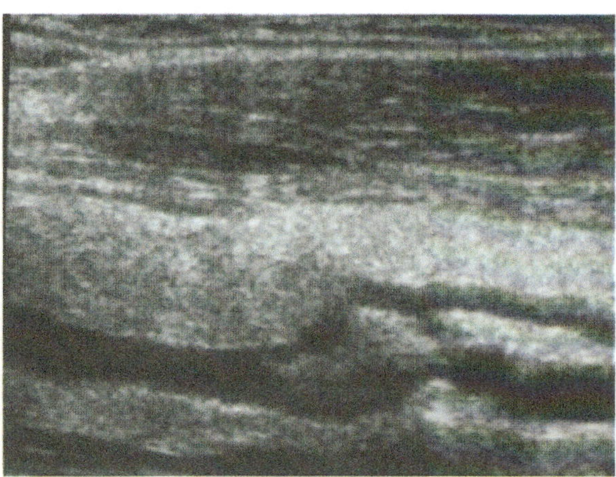

Fig. 1.6. Intrathyroid varicosity; on rare occasion, in the absence of any internal jugular vein thrombosis, an intrathyroid venous network may participate in cervicocephalic venous drainage. In this rare example, veins were spontaneously visible in the right thyroid lobe, without any notable hemodynamic modification during a Valsalva maneuver and without any sign of recent or long-standing cervical vein thrombosis

mucosal plexus of the trachea explains the tracheal involvement observed with certain thyroid cancers.

The normal lymph nodes can be visualized by US. Systematic exploration of the lateral neck regions is essential during thyroid workups, as detection of subclinical adenopathies may orient the etiological diagnosis towards malignancy. US suffices for exploration of the jugular chain, but the pretracheal nodes and drainage system of the superior mediastinum require examination by CT or MRI (Bruneton et al. 1994b).

Detection of one or more thyroid nodules requires analysis of their echotexture (solid with an echotexture comparable to that of the healthy thyroid tissue, fluid zones, calcifications) and contours and determination of the extent of the normal parenchyma and the various thyroid diameters. Locoregional examination must include a search for lymphadenopathy and tracheal compression. Thyroid mobility should be assessed during swallowing. Very high frequency transducers allow evaluation of the capsule and the visceral sheath (Bruneton et al. 1994a; Solbiati et al. 1995).

The presence of multiple nodular lesions requires determination of the quantity of residual normal tissue. Particular attention must be paid to the upper portion of the thyroid lobes, because their status determines the possibility of subtotal thyroidectomy.

If diving goiter is suspected, US may be insufficient, even if the patient is examined with the neck hyperextended (which is not always easy in the elderly). Thus, even though the anterior mediastinum can be correctly examined by US (Wernecke and Diederich 1994), disease staging should be supplemented by another imaging modality for the mediastinum, i.e., CT or MRI (Bruneton et al. 1998; Hopkins and Reading 1998; Naik and Bury 1998; Tessler and Tublin 1999).

1.1.2
Color Doppler (CD) and Power Doppler (PD)

Color Doppler (CD) and power Doppler (PD) provide comparable results for evaluation of thyroid disease. Naruo et al. (1999) performed vascular studies for diagnosis of thyroid nodules with both CD and PD; comparison of data provided by the two techniques did not reveal any significant difference, although PD demonstrated more details for tumor vessels.

Regardless of the method used, Doppler techniques are increasingly being used as complements to conventional US, especially when nodular or functional anomalies are detected. CD consistently identifies the superior and inferior thyroid arteries; sporadic signals are detected within the thyroid gland (Clark et al. 1995; Kerr 1994). Doppler study of the inferior thyroid artery allows determination of the peak flow velocity (Schweiger et al. 1996). Venous structures are generally well identified, especially in the perithyroid region. As for other anatomic sites, the thyroid is a source of intraobserver variations with CD (around 30% for color pixel density and nearly 10% for mean color value) (Delorme et al. 1995). Peak systolic velocity (PSV) in the thyroid arteries remains below 40 cm/s. The high diastolic velocity is consistent with the gland's secretory nature (Clark et al. 1995). Sponza et al. (1997) reported a mean PSV of 20±4 cm/s, a mean diastolic velocity of 8±1 cm/s, and a mean resistive index (RI) of 0.60±0.04.

Chan et al. (1999) investigated the relationship between the menstrual cycle and thyroid blood flow. Measurement of the pulsatility index (PI) in the superior thyroid artery suggested that estrogens influence thyroid function: The PI increases slightly during the first part of the cycle, then drops during ovulation and the second part of the cycle. Studies conducted during the prepubertal period and during menopause have not shown any cyclic modification, and the values recorded are similar to those measured during the ovulatory and luteal phases.

1.1.3 Ultrasound-guided Fine-needle Aspiration

Despite its simplicity, US-guided fine-needle aspiration (FNA) has been criticized because of the non-negligible frequency of uninformative results due to inadequate samples (Gharib et al. 1993; Hamburger 1994). In fact, the constant increase in the number of trained teams means that thyroid FNA will soon play the essential role that certain teams already give it today. Thyroid FNA does, however, require close cooperation between the sonographer and the cytologist. The efficacy of US-guided FNA both in adults and in children makes it the initial diagnostic procedure for management of nodular thyroid disease (Degnan et al. 1996; Ito et al. 1995; Lugo-Vicente et al. 1998; Raab et al. 1995).

1.1.3.1 Technique

A trajectory guidance device can be used to attach the needle to the transducer and guide it toward the target in the US beam. The trajectory of the needle shows up on the US unit screen. Such devices are available for use with linear-array, convex, or sector transducers. FNA can also be performed freehand, with the operator controlling the path of the needle in the ultrasonic beam. Although a guidance device facilitates learning, most experienced operators use the freehand technique (Fig. 1.7).

FNA is usually performed with a 21- to 26-gauge needle. To avoid altering the biopsy material, isotonic solution should be used as the coupling agent between the skin and the transducer, rather than gel. Although this reduces image quality during the procedure, the thyroid gland and the nodule or nodules to be biopsied have already been localized and mapped during prior US examination (Tramalloni et al.1997). Few teams continue to use an 18-G needle for core biopsy because of the need for local anesthesia. Taki et al. (1997), however, reported a sensitivity of 84%, a specificity of 95%, and an accuracy of 91% using an automated biopsy gun fitted with an 18-G needle. Incidents and hemorrhagic accidents have been reported with 18-G needles, whereas complications are very rare with

a 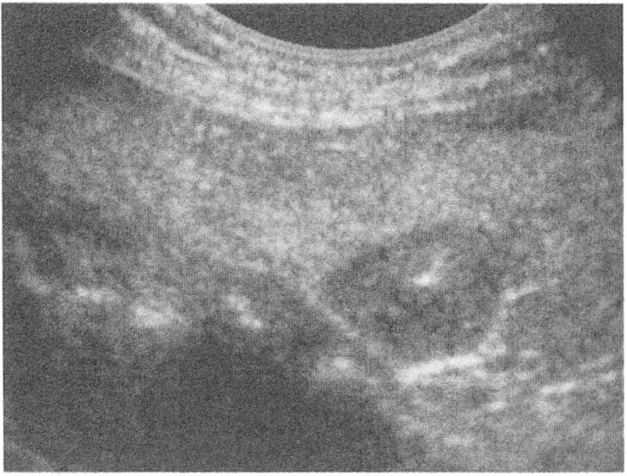

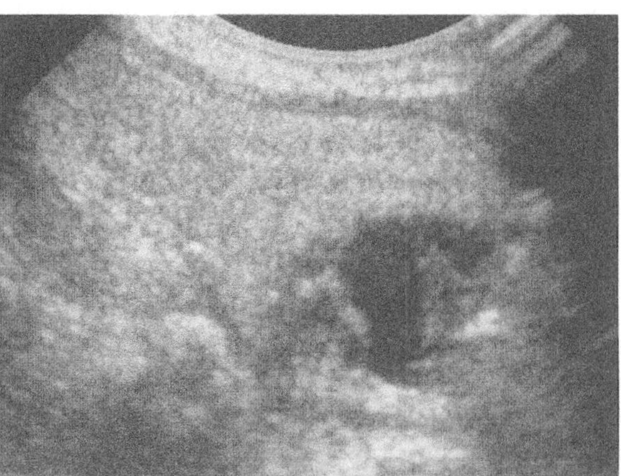 b

Fig. 1.7a,b. US-guided fine-needle aspiration biopsy. **a** FNA of a hypoechoic solid nodule (the tip of the needle is clearly visible as a small, highly echoic structure within the nodule). **b** FNA of the solid portion of an essentially fluid mixed nodule (the small, millimeter-sized echoic image corresponds to the tip of the biopsy needle)

FNA, especially when performed with US guidance.

1.1.3.2
Palpation-guided Aspiration and US-guided FNA

US guidance permits FNA of nonpalpable nodules (LEENHARDT et al. 1999). In the seven series of palpation-guided FNA (18,183 cases) reviewed by GHARIB and GOELLNER (1993), mean sensitivity was 83% (65%–98%), mean specificity was 92% (72%–100%), and the overall accuracy of cytology was greater than 90%. Table 1.1 lists the sensitivity and the specificity of palpation-guided FNA of the thyroid in the literature from 1997 to 1999, allowing comparison with the earlier review of GHARIB and GOELLNER (1993).

GHARIB (1997) recommends two to four aspirations at different sites in each nodule, and performs palpation-guided FNA without local anesthesia. This author considers a smear satisfactory if it contains at least six groups of well-preserved cells and each group contains at least ten cells. Inadequate smears may be related to aspiration biopsy of cyst fluid, excessive blood, excessive air-drying, or operator inexperience with FNA. Inadequate material for examination explains the false-negative findings observed in cystic carcinoma and neoplasms with an extensive calcified component (YOKOZAWA et al. 1996). In approximately 50% of cases, repeat aspiration provides diagnostic material (GHARIB 1997). In a series of 15,210 consecutive biopsies performed at the Mayo Clinic, aspiration was nondiagnostic in 21%; a malignancy was found in 4%, a benign lesion in 64%, and a suspicious cytodiagnosis in 11% (GHARIB 1997).

Thyroid FNA is an essential procedure for the management of nodular thyroid disease. FON et al. (1996) reported a sensitivity of 94% for FNA versus only 53% for US and 24% for radionuclide scanning. The specificity of FNA is not as good, however: 59% versus 72% for sonography and 58% for radionuclide scanning. Table 1.2 lists the sensitivity, specificity, and accuracy of palpation-guided FNA compared with US-guided FNA in the literature.

MOROSINI et al. (1996a) reported more nonsignificant results with US guidance but diagnosed more malignant lesions. TAKASHIMA et al. (1984) obtained better results with US guidance (3% initial failure rate versus 19% with palpation). ROSEN et al. (1993) used US guidance when initial palpation-guided biopsy had failed, as well as for nonpalpable nodules. Although the overall rate of nonsignificant results was 32%, these last authors obtained a cytologic response for 60% of the nodules. Finally, YOKOZAWA et al. (1996) used US guidance for repeat aspiration of nodules that had been considered benign by palpation-guided biopsy; 84.2% of the nodules were confirmed as benign, but 15.8% (n=107) were rediagnosed as malignant. The errors encountered with palpation-guided FNA appear related to nodules that are difficult to palpate and to necrotic or calcified neoplasms.

Evaluation of the true benefits of US guidance is often difficult because series are not comparable and a variety of methodologies have been used. Certain authors advocate US-guided FNA for all nonpalpable nodules, while others reserve it for cases where direct biopsy fails (ROSEN et al. 1993).

Table 1.1. Sensitivity and specificity of palpation-guided thyroid aspiration (1997–1999): review of GHARIB and GOELLNER (1993) concerns seven series (18,183 cases)

Author	Sensibility (%)	Specificity (%)
GHARIB and GOELLNER (1993)	65–98	72–100
GARCIA-MAYOR et al. (1997)	93.5	61.6
CHIU et al. (1998)	93	60
LUGO-VICENTE et al. (1998)	60	90
Baeza et al. (1999)	78	65

1.1.3.3
Results of US-guided FNA

US-guided FNA has a sensitivity of 79.8%–96%, a specificity of 77.7%–100%, an accuracy of 81.8%–94%, a positive predictive value of 95%–100%, a negative predictive value of 75%–91.7%, and a nonsignificant rate of 3%–32% (COCHAN-PRIOLLET et al. 1994; HORVATH et al. 1993; LIN et al. 1997b, MOROSINI et al. 1996a; ROSEN et al. 1993; TAKASHIMA et al. 1994; YOKOZAWA et al. 1996) (Table 1.3).

To better evaluate the efficacy of FNA and its utility for therapeutic decisions (surveillance versus sur-

Table 1.2. Sensibility (*Se*), specificity (*Sp*), and accuracy (*A*) of ultrasound-guided aspiration biopsy in the thyroid literature; all values are percentages

Author	Palpation-guided biopsy			US-guided biopsy		
	Se	Sp	A	Se	Sp	A
TAKASHIMA et al. (1994)	88	90	88	96	91	94
MOROSINO et al. (1996b)	86.6	77.7	81.8	85.1	78.1	80.6
CARMECI et al. (1998)	100	100		89	69	
DANESE et al. (1998)	97.1	70.9	75.9	91.8	68.8	72.6
HATADA et al. (1998)	62	74	68	45	51	48
MULTANEN et al. (1999)			52.4			40.6

Table 1.3. Sensibility and specificity of US-guided thyroid aspiration biopsy reported in the literature (1997–2000)

Author	Sensibility (%)	Specificity (%)
Kato et al. (1997)	88.3	100
Lin et al. (1997b)	79.8	98.7
Taki et al. (1997)	84	95
Avetis'ian et al. (1999)	98.1	94.7
Kimoto et al. (1999)	93	81
Mikoschi et al. (2000)	87.9	78.5

gery), several investigators have analyzed the outcome of thyroid nodules after biopsy. Hamburger (1987) repeated FNA for patients with lesions initially considered benign: 91% were confirmed as benign, but 6% were reclassified as suspicious and 3% were considered malignant. Kuma et al. (1994) followed up 134 patients for a mean of 10 years; 61 had undergone US-guided FNA. In their study, among the nodules for which cytology initially diagnosed a benign pathology, only one nodule was actually found to contain malignant cells.

In a personal study (Tramalloni et al. 1997), 311 patients were followed up for 2–7 years; 45% had undergone direct palpation-guided biopsy and 55% US-guided FNA. Palpation-guided biopsy gave nonsignificant results in 23% of cases; after repeat biopsy, this rate was reduced to 6%. None of the initially nonsignificant results were malignant at repeat FNA, but two suspicious results proved to be benign at surgery. In 3% of cases, the initially benign cytology became suspicious, and four cancers were found at histological examination.

1.1.3.4
Indications for US-guided FNA

Garcia Mayor et al. (1997) identified three periods between 1980 and 1993 during which the percentage of patients requiring surgery decreased owing to the increased use of thyroid FNA. Overall, the frequency of surgical indications dropped from 89.9% to 46.6% in 13 years. These authors observed a simultaneous increase in the percentage of malignant lesions coming to surgery (from 14.7% to 32.9%). The technical improvements in FNA and cytodiagnosis explain the marked decrease in the rate of inadequate material in recent publications (only 4.73% for Mikosch et al. 2000).

Two significant benign aspirates must be obtained at an interval of several months before a thyroid nodule can be definitively considered benign. This is an important consideration for management, especially because follicular carcinoma is difficult to diagnose histologically and FNA alone is not diagnostic. According to Okamoto et al. (1994), the sensitivity of FNA for follicular carcinoma is only 8%, versus 88% for papillary carcinoma.

Diagnosis of follicular carcinoma remains difficult, whether by FNA or intraoperative frozen-section examination (Multanen et al. 1999). For Tambouret et al. (1999), the 15% frequency of inadequate samples means that reaspiration is necessary under US guidance to differentiate macrofollicular lesions, which are not surgical indications, from microfollicular lesions that require surgery. Giovagnoli et al. (1998) also underscored the diagnostic difficulties for differentiation of adenoma and follicular adenocarcinoma.

US-guided FNA has not proven superior to palpation-guided FNA and is also more expensive. It should thus be reserved for nonpalpable nodules of sufficient size to allow accurate diagnosis (8 mm minimum). Khurana et al. (1998) reserve US-guided FNA for thyroid nodules where palpation-guided biopsy appears difficult, but they do not recommend US-guided FNA of nonpalpable thyroid nodules in patients without high-risk factors, preferring a more conservative approach limited to clinical surveillance. Use of US-guidance in cases where palpation was difficult reduced the rate of inconclusive biopsies (8.3% with palpation-guided biopsy versus 2.1% with US-guided FNA). Carmeci et al. (1998) performed US-guided FNA for nonpalpable and difficult-to-palpate nodules (75%), nodules discovered incidentally (14%), and previously failed palpation-guided FNA (11%). For Morosini et al. (1996b), repeat thyroid FNA is justified when the initial procedure is unsatisfactory, but also when a nodule that is apparently benign after the initial biopsy develops suspicious clinical or sonographic signs during follow-up. Woeber (1995) proposed that thyroid nodules considered benign after the initial biopsy be systematically rebiopsied 1 year later; regardless of the biopsy result. This author refers to a surgeon all patients with clinical signs of malignancy, all nodules discovered in patients with Graves' disease, and all nodules in patients with a history of irradiation. Lucas et al. (1995) consider routine reaspiration of cytologically benign thyroid nodules unnecessary because, in their experience, repeat procedures do not change nodule management. This attitude, shared by Gharib (1997), is adopted by most specialized teams. Merceron et al. (1997) advocate repeat biopsy after 2 or 3 years, as successive FNAs reduce the rate of nonsignificant findings to only 6%.

Multinodular goiters present a problem for selection of the nodule or nodules to be aspirated. GHARIB (1997) recommends FNA of the dominant nodule, an enlarging nodule in a patient under surveillance, and any firm or fixed nodule at palpation in patients with multinodular goiter. TOLLIN et al. (2000) performed FNA on 93 nodules in 61 patients with multinodular goiter; 23.6% of the nodules were suspicious and were managed surgically, and 22.7% of these lesions proved to be malignant.

US-guided FNA allows identification of those thyroid nodules that can merely be kept under surveillance and those warranting surgery. The resultant decrease in the number and percentage of surgical cases is associated with both a reduction in costs (GIMONDO et al. 1994) and an increase in the number of carcinomas coming to surgery (NG et al. 1990). LIN et al. (1997b) reported finding malignant lesions in 28.8% of surgical thyroid specimens. The frequency was even higher for KIMOTO et al. (1999), who found malignant tumors in 72% of all thyroid lesions that came to surgery following use of US-guided FNA.

1.1.4 Percutaneous Ethanol Ablation

SCHUMM-DRAEGER (1998) reviewed 17 literature reports published between 1990 and 1997 concerning percutaneous ethanol ablation (PEA) for autonomously functioning thyroid nodules (AFTN). PEA produces coagulative necrosis with eosinophilic ghost follicles, hemorrhage, thrombosis of the small vessels, and wedge-shaped hemorrhagic infarction. The directly induced irreversible damage to the central part of the lesion, related to the coagulative necrosis and vascular thrombosis with hemorrhagic infarction, is accompanied by potentially irreversible damage in the peripheral areas, with a reduction in intracellular enzyme activity and ultrastructural modifications (CRESCENZI et al. 1996).

Sterile 95% ethanol is injected using a 22-G needle, generally under local anesthesia. Most teams administer a total of four to eight sessions at intervals of 2 days to 2 weeks. The total amount of ethanol delivered corresponds to 1.5 times the pretreatment volume of the thyroid nodule. During the past 15 years, several technical improvements have helped to reduce the number of PEA sessions required and lowered the risk of ethanol spillage along the needle track, in particular, the use of CD for preferential ethanol injection into hypervascular areas and of special needles with a closed conical tip and three side holes (SCHUMM-DRAEGER 1998).

The indications for treatment of hot nodules by PEA include elderly individuals with an AFTN and contraindications for surgery, patients with AFTN and iodine-induced hyperthyroidism (in addition to medical treatment), pregnancy, overt hyperthyroidism due to AFTN, and large (>40 ml) nodules, for which PEA is performed to more rapidly induce euthyroidism.

PEA is generally well tolerated, and incidents are rare, although pain at the injection site is common during ethanol delivery. Overall, 70%–80% of patients experience mild pain for 1 or 2 days after the procedure. A number of infrequent incidents and accidents have been reported (BARTOS et al. 1999; FERRARI et al. 1997): transient dysphonia (3.9%–5%) due to vocal cord paresis (caused by mass effect or morphological alteration of the nerve by extracapsular leakage of ethanol), fever of short duration (5%–15%), cervical hematoma or ecchymosis (1.8%–2.5%), and aggravation of thyrotoxicosis (1.1%).

1.1.5 Differential Diagnosis

Sonography can differentiate a thyroid lesion from a nonthyroid pathology of the lateral neck such as lymphadenopathy or a cyst (FARWELL and BRAVERMAN 1996). Since the introduction of US, the only remaining differential diagnosis for nodular thyroid disease is intrathyroid parathyroid adenoma, a rare localization accounting for only 1%–2% of cases. In patients with primary hyperparathyroidism, the thyroid lobe containing the nodule must be explored surgically, even in the absence of a sharp separation between the nodule and the adjacent thyroid parenchyma. This is especially true if the remainder of the cervical examination is normal. Although there is no absolute surgical indication, US-guided FNA may be helpful (SOLBIATI et al. 1995). Hyperparathyroidism is frequently associated with thyroid nodules (48% of cases according to FUNARI et al. 1992); this is not surprising in light of the elevated incidence of thyroid nodules in the general population.

Hypopharyngeal diverticulae (Zenker's diverticulae) are potentially one of the rare instances in which it may prove difficult to distinguish a thyroid nodule from a nonthyroid etiology (KUMAR et al. 1994). Dynamic scanning during swallowing usually allows differential diagnosis. STRAUSS (1999) reported visualization of a thyroid pseudotumor on sagittal scans owing to a noncalcified cricoid cartilage (hypoechoic image with an anechoic halo and foci of calcifications); this type of pseudotumor image is never seen when the cricoid cartilage is calcified.

In practice, the difficulties encountered during sonographic evaluation of thyroiditis concern pseudonodular modifications in echotexture, particularly in chronic thyroiditis. The fibrous septa visualized as hyperechoic bands traversing the thyroid gland may create a pseudonodular appearance. Colloid-filled follicles may image sonographically as microlesions several millimeters in size, but they are not pathological (Bruneton et al. 1996; Solbiati et al. 1995).

1.2 Thyroid Nodules

The dilemma caused by the detection of one or more thyroid nodules is not new. From the very introduction of scintigraphy, the question arose as to whether surgery was indicated for one or more generally palpable nodules. In at least 90% of patients, systematic surgical intervention resulted in excision of a benign nodule; however, a wait-and-see attitude involves the risk that a possibly solitary, and thus curable, neoplasm might be overlooked.

Instead of providing the solution, ultrasonography has actually complicated the situation, because one or more thyroid nodules are commonly detected at cervical US performed for other purposes. The increased frequency of detection of thyroid nodules is attributable to better familiarity with their sonographic features and to CD, which is used increasingly to analyze the cervical arteries. US has become indispensable for thyroid examination, with a clearly recognized superiority over physical examination and scintigraphy both in adults (Brander et al. 1992) and in children (Aghini-Lombardi et al. 1997). In addition, although palpation can detect nodules of at least 1 cm, only half of all palpable nodules are truly solitary, as clearly demonstrated by US (Tan et al. 1995).

The high prevalence of thyroid nodules was initially a source of controversy between advocates of a wait-and-see attitude and proponents of systematic surgical management. More recently, a consensus has been reached based on the results of US-guided FNA (Cannoni and Demard 1995; Sadoul 1995; Singer et al. 1996). Gharib (1997) performed a Medline search of publications on thyroid nodule diagnosis and management; comparison of findings published between 1970 and 1975 with articles published from 1990 to 1995 revealed a threefold increase in the number of publications concerning nodular disease, a 35-fold increase concerning thyroid FNA, and a fivefold increase for thyroid suppressive therapy. Currently, most investigations concerning thyroid nodules deal with the use of FNA, the role of TSH assays, and the indications for levothyroxine (LT4) suppressive therapy.

1.2.1 Frequency of Thyroid Nodules

The frequency of thyroid nodules depends on the study population and the investigation technique (palpation, sonography). The prevalence of thyroid nodules increases with age, exposure to ionizing radiation, and iodine deficiency. Generally speaking, women are affected more often than men, and the annual incidence is evaluated at 100 cases per 100,000 persons (Burch 1995; Gharib 1997).

In a study performed in an adult population using a 13 MHz transducer, one or more thyroid nodules were discovered in 34% of the subjects (Bruneton et al. 1994a). This rate of detection is much higher than in epidemiological studies, which estimate the incidence of thyroid nodules at only 5% (Danese and Schiacchitano 1993; Rifat and Ruffin 1994). However, the prevalence of thyroid incidentalomas varies greatly in the literature. Ezzat et al. (1994) found one or more thyroid nodules in 67% of patients (physical examination was positive in only 21%), whereas Miki et al. (1993) discovered a thyroid nodule in less than 21% (physical examination was positive in under 2%). These two series probably represent the extremes concerning the sonographic frequency of thyroid nodules.

Sonographic examination is more accurate than palpation for the detection of thyroid nodules, particularly in individuals with a short, fat neck (Witterick et al. 1993). Although manual palpation is satisfactory for quantitative evaluation of thyroid volume (Nordmeyer et al. 1997), it gives numerous false-negative findings in cases where US reveals one or more lesions. For Wiest et al. (1998), physical examination detected only 48.2% of nodules larger than 2 cm and only 6.4% of those smaller than 0.5 cm.

Postmortem studies, some of which were performed years ago, report discovery of benign or malignant thyroid nodules in 8%–45.6% of cases (Vidone and Silverberg 1966). Mortensen et al. (1955) found one or more thyroid nodules in 50% of autopsies (37% multiple, 13% solitary), with a prevalence of cancer of 4.2%. Overall, it should be remembered that slightly over one third of the general population, and in particular women over the age of 40, have one or more thyroid nodules (Horlocker et al. 1986).

Thyroid carcinoma is rare. Papillary carcinoma, the main variant, has an indolent course and an excellent prognosis. In light of the anatomic frequency of thyroid nodules, management strategies require an approach that limits the risks of overlooking a carcinoma while also limiting morbidity and the cost of treatment. The annual rate of detection of clinically significant thyroid cancer in the general population is only 0.004% (Gharib 1994), and thyroid carcinoma accounts for only 0.5%–1.3% of all neoplasms (Gandon and Ledoux-Robert 1995).

The incidence of cancers was evaluated at 2.98% by Lin et al. (1997b) in a series of 3657 cases seen in 1 year. Age is an important factor when evaluating the risk of malignancy; the risk is increased in young people under 20 years and in individuals over 60 years (Burch 1995; Singer 1996). Likewise, a nodule discovered in a male subject has a greater risk of being malignant than one detected in a female.

This low clinical frequency of thyroid carcinoma contrasts with postmortem rates of up to 38% (Ross 1991). Most lesions found at autopsy, however, are microcancers. Nevertheless, establishment of guidelines remains difficult, because the arguments used to support a wait-and-see attitude also apply to surgical management.

Although thyroid nodules may be incidental discoveries at cervical US performed for other reasons (particularly vascular studies), systematic sonographic search for thyroid disease is essential in patients with recognized risk factors: (a) accidental irradiation, as at Chernobyl, where there has been an increase in the frequency of thyroid abnormalities (essentially thyroiditis and cystic lesions) and where the incidence of cancer is higher than in the normal population (Hancock et al. 1995; Ito et al. 1995; Kumpusalo et al. 1996); and (b) a history of therapeutic irradiation of the head and neck in childhood (Crom et al. 1997; Healy et al. 1996). Shafford et al. (1999) followed-up patients treated for Hodgkin's disease in childhood; these authors consider palpation insufficient for detection of possible thyroid anomalies. Three of the 47 patients in their series were found to have cancer. Young age at irradiation and the duration of TSH elevation were identified as risk factors. The irradiation dose also plays a role. Among patients who had received cervical irradiation at doses greater than 15 Gy during childhood, 44% were found to have essentially benign anomalies (Crom et al. 1997).

Nodular thyroid disease can be approached in two manners. A first classification distinguishes between benign and malignant lesions:

- Benign lesions: multinodular goiter, Hashimoto's thyroiditis, simple or hemorrhagic colloid cyst, vesicular adenoma (orthoplastic, macrovesicular or colloid vesicular, microvesicular or fetal, solid microtrabecular) oxyphilic Hürthle cell adenoma
- Malignant lesions: papillary carcinoma (follicular variant, sclerosing, cystic adenocarcinoma), vesicular carcinoma (with minimal or massive invasion, oxyphilic), medullary carcinoma, undifferentiated carcinoma (anaplastic), non-Hodgkin's lymphoma (NHL), metastasis, malignant hemangioendothelioma

The second approach is based on the solitary or multiple nature of nodules:

- Single thyroid nodule: carcinoma, adenoma (including toxic adenoma), rarely a cyst
- Multinodular lesions: multinodular goiter, Basedow's goiter, anaplastic carcinoma, lymphoma

1.2.2 Ultrasound Patterns

1.2.2.1 Gray Scale

Ultrasonography can demonstrate the location, size, number, echotexture and margins of thyroid nodules. Very high frequency transducers improve analysis of nodule contours and can demonstrate parietal anomalies suggestive of a neoplastic process.

A peripheral halo is almost unanimously considered a sign of benignity, although only when complete (Fig. 1.8); a nodule with an incomplete halo may correspond to a neoplasm (Seya et al.1990). The completeness of any halo must be sought systematically, both at gray-scale imaging and with CD, to avoid diminishing the complete halo's justified reputation of benignity. Rago et al. (1998) consider absence of the halo sign the sonographic pattern most predictive for malignancy (sensitivity 66.6%, specificity 77%). For these authors, the combination of an absent halo sign and the presence of microcalcifications on US had a low sensitivity (26.6%) but a very high specificity (93.2%). Pacella et al. (1998) underscored the low specificity of blurred nodular margins. Although in their study 80% of papillary carcinomas with a diameter less than or equal to 1.5 cm had blurred margins, 33% of benign nodules also showed this finding.

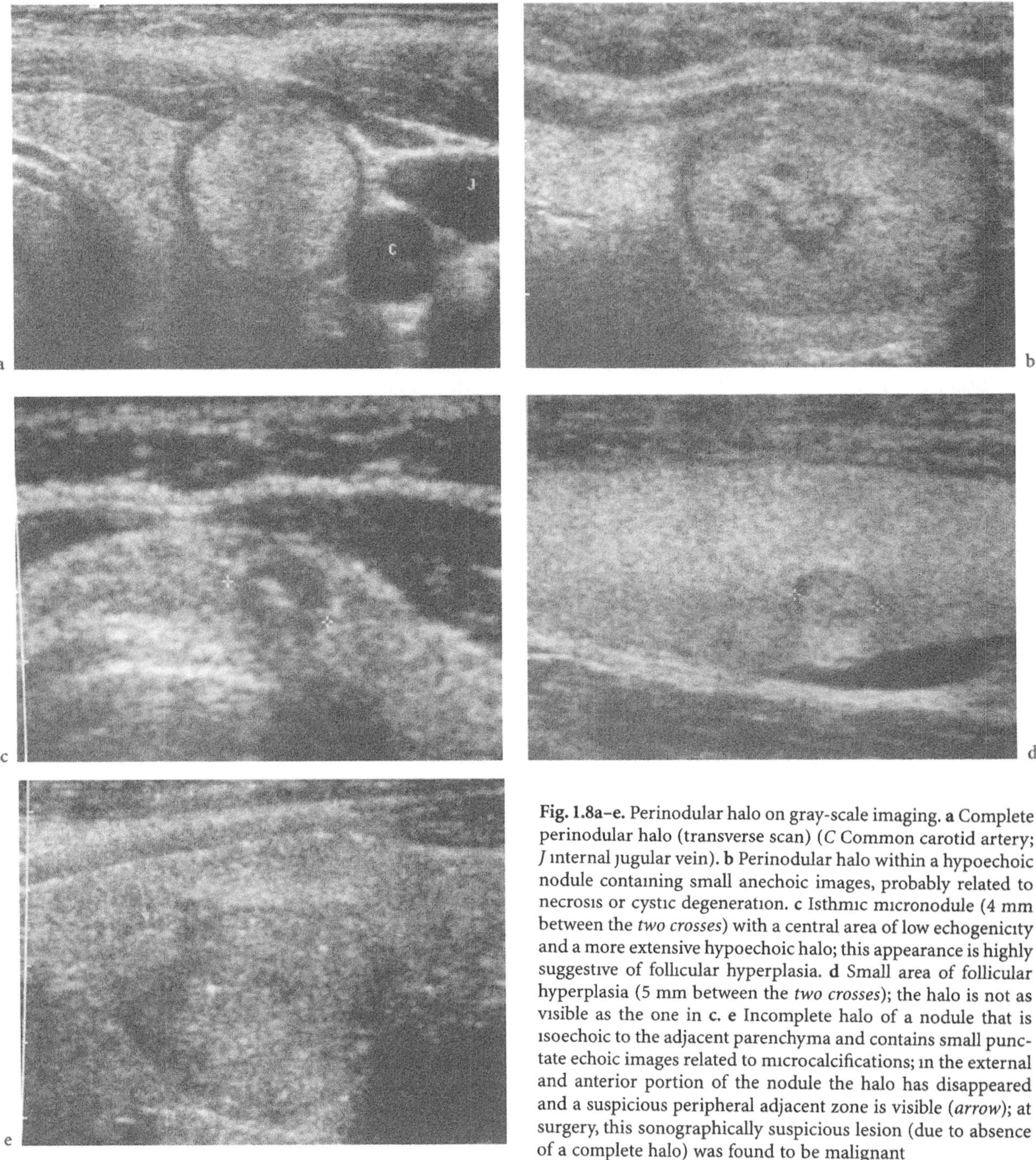

Fig. 1.8a–e. Perinodular halo on gray-scale imaging. **a** Complete perinodular halo (transverse scan) (*C* Common carotid artery; *J* internal jugular vein). **b** Perinodular halo within a hypoechoic nodule containing small anechoic images, probably related to necrosis or cystic degeneration. **c** Isthmic micronodule (4 mm between the *two crosses*) with a central area of low echogenicity and a more extensive hypoechoic halo; this appearance is highly suggestive of follicular hyperplasia. **d** Small area of follicular hyperplasia (5 mm between the *two crosses*); the halo is not as visible as the one in **c**. **e** Incomplete halo of a nodule that is isoechoic to the adjacent parenchyma and contains small punctate echoic images related to microcalcifications; in the external and anterior portion of the nodule the halo has disappeared and a suspicious peripheral adjacent zone is visible (*arrow*); at surgery, this sonographically suspicious lesion (due to absence of a complete halo) was found to be malignant

When examining large lesions, care must be taken to search for invasion of adjacent structures, and in particular the prethyroid and sternocleidomastoid muscles. Examination must be performed in real time, care being taken to obtain scans while the patient moves his neck and during swallowing. However, US does not always permit visualization of spread towards the muscular structures and the tracheo-esophageal axis. For Shimamoto et al. (1998), sonography had a sensitivity of only 77.8% for detection of tumor extension to muscle, 42.9% for invasion into the trachea, and just 28.6% for spread to the esophagus.

Certain rare thyroid nodules have a completely fluid-like echotexture (Fig. 1.9). Meticulous methodology is required to demonstrate an anechoic struc-

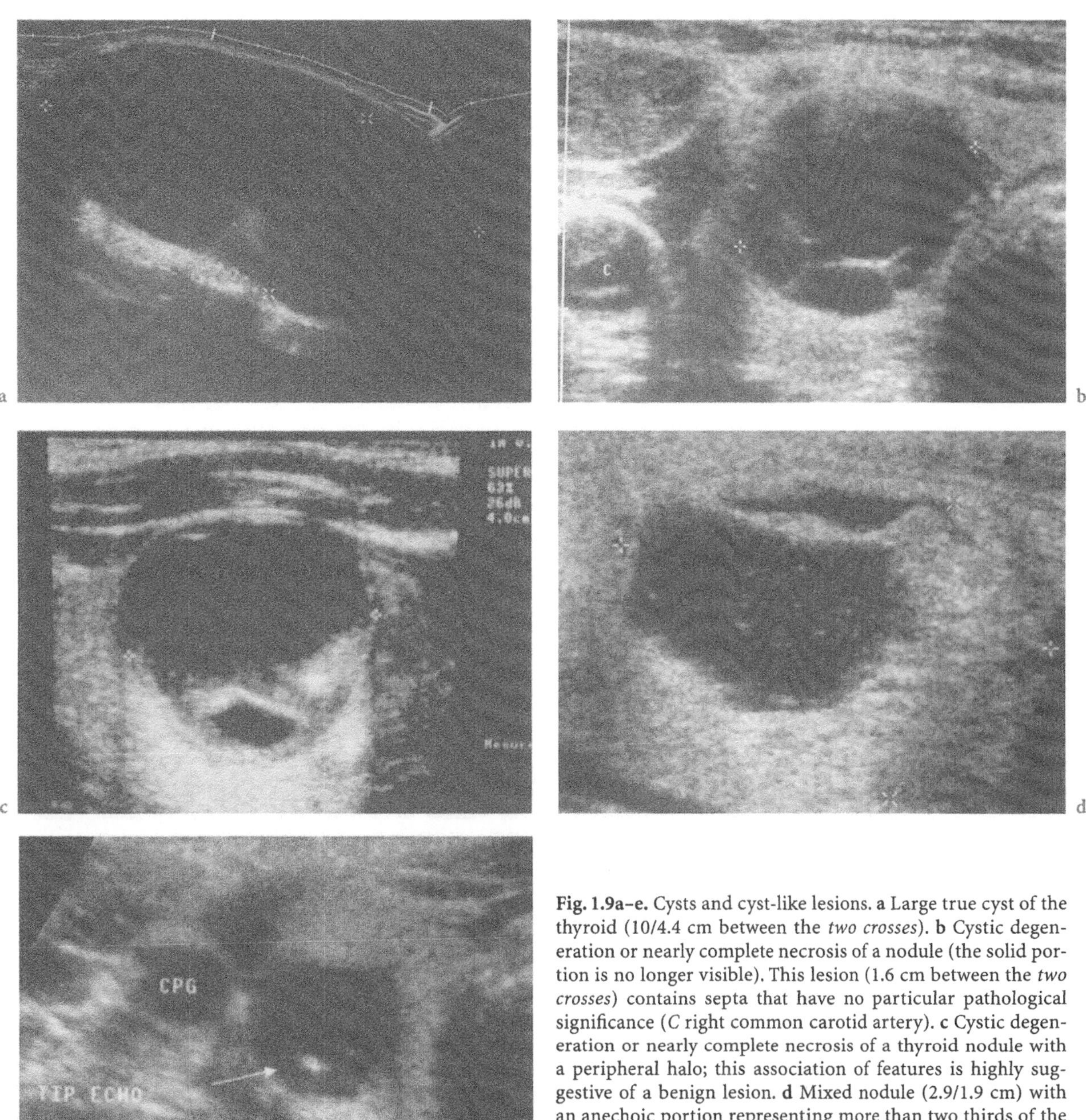

Fig. 1.9a–e. Cysts and cyst-like lesions. **a** Large true cyst of the thyroid (10/4.4 cm between the *two crosses*). **b** Cystic degeneration or nearly complete necrosis of a nodule (the solid portion is no longer visible). This lesion (1.6 cm between the *two crosses*) contains septa that have no particular pathological significance (*C* right common carotid artery). **c** Cystic degeneration or nearly complete necrosis of a thyroid nodule with a peripheral halo; this association of features is highly suggestive of a benign lesion. **d** Mixed nodule (2.9/1.9 cm) with an anechoic portion representing more than two thirds of the entire volume of the nodule; this appearance is very suggestive of benignity. **e** FNA of a nearly completely necrotic or cystic nodule (*arrow* indicates the needle tip; *CPG* left common carotid artery)

ture with posterior reinforcement and thin margins. Cysts may contain diffuse echoes; viscous fluid typically has a homogeneous echotexture. Actually, fluid-like nodules are usually not cysts at all; most correspond to solid lesions that have undergone necrosis or cystic degeneration. Rapid enlargement of a thyroid mass has several possible causes. In the series of 42 thyroid nodules investigated by King et al. (1997), an increase of more than 3 cm in less than 2 months corresponded to hemorrhage in 31 cases and to cancer in only 11 cases. Hemorrhage produces a cystic pattern with small internal echoes that move with changes in position; septa are present occasionally (Fig. 1.10). Neoplasms, which image as well-limited hypoechoic nodules, have a number of etiologies: thyroid metastasis of end-stage disease, anaplastic

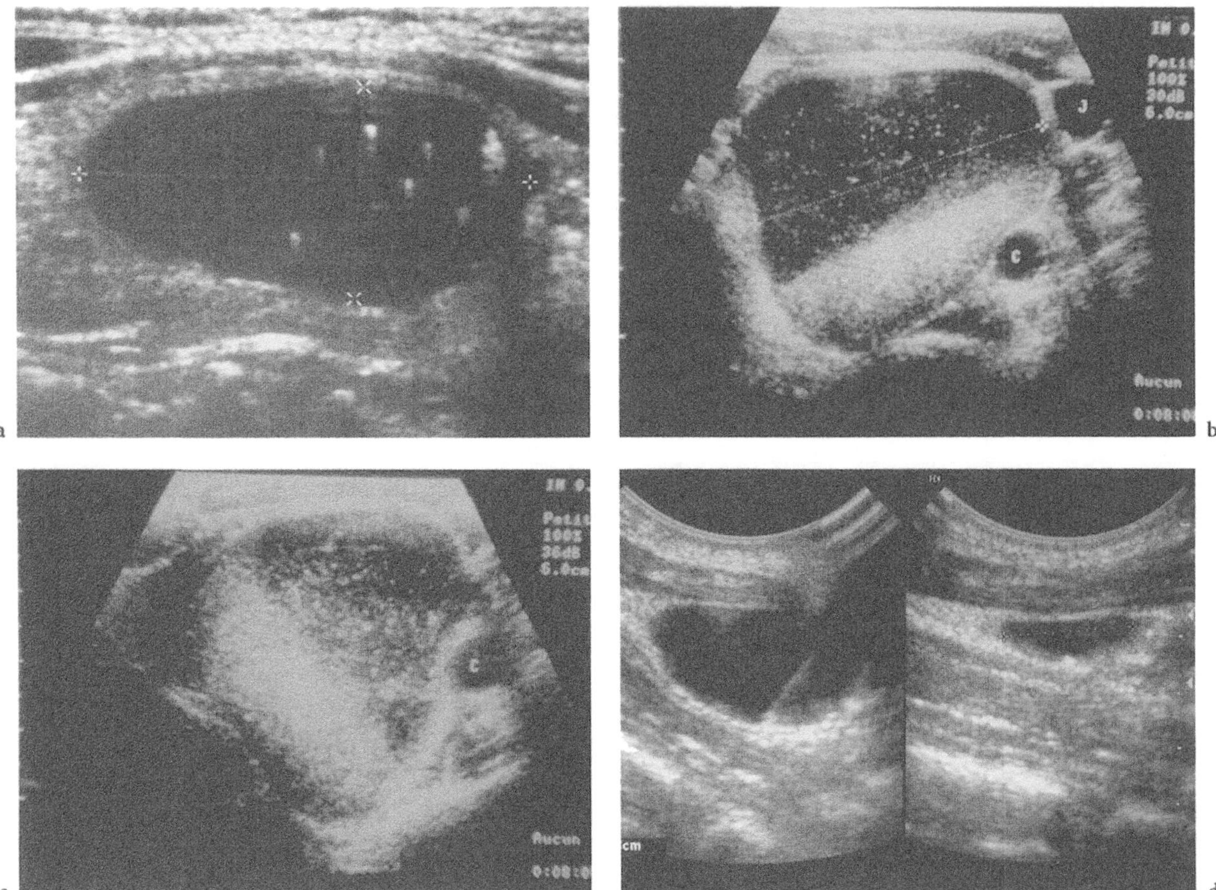

Fig. 1.10a–d. Hematocele in a thyroid nodule. **a** Hematocele complicating a thyroid nodule (2.4/1.1 cm), the small echogenic images were mobile with changes in position. This compressive hematocele was drained percutaneously. **b** Left thyroid hematocele involving the entire lobe (4.4 cm between the *two crosses*). Note the numerous echoic images and a declivitous echoic level (*C* common carotid artery, *J* internal jugular vein). **c** Same patient as in **b**: Imaging performed after the patient was placed in left lateral decubitus revealed migration of the echoic images (*C* common carotid artery). **d** Evacuation of a small but painful hematocele (the needle used for aspiration is visible) and follow-up sonogram (1.2 cm between *the crosses*)

cancer, lymphoma. For King et al. (1997), any asymmetrical cervical swelling, especially when rapid, justifies sonographic examination in search of a hematocele that may be amenable to drainage.

Solid nodules, which predominate, may be hypoechoic, hyperechoic, or isoechoic to the normal thyroid tissue. Hypoechoic nodules are most common (Fig. 1.11); isoechoic and hyperechoic nodules occur at similar frequencies (Brkljacic et al. 1994; Solbiati et al. 1995; Viateau-Poncin 1992). Hyperechogenicity is highly suggestive of benignity (Gooding 1993) because hyperechoic nodules are rarely malignant (only 2%–4% of cases, according to Messina et al. 1998a) (Fig. 1.12).

Certain apparently hyperechoic nodules actually contain microcalcifications that have gone undetected by the examiner (Fig. 1.13). These small echoic foci are too small to have an acoustic shadow. An inexperienced sonographer may be misled by the reassuring sonographic pattern of the apparently hyperechoic nodule, because microcalcifications are a characteristic feature of papillary carcinoma (Lee et al. 1993). Hyperechoic nodules often correspond to colloid-type follicles, whereas hypoechoic nodules frequently correspond to an adenoma composed of embryonal-type follicles (Chang et al. 1990). According to Ahuja et al. (1996), the comet-tail artifact is correlated in 85% of cases with the presence of colloid. Complex nodules with an inhomogeneous echotexture (mixed pattern) account for approximately 25% of all thyroid nodules. A fluid component of variable size may be present. Complex nodules in which fluid accounts for at least two thirds of the volume are almost always necrotic, solid benign lesions (Viateau-Poncin 1992).

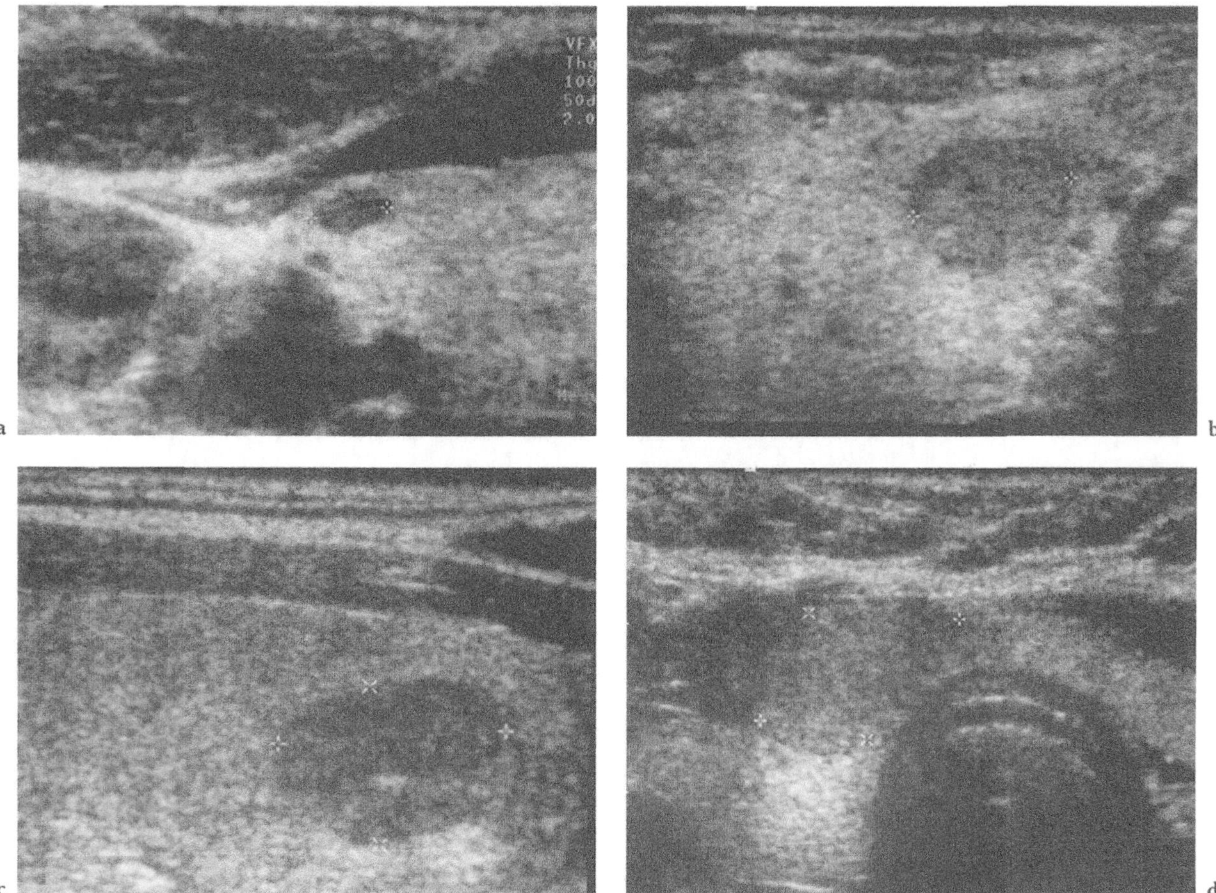

Fig. 1.11a–d. Hypoechoic nodule. **a** Small (3 mm) hypoechoic nodule that merely requires surveillance. **b** Well-delimited hypoechoic nodule (8 mm between the *crosses*) associated with other millimeter-sized nodular elements. The absence of US specificity for this nodular mass is an indication for US-guided FNA. **c** Hypoechoic nodule containing a small central calcification without any associated acoustic shadow and without any particular pathological significance owing to its solitary nature; despite the absence of any associated anomalies, this nodule (1.5/1 cm between the *two crosses*) requires US-guided FNA for histological confirmation. **d** Right-sided palpable hypoechoic nodule near the isthmus (1.4/0.9 cm between the *two crosses*) surrounded by an incomplete, very thin peripheral halo; US-guided FNA is advisable

Other architectural modifications may also be detected, in particular calcifications. Macrocalcifications are readily identified as highly echoic zones with an acoustic shadow (Fig. 1.14). Microcalcifications often escape detection by US with a 7.5-MHz transducer. It was not until the introduction of higher frequency probes with a better sensitivity that microcalcifications were visualized as small, often punctate echoic foci, on rare occasion associated with an acoustic shadow. As emphasized previously, the detection of microcalcifications is important because they are highly suggestive of malignancy (specificity 93%, positive predictive value 70%). However, the overall sensitivity of US for the detection of microcalcifications is low (36% according to Takashima et al. 1995a).

1.2.2.2 Color Doppler and Power Doppler

Solbiati et al. (1995) described attempts to differentiate between benign disease and malignancy with CD and PD; they described three different patterns: (a) avascular lesion, (b) peripheral vascularity, and (c) peripheral and central vascularity. Pacella et al. (1998) described four vascular patterns, using a scoring system of 0–3: 0 absence of flow signals; 1 a few peripheral vessels; 2 peripheral vascularity (flow signals in the peripheral rim); 3 intranodular flow associated with perinodular signals. In their prospective study of hypoechoic thyroid nodules measuring less than 15 mm, CD did not allow unequivocal differentiation of benign lesions (adenomas and benign

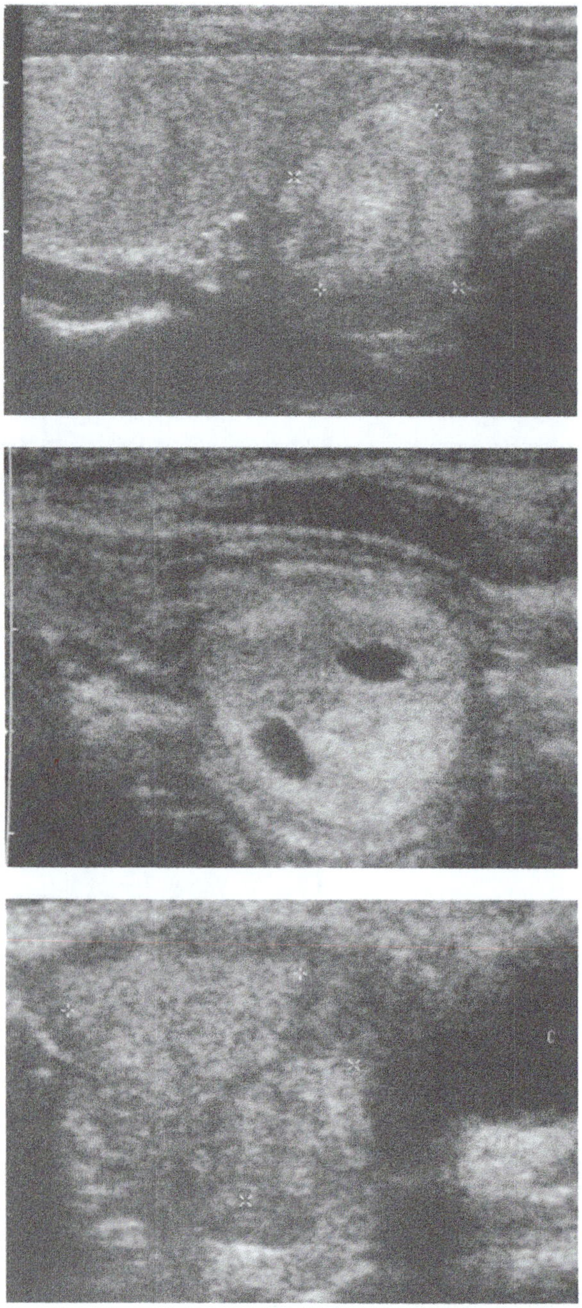

Fig. 1.12a–c. Hyperechoic nodule. **a** Discretely inhomogeneous hyperechoic nodule (1.5/1.4 cm between the *two crosses*). **b** Nodule in the left lobe (3 cm in length) containing two central areas of necrosis. **c** Two hyperechoic nodules (1.1 and 0.8 cm between the *crosses*) in the left thyroid lobe (transverse scan, *C* common carotid artery)

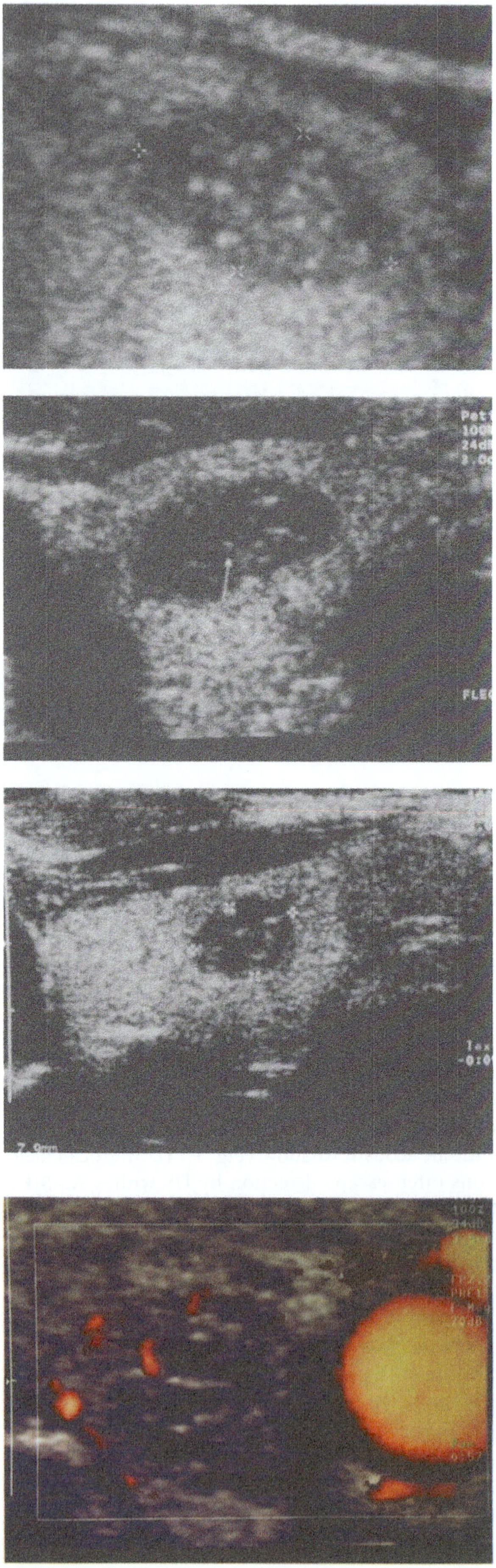

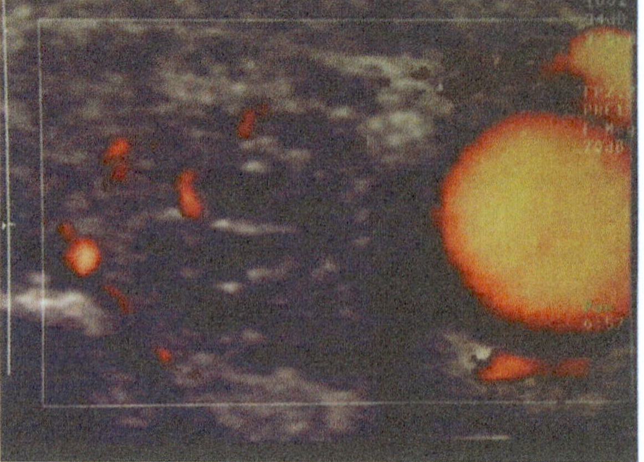

Fig. 1.13a–d. Microcalcifications. **a** Diffuse intranodular microcalcifications (0.9/0.5 cm between the *crosses*) without any acoustic shadow. The large number of microcalcifications, associated with the hypoechoic US pattern of the nodule, mandates histological examination (*C* common carotid artery) **b** Presence of several microcalcifications (*arrow*) within a hypoechoic nodule. **c** Micronodule (0.7/0.4 cm between the *crosses*) containing three microcalcifications. **d** Differential diagnosis of microcalcifications. The thyroid micronodule contains small punctate linear echoic images that actually correspond to microcysts rather than to microcalcifications (power Doppler study)

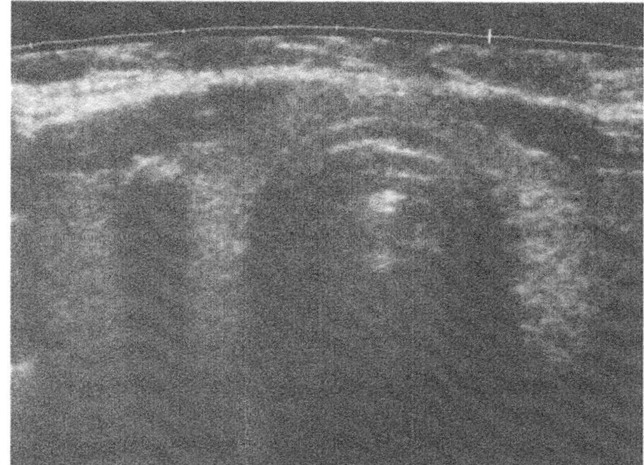
a

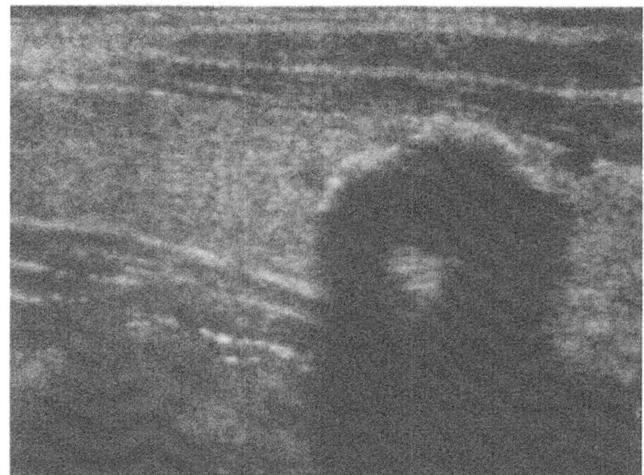
b

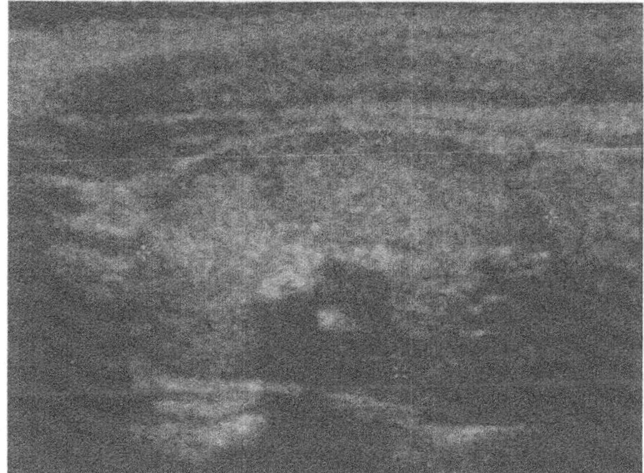
c

Fig. 1.14a–c. Macrocalcification. **a** Centimeter-sized macrocalcification with posterior acoustic in the right thyroid lobe (transverse scan). **b** Macrocalcification in an 11-mm nodule creating a posterior acoustic shadow. **c** Thyroid adenoma with a central macrocalcification (2.5/1.4 cm between the *crosses*)

nodules) and papillary carcinomas. The malignant lesions (representing 23% of the hypoechoic nodules under 15 mm) were type 1 (avascular) in 10% of cases (versus 20%–33% of the benign lesions). Thirty percent of the papillary carcinomas were type 3; this vascular pattern was never seen for benign lesions, and high-grade vascularization at CD thus had an elevated positive predictive value for malignancy.

While an intranodular vascular pattern is associated with a high risk of malignancy (Messina et al. 1998a), certain adenomas also show internal hypervascularity. This pattern thus cannot be used to predict whether a nodule is benign or malignant. Avascular nodules are the only consistently benign lesions and generally correspond to follicular hyperplasia (Argalia et al. 1995). The other two patterns of vascularity defined by Solbiati et al. (1995) do not allow differentiation between benign and malignant lesions (Argalia et al. 1995; Clark et al. 1995; Holden 1995, Shimamoto et al. 1993).

CD demonstration of a complete halo containing vascular structures (usually venous rather than arterial) around an adenoma is highly suggestive of benignity (sensitivity 96%, specificity 93% for Stern et al. 1994) (Fig. 1.15). According to Rago et al. (1998), absence of the halo sign associated with both perinodular and intranodular blood flow at CD had a sensitivity of 50% and a specificity of 89% for diagnosis of cancer. The combination of an absent halo sign, microcalcifications on US, and marked intranodular blood flow had a very high specificity for malignancy (97.2%) but a sensitivity of only 16.6%. Predictive value for malignancy is high only if multiple sonographic signs are present in a thyroid nodule at gray-scale imaging and CD. In practice, there are thus few cases in which sonography, including CD, can affirm a diagnosis of malignancy (Fig. 1.16).

Awareness of the position of these vessels is helpful when FNA is scheduled: Small-caliber needles are required for hypervascular nodules, whereas poorly vascularized nodules can theoretically be biopsied with a large-caliber needle without any major risk of hemorrhage. This point is especially important for the minority of investigators who use 18-G needles.

Hot thyroid nodules are always hypervascular (Becker et al. 1997; Clark et al. 1995) (Fig. 1.17). According to Lupi et al. (1999), CD cannot replace scintigraphy for determination of the functional or nonfunctional nature of a nodule. Hyperfunctional nodules have a halo in 70.2% of cases and intranodular vascularity in 18.9% of cases. Isofunctional nodules have a halo in 63.6% of cases and intranodular vascularity in 9% of cases. Hypofunctional nodules

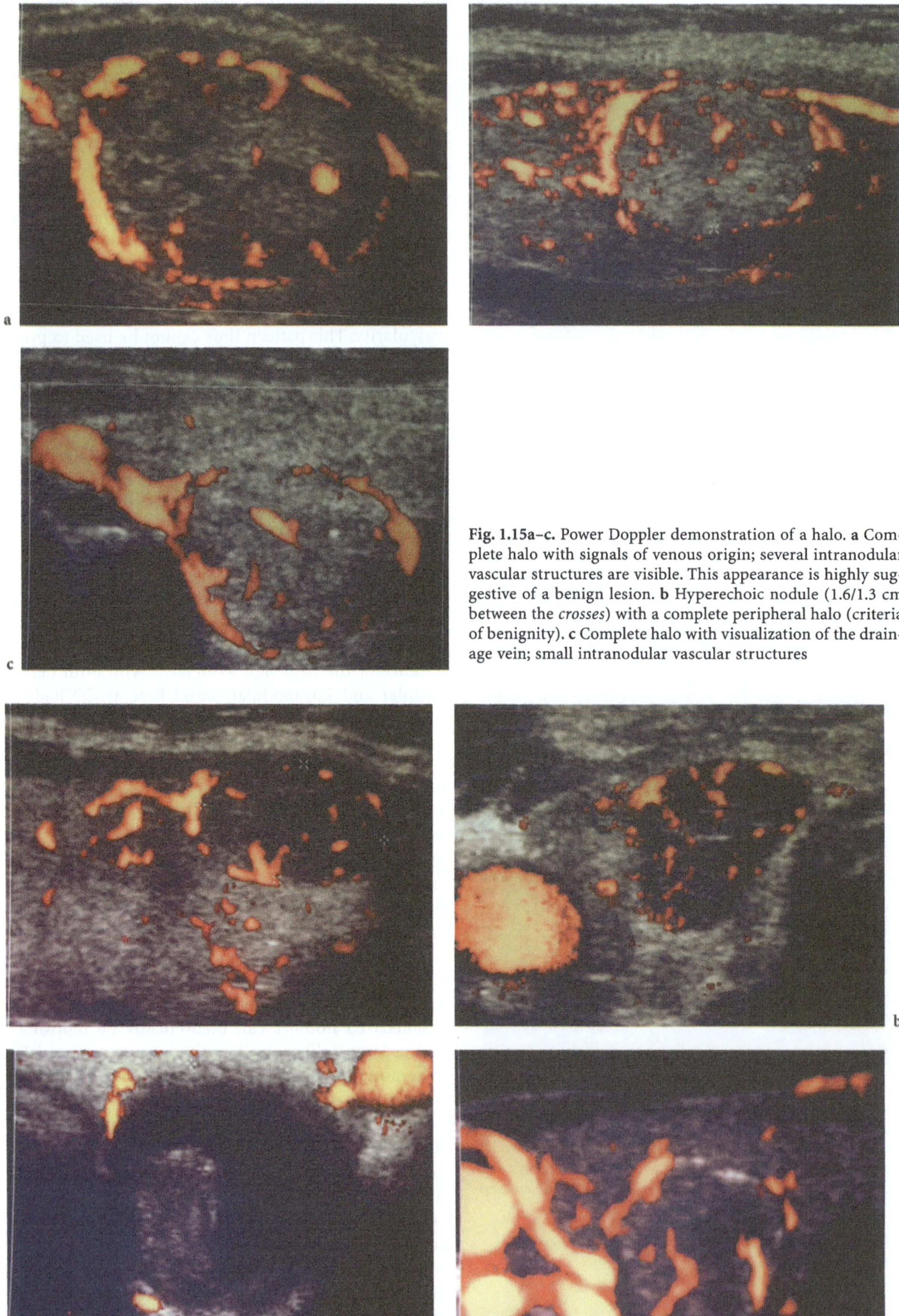

Fig. 1.15a–c. Power Doppler demonstration of a halo. **a** Complete halo with signals of venous origin; several intranodular vascular structures are visible. This appearance is highly suggestive of a benign lesion. **b** Hyperechoic nodule (1.6/1.3 cm between the *crosses*) with a complete peripheral halo (criteria of benignity). **c** Complete halo with visualization of the drainage vein; small intranodular vascular structures

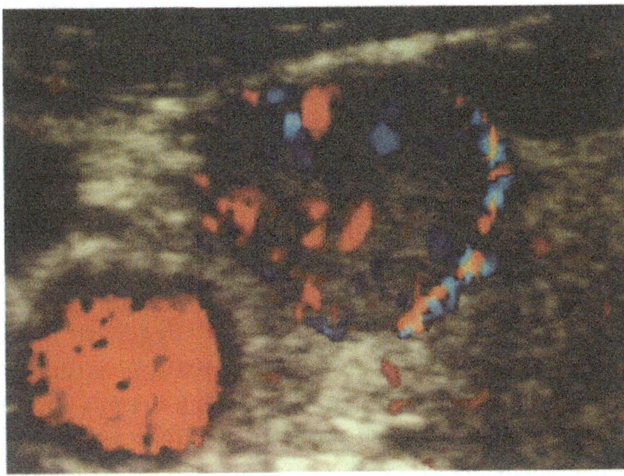

Fig. 1.17. Hot nodule: central and peripheral hypervascularity (CD)

have a halo in 59.3% of cases and intranodular vascularity in 21.8% of cases. There are thus no significant differences in vascularity or morphology allowing determination of whether or not a thyroid nodule is functionally active (LUPI et al. 1999).

There is no correlation between sonographic patterns, hypervascularity detected by CD or PD, and scintigraphic and laboratory data. Similarly, there is no correlation between increased flow demonstrated by Doppler studies and locoregional spread of a cancer (SHIMAMOTO et al. 1998).

Furthermore, 5 mm nodules are often poorly vascularized, and etiologic diagnosis remains difficult. Thus, although a peritumoral halo containing venous or arterial structures is highly suggestive of a benign process, biopsy or exeresis is indicated for all lesions with central hypervascularity (MESSINA et al. 1998a). Spectral analysis of nodule vascularity does not appear to have any practical value (ARGALIA et al.1995; HOLDEN 1995).

1.2.2.3
Reporting Results

As previously emphasized for CD and PD, interobserver differences must be taken into account when deciding to monitor thyroid nodules. In addition to the written report, an accurate map of the thyroid should be prepared, indicating all pertinent volumetric data and the position and maximum diameter of all nodules. This easily prepared document is an excellent means of conveying information during follow-up (BRUNETON et al. 1987; JARLOV et al. 1993; MEYER 1991) and a valuable perioperative aid for the surgeon when lesions are not palpable (KRAIMPS and BARBIER 1993).

1.2.3
Sonographic Features Suggestive of Benignity or Malignancy

Ultrasonography can accurately localize thyroid nodules and determine whether or not they are solitary. Criteria exist in favor of benignity and malignancy, but each criterion taken separately has little predictive value. In contrast, a constellation of findings is helpful for patient management:

- A benign etiology is suggested by a hyperechoic or extensively cystic nodule (over two thirds of the nodule volume), presence of a complete halo, absence of hypervascularity, and absence of laterocervical lymphadenopathy.
- Features in favor of a malignant process include a solitary hypoechoic nodule (LIN et al. 1997a), microcalcifications, ill-defined margins, an incomplete halo, cervical lymphadenopathy, central hypervascularity on CD or PD, a history of cervical irradiation, existence of a metastasis that should prompt a search for a primary cancer, young age, and male sex.

For Katagiri et al. (1994), presurgical diagnosis based on US patterns has a sensitivity of 82%, a specificity of 78%, and an accuracy of 80% for malignancy.

1.2.4
Benign Lesions

1.2.4.1
Thyroid Adenomas

These typically solitary and follicular benign lesions can involve difficulties for differentiation from adenocarcinoma by FNA. Thyroid adenomas are less frequent than hyperplastic lesions, accounting for under 10% of all nodular thyroid lesions. Half of all follicular lesions are isoechoic, whereas nonfollicular adenomas are usually hypoechoic. Regardless of the histological type, other solid patterns can also be encountered. CD and PD demonstrate mixed vascu-

Fig. 1.16a–d. Vascular patterns of solid nodules. **a** Incomplete peripheral and partially central vascularity of a benign lesion. **b** Peripheral vascularity communicating with the central vascularity of a hypoechoic nodule. **c** Extensively necrotic nodule (2.3 cm between the *two crosses*); the apparently solid portion was actually not vascularized at power Doppler analysis (posthemorrhage sequela). **d** Internal and perinodular vascularity without any particular etiological significance; nodule containing a peripheral parietal calcification

larity (both peripheral and central), and there are thus no characteristic features suggesting the diagnosis (Fig. 1.18).

Functional thyroid adenomas have no typical sonographic features, but exhibit marked central hypervascularity and an increased peak systolic velocity (Solbiati et al. 1995). For nonsurgical adenomas that are merely kept under surveillance (possibly under suppressive therapy), US can usefully evaluate modifications in echotexture and especially size (Viateau-Poncin 1992).

1.2.4.2
Cystic Lesions

True thyroid cysts are exceptional. Most cystic lesions in the thyroid are adenomas or hyperplastic lesions that have undergone hemorrhagic degeneration or necrosis. Cho et al. (2000) recommend PEA for both complex and purely cystic lesions. After aspiration of cyst contents, ethanol sclerotherapy is performed using absolute alcohol (99.9%) (volume ranges from 40%–100% of the aspirated fluid). One to three sessions are necessary. These authors observed greater than 50% reduction in size in more than half of cases and noted a relationship between the volume of ethanol injected and the extent of regression.

1.2.4.3
Multinodular Goiter

Multinodularity is best evaluated by US, particularly because 70% of scintigraphically solitary lesions are multiple on sonograms, and because nearly one third of all thyroid cancers are discovered within multinodular goiters (Solbiati et al.1995). Histologically, multiple nodular lesions correspond to benign growth; cycles of hyperplasia and involution of the thyroid tissue with fusion of regions of colloid-filled follicles and the thyroid parenchyma create the nodular lesions. Tollin et al. (2000) estimated the risk of malignancy for multiple nodules at 50%, which is similar to the risk for solitary nodules.

Multinodular goiters are generally composed of hyperechoic areas that are highly suggestive of a benign process. This hyperechoic pattern is due to their macrofollicular structure, which creates interfaces between the cells and the colloid substance (Muller et al. 1985; Solbiati et al. 1995). Hypoechoic multinodular goiters with high cellularity are less frequent. There are no signs of invasion of adjacent structures, but areas of cystic or hemorrhagic degeneration may be present. Cystic degeneration may be complete or create a fluid-fluid level due to the echotexture of the colloid substance. Coarse or "eggshell" calcification may be observed (Fig. 1.19).

CD often reveals anarchic vascularity (Fig. 1.20). Peak systolic velocities remain within normal limits, except in patients with thyrotoxicosis (Kerr 1994; Solbiati et al. 1995).

Accurate mapping of lesions is essential prior to therapy. Multinodular goiter is usually bilateral and diffuse. The surgeon must keep this in mind before deciding to operate on a small and apparently unilateral lesion. Sonography should be performed to evaluate the status of the upper portion of the thyroid lobes, as this determines the possibilities for subtotal or total thyroidectomy (Bruneton et al. 1987) (Fig. 1.21). If surgery seems advisable owing to the volume of the thyroid and clinical symtoms of com-

a
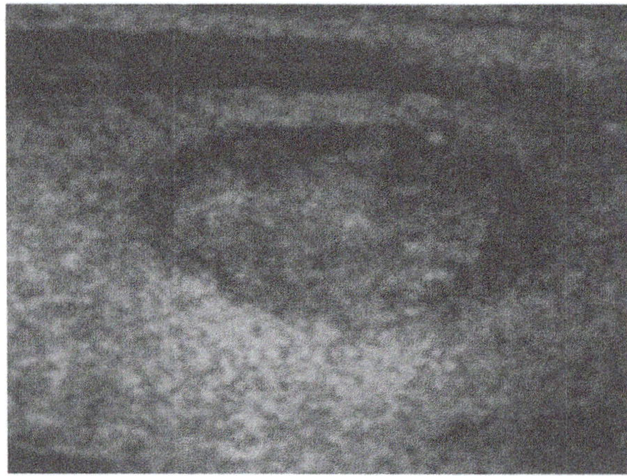
b
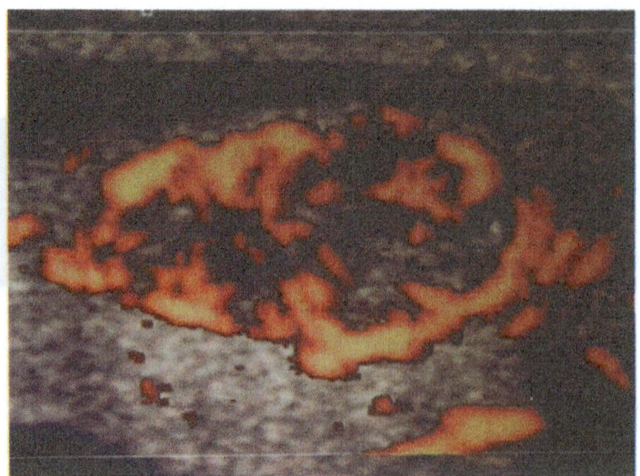

Fig. 1.18a,b. Thyroid adenoma. **a** This nodule was almost isoechoic to the healthy parenchyma but was identified owing to the presence of a less echoic peripheral structure. **b** Mixed (peripheral and central) hypervascularity (PD)

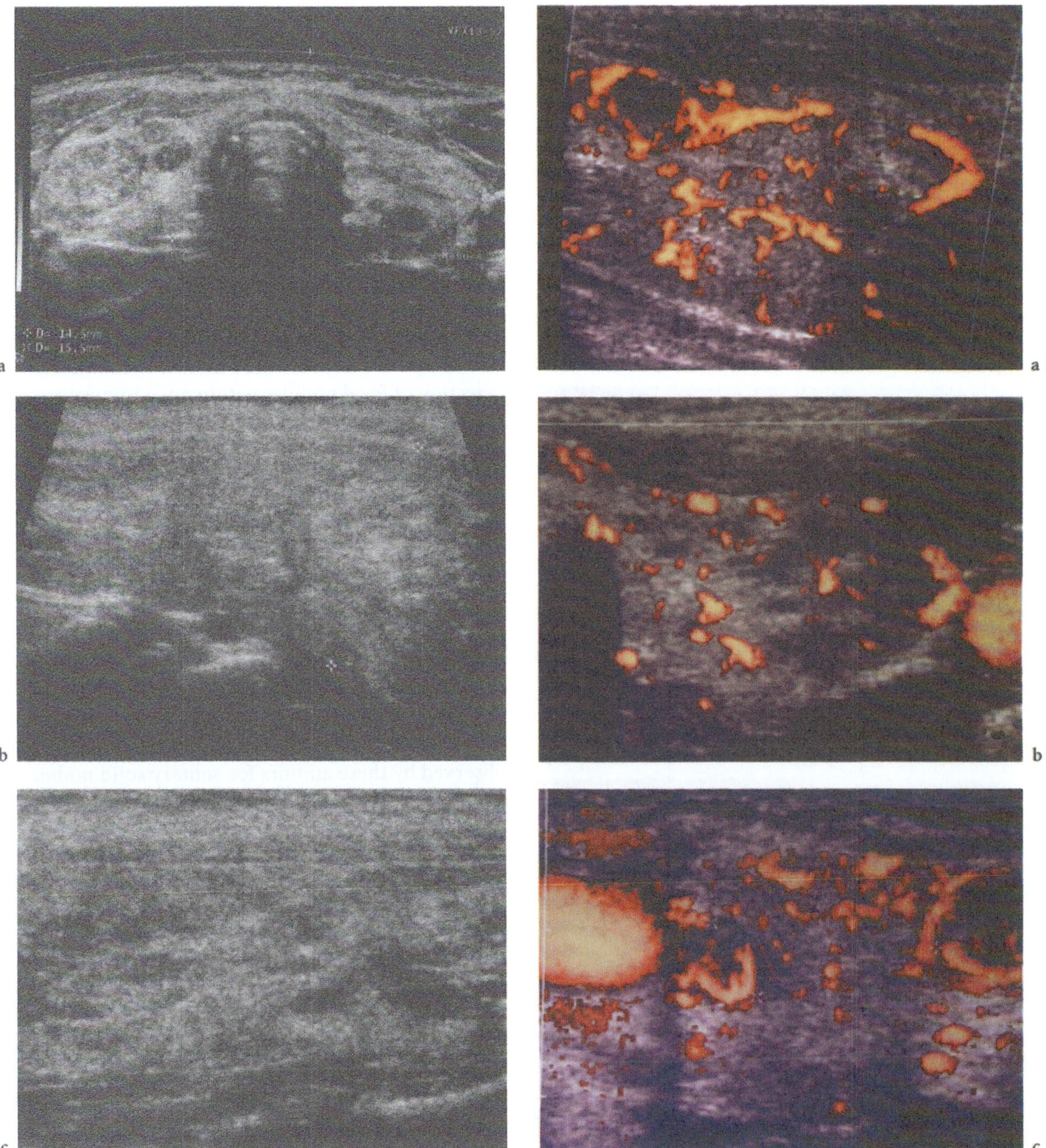

Fig. 1.19a–c. Multinodular goiter. **a** Examination of the entire thyroid revealing nodules of varying size throughout the lobes, but partially sparing the isthmus (thickness of the right lobe: 1.5 cm between the *crosses*; thickness of the left lobe: 1.6 cm between the *crosses*). **b** Echo pattern of diffuse multinodular disease with thickening of the lobe (2.5 cm between the *two crosses*). **c** Hypoechoic millimeter-sized nodules throughout the entire thyroid gland

Fig. 1.20a–c. Power Doppler analysis of a multinodular goiter. **a** Hypoechoic multinodular goiter with increased vascularity suggesting Basedow's goiter. **b** Anarchic vascularity of multinodular thyroid lesions, without any particular features indicating etiological diagnosis. **c** Mixed (peripheral and central) vascularity of micronodules in a multinodular goiter (0.6 and 0.8 cm between the *crosses*)

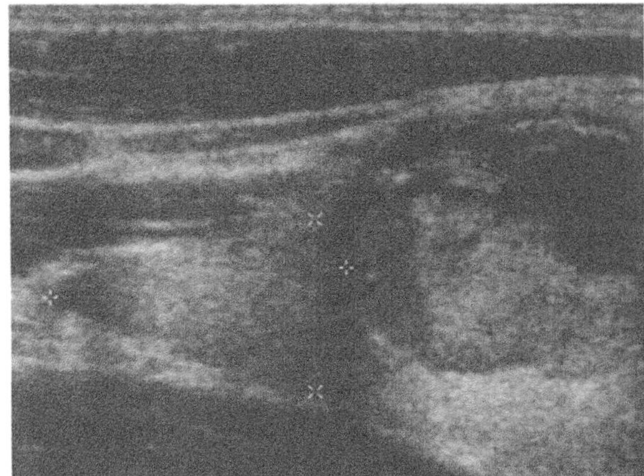
a

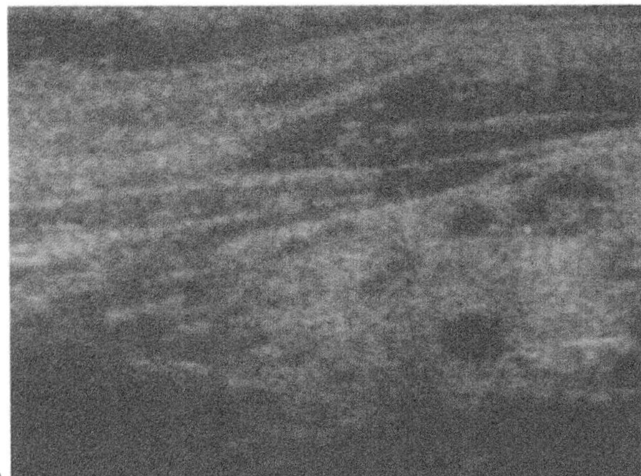
b

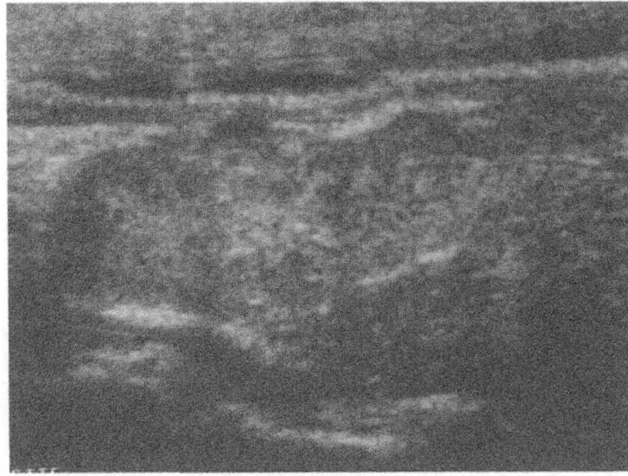
c

Fig. 1.21a–c. Analysis of the upper portion of the thyroid lobes. **a** Normal dome (1.7/1 cm between the *crosses* at the level of the nodular lesions in the thyroid). **b** Micronodular disease in the left apical dome related to diffuse thyroid disease that also involves the upper portions of the lobes. **c** Sonographically ill-defined multinodular disease; identification is easy, however, owing to the morphological modifications of the anterior wall and the summit of the dome

pression, CT or MR imaging should be performed first.

Although multinodular goiter carries less risk of malignancy than a solitary nodule, US alone usually cannot suggest the presence of cancer within a poly-adenomatous goiter unless it is accompanied by laterocervical lymphadenopathy (Brkljacic et al. 1994). As mentioned previously, sonographic depiction and FNA of follicular cancers are difficult. Additional studies are required to determine whether focal zones of hypervascularity in a polyadenomatous goiter have any predictive value for malignancy. The "dominant nodule" concept was developed in an attempt to overcome the problem encountered in detection of focal nodules within an inhomogeneous thyroid. This nodule corresponds to the largest thyroid mass or to the mass that differs the most from the remainder of the thyroid at US (Fig. 1.22). This is the nodule that should be biopsied with priority in search of a possible malignancy (Tessler and Tublin 1999).

Literature results concerning levothyroxine suppressive therapy vary considerably. For Lima et al. (1997), administration of 200 µg of LT4 daily for 1 year reduced thyroid volume by 50% in approximately one third of patients with multinodular goiter. However, 46.8% of patients failed to respond to such therapy; this corresponds to the same efficacy observed by these authors for solitary solid nodules. Papini et al. (1998) followed up 83 patients with multinodular goiter for 5 years and observed only a nonsignificant reduction in thyroid volume in treated patients. For these authors, long-term LT4 therapy is indicated essentially to prevent the appearance of new nodular lesions, and they proposed that it be reserved for small nodules in younger subjects.

Acromegaly is frequently associated with multinodular goiter (92% of cases, including 72% with nodules or heterogeneous structures). While specific treatment permits regulation of excess growth hormone secretion and reduces thyroid volume, it has no influence on nodules (Cheug and Boyages 1997).

1.2.5 Malignant Lesions

1.2.5.1 *Papillary Carcinoma of the Thyroid*

The most frequent thyroid malignancy (>70% in all series), papillary carcinoma usually affects young females. This carcinoma has three main features:

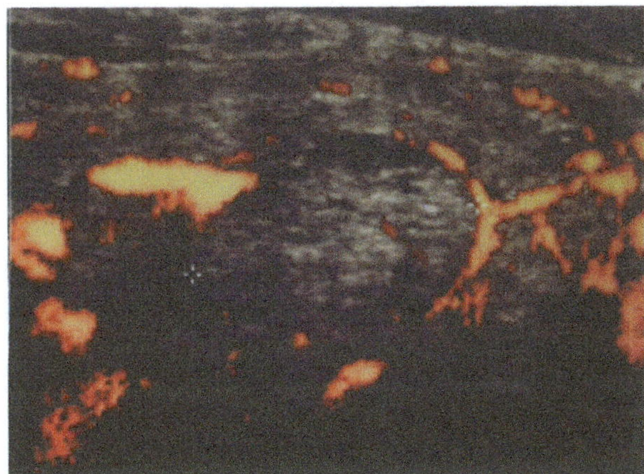

Fig. 1.22. This 1.6-cm nodule is the largest in this patient with diffuse multinodular disease of the thyroid. If FNA is envisaged, this dominant nodule should be aspirated

(a) it has a propensity for lymphatic spread, (b) its growth rate is slow, and (c) it is often multifocal. It rarely metastasizes (to the lung) and is often curable; the prognosis is often excellent.

Witterick et al. (1993) analyzed the pathological significance of occult carcinomas of the thyroid, for which the prevalence in the literature varies from 0.5% to 35.6%. Most occult papillary carcinomas remain small and circumscribed, without a tendency to increase in size. Although Hazard (1960) underscored the fact that 23% of occult cancers are accompanied by adenopathies, the risk of regional spread remains low. These observations explain the different management strategies proposed in the literature, ranging from systematic total thyroidectomy to lobectomy, depending on lesion size, in particular for occult microcancers. For Witterick et al. (1993), surgical planning must take into account not only the significance and risk of occult microcarcinomas, but also the increased risk to the recurrent laryngeal nerves and the parathyroid glands that is inherent in total thyroidectomy.

The possibility of multifocal disease spread explains the risk of recurrence in patients not treated by total thyroidectomy; the reported recurrence rate is less than 10%, however, and such recurrences do not influence survival.

The most common US finding is a hypoechoic nodule (86.7% of cases for Lu et al. 1994) (Fig. 1.23). These nodules are always inhomogeneous once they reach 1 cm. Margins are poorly defined in 80% of patients (Pacella et al. 1998) (Fig. 1.24); less than half contain sonographically visible microcalcifications (Fig. 1.25). Less frequent features include cystic degeneration (28.3%) and the halo sign (13.2%). Isoechoic and hyperechoic nodules (2%) are much rarer (Lu et al. 1994). According to Lin and Huang (1998), solid sonographic patterns predominate (85.5%); mixed patterns (11.7%) and cystic patterns (2.8%) are less common (Fig. 1.26).

In addition to solitary hypoechoic lesions (Garretti et al. 1994), papillary carcinoma on rare occasion manifests as a subcentimeter tissue mass within an apparently cystic lesion (Hiromura 1994). For diagnosis of these rare cystic lesions, it must be remembered that FNA of an extensively cystic lesion should target the solid portion of the lesion (Lin and Huang 1998). Hatabu et al. (1991) reported that analysis of the solid portion of an essentially cystic

a

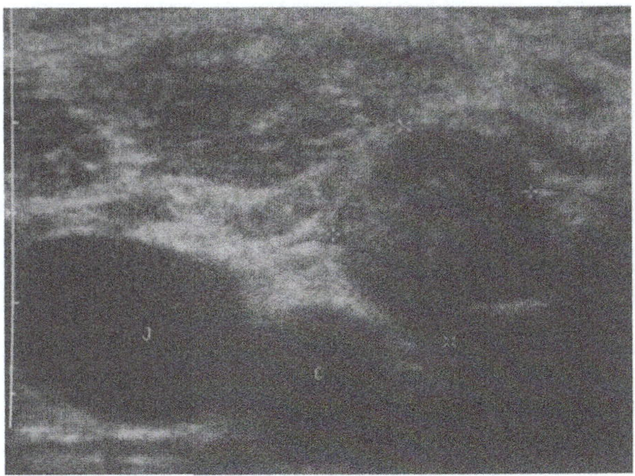

b

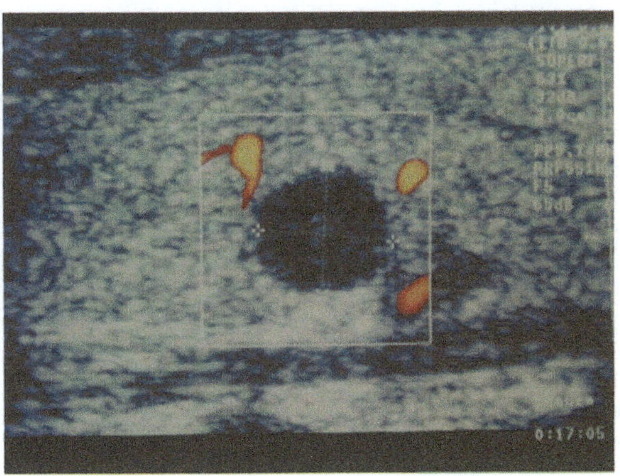

Fig. 1.23a,b. Papillary thyroid carcinoma. **a** Solitary hypoechoic nodule (1.2/1.1 cm; *C* common carotid artery; *J* internal jugular vein). **b** Hypoechoic nodule (0.7/0/6 cm between the crosses) without any hypervascularity at PD; nevertheless, this was a small papillary carcinoma

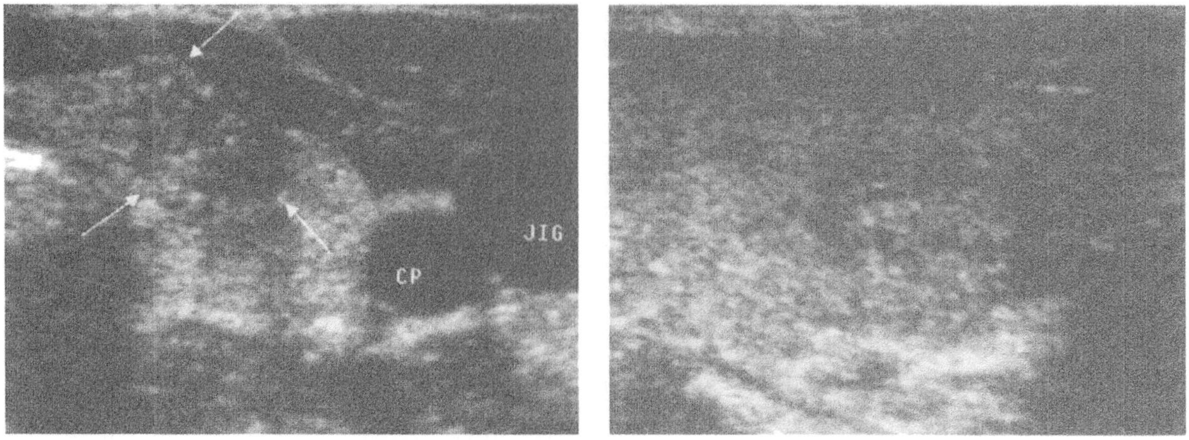

Fig. 1.24a–c. Analysis of the margins of a papillary carcinoma. **a** Hypoechoic papillary carcinoma with ill-defined (and thus suspicious) margins corresponding to the early stage of invasion of the anterior muscles (*arrows*) (*CP* common carotid artery; *JIG* left internal jugular vein). **b** Nearly isoechoic nodule; the small puctate echoic images correspond to microcalcifications that are better visualized in real-time than on static images. The margins of this nodule (papillary carcinoma) were ill-defined. **c** Papillary carcinoma with irregular margins

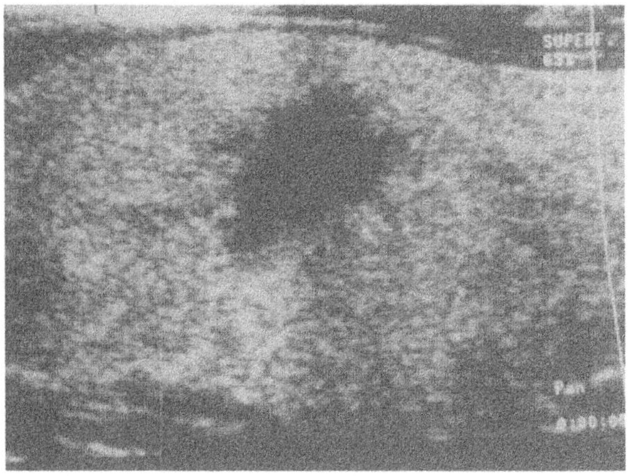

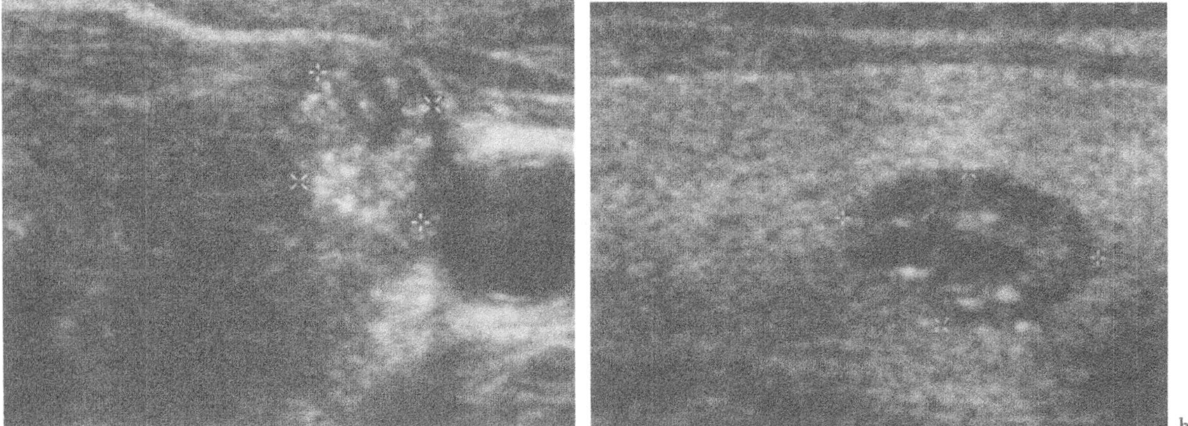

Fig. 1.25a,b. Microcalcifications of papillary carcinoma. **a** Left-sided thyroid micronodule (0.8/0.7 cm between the *crosses*). This nodule, which could erroneously be considered hyperechoic, is actually a hypoechoic nodule nearly completely filled with hyperechoic microcalcifications without any acoustic shadow owing to their small size. The sonographic pattern is suspicious and should suggest the possibility of a papillary carcinoma. **b** Hypoechoic nodule with several microcalcifications

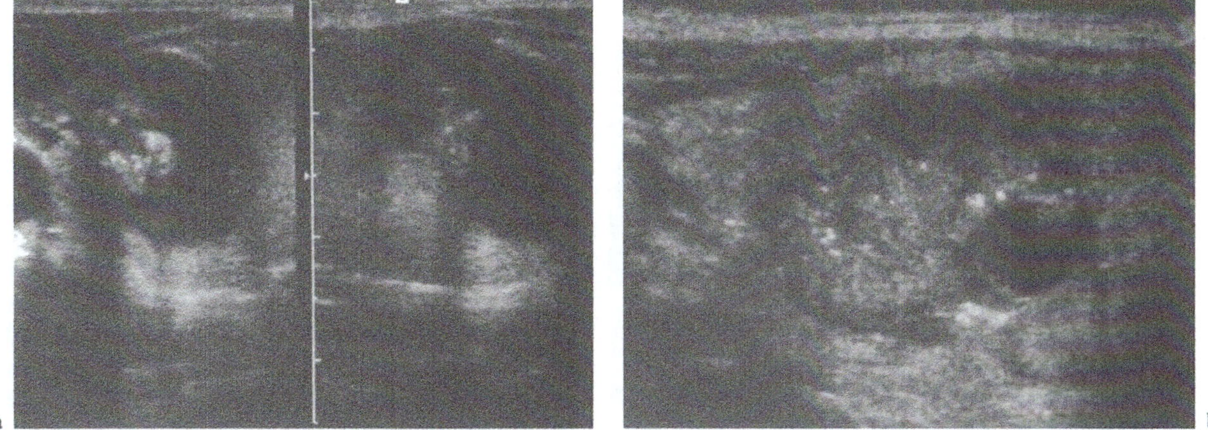

Fig. 1.26a,b. Cystic form of papillary carcinoma. **a** Endocystic mass with microcalcifications. **b** Partially necrotic mass; the solid portion contains numerous calcifications (small hyperechoic punctate images)

mass may prove helpful when microcalcifications are present; microcalcifications are frequent and should be sought systematically, owing to their high specificity for malignancy.

A solitary cervical adenopathy in a young patient is another rare but classical clinical presentation (Fig. 1.27). Ultrasonography may reveal a small homolateral and nonspecific intrathyroid lesion; in other instances, thyroid sonography is strictly normal. US-guided FNA is indispensable in such cases and generally yields neoplastic tissue that confirms the need for surgery (Lee et al. 1993; Solbiati et al. 1995).

Laterocervical exploration, which must be performed systematically, may depict various forms of lymphadenopathy: round rather than oval nodes, or disappearance of the central echoic hilum in small lesions. Nodal metastases are often hyperechoic to adjacent muscle and are usually homogeneous (81.2%, according to Ahuja et al. 1995). Punctate peripheral calcifications are seen in over two thirds of patients (Fig. 1.28). These calcifications, correlated with psammoma bodies, are characteristic of papillary carcinoma. Sugino et al. (1998) reported lymph node metastases in 63.8% of papillary carcinomas with a diameter less than or equal to 10 mm. In the study of Shimamoto et al. (1998), US had a sensitivity of only 36.7% for the detection of regional lymph node metastases, and, even when detected,

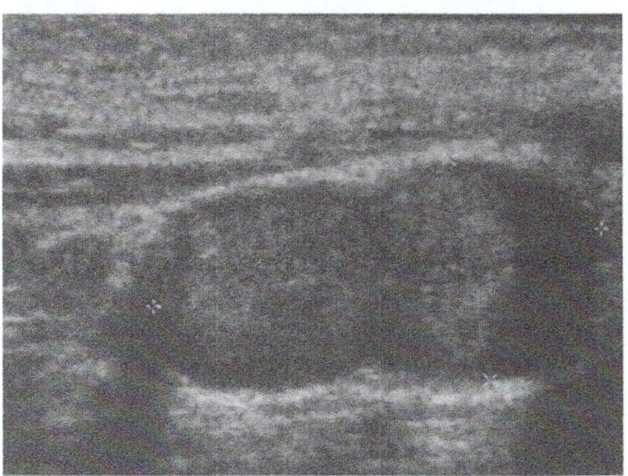

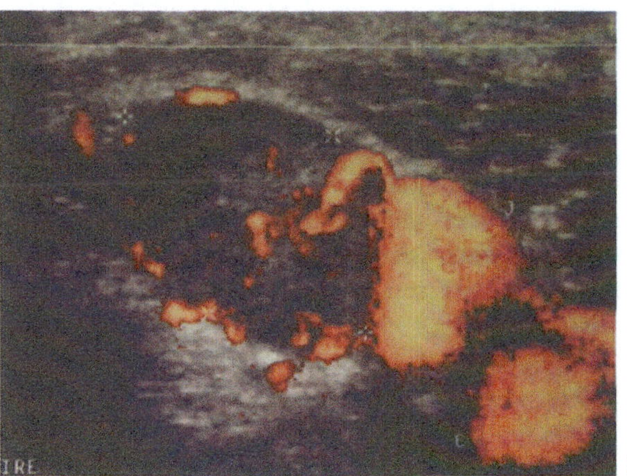

Fig. 1.27a,b. Dominant nodule of a papillary carcinoma. **a** The presence of two confluent adenopathies creates a pseudo mass syndrome (oval mass) (2.7/1.3 cm between the *two crosses*). These two confluent nodules have completely lost their normal echotexture. **b** Same patient as in **a**: PD analysis of the vascularity of these adenopathies; visualization of the drainage vein that pierces the capsule of the node to join with the internal jugular vein (*J*). Capsular effraction is an additional sign of the malignant nature of this node (1.9/1.3 cm between the *two crosses*); (*C* internal carotid artery)

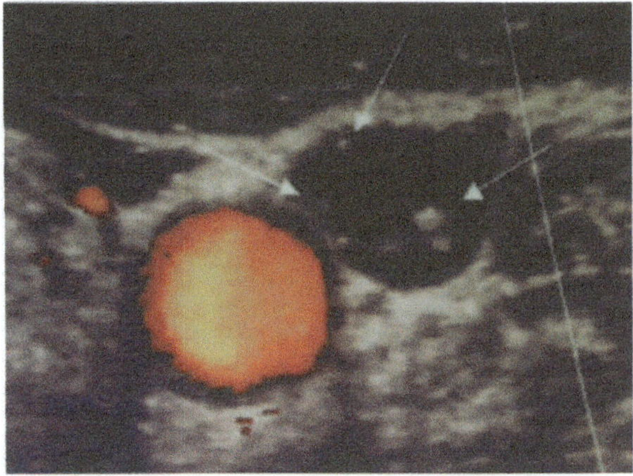

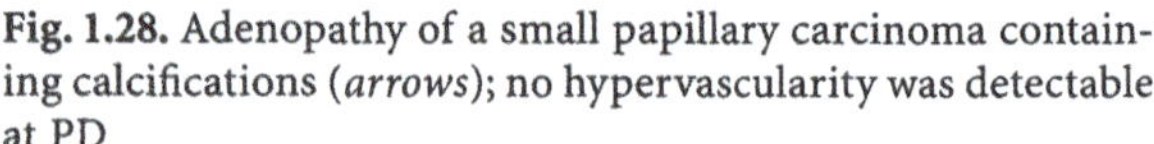

Fig. 1.28. Adenopathy of a small papillary carcinoma containing calcifications (*arrows*); no hypervascularity was detectable at PD

such nodes were underestimated in 48.1% of cases. These last authors emphasized the limitations of sonography for accurate determination of the depth of spread, in particular towards the trachea and the esophagus. Frasoldati et al. (1999) advocate US-guided FNA for all laterocervical nodal masses, with both histological examination and thyroglobulin (Tg) measurement in the needle wash-out. This combination of cytology and Tg assays has a sensitivity of 92%, and may thus be a valuable technique for pretherapy workup and post-treatment follow-up in search of metastasis.

The rare lesions revealed by a necrotic node with a pseudocystic appearance involve problems for management: They may be merely a branchial cleft cyst, especially as these cysts, often superinfected, may have a misleading sonographic pattern. Cysts generally have a thin wall, but they may contain homogeneous echogenic material if infection and bleeding have occurred (Ahuja et al. 1998; Loughran 1991). In such cases, the association of histological data and Tg assay in the needle wash-out may provide conclusive diagnostic information.

Regardless of the presentation of papillary carcinoma, CD can demonstrate nonspecific central hypervascularity (Fig. 1.29). Particular care should be paid to recognition of this feature, especially in predominantly cystic tumors (small, hypervascular parietal zone).

Accurate evaluation of the contralateral thyroid lobe is essential, because the thyroidectomy specimen often contains coexistent tumor, even though US is negative (Price et al. 1993). Contralateral can-

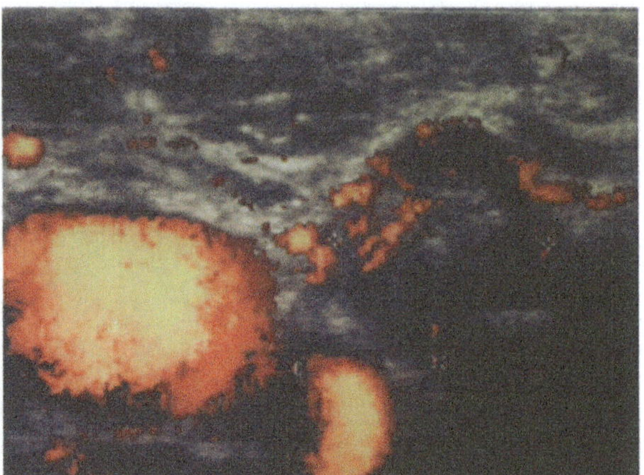

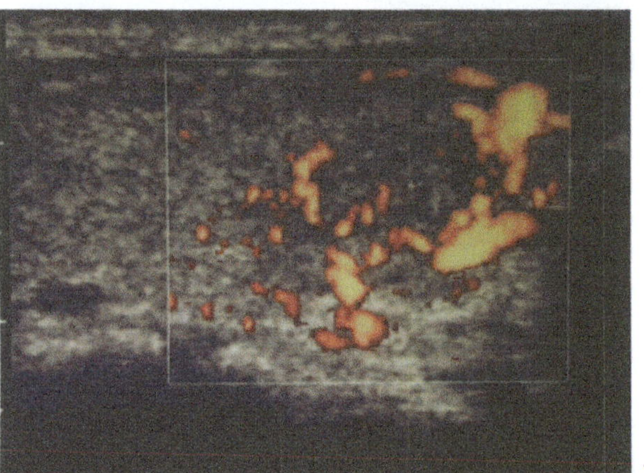

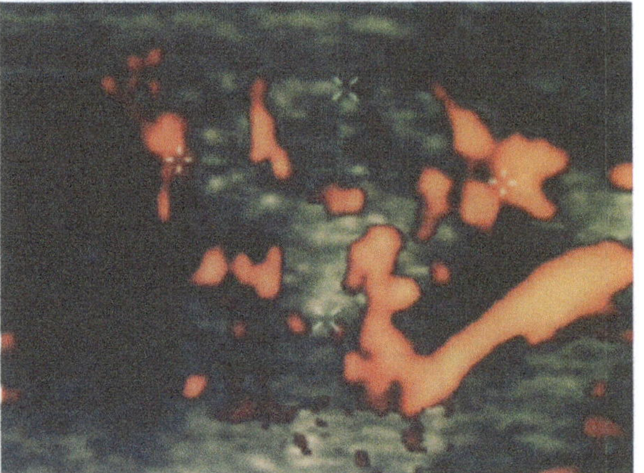

Fig. 1.29a–c. PD analysis of the vascularity of a papillary carcinoma. **a** Same patient as in Fig. 1.23a: nonspecific anarchic vascularity within a hypoechoic nodule (*J* jugular vein; *C* common carotid artery; 1.3/1.2 cm between the *crosses*) **b** Same patient as in Fig. 1.24b: This lesion detected by US shows anarchic vascularity and especially poorly defined limits. **c** Same patient as in Fig. 1.25a; the mixed (peripheral and central) vascular pattern is a secondary but supplemental feature in favor of a malignant etiology

cers were recognized sonographically in only 12.8% of cases by Lu et al. (1994).

Although the sonographic patterns are varied and the clinical presentation is not very suggestive, histological diagnosis of papillary carcinoma is usually facilitated owing to the presence of a characteristic papillary configuration and large, irregularly shaped nuclei (Gharib 1997). All of these data underscore the utility of routine FNA cytology for all centimeter-large thyroid nodules.

1.2.5.2
Follicular Carcinoma

Follicular carcinoma represents less than 15% of all thyroid cancers. If the entire surgical specimen is not available for examination, a well-differentiated tumor may be confused with an adenoma because sparse tumoral emboli in peripheral veins may be the only signs of malignancy. Follicular carcinomas often have a slow growth pattern and rarely spread to the lymph nodes.

Two thirds of all follicular thyroid carcinomas are associated with goiter, and this creates problems for detection. If the tumor is hypervascular, CD and PD can theoretically suggest the etiologic diagnosis by demonstrating a suspicious area within a multinodular goiter. This finding may indicate US-guided FNA.

This rare carcinoma may be isoechoic or, less often, hypoechoic (Fig. 1.30). Neither calcification nor lymphadenopathy is present. Diagnosis of follicular thyroid cancer is thus particularly difficult; US-guided FNA rarely provides useful information (Okamoto et al. 1994), and these tumors often develop within benign multinodular lesions. According to Lin et al. (1997a), follicular tumors, whether benign or malignant, represent 3.2% of all FNA findings; for these authors, the sonographic pattern of follicular tumors allows evaluation of the risk of malignancy. In their series, 76.2% of all follicular cancers that came to surgery presented as a hypoechoic nodule, whereas only 23.8% of benign follicular tumors exhibited this hypoechoic nodular character. Visualization of a hypoechoic nodule and demonstration of a follicular pattern by FNA are findings strongly in favor of malignancy, especially in males. The difficulties for histological diagnosis have been mentioned previously. Differentiation of benign and malignant tumors is generally not possible, as these lesions produce hypercellular aspirates with the cells arranged in microfollicular patterns, decreased or absent colloid, and nuclear atypia. This underscores the importance of surgery for all patients with such nondiagnostic aspirates.

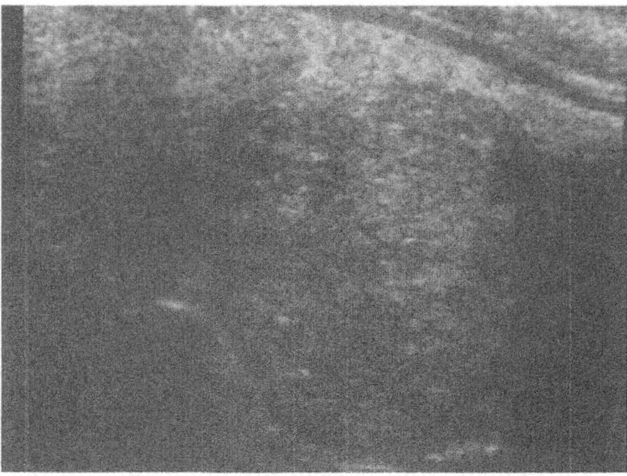

Fig. 1.30. Solid nodule with an incomplete halo (follicular carcinoma)

1.2.5.3
Medullary Carcinoma

Medullary carcinoma arises from the parafollicular cells that secrete calcitonin, which is thus the marker for this malignancy. Medullary carcinomas account for approximately 4% of all thyroid carcinomas (Baeza 1999; Lukomskii et al. 1999). Owing to the pathognomonic diagnostic role of serum calcitonin assays, Mayr et al. (1999) proposed routine use of the technique to screen for nodular thyroid disease. Such assays are all the more contributory owing to the relatively low accuracy of FNA cytology. In the series of 19 cases described by Ho et al. (1996), only one of which was familial, FNA had an accuracy of only 42%. Generally speaking, sporadic forms tend to be solitary, whereas multinodular involvement is seen essentially in familial disease.

Sonographically, medullary carcinomas tend to be hypoechoic. Isoechoic tumors recognizable by a halo are rare. Microcalcifications exist in 80%–90% of cases (Gorman et al. 1987) and are correlated with the presence of amyloid substance. The simultaneous presence of central calcifications (corresponding to amyloid deposits) and hyperechoic areas due to fibrosis creates a suggestive sonographic pattern within a hypoechoic nodule. CD and PD demonstrate peripheral and central hypervascularity (Figs. 1.31, 1.32). Laterocervical lymphadenopathy is frequent. Ho et al. (1996) found cervical adenopathies in seven of 19 medullary tumors at least 3 cm in diameter. In contrast, except for familiar forms, medullary carcinomas are rarely revealed by a cervical adenopathy (Sironi et al. 1999).

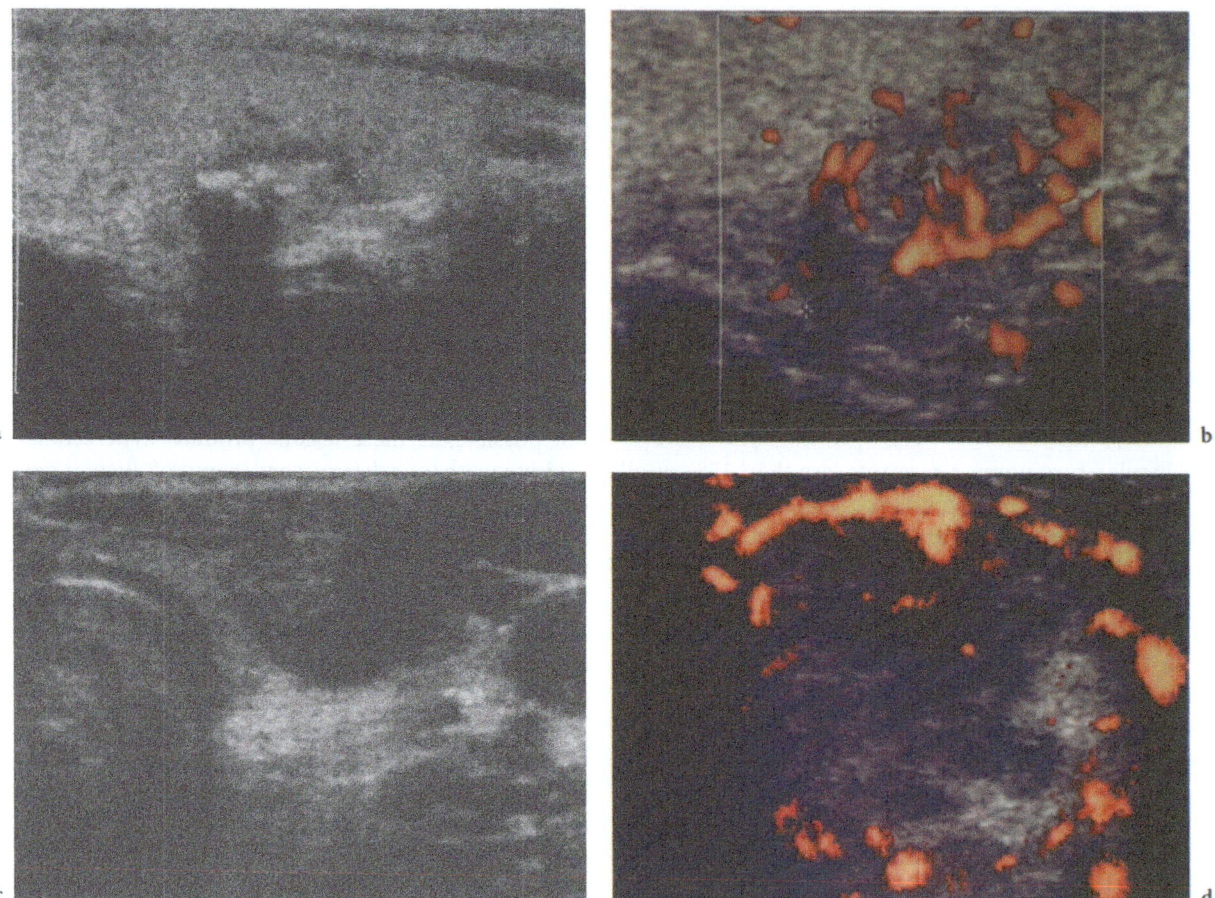

Fig. 1.31a–d. Medullary thyroid carcinoma. **a** Hypoechoic nodule; the central calcifications have low specificity. **b** Power Doppler study of the same patient as in **a**, allowing analysis of the nodules' peripheral and central vascularity. **c** Medullary carcinoma was suspected in this patient with hypercalcitonemia: mixed nodule with an essentially cystic appearance; surgery confirmed the diagnosis of medullary carcinoma. This unusual appearance emphasizes the importance of systematic calcitonin assays in patients with thyroid nodules. **d** Medullary carcinoma in the left thyroid lobe: essentially peripheral hypervascularity

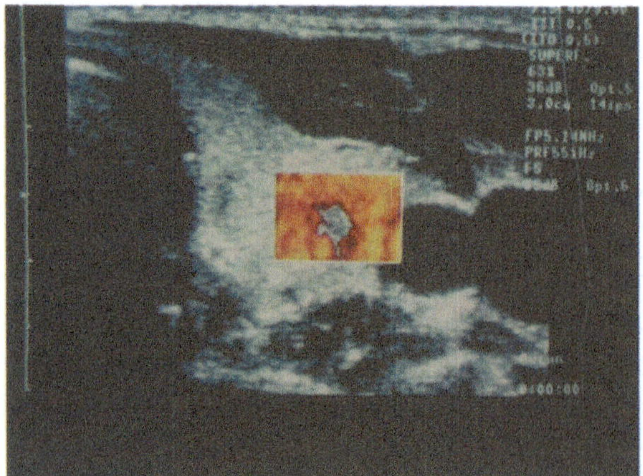

Fig. 1.32. Systematic screening for familial medullary carcinoma. PD analysis of this hypoechoic micronodule detected in a young subject failed to reveal any hypervascularity, yet the final diagnosis after surgery was medullary carcinoma

CT and MRI are helpful for demonstration of lymphatic spread to the mediastinum. CT can be performed with iodinated contrast material because medullary carcinoma is not treated by radioactive iodine.

Although most cases of medullary thyroid carcinoma are sporadic, 15% are autosomal dominant familial forms. Systematic familial screening by laboratory tests and US is thus indicated for the relatives of affected patients.

1.2.5.4 *Anaplastic Carcinoma*

Anaplastic carcinoma of the thyroid usually involves the entire gland and is seen predominantly in the elderly. Despite several reports of solitary anaplastic lesions, most patients have more or less diffuse invasion of the thyroid, and the course is rapidly unfavorable.

Sonographically, anaplastic carcinoma manifests as a weakly echoic mass with a complex echotexture infiltrating the thyroid and spreading towards the adjacent muscle (and sometimes the vascular structures; Fig. 1.33).

Extension to the trachea is difficult to assess sonographically, and is best evaluated by other techniques, in particular CT. Laterocervical lymphadenopathy is nearly constant. CD and PD reveal variable degrees of vascularity, which often appears poor compared with the extensive nature of the thyroid lesion (unless metastatic jugular thrombosis has resulted in creation of intrathyroid venous bypasses). US is performed primarily to confirm the findings of physical examination and to guide FNA of non-necrotic areas.

1.2.5.5 Primary Thyroid Lymphoma

Primary thyroid lymphoma accounts for approximately 4% of all thyroid cancers and is most prevalent in elderly women. All thyroid lymphomas are of the B-cell type (Podoloff 1966). Nearly all patients with thyroid lymphoma have coexistent Hashimoto's thyroiditis, but only a small percentage of individuals with Hashimoto's disease have lymphoma (Burke et al. 1977; Hamburger et al. 1983). The tumor generally invades the adjacent structures (esophagus, muscles, vessels). Weakly echoic enlarged nodes are common.

The sonographic patterns of primary thyroid lymphoma vary considerably (Figs. 1.34, 1.35). According to Takashima et al. (1995c), the predominant pattern is a solitary hypoechoic mass; multinodular disease is much less common (two of 11 cases for these authors). Multiple, very hypoechoic nodules, occasionally with posterior reinforcement, may be associated with bilateral laterocervical lymphadenopathy (Komatsu et al. 1994; Tatsuno et al. 1994). Involvement of the sternohyoid and sternocleidomastoid muscles is more frequent than vascular or esophageal involvement. The differential diagnosis for multiple lesions is anaplastic carcinoma, especially when the disease has invaded the muscular structures (Kasagi

a
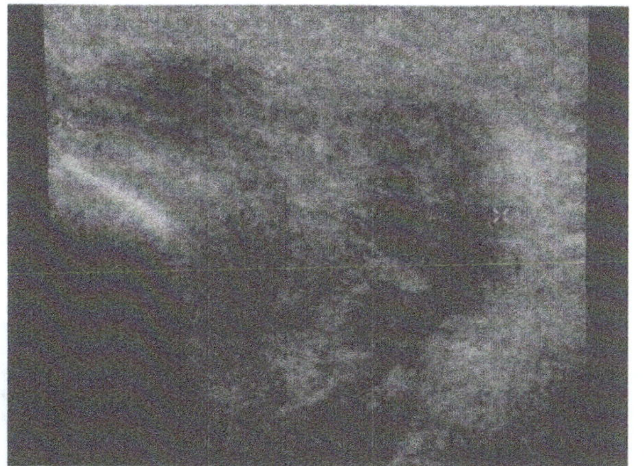

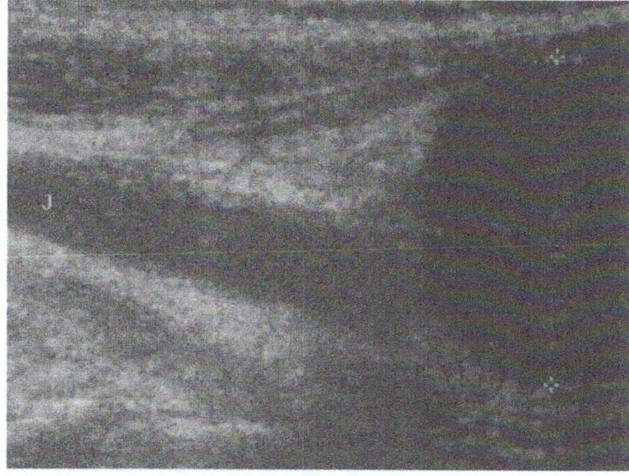

b

c
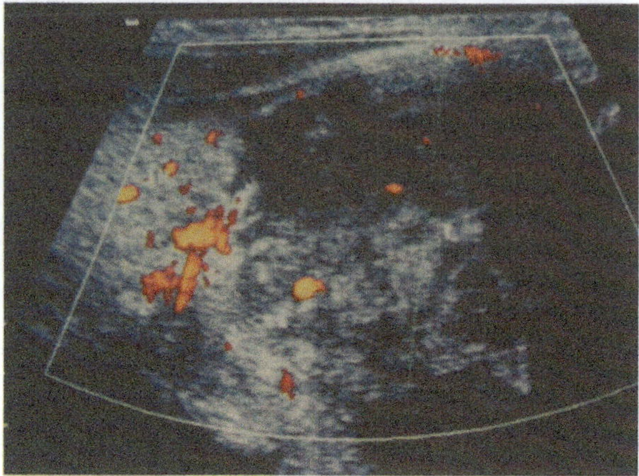

Fig. 1.33a–c. a Massive infiltration of the left thyroid lobe in the form of a weakly echoic, ill-defined lesion. **b** Same patient as in **a**: The sagittal scan reveals the internal jugular vein (*J*) encased by the diffuse tumoral process of the thyroid. **c** Analysis of the vascularity of an anaplastic thyroid carcinoma involving nearly the entire left lobe, but sparing the apical dome. The hypovascularity of this lesion (4.2 cm between the *two crosses*) has low specificity

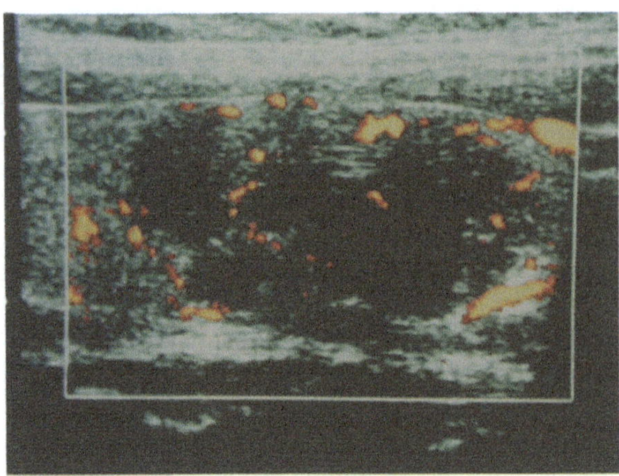

Fig. 1.34. Nodular lymphoma: hypoechoic nodule with both peripheral and central hypervascularity. Detection of a nodule in a patient with chronic thyroiditis should initially suggest lymphoma

et al. 1991). For focal lesions without signs of invasion, sonographic features suggestive of malignancy include irregular margins (90%) and constant absence of a halo. Cystic degeneration and areas of calcification are observed in less than 10% of cases (Takashima et al. 1992).

A weakly echogenic or fluid-like mass in a patient with Hashimoto's disease suggests the diagnosis and indicates FNA. In the opinion of Takashima et al. (1995c), US is more accurate than CT or MRI for diagnosis of lymphoma during follow-up of patients with Hashimoto's thyroiditis, but it is less effective for detection of tumor spread to adjacent structures.

1.2.5.6 Thyroid Metastases

Thyroid metastases are rare entities that occur late in the course of 2%–17% of all cancers (Shimaoka et al. 1962). Ferrozzi et al. (1998) reported a low clinical incidence of thyroid metastases (3%) as opposed to the 17% rate in autopsy series (this higher frequency is attributable to the extensive vascularity of the thyroid). Regardless of the type of cancer, thyroid metastases are always metachronous. In a series of 1013 thyroid cancer patients reviewed by Lin et al. (1998), only 1.4% had thyroid metastases, which are associated with a very short survival times.

The most frequently implicated primaries are melanoma, breast cancer, and lung cancer. Thyroid metastases may be solitary or multiple (Fig. 1.36). They are often large (up to 6 cm) but do not undergo cystic degeneration and are commonly associated with cervical lymphadenopathy and metastatic spread to the liver or lungs (Ahuja et al. 1994). Barczynski et al. (1998) described two patients with renal cancer who developed a thyroid metastasis presenting as a hypoechogenic nodule that appeared highly vascular on PD.

1.2.6 Management Strategy

Since the 1980s, a number of teams have addressed the problem of sonographic detection of one or more thyroid nodules (Brander et al. 1989; Carrol 1982).

a

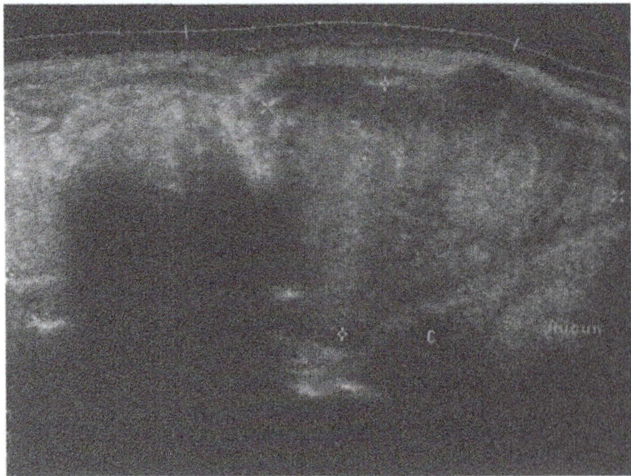

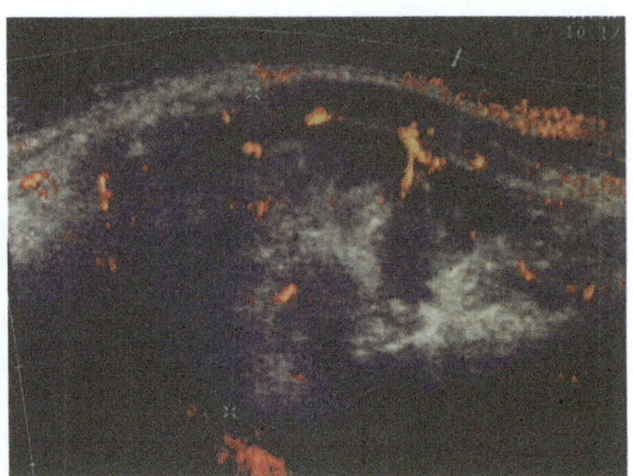

b

Fig. 1.35a,b. Diffuse thyroid lymphoma. **a** The transverse scan reveals bilateral enlargement, predominantly at the level of the left lobe (on the *right*, thickness 2.3 cm between the *two crosses*; massive infiltration of the left lobe in the form of a lesion measuring 5.5/3.8 cm between the *two crosses*); anteriorly, early infiltration of the muscles is visible (*C* common carotid artery). **b** Analysis of the left lobe revealed moderate tumor vascularity and confirmed the anterior muscle infiltration (6.7/3.3 cm between the *two crosses*)

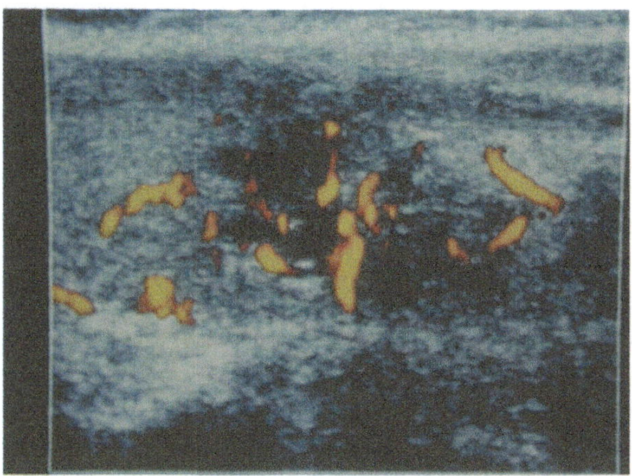

Fig. 1.36. Thyroid metastasis of breast cancer; PD revealed the anarchic vascularity of this poorly delineated nodule

Clinically, these incidentalomas (TAN and GHARIB 1997) have been associated with widely variable risks of malignancy; rates of 0.45%–13% have been cited in the literature over the past 15 years (TAN and GHARIB 1997). More recently, however, LIN et al. (1997b) reported a rate of only 2.98%. Owing to the indolent course of papillary cancer and its favorable prognosis, search for features that can aid treatment planning (follow-up versus surgery) appears justified. Clinical factors in favor of malignancy include young age, male sex, rapid nodule growth, hard and fixed nodule, cervical adenopathy, and a history of irradiation (HOPKINS and READING 1998).

In over 90% of cases, sonographic findings are accurately correlated with the gross features of these lesions. However, there are no pathognomonic signs of benignity or malignancy except, of course, in advanced cancers (cervical lymphadenopathy, anaplastic cancer, metastases). CD provides no conclusive elements for differentiation of benign and malignant tumors, even though central hypervascularity in a nodule suggests a neoplastic process. Scintigraphy has clearly seen its indications decrease, and there do not seem to be any broad diagnostic indications for CT or MRI.

US is the first and often the only morphological examination required for assessment of nodular thyroid disease, but all nodules larger than 8 mm should also be subjected to US-guided FNA. GHARIB (1997) recommends FNA biopsy as the initial procedure for thyroid nodules, because over 75% are benign and may be amenable to medical management. For this author, only 15% of nondiagnostic nodules after palpation-guided FNA require a second biopsy under US guidance. CASTRO and GHARIB (2000) proposed routine serum TSH assay to guide management; they propose FNA if the TSH concentration is normal and radionuclide scanning if the serum TSH level is below normal.

Numerous management strategies have been proposed. Certain of these are based on the palpable or nonpalpable nature of the thyroid nodule (PROYE 1993). The utility of complementary techniques can be evaluated by determining the cost, the frequency of cancers, the death rate, and iatrogenic postoperative complications (EECKHOUDT et al. 1993). GIUFFRIDA and GHARIB (1995) suggested mere US surveillance for nodules smaller than 1.5 cm; they reserved US-guided FNA for nodules larger than 1.5 cm. US-guided FNA can be performed in the office setting (RIFAT and RUFFIN 1994). Incidentalomas must be distinguished from lesions requiring aggressive management, in particular in patients with a history of neck irradiation. FNA cytology should be performed systematically for solitary nodules in such patients (VISSET 1999).

GHARIB (1997) proposed subtotal thyroidectomy with LT4 therapy for patients with multinodular disease. For clinically asymptomatic and moderate nontoxic goiters, HURLEY and GHARIB (1996) proposed biological surveillance; if TSH assays reveal euthyroidism, FNA is performed on the dominant nodule. Benign nodules are monitored by clinical examination and annual TSH assays. US is indicated for symptomatic patients (cervical swelling of rapid onset) and may demonstrate cystic change or hemorrhage in a nodule. Surgery remains indispensable for thyroid nodules larger than 3–4 cm, especially when signs of compression are present.

BURCH (1995) questioned the efficacy of LT4, because fewer than 20% of patients respond to such therapy; this author proposed LTA administration for 6–12 months, followed by sonographic evaluation of the size of the nodule or nodules. Surveillance alone is offered when no modification is visualized, but any increase in size prompts biopsy. In addition, GHARIB (1997) emphasized the high frequency of thyroid nodules that regress spontaneously. The potential adverse effects of long-term suppressive therapy, and in particular aggravation of postmenopausal osteoporosis, must be assessed before offering such treatment.

In addition to these diagnostic approaches, a nonsurgical and nonhormonal therapeutic alternative has been developed for hot nodules, i.e., PEA. This increasingly common technique is indicated whenever diagnostic aspiration has conclusively identified a benign lesion. PEA has also proven effective for predominantly cystic lesions, which are unlikely to be malignant (Kim et al. 1997; Verde et al. 1994; Zingrillo et al. 1996b). PEA in one or more sessions successfully reduces nodule volume in over 80% of cases and is associated with a much lower recurrence rate than cyst fluid aspiration only (Verde et al. 1994). Fewer trials have been conducted on cold nodules, which are much less common (Goletti et al. 1993). Owing to the fact that LT4 does not modify the size of lesions, Caraccio et al. (1997) proposed PEA for benign cold thyroid nodules. These authors obtained significant nodule shrinkage in 4–13 weekly sessions (mean lesion volume 21 ml before PEA versus 4.4 ml 1 year later). Applicable to all nodular lesions (Komorowski et al. 1998), PEA can be also given as a single injection. Bennedbaek et al. (1998) administered a single intranodular injection of sterile 98% ethanol corresponding to a mean dose of 21% of the pretreatment volume of the nodule; median reduction in nodule volume was 47% after 1 year, without any change in the perinodular thyroid volume, and complete relief of symptoms was obtained in 56% of patients. For these authors, single-session PEA was more effective than LT4 suppressive therapy. Zingrillo et al. (1998) treated 41 patients with a benign cold thyroid nodule larger than 10 ml by PEA; thyroid volume decreased by more than 50% in 92.7% of patients and this was accompanied by disappearance or reduction of the tracheal displacement caused by large nodules. These authors consider PEA most effective for nodules with only necrotic material or cystic changes at cytology.

1.3 Ultrasonography of Inflammatory and Functional Thyroid Disorders

In addition to its essential role for nodular thyroid disorders, ultrasonography has progressively demonstrated its value for the management of inflammatory and functional diseases of the thyroid. As for thyroid nodules, US is increasingly becoming the first-line imaging modality for these pathologies (Tranquart et al. 1996).

1.3.1 Sonographic Features

Ultrasonographic evaluation of non-nodular thyroid disease may demonstrate modifications in gland volume and/or echotexture.

1.3.1.1 Normal or Enlarged Thyroid Gland

Isoechoic Parenchyma. The thyroid parenchyma is usually isoechoic in simple goiters; nodules or modifications in echotexture suggest progression to autoimmune or nodular thyroiditis (Clark et al. 1995).

Hypoechoic Parenchyma. Regardless of the etiology, inflammatory processes are often associated with a hypoechoic parenchyma (Viateau-Poncin 1992). Hypoechogenicity can be evaluated qualitatively by comparison with adjacent muscle, but quantitative evaluation is of no practical benefit for routine management (Benson et al. 1983).

Focal hypoechogenicity may correspond to an infrequent form of subacute thyroiditis for which the differential diagnosis is nodular thyroid disease.

Diffuse hypoechogenicity is encountered in three clinical situations that are usually associated with a functional goiter: subacute thyroiditis, chronic lymphocytic thyroiditis, and Basedow's goiter. Basedow's goiter never exhibits extensive hypoechogenicity, whereas this pattern is possible in subacute thyroiditis. If the clinical picture is not very suggestive (especially during early disease), US depiction of goiter associated with hypoechogenicity does not suggest the diagnosis. CD analysis of flow velocities in the inferior thyroid artery may allow diagnosis on the basis of vascular characteristics; Basedow's goiter is highly vascular as opposed to subacute thyroiditis and chronic lymphocytic thyroiditis, which are not, at least initially.

Inhomogeneous Parenchyma. An inhomogeneous echo pattern may be encountered in chronic lymphocytic thyroiditis, particularly during the early phase, before thyroid dysfunction becomes apparent. During this initial stage, the gland is enlarged and vascularity is at the upper limit of the normal range, probably due to inflammation.

1.3.1.2 Thyroid Gland of Reduced Volume

A thyroid of reduced volume is frequently observed in progressive hypothyroidism of the adult, whether idiopathic or the final stage of chronic lymphocytic thyroiditis. Echogenicity is extremely variable, but is usually normal or discretely diminished. Sonographic features often include a reduction in thyroid dimensions (especially the anteroposterior diameter), ill-defined contours, and poor differentiation from adjacent structures (difficulty in identifying the thyroid gland is suggestive of hypothyroidism).

1.3.2 Inflammatory Thyroid Disease

1.3.2.1 Subacute Granulomatous Thyroiditis (de Quervain's Thyroiditis)

A painful, self-limited inflammatory disease, subacute granulomatous thyroiditis develops after a viral infection of the upper respiratory tract and is often diagnosed clinically (FARWELL and BRAVERMAN 1996). Women in the second to fifth decades of life are affected most often. Clinical presentations vary between focal and diffuse disease.

RAJKOVACA et al. (1999) described three sonographic patterns: hypoechoic, multiple hypoechoic areas, and pseudocystic. US generally demonstrates extensive and diffuse hypoechogenicity (over 75% of the entire thyroid) with an increased mean thyroid volume. The hypoechoic zones are poorly delimited and do not appear nodular (Fig. 1.37).

A rare form of de Quervain's thyroiditis presents as a painful but regressive solitary nodule; differential diagnosis from a true nodular pathology (which is more frequent) can be difficult, but US-guided FNA is diagnostic (HARDOFF et al. 1995).

Serial US studies performed by RAJKOVACA et al. (1999) failed to reveal any correlation between sonographic findings and T3, T4, and TSH levels during the first 6 months of the disease (acute phase). In contrast, sonographic findings were closely correlated with the Tg level during both the acute and the recovery phase.

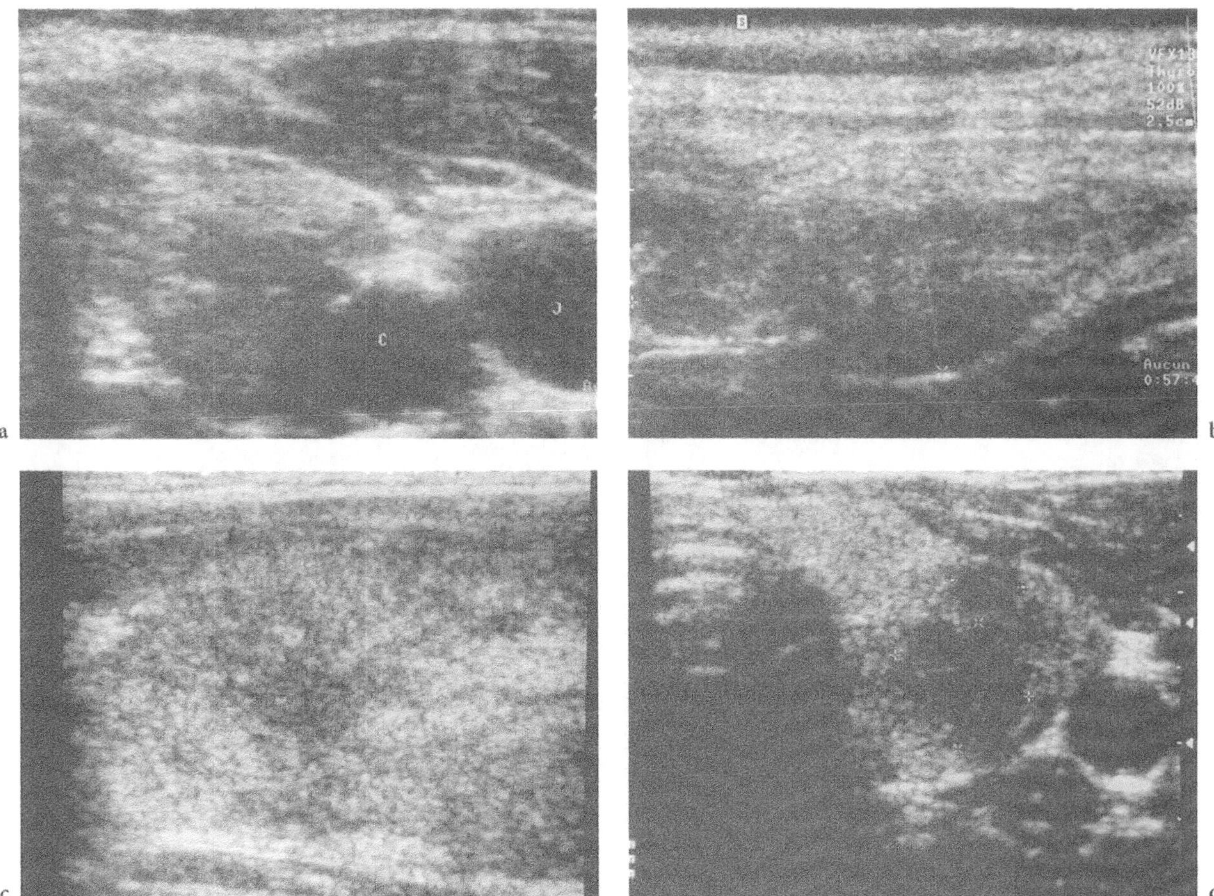

Fig. 1.37a–d. Subacute thyroiditis. **a** Transverse scan: very hypoechoic and ill-defined appearance of the posterior two thirds of the left thyroid lobe (axial scan) (*C* common carotid artery; *J* internal jugular vein). **b** Sagittal scan of the left thyroid lobe (same patient as in **a**): hypoechoic appearance of nearly the entire gland; only the superficial portion has a normal sonographic appearance (3.2/1.2 cm between the *two crosses*). **c** Minor form of subacute thyroiditis; the hypoechoic areas are less extensive than the sonographically-normal areas. **d** Pseudonodular focal appearance of subacute thyroiditis (1/0.9/0.5 cm between the *crosses*)

Vascularity may appear normal or decreased on CD, especially in hypoechoic zones (Solbiati et al. 1995). According to Hiromatsu et al. (1999), the areas of hypovascularity correspond to the hypoechoic zones seen at gray-scale imaging; such features are helpful for differential diagnosis from Graves' disease, which is constantly hypervascular. Hiromatsu et al. (1999) reported an increase in vascularity during the recovery phase, as the affected zones gradually became isoechoic, with a return to vascular normality after 1 year (Fig. 1.38).

Examination of the laterocervical neck may reveal lymphadenopathy (Bennedbaek and Hegedus 1997; Birchall et al. 1990; Horvath et al. 1997). Juxtajugular and supraisthmic node enlargement is highly suggestive of inflammatory thyroid disease (Solivetti et al. 1998), even if there are no objective sonographic signs at the level of the gland itself. In the experience of these authors, 91% of all patients with subacute thyroiditis have inflammatory juxtajugular or supraisthmic nodes.

Subacute thyroiditis usually responds completely to treatment. Possible recurrences image as an increase in the hypoechoic zones and thyroid volume (Fig. 1.39). The risk of recurrence is not correlated with the extent of sonographic anomalies (hypoechogenicity) seen at initial diagnosis (Bennedbaek and Hegedus 1997).

1.3.2.2 Chronic Lymphocytic Thyroiditis (Hashimoto's Thyroiditis)

Chronic lymphocytic thyroiditis is an autoimmune syndrome with a predilection for middle-aged women that manifests in several ways: fibrous, atrophic or asymptomatic thyroiditis, idiopathic myxedema, and an adolescent lymphocytic variety. Circulating antithyroglobulin or antimicrosomal antibodies are an almost constant finding. In the series of 437 patients with chronic thyroiditis investigated by Takamatsu et al. (1998), 72.3% had both antithyroglobulin antibodies (TgAb) and antithyroid peroxidase (PO) antibodies, 7.1% had only TgAb, and 2.4% had only PO; the remaining 8.2% had neither TgAb nor PO. Giusti et al. (1999) suggested a possible role for prolactin in the development of thyroid

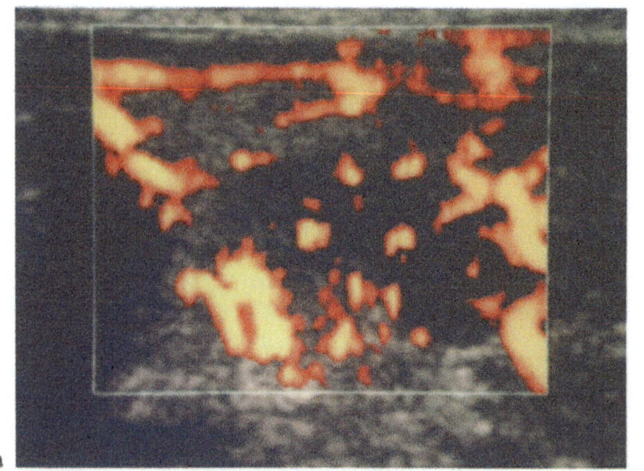
a

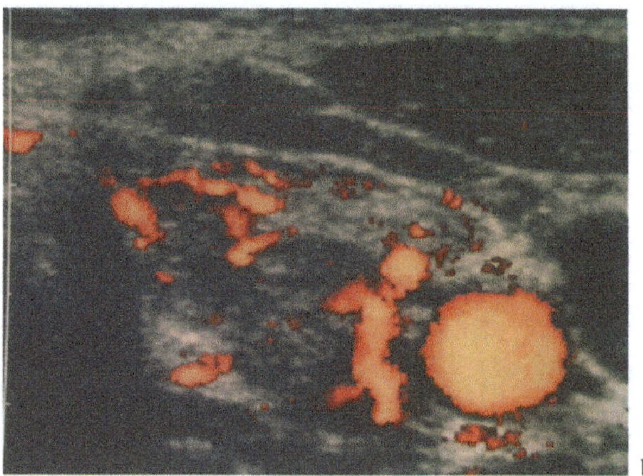
b

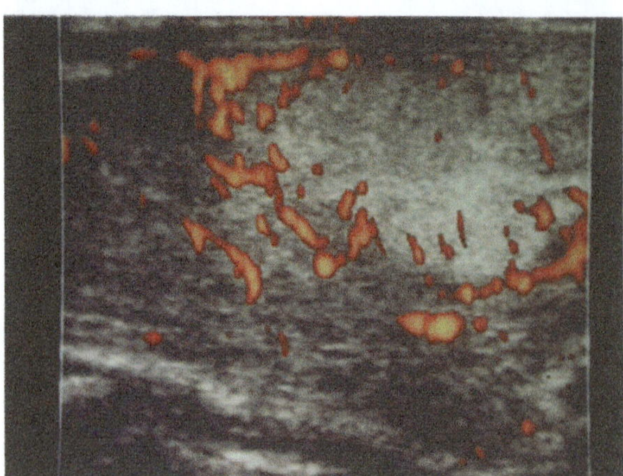
c

Fig. 1.38a–c. PD analysis of subacute thyroiditis. **a** The hypoechoic areas exhibit normal or decreased vascularity. **b** Reduced vascularity within the hypoechoic zones. **c** The hypoechoic portion actually corresponds to normal tissue; the less echoic portion is hypovascular

a 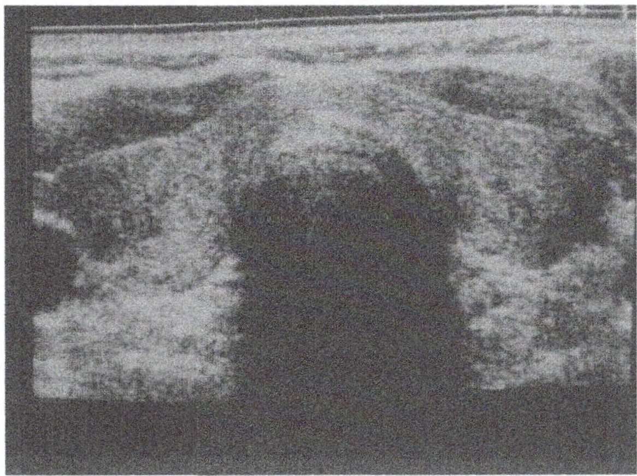

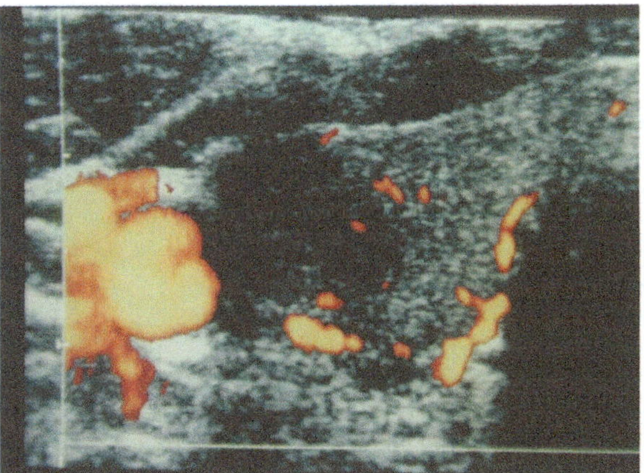 b

Fig. 1.39a,b. Evolution of subacute thyroiditis. **a** Transverse scan of the thyroid revealing residual peripheral areas of low echogenicity. **b** Same patient as in **a**; PD study of the right lobe reveals hypovascularity of the residual hypoechoic zone

diseases, and in particular chronic lymphocytic thyroiditis. They found that women treated for hyperprolactinemia had a higher prevalence of thyroid disease than controls (30.8% versus 15.5%) and were more apt to have autoantibodies (29.6% versus 14.3%). One third of patients have an associated functional disorder such as hypo- or hyperthyroidism. The clinical presentation depends on the stage of the disease, varying from thyrotoxicosis in the early phase to atrophy.

Early sonographic reports described almost constant and durable hypoechogenicity that appeared homogeneous with the sonographic equipment available at the time (HAYASHI et al. 1986; VIATEAU-PONCIN 1992). Today's state-of-the-art high-resolution transducers can depict micronodules as small as 1–6 mm in diameter (SET et al. 1996). These hypoechoic micronodules are surrounded by an echoic halo (SOSTRE and REYES 1991) and are correlated with increased lobulation. Such micronodules have a predictive value of 94.7% for diagnosis of Hashimoto's disease (YEH et al. 1996). According to RUBELLO et al. (1996), even though there is no absolute correlation between hypothyroidism and hypoechogenicity, the prevalence of hypothyroidism increases with the extent of hypoechogenicity.

MESSINA (1999) classified thyroid US patterns in four groups: group I corresponds to an enlarged thyroid with diffuse hypoechogenicity; group II corresponds to multiple foci of hypoechogenicity; group III presents as a hypoechoic thyroid gland with scattered hyperechoic areas and one or more nodules; group IV corresponds to a small, isoechoic thyroid characterized by numerous spots and hyperechoic spots and lines. Groups I and II always corresponded to chronic autoimmune thyroiditis, whereas patients with group III and IV patterns had extensive thyroid fibrosis (which explains why FNA is often inconclusive) (Fig. 1.40).

Size data are related to the duration of thyroiditis. Although gland enlargement and surface irregularity, associated or not with heterogeneities in echotexture, are suggestive of chronic thyroiditis, problems may exist for differentiation from simple goiter, adenomatous goiter, or lymphoma (YASUDA et al. 1998). According to TAKAMATSU et al. (1998), the presence of PO alone is associated with an elevated risk of hypothyroidism, even if the echotexture of the gland is normal. The presence of TgAb alone, even if associated with thyroid micronodules, is associated with a lower risk of hypothyroidism. In the series of 18 children studied by SET et al. (1996), the thyroid was often more echoic than the muscles, and micronodules ranging from 2 to 5 mm were found within poorly delimited areas of hypoechogenicity.

CD and PD are useful for examination of an enlarged thyroid that appears hypoechoic on sonograms, and when problems exist for differentiation of Hashimoto's disease and Graves' disease. VITTI et al. (1995) defined four CD flow patterns ranging from normal to extensive hypervascularity. In Hashimoto's disease, the flow is normal in 49% of cases and slightly increased in 44%. This clearly distinguishes Hashimoto's disease from untreated Graves' disease, which always exhibits markedly increased vascularity. CD can thus easily distinguish Hashimoto's disease and Graves' disease in their initial stages. BOGAZZI et al. (1999) suggested that the moderate increase in vascularity and blood velocity observed in patients with Hashimoto's thyroiditis might be

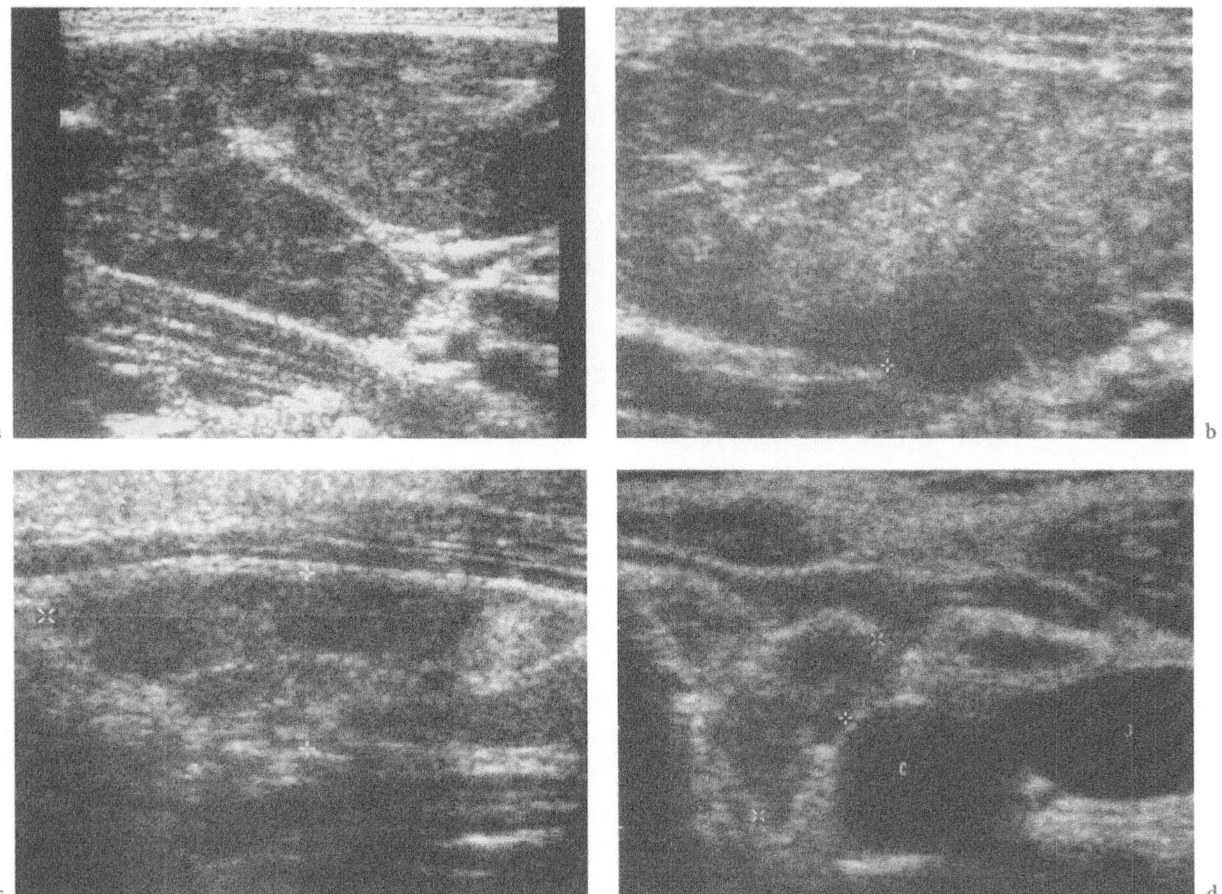

Fig. 1.40a–d. Sonographic patterns of Hashimoto's disease **a** Inhomogeneous appearance of the thyroid, with the presence of small, ill-defined structures of variable echogenicity **b** Discrete increase in the size of the thyroid (1.8 cm between the *crosses*) that has an inhomogeneous echotexture (sagittal scan). **c** Reduction in the size of the thyroid that appears globally hypoechoic, with hyperechoic linear septa (sagittal scan) (3.1/1 cm between the crosses). **d** Same patient as in **c** (transverse scan, 1 2/1 cm between the *crosses*, *C* common carotid artery, *J* internal jugular vein)

related to thyroid stimulation by TSH-receptor antibodies (Figs. 1.41, 1.42).

Yarman et al. (1997) compared US and scintigraphic findings for 48 patients with Hashimoto's disease. Radionuclide scanning revealed diffuse hyperplasia in 12 cases, multinodular goiter in 20 cases, and a solitary nodule in 16 cases. These findings corresponded sonographically to areas of hyperplasia in 19 cases, multinodular involvement in 20 cases, and a solitary nodule in nine cases. The variability of morphological features seen on imaging studies underscores the utility of thyroid antibody assays (Yarman et al. 1997).

Serial studies reveal a decrease in gland volume that is directly correlated with the extent of hypothyroidism. At this stage, CD and PD may demonstrate increased vascularity, especially in the fibrous septa (Romaldini et al. 1996; Solbiati et al. 1995).

The possibility of progression to hypothyroidism is complicated by the risk of lymphoma (Podoloff 1996). Detection of a thyroid nodule in a patient with Hashimoto's disease warrants particular attention (Takashima et al. 1992); hyperechoic masses are usually benign, but hypoechoic nodules may correspond to a papillary carcinoma (Fig. 1.43). Lymphoma nearly always images as a markedly hypoechoic mass but is sonographically indistinguishable from pseudotumor or adenomatous hyperplasia (Fig. 1.44). This underscores the utility of US-guided FNA. Although routine follow-up is not feasible, any cervical swelling in a patient with Hashimoto's thyroiditis should prompt sonography and US-guided FNA. Zardo et al. (1999) reviewed the literature to analyze the relationship between papillary thyroid carcinoma and chronic autoimmune thyroiditis. A relationship was noted in 0.5%–22.5% of cases. Pisani et al. (1999a)

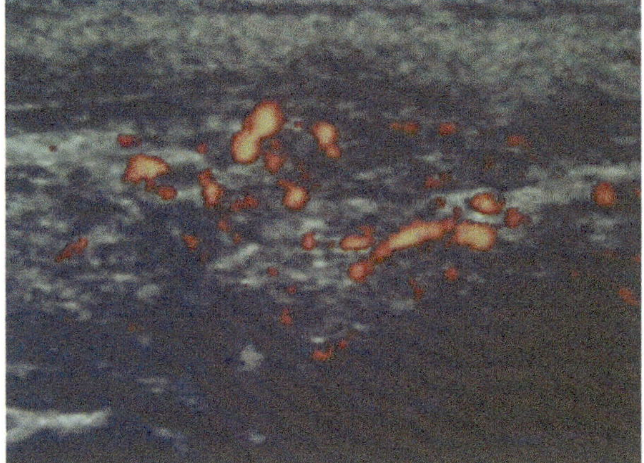

Fig. 1.41. PD appearance of Hashimoto's disease

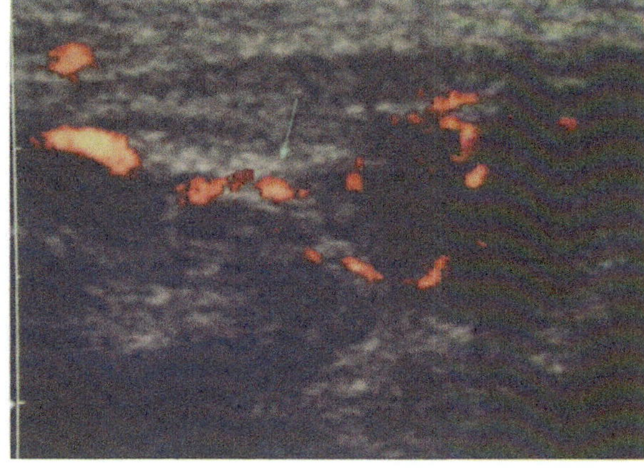

Fig. 1.42. Hashimoto's disease with hypothyroidism; PD study revealing the presence of vascular structures within the hyperechoic bands

also underscored the role of chronic lymphocytic thyroiditis as a risk factor for the development of papillary carcinoma of the thyroid.

1.3.2.3 Invasive Fibrous Thyroiditis (Riedel's Thyroiditis)

Riedel's thyroiditis is a chronic inflammatory disease corresponding to an invasive fibrotic process that destroys all or part of the thyroid gland and invades the adjacent structures. Although its origin remains unclear, an association seems probable with other fibrosing conditions (retroperitoneal fibrosis, sclerosing cholangitis, mediastinal fibrosis). This rare disorder is responsible for less than 0.1% of all thyroidectomies (Mallote et al. 1991). Middle-aged women are affected predominantly. Pressure in the neck and pain may suggest carcinoma, and especially anaplastic cancer. One third of all cases of Riedel's thyroiditis progress to hypothyroidism.

Sonography visualizes a hypoechoic mass in one of the thyroid lobes that often invades the adjacent muscle (Fontan et al. 1993) or, occasionally, the vascular structures (James et al. 1991).

1.3.2.4 Other Types of Thyroiditis

Suppurative thyroiditis is rare, and should prompt a search for immunodepression or, in young subjects, a piriform sinus fistula. The lesion may manifest as a collection of viscous fluid (Viateau-Poncin 1992)

a

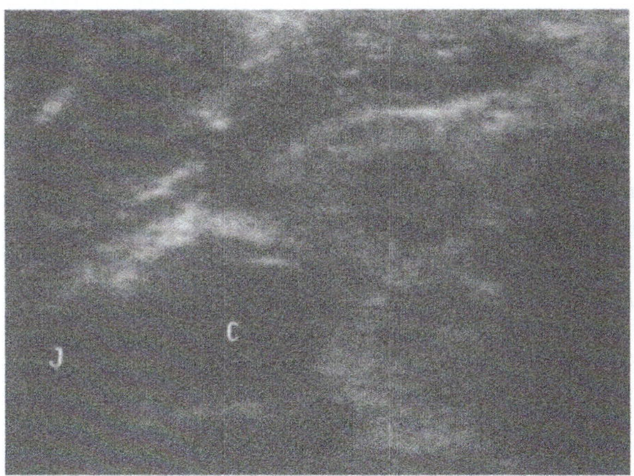

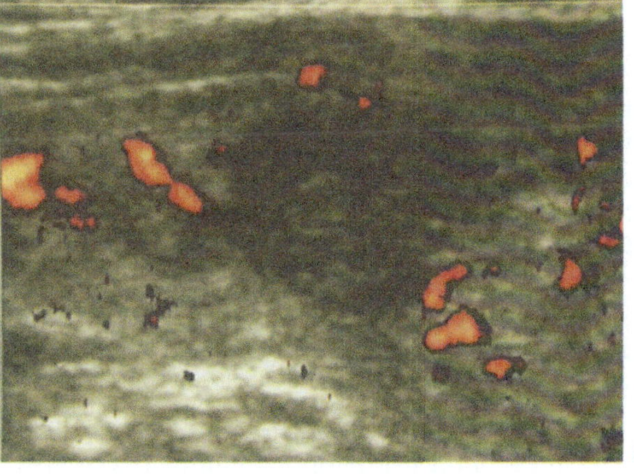

b

Fig. 1.43a,b. Papillary carcinoma in Hashimoto's disease. **a** Small, centimeter-sized nodule detected during surveillance of a patient with Hashimoto's disease. Aspiration biopsy revealed malignant cells; a papillary carcinoma was discovered at surgery (*C* common carotid artery; *J* internal jugular vein). **b** Color Doppler study of a small papillary carcinoma detected in a patient with Hashimoto's disease; no notable hypervascularity is visible in the nodule

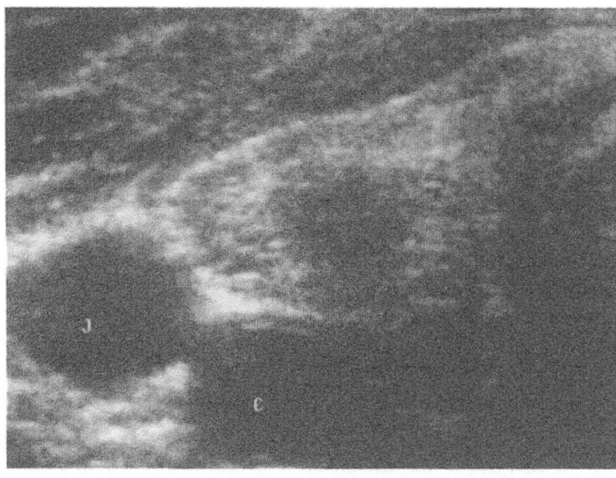

Fig. 1.44. Lymphoma in a patient with Hashimoto's disease; ill-defined nodule in the right thyroid lobe. Biopsy of cervical adenopathies led to diagnosis of lymphoma (*C* common carotid artery; *J* internal jugular vein)

or a complex nodule, occasionally containing hyperechoic trabeculae, whereas the remainder of the thyroid is diffusely hypoechoic (Gimondo et al. 1996). A hypoechoic perithyroid mass may be demonstrated by US (Diez et al. 1998).

Owing to the difficulties in differential diagnosis from focal subacute thyroiditis (because of the associated pain), a hemorrhagic cyst, carcinoma, or lymphoma, FNA is required for definitive diagnosis.

Silent or painless thyroiditis and postpartum thyroiditis are subacute forms of lymphocytic thyroiditis (Loevner 1996). The presence of antithyroid antibodies suggests an autoimmune origin. Early thyrotoxicosis usually progresses to transient hypothyroidism before ultimate return to the euthyroid state. One of 20 women who develop postpartum thyroiditis has a recurrence during subsequent pregnancies. Progression to a chronic form is possible. According to Premawardhana et al. (2000), postpartum thyroiditis affects 5% of women, 23% of whom develop hypothyroidism 3–5 years later. PO concentrations are increased, and these authors identified hypoechogenicity as an important risk factor for hypothyroidism.

Sonography reveals ill-defined patches of hypoechogenicity. A diffuse hypoechoic form is associated with an increase in the size of the multiple hypoechoic nodules.

The extent of these sonographic images allows assessment of the degree of thyroiditis (Adams et al. 1992; Parkes et al. 1996). Mitteldorf et al. (1999) described a multicystic autoimmune thyroiditis-like disease associated with HIV infection. The multicystic appearance of the thyroid in this pathology is similar to the multiple lymphoepithelial cysts described in the parotid gland and the thymus. The return to normal is associated with a reduction in the volume of the thyroid (Adams and Jones 1990).

1.3.3 Functional Thyroid Disease

1.3.3.1 Basedow's Goiter

General Features. Basedow's goiter is the most frequent autoimmune disorder. In the United States, for example, it affects 0.4% of the general population (De Lellis 1989). Women in the fourth decade of life are affected most often, and a familial predisposition has been observed. Diffuse enlargement of the gland is associated with hypervascularity. Coexistence of other autoimmune disorders is possible. Treatment is based on synthetic antithyroid drugs, radioactive iodine treatment, and surgery.

Ultrasound Patterns. US depicts thyroid enlargement and hypoechogenicity in 86% of cases (Vitti et al. 1995). The echotexture is homogeneous and discretely heterogeneous (Bogazzi et al. 1999); small vascular structures are visible within the thyroid tissue as small tubular structures (Fig. 1.45); unilateral involvement is exceptional (Dimai et al. 1999). Lucas (2000) adapted the dose of radioactive iodine for treatment of hyperthyroidism to thyroid volume.

Increased flow is demonstrated in the inferior thyroid artery. Schweiger et al. (1996) reported a correlation between the peak velocity and free triiodothyroxine (fT3) and free thyroxine (fT4). In the view of these authors, a velocity of less than 0.3 m/s corresponds to hypothyroidism, while a flow greater than 1.2 m/s is indicative of hyperthyroidism.

CD depicts gland hypervascularity as the "thyroid inferno" described by Ralls et al. (1988). This increased vascularity is due to arteriovenous shunts (Fig. 1.46); the flow rate is generally over 70 ml/min (Hodgson et al. 1988). According to Baldini et al. (1997), hypervascularization is not related to the level of circulating hormones but probably to autoimmune processes. This opinion is shared by Arslan et al. (2000), who failed to observe any correlation between thyroid hypervascularization in Graves' disease and circulating thyroid hormone levels or the severity of the disease. The latter authors used a subjective grading system of 0 (normal thyroid vascularization) to 3 (markedly increased hypervascularization).

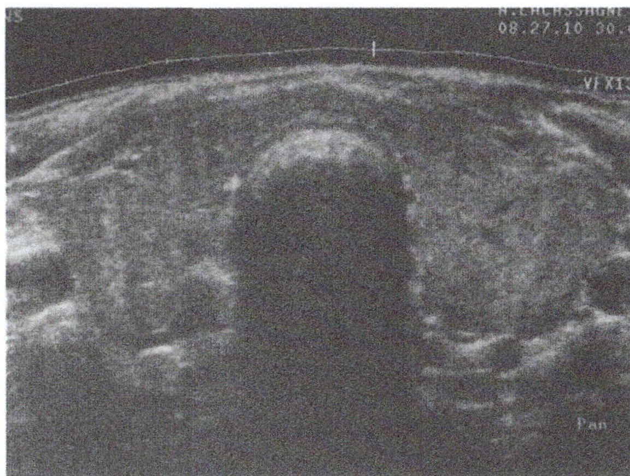
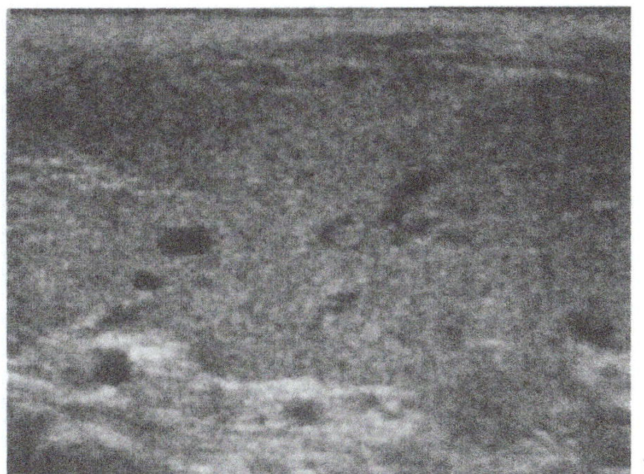

a b

Fig. 1.45a,b. Sonographic features of Basedow's disease. **a** Transverse scan revealing discretely inhomogeneous enlargement of the thyroid and numerous dilated vascular structures throughout the parenchyma. **b** Sagittal scan revealing a discrete inhomogeneity in the echotexture, and especially the presence of vascular elements

CASTAGNONE et al. (1996) did not observe any correlation between normalization of thyroid vascularity and reduction of hormone secretion in response to treatment. However, patients in remission are at increased risk of recurrence if the number of vessels per square centimeter is high and if the flow velocity increases in the inferior thyroid artery (Fig. 1.47). SPONZA et al. (1997) proposed use of CD and PD for post-therapy follow-up. In a series of 21 patients with Graves' disease, the mean PSV was 51±12 cm/s and the mean RI was 0.71±0.04. Re-evaluation at 6 or 8 months following medical treatment demonstrated normalization of flow velocities but not the hypervascularization; these authors concluded that flow-velocity data are more useful than morphological data. VERSAMIDIS et al. (2000) consider Doppler examination of the inferior thyroid artery the most effective means of detecting post-treatment recurrence.

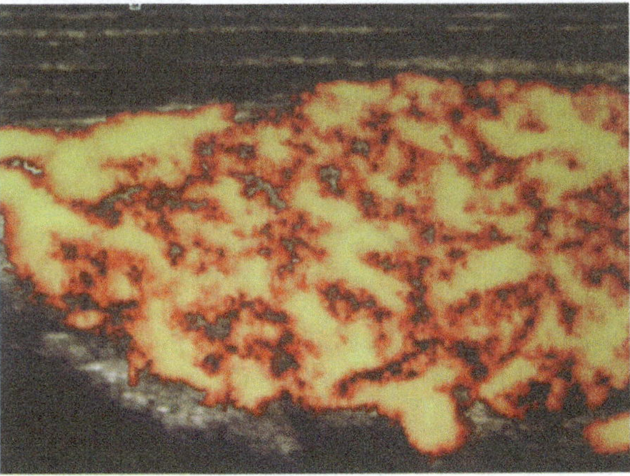

Fig. 1.46. PD study of a patient with Basedow's goiter: extensive hypervascularity

Graves' disease may recur in two rarely associated histological forms (MOROSINI et al. 1998): prevalent endothelial hyperplasia, seen as intraparenchymal homogeneous vascular color spots (diffuse or focal), and prevalent intimal hyperplasia that images as vascular bands, with vascular or poorly vascularized parenchymal areas corresponding to fibrous septa.

Follow-up of patients treated with methimazole must include a search for hypoechogenicity, which may exist early in the disease but is absent in overt Basedow's goiter. The absence of hypoechogenicity during treatment appears to be a favorable prognostic indicator of remission for hyperthyroidism, even though hypoechogenicity is not an indicator of recurrence (GEMMA et al. 1996; ZINGRILLO et al. 1996a). BENKER et al. (1998) used US to follow up patients with Graves' disease treated with methimazole and failed to observe any modification in gland size in patients in remission or in those with recurrent disease.

After subtotal thyroidectomy, sonography permits analysis of the residual thyroid tissue; KIRILLOV et al. (1997) reported a 90% increase in the volume of the remaining tissue after 1 month and a 186% increase after 1 year. Volumetric data can be helpful for surgical planning if the patient refuses secondary treatment with radioactive iodine (HERMANN et al. 1999).

Graves' Disease and Cancer. Coexistent Graves' disease and thyroid carcinoma is reported in 0.3%–16.6% of patients, with a higher incidence in toxic nodular goiter than in Graves' disease. The neoplasm is generally a small papillary carcinoma (follicular carcinomas are less common) that is identified only in the surgical specimen. The prognosis does not appear to be influenced by this association (NICOLOSI et al. 1994).

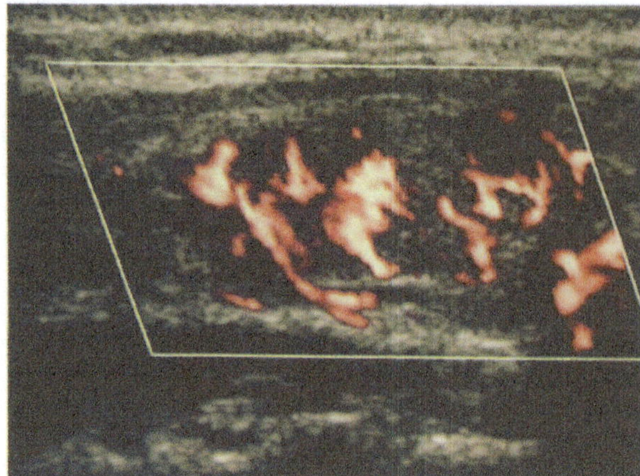
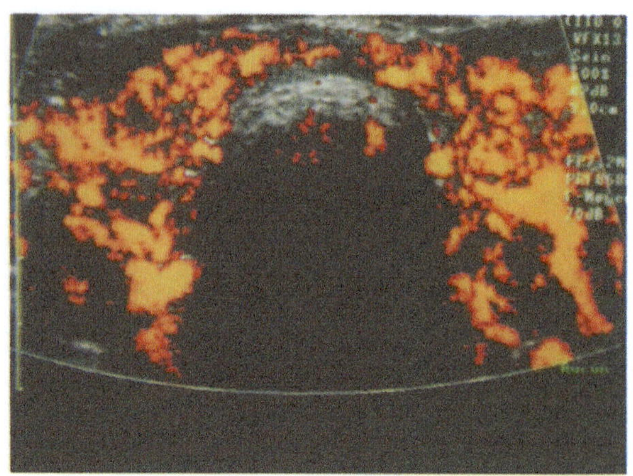

Fig. 1.47a,b. Recurrence of treated Basedow's goiter. **a** Recurrence on residual thyroid tissue after subtotal thyroidectomy for Basedow's goiter; PD analysis revealed extensive hypervascularty of the residual thyroid tissue. **b** Recurrence of a Basedow's goiter treated medically; PD demonstrates the diffuse hypervascularity

No consensus exists regarding the management of nodules discovered in patients with Graves' disease. As reported by Cantalamessa et al. (1999), 33.7% of their 315 patients with Graves' disease had one or more nodules with a diameter of at least 8 mm; the nodules were discovered with equal frequency at diagnosis and during follow-up. Only one patient in their series had cancer (0.3%), which led the authors to conclude that when FNA is in favor of benignity, there is no need to be more aggressive when a nodule is visualized or appears during the course of Graves' disease. In contrast, Kraimps et al. (1998) estimate the risk of papillary carcinoma at 5.5% in patients with Graves' disease; when associated with nodules, this risk rises to 21.4%. These authors therefore advocate systematic surgery for all thyroid nodules discovered in patients with Graves' disease.

Thyrotoxicosis factitia (Bogazzi et al. 1996), caused by use of exogenous thyroid hormones, can be diagnosed by elevated fT3 and fT4 levels, very low TSH and serum Tg, the absence of antithyroid antibodies, and absent or markedly decreased radionuclide uptake. US reveals a gland of normal volume and echotexture. CD and PD may reveal several vascular foci without hypervascularity. The PSV is at the lower limit of normal, a feature that differentiates this pathology from Graves' disease. When findings are equivocal, CD or PD can easily suggest the etiologic diagnosis (Bogazzi et al. 1999).

Two types of amiodarone-induced thyrotoxicosis were classified by Bogazzi et al. (1997); one occurs in abnormal thyroid tissue while the other develops in an apparently normal gland. CD may facilitate diagnosis because the first type is characterized by variable degrees of hypervascularization detectable by CD, whereas the second type is avascular on CD. This ready differentiation by CD permits more rapid therapeutic management: The first type of thyrotoxicosis is treated with methimazole and potassium perchlorate while the second type is managed with glucocorticoids.

1.3.3.2
Autonomous Thyroid Nodules and PEA

A thyroid nodule that appears hypervascular on CD or PD and is associated with reduced circulating TSH levels is an indication for scintigraphy, which usually reveals an autonomous thyroid nodule. On scintigrams, 74.4% of autonomous adenomas (hot nodules) are solitary, but 25.6% occur in a multinodular goiter (Van Espen et al. 1997).

Gimondo et al. (1998) observed a hypoechoic solid nodular lesion in 59.8% of cases, and simple hyperplasia was the most frequent cytologic finding. A mixed US pattern, often noted in the toxic phase and in large nodules, generally corresponded to a hemorrhagic pseudocyst. Calcifications are infrequent (4.3%–8.6%). For these authors, CD allows classification of these lesions in two categories: 75% of nodules with extensive peripheral and internal vascularization corresponded to the toxic phase, whereas 85.7% with predominantly perilesional flow were partially autonomous nodules. The flow velocity is increased, with a mean PSV of 11±2.4 cm/s (Bogazzi et al. 1999).

Italian investigators were the first to propose therapeutic intratumoral injection of ethanol for these lesions. The efficacy of PEA markedly reduces the incidence of post-therapy hypothyroidism compared with other methods, including surgery and especially radioactive iodine treatment.

LIPPI et al. (1996) reviewed a series of 429 patients, 56.4% of whom had a toxic adenoma treated by PEA. Patients underwent a mean of four sessions and received 1–8 ml per session for a cumulative dose of 2–50 ml. Surveillance was conducted with sonography (including CD), isotopic studies, and laboratory tests (TSH, fT3, fT4). After more than 1 year, they reported a success rate of 66.5% for toxic adenomas and 83.4% for pretoxic adenomas. All of the thyroid nodules had decreased in volume, but the efficacy of the technique decreased with nodule size. The authors consider PEA an excellent alternative to surgery for nodules smaller than 15 ml.

CD and PD may optimize ethanol injection techniques. For SPIEZIA et al. (2000), the improved visualization of blood flow, even in small vessels (and thus the areas to be treated with priority), achieved with PD sonographic guidance makes it possible to monitor ethanol diffusion and its effect on nodular vascularization. This, in turn, permits a reduction in the number of ethanol injection sessions.

SCHUMM-DRAEGER (1998) reviewed the results achieved with PEA as reported in the literature. The response is considered complete when the TSH level returns to normal and radionuclide scanning reveals reactivation of the normal tissue. Normalization is achieved in 68%–100% of patients with subclinical hyperthyroidism and AFTN, but a complete response is observed in only 36%–89% of symptomatic patients. A partial response (detectable TSH and partial reactivation at radionuclide scanning) is observed in 0%–50% of patients, regardless of the clinical picture. First pointed out by LIPPI et al. (1996), the more favorable response obtained with PEA for large nodules was confirmed by the review of SCHUMM-DRAEGER (1998).

CD and PD are helpful for evaluation of response to therapy because toxic adenomas are always hypervascular (BECKER et al. 1997; BRAUN and BLANK 1994). Decreased echogenicity and modifications in nodule shape and volume have been observed after PEA (GONSORCIKOVA et al. 1996). The sensitivity of CD may be improved by injection of an echo-enhancing agent allowing detection of arterial signals corresponding to residual viable tissue (LAGALLA et al. 1998; SOLBIATI et al. 1999). For SOLBIATI et al. (1999), when TSH is not detectable, a second cycle of PEA is performed. The decison to use an ultrasound contrast agent is based on hormone anomalies and absence of nodule vascularity at CD; this approach improves sonographic depiction of areas of recurrence requiring repeat PEA.

PEA preserves the function of the residual thyroid tissue and reduces the risk of post-therapy hypothyroidism (LIVRAGHI et al. 1994; OZDEMIR et al. 1994). The technique can also be proposed for larger hot nodules (even those over 30 ml). A mean of six sessions is required, and the total ethanol volume administered may exceed 50 ml. Nodules may regress by 40%–80% in 6–9 months. Autonomous nodules do not recur, but PEA is always painful (TARANTINO et al. 1997). More recently, TARANTINO et al. (2000) presented their results for large (>30 ml) hot nodules followed-up from 6 to 48 months; no recurrences were seen in their series (Figs. 1.48, 1.49).

MESSINA et al. (1998) recommend PEA for all small-diameter AFTN; in their opinion, the respective advantages of surgery, radioisotope treatment, and increasingly PEA need be evaluated only for large nodules.

1.3.3.3
Hypothyroidism

Ultrasonography can assess the therapeutic response of reversible hypothyroidism of chemical, immunological, mixed, or postpartum origin (SATO et al. 1996). Response corresponds to a decrease of at least 50% in the initially elevated TSH concentration during iodine restriction over a 2- to 15-week period without replacement therapy. Sonographically, the preexistent hypoechogenicity disappears more rapidly in chemically induced hypothyroidism than in other etiologies. If imaging is required, US is sufficient for atrophic thyroiditis; sonograms demonstrating hypoechogenicity and a more or less constant reduction in thyroid volume obviate the need for scintigraphy (VITTI et al. 1994) (Fig. 1.50).

1.3.3.4
Role of Ultrasound in the Management of Functional Thyroid Disease

FELDKAMP and HORSTER (1995) defined the role of ultrasonography in various clinical settings:

- Thyroid dysfunction can be ruled out if sonography and the TSH level are normal
- Hyperthyroidism can be confirmed with 98% confidence if TSH is suppressed and triiodothyroxine (T3) and fT3 are elevated. If Graves' disease is suspected, US supplements laboratory tests (thyroxine (T4), TSH antibody receptors, and thyroid peroxidase (PO) antibodies). Scintigraphy and US are indicated if focal or diffuse autonomy is suspected.

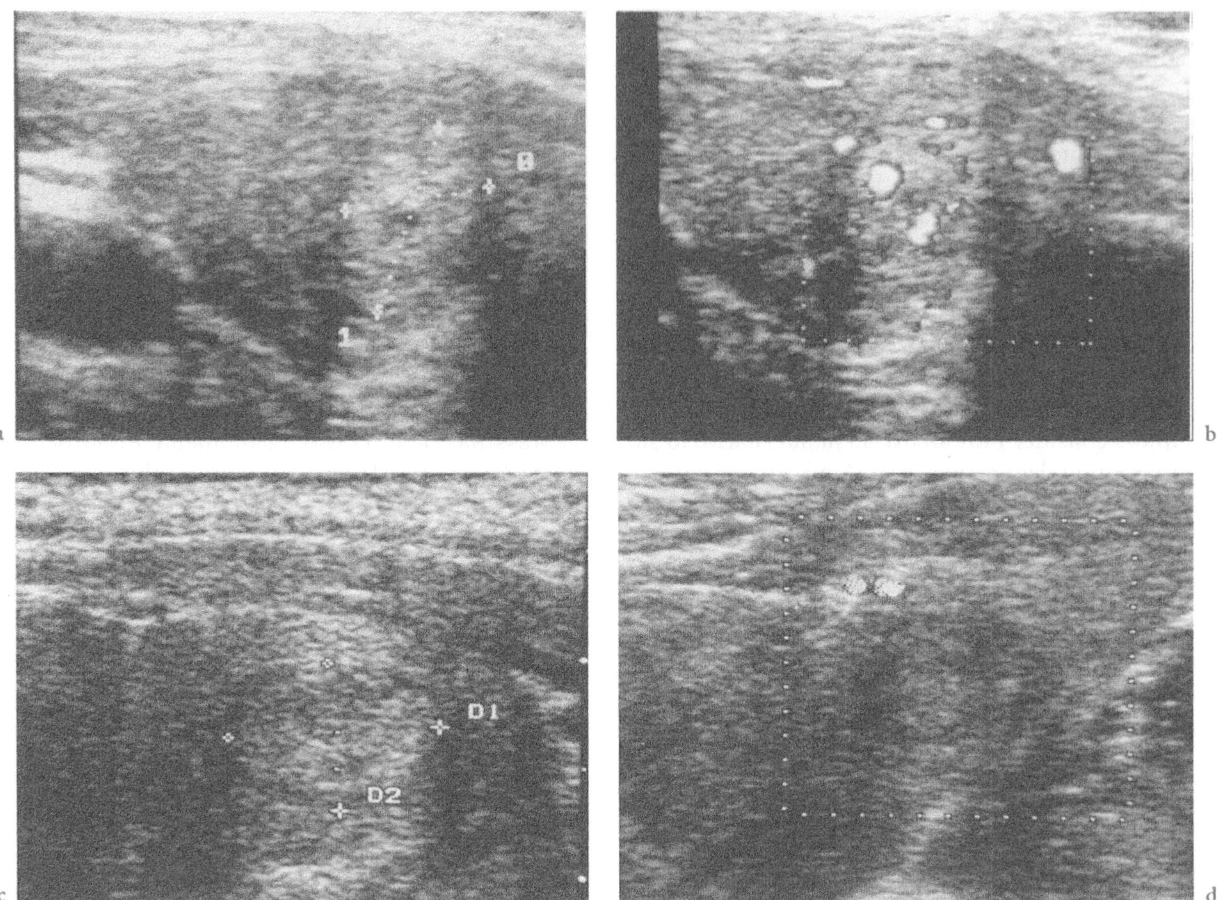

Fig. 1.48a–d. PEA of a hot nodule. **a** Hyperechoic nodule (1.6/1.2 cm). **b** PD study revealing the central hypervascularity of the nodule. **c** Follow-up 3 months after PEA revealed a reduction in size (1/0.7 cm between the *crosses*) and appearance of a peripheral halo. **d** PD revealed a reduction in lesion vascularity after PEA

- Hypothyroidism can be diagnosed with 98% confidence if the TSH concentration is elevated and the T4 concentration is low. In congenital hypothyroidism, US suffices in 50% of patients (Takashima et al. 1995d). If ectopia is suspected, scintigraphy is more effective (Yoshimura et al. 1995). For patients with symptoms of acquired hypothyroidism, thyroid PO antibody assays are required along with US and possibly FNA to rule out de Quervain's thyroiditis or Hashimoto's disease.

1.4 Nonultrasonographic Imaging of Thyroid

The introduction of new imaging modalities and refinement of laboratory techniques that today permit indirect and highly accurate analysis of thyroid disorders have markedly reduced the indications for diagnostic thyroid scintigraphy. Recent research has been successful in cloning the thyroid iodine transporter, thereby helping to elucidate the mechanisms of iodine transport in healthy and diseased tissues. Similar clarification is under way concerning the mechanisms of regulation of thyroid hormone biosynthesis (Cavalieri 1997).

1.4.1 Nuclear Medicine

1.4.1.1 Current Techniques

Technetium (^{99m}Tc), used in the form of pertechnetate ^{99m}Tc-04, is taken up by the thyroid but is not

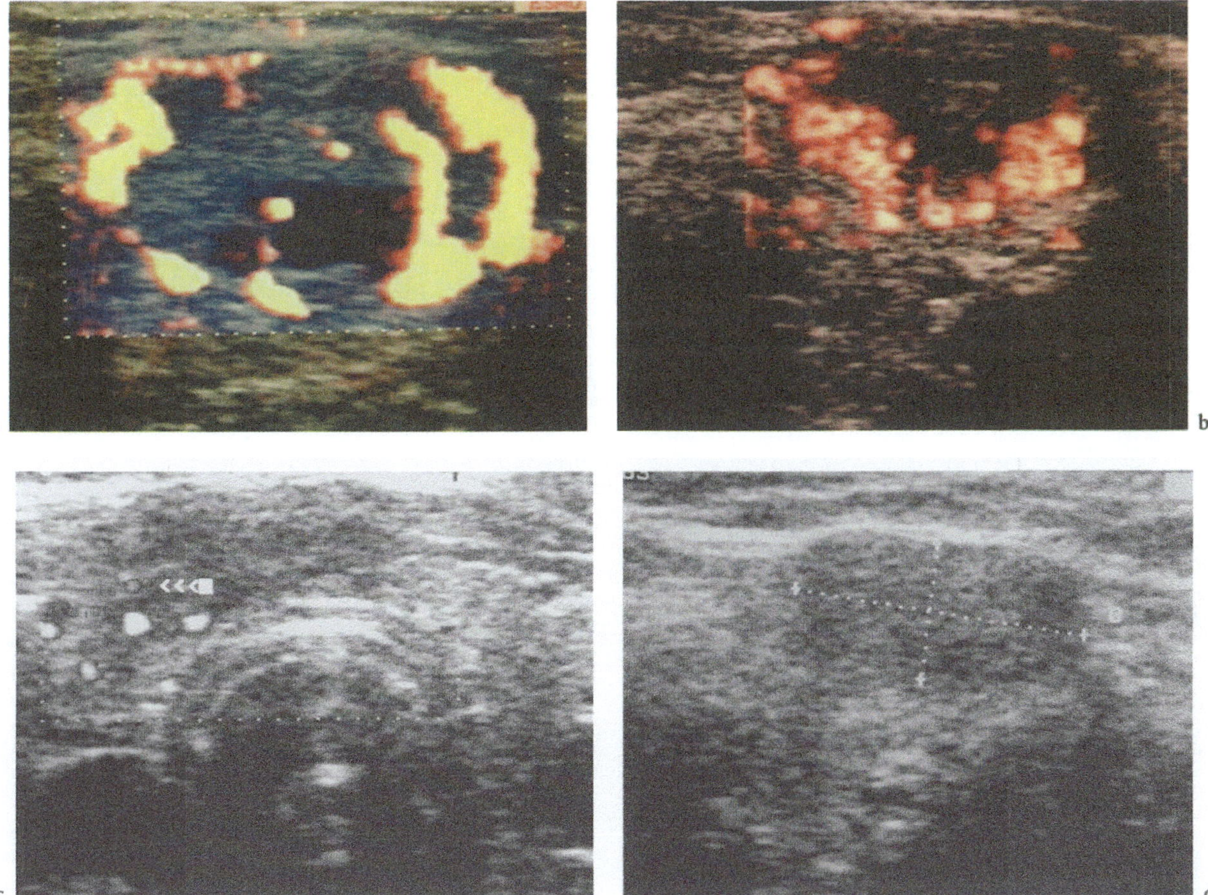

Fig. 1.49a–d. PEA of a hot nodule. **a** Hypervascularity of a hot nodule. **b** Follow-up 2 years after PEA revealed a recurrence, manifesting on PD as hypervascularity of nearly half of the nodule. **c** Two years after the second PEA treatment, residual appearance without hypervascularity on PD. **d** Morphological analysis of the nodule revealing the hypoechoic pattern and especially a decrease in size (1.8/0.9 cm between the *crosses*)

organified. The ready availability of this radionuclide explains its widespread use.

Owing to its similarity to natural iodine and its favorable dosimetric properties, iodine-123 is the nearly ideal tracer for assessment of thyroid function. However, the short half-life (13 h) of this relatively expensive product precludes long-term storage.

Iodine-131, another analogue of natural iodine, is much less expensive but is currently reserved for certain indications because its involves non-negligible radiation exposure. Owing to its long half-life (8 days), iodine-131 can be used to assess long-term uptake kinetics prior to treatment and for whole-body scanning of patients with thyroid cancer. Iodine-131 is also used for therapeutic metabolic irradiation of hyperthyroidism and thyroid cancer (Tranquart et al. 1996).

1.4.1.2 Results

Elements Interfering with Iodine Uptake. The quality of scintigraphy and accurate interpretation of data are affected by several factors that interfere with iodine uptake by the thyroid:

- Prior overload with iodine must be taken into consideration. Scintigraphy should be performed before radiological examinations requiring injection of iodinated contrast material. If this is not possible, an interval of at least 3 weeks is necessary after the radiological examinations before scintigraphy is performed. Potential problems include isotope dilution, blockage of iodine organification due the Wolff-Chaikoff effect, which causes hypothyroidism with elevation of TSH, and iodine saturation with complete blockage

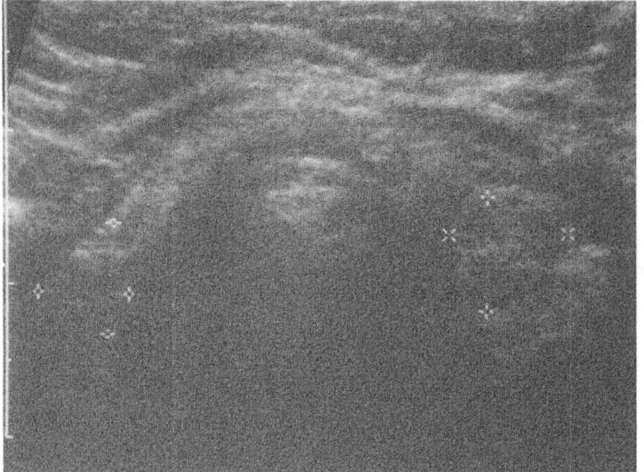
a

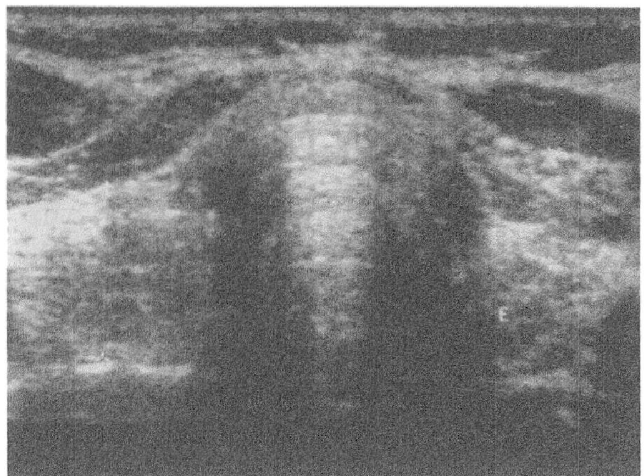
b

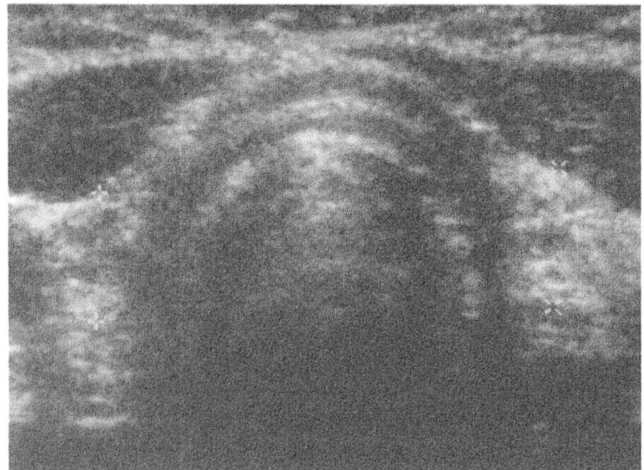
c

Fig. 1.50a–c. Hypothyroidism. **a** Significant reduction in the size of both thyroid lobes (on the *right*, 0.8/0.8 cm between the *crosses*; on the *left*, 0.7/0.6 cm between the *crosses*); the echotexture of the residual parenchyma is indistinguishable from the adjacent structures. **b** Chronic post-thyroiditis hypothyroidism (lobe thickness 1 cm between the *crosses* on the right and 0.6 cm on the left; *E* esophagus). **c** Hypothyroidism with severe thyroid atrophy following radiotherapy (lobe thickness 0.6 cm between the *crosses* on the *right* and 0.7 cm on the *left*)

of uptake (usually accompanied by hyperthyroidism).

- Numerous drugs (e.g., propylthiouracil, methimazole) interfere with thyroid metabolism of iodine and reduce the gland's uptake capacity (Albert et al. 1987).
- An elevated TSH level may produce a biphasic uptake curve.

Results with Iodine-123. A number of anomalies are associated with suppressed iodine-123 uptake, i.e., subacute thyroiditis, thyrotoxicosis factitia (Cohen et al. 1989), hyperthyroidism due to excess iodine (particularly after amiodarone administration) (Albert et al. 1987), certain forms of non-Basedow autoimmune thyroiditis, and postpartum thyroiditis.

Uptake is lowered, and usually accompanied by hypothyroidism, in chronic lymphocytic thyroiditis and hypothyroidism in the elderly. Increased uptake is often seen in diffuse hypertrophy of the entire gland. Homogeneous uptake is suggestive of Graves' disease, whereas inhomogeneous uptake suggests chronic lymphocytic thyroiditis.

Elevated uninodular uptake corresponds to a hot nodule that may be asymptomatic. Evaluation of uptake by the adjacent parenchyma can demonstrate the extinctive nature of such nodules. Although the presence of a hot nodule is usually a sign of benignity, it does not exclude the possibility of a malignant nodule elsewhere in the thyroid (Shamma and Abrahams 1992).

Absent or markedly decreased uninodular uptake corresponds to a cold nodule. This feature may be difficult to determine for posterior or isthmic nodules. The term "cold nodule" actually refers to a variety of entities ranging from a colloid nodule to cancer (Tennvall et al. 1981).

Scintigraphic evaluation of thyroid volume (using the ellipsoid formula or Himanka formula) may underestimate actual gland size in case of diffuse goiter (Wesche et al. 1998). According to Galloway and Smallridge (1996), causes of false-positive findings with iodine scans of the head and neck include meningioma, chronic sinusitis, dacryocystitis, ocular prosthesis, sialadenitis, carotid ectasia, saliva in the esophagus, and Zencker's diverticulum.

1.4.1.3
Scintigraphy vs Ultrasonography

Until recently, scintigraphy was sometimes still considered the next logical step following US. Owing to the efficacy of sonography and the accuracy of laboratory tests, the indications for radionuclide studies have declined considerably, especially because they usually prove unnecessary.

The "maximalist" approach for subcentimeter lesions that resulted in unnecessary scintigraphy (unnecessary because it is consistently negative) is increasingly being replaced by a "minimalist" approach consisting in US-guided FNA followed by adaptation of the indications for scintigraphy to the circulating TSH level. If the TSH concentration is low, scintigraphy is performed to search for a hot nodule (TOURNIAIRE et al. 1997); this allows differentiation of a toxic adenoma from a cold nodule in Graves' disease (DUQUENNE et al. 1997). Scintigraphy may be unnecessary if the nodule is smaller than 1 cm, if it is not extinctive, or if sonograms demonstrate cystic changes in at least one half the volume of the nodule.

Scintigraphy does not provide any fundamental data for assessment of inflammatory thyroid disorders, which are diagnosed by laboratory tests. The required morphological information is provided by sonography. The results of recent scintigraphy studies concerning acute and chronic inflammatory thyroid disease are too variable for establishment of diagnostic guidelines (LOEVNER 1996; PRICE 1993).

US, associated with CD and PD, even appears capable of replacing scintigraphy for differential diagnosis of thyroid gland dysfunction (Graves' disease versus an inflammatory pathology), especially because it is faster and more economical. For GHARIB (1997), appropriate use of thyroid scintigraphy includes diagnosis of a hot nodule, determination of goiter size (in particular in case of mediastinal spread), detection of ectopic tissue (sublingual, struma ovarii), and postoperative surveillance of differentiated thyroid carcinoma. KRAIMPS (1999) suggests that scintigraphy may be beneficial for patients who have had previous thyroid surgery to search for residual fixation on the operated side or for a pyramidal lobe left in place during the initial procedure.

1.4.1.4
Recent Applications of Scintigraphy

GALLOWAY and SMALLRIDGE (1996) reviewed the sensitivity and the specificity of commonly used radioisotopes reported in the literature. For detection of recurrent thyroid carcinoma by I-123 or I-131, sensitivity ranged from 48%–84% and specificity from 96% to 100%. The use of thallium 201 is more recent; thallium scanning has a sensitivity of 17%–100% and a specificity of 37%–100% for evaluation of thyroid nodules, and a sensitivity of 45%–94% and a specificity of 82%–97% for detection of recurrent thyroid carcinoma.

Thallium-201 scintigraphy has proven disappointing for demonstration of nodule malignancy. DEREBEK et al. (1996) concluded that early and delayed thallium-201 imaging have no utility for determination of the benign or malignant nature of a cold nodule. For KUME et al. (1996), delayed thallium-201 scans reflect proliferative tumor activity, but delayed thallium uptake is also seen in thyroiditis and parathyroid pathologies, and few teams currently use this technique routinely.

^{99m}Tc-methoxyisobutylisonitrile (MIBI), using a dual-phase acquisition protocol (at 30 min and 2 h), has also been employed in attempts to determine the etiology of cold nodules (KRESNIK et al. 1997). Prolonged retention of MIBI is generally not considered specific for cancer because it is even more frequent in adenomas, although this is debated by some authors (ALONSO et al. 1996).

Although MIBI apparently cannot determine the nature of a nodule, it may be helpful for cervical lymph node involvement by a differentiated cancer, and in particular for Hürthle cell tumors (GALLOWAY and SMALLRIDGE 1996).

Owing to its high resolution (up to 6–7 mm), single photon emission CT (SPECT) can accurately depict cold nodules, which are usually surrounded by more intense peripheral activity (WANET et al. 1996). Thyroid volumetry appears more accurate than planar imaging (ZAIDI 1996).

For GALLOWITSCH et al. (1999), the validity of the sentinel lymph node technique remains to be proven and warrants additional investigations.

Future applications may develop, thanks to new contrast agents such as octreotide or fluorodeoxyglucose (FDG). The mechanism behind diffuse thyroid FDG uptake remains unclear (YASUDA et al. 1998). HIROMATSU et al. (1998) performed ^{99m}Tc-tetrofosmin scintigraphy for patients with subacute thyroiditis; the diffuse and marked uptake reflecting the inflammatory process allowed quantitative assessment of disease severity. GUERRA et al. (1988) evaluated the efficacy of pentavalent technetium dimercaptosuccinic acid [Tc (V) DMSA] for imaging medullary carcinoma; the diagnostic sensitivity was 66% for metastases and 77% for the primary tumor, while the specificity was 100%. James et al. (1999) used ^{99m}Tc-DMSA and somatostatin receptor scintigraphy to investigate recurrent medullary thyroid carcinoma.

These radiopharmaceuticals are currently reserved for the detection of metastases of thyroid cancer and are not used for pretherapy disease staging (Reinhardt and Moser 1996).

1.4.2 Computed Tomography (CT)

1.4.2.1 Indications and Limitations of CT

Injection of an iodinated contrast material compromises the efficacy of subsequent radioiodine therapy for differentiated thyroid carcinoma by saturating the thyroid gland and any metastases with iodine. Iodinated injections should therefore be avoided during thyroid investigations unless the diagnosis has already been established (anaplastic carcinoma, medullary carcinoma).

CT has the advantage of permitting cervicomediastinal assessment (along with subdiaphragmatic evaluation in case of medullary carcinoma) and, thanks to the use of thin slices, three-dimensional image reconstruction. However, the spatial resolution of CT is lower than that of high-resolution US. In addition, there are no CT features allowing differentiation of benign and malignant nodules except for indirect signs such as lymphadenopathy and muscle or vascular invasion.

CT is not reliable for characterization of thyroid nodules (Hopkins and Reading 1995). However, unenhanced CT with contiguous, 5-mm-thick slices allows determination of thyroid volume (mean error compared with surgical specimens ±12%), based on the assumption that 1 cm^3 of thyroid tissue weighs 1 g (Hermans et al. 1997). This information is beneficial when adjusting radioiodine therapy to the volume of the gland.

1.4.2.2 CT Features of Thyroid Disease

CT characterization of thyroid nodules is not routine practice, even though certain authors emphasize the value of the technique for helping to suggest benignity or malignancy (Sashi et al. 1997). Cervical lymphadenopathy, with or without venous thrombosis (visible by ultrasound), and tracheal, esophageal, or bone invasion are the only signs of a malignant process. CT thus is not indicated for the workup of differentiated, curable carcinomas, which account for the majority of thyroid cancers.

Anaplastic carcinomas, which represent approximately 10% of all thyroid cancers (Bittman et al. 1992), are diagnosed clinically in cases of diffuse involvement that manifests as rapid swelling of the neck, sometimes accompanied by lung or bone metastases. US can confirm the highly suspicious nature of these lesions (tumor mass and cervical lymphadenopathy, invasion of adjacent structures) and be used to guide FNA. Subsequent CT is indicated for rapid assessment of cervicomediastinal spread in patients with symptoms of respiratory compression, because it can demonstrate locoregional extranodal invasion more accurately than US (Hopkins and Reading 1995).

If thyroid NHL is diagnosed, thoracic and abdominopelvic CT are indicated. Contrast-enhanced cervical CT may demonstrate isodense or hypodense zones corresponding to the hypoechoic areas seen on sonograms (Takashima et al. 1995c).

CT is of no practical value for workup of thyroiditis unless sonograms or clinical findings suggest malignancy (Kamijo 1994), as in Riedel's thyroiditis that has invaded adjacent structures (Fontan et al. 1993). Except for the evaluation of exophthalmos, CT has no diagnostic value for Basedow's goiter.

If US demonstrates mediastinal involvement in a patient with multinodular goiter, CT may be helpful when surgery is envisaged because it can accurately demonstrate relations with the trachea, anterior or posterior mediastinal spread, and the generally symmetrical displacement of the vessels, without infiltration (Galloway and Smallridge 1996; Rodriguez et al. 1999).

1.4.3 Magnetic Resonance Imaging

MRI has an advantage over CT because it does not require injection of iodinated agents and allows multiplanar imaging as well as cervicomediastinal workup. However, its more limited availability, higher cost, and the duration of acquisition times together with a number of contraindications and artifacts restrict the indications for pretherapy MRI of thyroid disorders.

On T_1-weighted sequences, the thyroid appears homogeneous and discretely hyperintense to muscle. On T_2-weighted sequences, the gland appears hyperintense to muscle; gadolinium injection results in diffuse homogeneous enhancement (Loevner 1996).

1.4.3.1
MRI and Nodular Thyroid Disease

To date, MRI has not proven conclusive for differential diagnosis of benign and malignant lesions. Renard et al. (1991) described features associated with benign thyroid nodules, and absence of these features is suggestive of a malignant process. However, the frequency of false-positive findings (linked to the cystic or hemorrhagic nature of a nodule) and false-negative results (encapsulated cancer, lymphoma associated with thyroiditis) continues to render histological examination indispensable.

In addition, MRI cannot detect the microcalcifications that are typical of papillary carcinoma. Kusunoki et al. (1994) studied "uncomplicated" nodules without any secondary modifications such as hemorrhage, necrosis, calcification, or fibrosis. While the grade of differentiation and proliferative cellular activity was recognizable on T_1- and T_2-weighted images, these features did not establish the benignity or malignancy of nodules.

Adenomas may appear hyperintense on T_1-weighted images and be enhanced after gadolinium administration. Thyroid carcinoma is also enhanced with gadolinium, but it may have irregular margins (Stern et al. 1994). Nakahara et al. (1997) failed to observe any difference between benign and malignant nodules on T_1- and T_2-weighted images or gadolinium-enhanced scans (King et al. 2000).

MRI has an accuracy of 80% for detection of lymphadenopathy (Takashima et al. 1997). For Som et al. (1994), nodal metastases have an intermediate signal on T_1-weighted images and a high-intensity signal on T_2-weighted images. According to them, areas of high attenuation on T_1-weighted images reflect an elevated thyroglobulin concentration.

If medullary carcinoma has been diagnosed preoperatively, MRI may be useful for pretherapy staging. These lesions are isointense or hyperintense on T_1-weighted images and hyperintense on T_2-weighted sequences. Malignant nodes are hypointense to fat on T_1-weighted sequences and hyperintense on T_2-weighted sequences. Medullary carcinoma is enhanced discretely after gadolinium injection. Increased amyloid deposits and tissue cellularity appear to increase the T_2 signal (Wang et al. 1997).

Data in the literatureconcerning primary thyroid lymphoma are rather variable. The lesions are often isointense on T_1-weighted sequences and half enhanced after gadolinium injection. On T_2-weighted images, thyroid lymphomas are hyperintense in 50% of cases, but they may also have a complex or isointense signal (Nakahara et al. 1997; Takashima et al. 1995c). MRI has not proven more contributory than CT in thyroid lymphoma.

1.4.3.2
Other Applications of MRI

MRI appears more accurate than scintigraphy for analysis of tumor volume in patients with a large goiter (Huysmans et al. 1994).

It can also optimize assessment of ophthalmologic involvement in Graves' disease. Laitt et al. (1994) used short tau inversion recovery (STIR) sequences in addition to visual assessment of muscle size. The increased signal intensity is due to edema secondary to inflammation. STIR sequences with retro-orbital fat suppression permit excellent analysis of modifications in the muscles. In the opinion of Laitt et al., this technique can predict which patients will respond to anti-inflammatory therapy. Onishi et al. (1994) investigated measurement of the T_2 relaxation time; in their study, the probability of response to treatment increased with augmentation of the mean T_2 relaxation time of the extraocular muscles.

Examination of thyroiditis by MRI does not provide any truly valuable information, in particular for subacute thyroiditis and Riedel's thyroiditis, because MRI has the same limitations as other techniques for morphological analysis (Fontan et al. 1993; Otsuka et al. 1994). However, Takashima et al. (1995b) reported that signal-intensity ratios were helpful for evaluation of Hashimoto's thyroiditis. For these authors, a proton density-weighted signal intensity ratio of 1.54 or higher suggests hypothyroidism, while a T_2-weighted signal-intensity ratio of 5.8 or higher corresponds to advanced glandular destruction.

1.4.4
Conclusion

Owing to the efficacy of laboratory tests and the morphological data provided by US, other imaging modalities remain second-line techniques. Scintigraphy, previously the sole morphological examination, has seen its indications decrease, even though the examination is still often performed merely out of habit. Following TSH assays and US, scintigraphy can be used to search for a hot nodule. Scintigraphy can also be used to determine the efficacy of PEA, which is increasingly proposed as an alternative to surgery. Outside of clinical trials and research on new contrast agents, scintigraphy often serves merely to confirm the diagnostic hypotheses formulated by US techniques (including CD, PD, and US-guided FNA). The indications for CT and MRI are similar, and either technique may be used, depending on equipment availability. Contrast-enhanced CT or MRI is indicated for preoperative staging of recognized medullary carcinoma (analysis of mediastinal nodes and abdominal examination in search of multiple endocrine neoplasia: adrenals, pancreas) and anaplastic thyroid carcinoma. Unenhanced CT or MRI may be useful for goiters with mediastinal involvement if surgery is being planned.

1.5 Post-therapy Follow-up of Thyroid Tumors

1.5.1 Benign Thyroid Pathologies

1.5.1.1 Nonsurgical Thyroid Disease

Nonsurgical thyroid pathologies include lesions that are merely followed up after FNA and thyroid disease managed by hormone therapy. Using the thyroid map established during initial workup for comparative purposes, US can reveal progression or regression in nodule size.

As mentioned previously, the role of LT4 remains controversial. Miccoli et al. (1993) consider LT4 effective for prevention of nodular recurrences after subtotal surgery, but they pointed out that Italy is an iodine-deficient region. Bennedbaek et al. (1998) noted a decrease in the perinodular volume in 20% of patients, a decrease in nodule diameter in 9%, and above all disappearance of clinical signs in 32%. Gordon et al. (1999) emphasized the fact that changes in the size of thyroid nodules may occur at any time up to 6 months after FNA; such changes must be taken into account when evaluating the efficacy of TSH suppression therapy for thyroid nodules.

PEA of cold nodules leads to a reduction in the size of nearly half of all solid nodules and 68.9% of cystic nodules (Komorowski et al. 1998).

In patients with multinodular nontoxic goiter, iodine-131 therapy reduces thyroid volume by about 50% within 12–18 months (Nygaard et al. 1997) and by up to 50%–60% after 3–5 years (Huysmans et al. 1997). However, after 5 years, the incidence of post-therapeutic hypothyroidism is 20%–30%. Surgery rather than radioactive iodine therapy should thus be proposed to young patients with multinodular nontoxic goiter (Huysmans et al. 1997).

1.5.1.2 Post-surgical Follow-up

After loboisthmectomy or nodule enucleation, US can demonstrate the appearance of any new nodules (Fig. 1.51). This is particularly helpful after surgery for colloid goiter or multinodular goiter. Optimum diagnostic accuracy is obviously required to avoid repeat surgery that would result in subtotal or total thyroidectomy for benign disease. US is not indicated for follow-up of total thyroidectomy performed for a nonmalignant lesion.

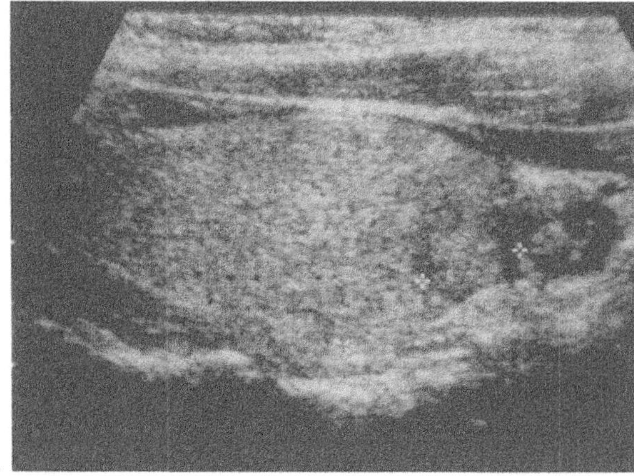
a

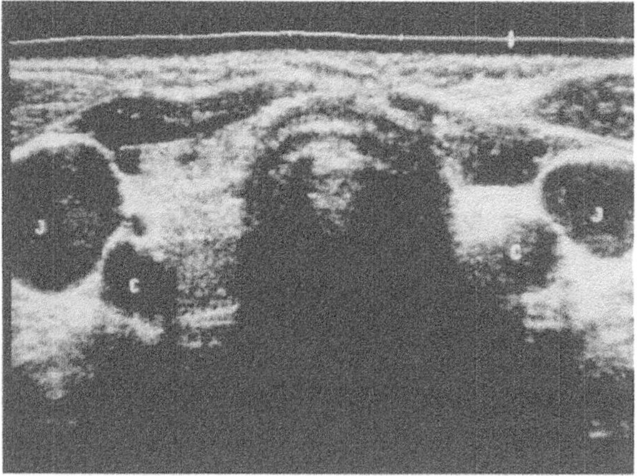

b

Fig. 1.51a,b. Nodular recurrence after surgery. **a** Nodular recurrence on the tumorectomy margin in the right lobe (sagittal scan, 1.2/0.7 cm between the *crosses*). **b** New nodules developed in the right lobe after left thyroidectomy (*C* common carotid artery; *J* internal jugular vein)

After subtotal lobectomy, the mean remaining volume, determined sonographically, does not exceed 0.8 ml (Mann et al. 1996). After lobectomy, the volume of the remaining thyroid tissue generally increases, whether or not the patient is placed on postoperative LT4 suppressive therapy. This increase in gland size, which may amount to 30% as early as the first month, persists the entire first year (Berglund et al. 1998) (Fig. 1.52).

1.5.2 Curable Differentiated Thyroid Cancers

1.5.2.1 Natural History of Differentiated Thyroid Cancer

Papillary carcinomas have a propensity for lymphatic spread. Their main risk is local recurrence in the form of neoplastic grafts in the thyroidectomy bed.

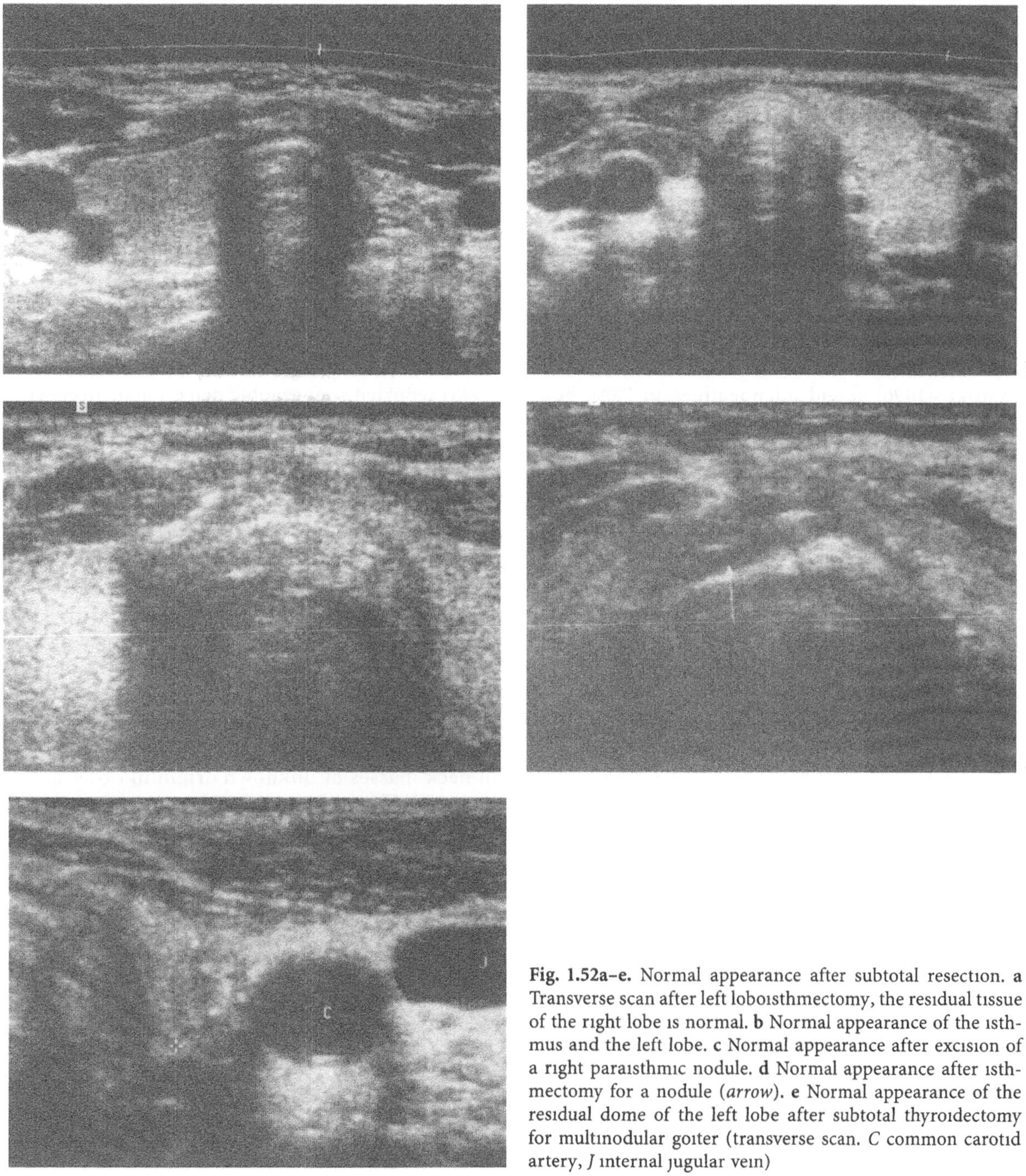

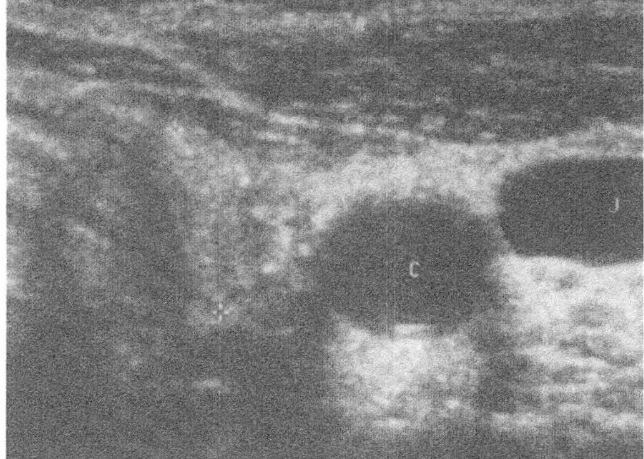

Fig. 1.52a–e. Normal appearance after subtotal resection. **a** Transverse scan after left loboisthmectomy, the residual tissue of the right lobe is normal. **b** Normal appearance of the isthmus and the left lobe. **c** Normal appearance after excision of a right paraisthmic nodule. **d** Normal appearance after isthmectomy for a nodule (*arrow*). **e** Normal appearance of the residual dome of the left lobe after subtotal thyroidectomy for multinodular goiter (transverse scan. *C* common carotid artery, *J* internal jugular vein)

Recurrence is most common in elderly patients with an aggressive tumor.

Simon et al. (1996) reported a rate of recurrence of 31% after total thyroidectomy, with recurrences being more frequent in the absence of systematic nodal dissection. For Sophocleous et al. (1997), recurrence was seen in 8% of cases a mean of 4.7 years after treatment. For these authors, tumors smaller than 2 cm in diameter had a favorable prognosis; the 10-year survival rate was 91% for papillary carcinoma and 84% for follicular carcinoma. For Pelizzo et al. (1998) the 20-year survival rate for papillary thyroid carcinoma was 88.7%, and no tumor smaller than 1.5 cm in their study recurred.

Nodal recurrence (less than 10% of cases) occurs secondarily if a micrometastasis is left in situ; nodes at the limits of high cervical, spinal, and superior mediastinal curettage are involved most often (Cannoni and Demard 1995). Visceral metastases are rare; miliary and micronodular pulmonary metastases predominate. These lesions take up iodine and have a favorable prognosis (Schlumberger et al. 1988; Witterick et al. 1993).

In a series of 1916 thyroid carcinomas, Shah and Samuel (1996) found adenopathies in 78%, bone metastases in 21%, and lung metastases in 13%. In contrast, there were only 11 cases of hepatic metastases, the majority of which occurred in a context of rapidly fatal multimetastatic disease.

Pachucki and Burmeister (1997) reported 17 patients with an increased Tg level and normal whole-body scintigraphy (WBS); seven of these patients had a malignant cervical mass of 1–4 cm, but no etiology was found in the other ten cases (complementary treatment by I-131 revealed post-therapeutic uptake in seven of these ten patients).

Local recurrence of follicular cancer is exceptional and is usually due to incomplete resection of extracapsular lesions. The prognosis is determined primarily by the existence of visceral metastases, which are present in 20% of cases (Zohar and Strauss 1994). These lung and bone metastases inconstantly exhibit intense uptake and hypervascularity. The mortality at 5 years is 60% despite radioiodine therapy or external irradiation.

1.5.2.2 Follow-up of Differentiated Thyroid Cancers

In the post-surgical setting, the extent of thyroid ablation can usefully be evaluated by quantification of neck uptake. Follow-up is based on iodinated WBS combined with Tg assays. The association of these two methods has an estimated diagnostic accuracy of 96.7% (Ronga et al. 1990). WBS can localize histologically well-differentiated metastases in a two-dimensional plane after suppressive therapy. Doses (usually 5–10 mCi) can reach 100–150 mCi (Schlumberger et al. 1988); this has the advantage of being both diagnostic and therapeutic.

Tg should be undetectable after thyroidectomy and radioiodine treatment. Any elevation should be considered indicative of locoregional or metastatic recurrence (Cavalieri 1996; Sweeney and Johnston 1995).

1.5.2.3 Ultrasound

Ultrasonography is increasingly being used for post-operative follow-up of curable differentiated thyroid cancer (Figs. 1.53–1.55), owing to its efficacy for cervical examination (Bolland et al. 1993; Simeone et al. 1987; Solbiati et al. 1992). Franceschi et al. (1996) reported that post-therapy cervical US visualized 23 lesions even though Tg levels were negative in 52% and WBS was negative in 83%. Antonelli et al. (1995) reported sonographic detection of 16 cervical anomalies (12 recurrences, four cases of lymphadenitis) after surgery and radioiodine therapy despite normal WBS.

In the study by Rodriguez et al. (1997), US follow-up of 89 patients with differentiated thyroid carcinoma detected 22 anomalies (16 adenopathies, six lesions in the thyroid bed), 59% of which were malignant. US screening thus had a sensitivity of 65%, a specificity of 86%, and an accuracy of 82% for detection of neoplastic disease. These authors recommend use of US as an integral part of the follow-up protocol for curable thyroid cancers. Pisani et al. (1999b) advocate routine US-guided FNA of all neck masses of unknown origin in order to differentiate between nonspecific lymphadenitis and nodal metastases. Like Frasoldati et al. (1999), these authors recommend immunocytochemical assay of Tg in the needle wash-out.

1.5.2.4 Other Imaging Modalities

Few studies have been published on the routine use of MRI for surveillance of curable differentiated cancers. According to Cyna-Gorse et al. (1996), MRI has a sensitivity of 100%, a specificity of 66.6%, and an overall accuracy of 82.6% for detection of recurrences of differentiated thyroid cancers.

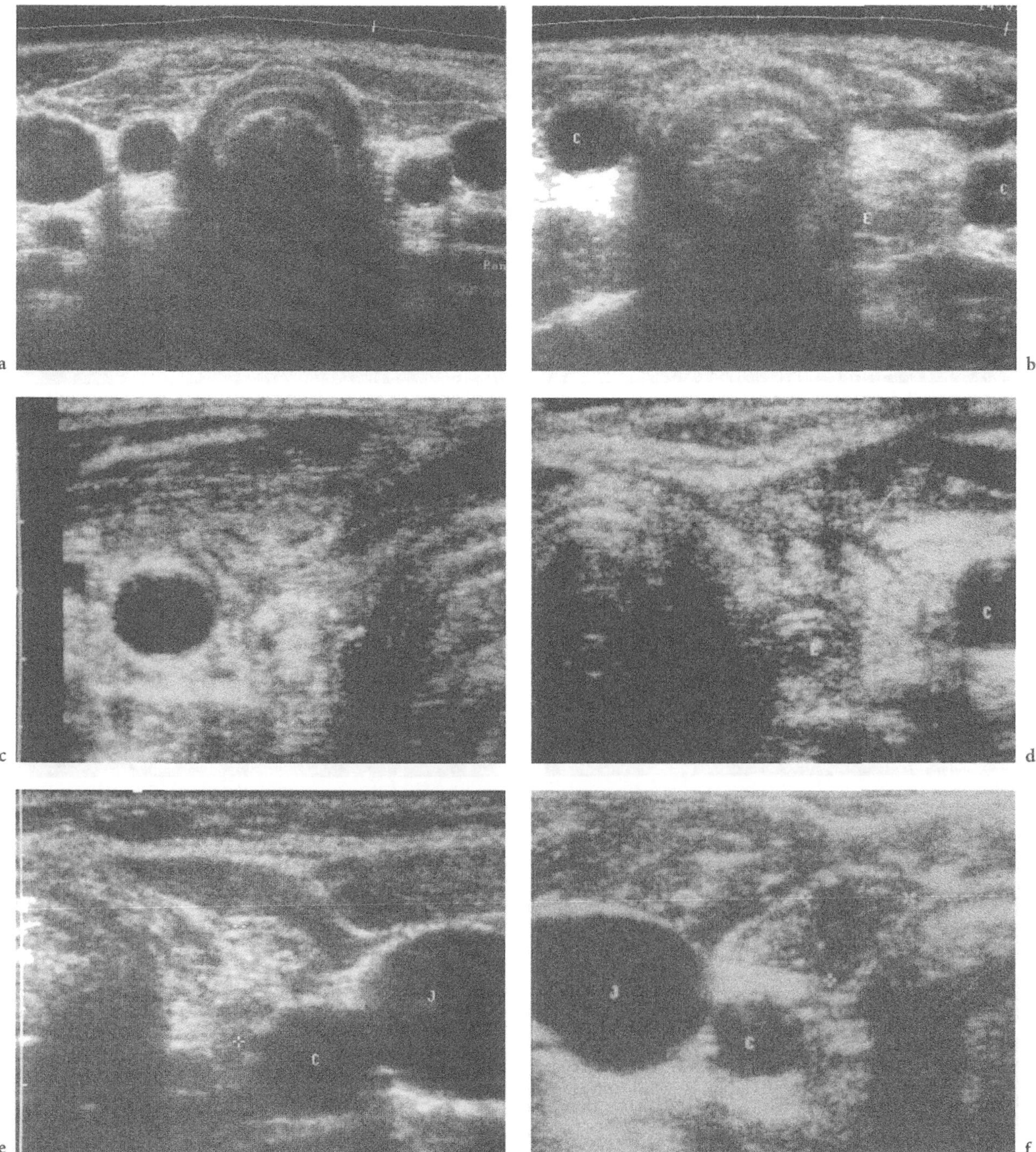

Fig. 1.53a–f. Total thyroidectomy **a** Normal appearance with symmetry of the laterocervical regions (after thyroid surgery, the internal carotid artery and the internal jugular vein are now located closer to the aerodigestive axis) **b** Asymmetry of the fibrotic zones, the right common carotid artery is located closer to the aerodigestive axis, the projection of the esophagus is clearly visible on the left (*C* common carotid artery, *E* esophagus) **c** Area of fibrosis corresponding to an involuted hematoma 21 days after total thyroidectomy **d** Extensive fibrosis following thyroidectomy for cancer, PD failed to reveal any hypervascularity (*C* common carotid artery, *E* esophagus) **e** Pseudonodular appearance of a fibrotic zone without any particularities in the left lateral neck (0 8 cm between the *crosses*) (*C* common carotid artery, *J* internal jugular vein) **f** Differential diagnosis of tumor recurrence, this suspicious image actually corresponds to a section of the sternocleidohyoid muscle (1 2/0 7 cm between the *crosses*) (*C* common carotid artery, *J* internal jugular vein)

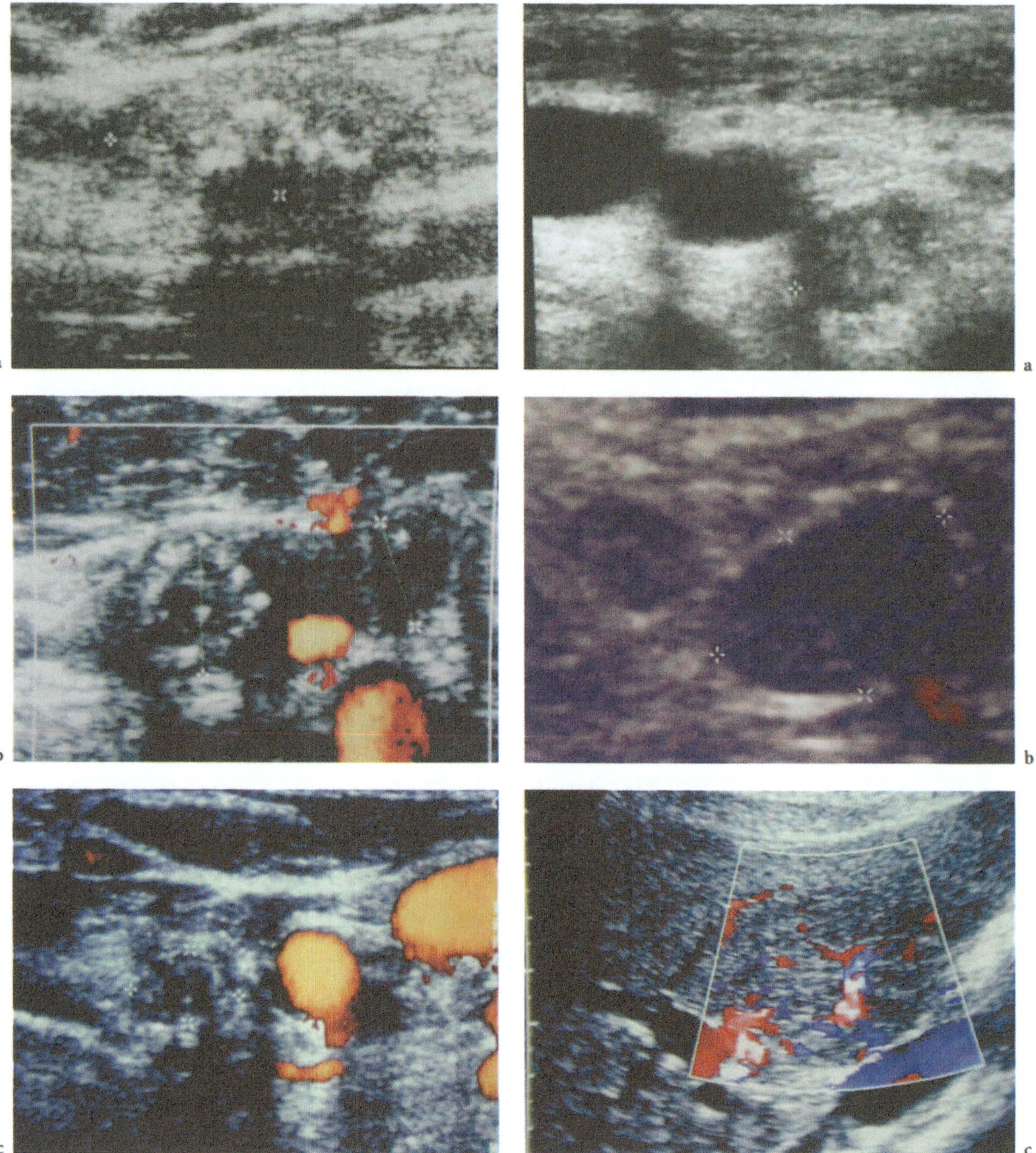

Fig. 1.54a–c. Post-treatment imaging of papillary carcinoma. **a** metastasis treated by radioiodine therapy in a patient with thyroid cancer. The area of calcification involves two thirds of the node, no change in appearance over 2 years and no notable vascularity on PD (1.6/0.8 cm between the *crosses*). **b** Residual lesion in the lateral neck unchanged over 4 years, corresponding to calcified and involuted nodal metastases (0.8 and 0.7 cm between the *crosses*). **c** Post-therapy residual image of the thyroidectomy bed; appearance unchanged over 3 years (0.8/0.6 cm between the *crosses*)

Fig. 1.55a–c. Sonographic detection of recurrence during follow-up of papillary carcinoma. **a** This solid nodule (1 cm between the *crosses*) appeared during follow-up of a treated thyroid cancer; radionuclide scanning was negative, but US-guided aspiration biopsy revealed malignant tissue. **b** Nodal recurrence in the form of two morphologically suspicious hypoechoic elements (round shape, hypoechogenicity without image of a hilus), these lesions were not detected by scintigraphy. PD did not reveal any hypervascularity, but US-guided FNA confirmed the diagnosis of malignancy (0 7/0.5 cm between the *crosses*). **c** Hepatic metastasis, imaging as an isoechoic lesion with central hypervascularity surrounded by a hypoechoic halo (CD)

Although US appears to be the sole nonscintigraphic technique of any practical complementary value owing to its sensitivity and availability, a number of investigations have been conducted with new isotopic techniques in an attempt to improve the efficacy of WBS.

Quantification of neck uptake appears superior to visual assessment. Ablation is considered complete when uptake is under 1%. This is all the more useful because visual evaluation overestimates uptake in 22% of cases (Chopra et al. 1996).

Although not yet widely available, diagnostic scanning using new radioisotopes such as octreotide, FDG (F18 FDG-PET), and ^{99m}Tc-tetrofosmin reportedly reveals metastases even when iodinated scintigraphy is normal (Conti et al. 1997; Fridrich et al. 1997; Lind et al. 1997; Reinhardt and Moser 1996; Seabold et al. 1997).

According to Kobayashi et al. (1997), MIBI markedly improves the sensitivity of conventional scintigraphic techniques for the detection of recurrence, especially when coupled with SPECT. In addition to searching for means of improving results, Reynolds and Robbins (1997) investigated ways to reduce the discomfort caused by the symptoms of hypothyroidism. Scott et al. (1995) demonstrated the interest of sensitive isotopic imaging combined with morphological analysis by CT or MRI.

Overall, follow-up of curable differentiated cancers has changed very little. The main source of progress concerns complementary cervical US. The role of new contrast agents has not yet been conclusively established, but F18 FDG-PET and MIBI have recently proven superior to the conventional technique for patients with increased Tg levels not explained by scintigraphy. Finally, Casara et al. (1999) recommend a combination of ^{99m}Tc-MIBI scanning and sonography for patients with elevated serum Tg levels and a normal WBS.

1.5.3 Medullary Thyroid Carcinoma

1.5.3.1 Course of Disease

Whether sporadic, familial, an isolated form, or associated with a multiple endocrine neoplasia (MEN) syndrome (IIa or IIb), medullary carcinoma does not take up iodine and can be treated only by surgery (primary cancer, metastases). Medullary carcinoma metastasizes to the lymph nodes and the liver; metastases are often calcified by amyloid deposits and calcium. Optimum follow-up is based on assays of calcitonin, an excellent marker of locoregional and distant tumor progression. Any elevation in calcitonin should prompt imaging studies (Bourguignat et al. 1997).

1.5.3.2 Post-therapy Imaging Follow-up

While scintigraphic methods using various isotopes may detect subradiologic and subclinical metastases, they are less accurate than selective venous sampling (Abdelmoumene et al. 1994; Dorr et al. 1993; Lupoli et al. 1991). ^{99m}Tc-(V)-DSMA is reportedly more accurate than MIBI and thallium-201 for diagnosis of secondary disease sites (Ugur et al. 1996).

Cervicomediastinal examination in search of nodal lesions can be performed with MRI, which can differentiate tumor recurrence from fibrosis (Aufferman et al. 1988; Som 1992; Van Den Brekel et al. 1990).

Hepatic metastases are identified by US and characterized by CT or MRI. Sonographically, hepatic metastases of medullary thyroid cancer image as one or more homogeneous hyperechoic nodules that may suggest an angioma (frequency, 91.3%; Leclere et al. 1996). T_2-weighted sequences can distinguish the increasing hypersignal of hemangioma from the stable and less intense signal of a metastasis.

Follow-up of medullary thyroid carcinoma is essentially performed using tumor markers, i.e., calcitonin and carcinoembryonic antigen (CEA) assays. Depending on results, imaging studies may be indicated. US usually suffices for cervical and hepatic examination, but CT or MRI are required for thoracoabdominal workup (Figs. 1.56, 1.57).

1.5.4 Undifferentiated Thyroid Carcinomas

These lesions have a very poor prognosis, and examinations should be kept to a minimum. Cervicomediastinal CT appears the best approach. Other investigations in search of secondary localizations are dictated by clinical symptoms.

1.6 Congenital Malformations

Aside from thyroid agenesis and ectopia in children (cf. Chap. 9), thyroid anomalies are basically limited to agenesis or hypoplasia of a lobe.

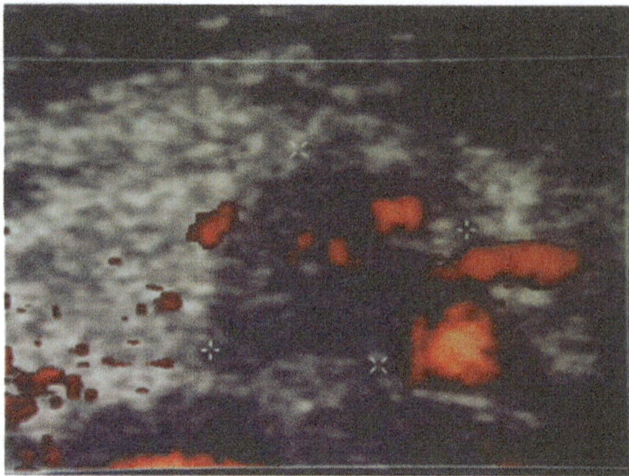

Fig. 1.56. Local recurrence of a medullary carcinoma (0.7/0.6 cm between the *crosses*). PD revealed lesion hypervascularity (the examination had been prompted by the appearance of hypercalcitonemia during post-therapy follow-up)

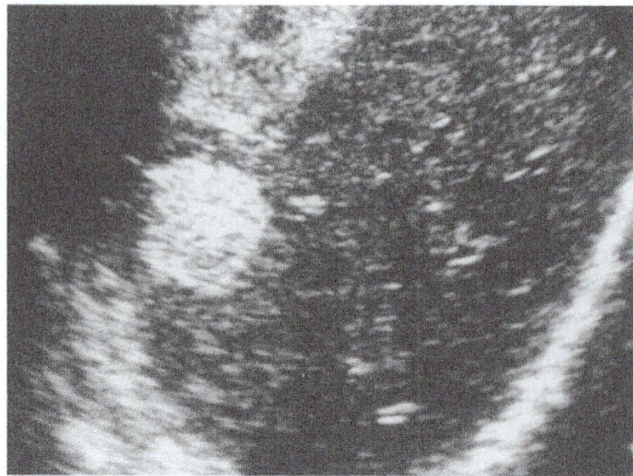

Fig. 1.57. Hyperechoic metastasis of a medullary carcinoma; the sonographic appearance does not permit determination of the benign (i.e., hemangioma) or malignant nature of this hepatic lesion

Lobe agenesis occurs in less than 0.1% of the population (GREENING et al. 1980). The malformation is an incidental discovery during cervical examinations for another pathology or when the existing lobe is the site of an anomaly. On sonograms, the fat tissue that replaces the absent lobe is imaged as an area of dense, irregular echoes; the common carotid artery and the internal jugular vein lie near the trachea. Females are affected more often than males, and the left lobe is more apt to be missing than the right lobe. Apart from the possibility of an anomaly induced by the existing lobe, agenesis of a thyroid lobe has no functional implications.

Hypoplasia of a thyroid lobe is more frequent, and is easily recognizable sonographically by the asymmetry of images on transverse scans (difference of at least 50% between the size of the two lobes). This malformation has no impact on gland function (Fig. 1.58).

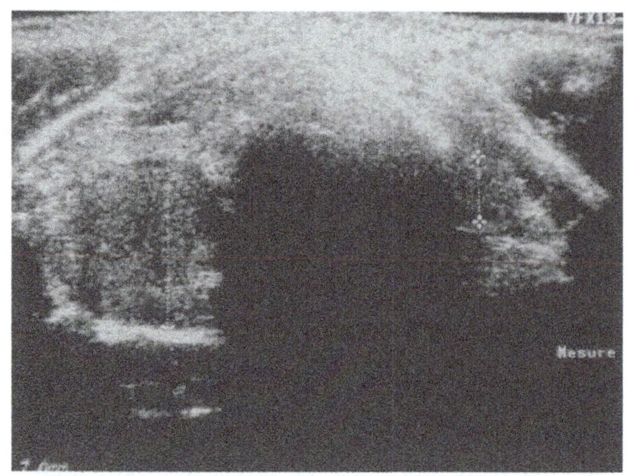

Fig. 1.58. Hypoplasia of a thyroid lobe; the left lobe measures 0.7 cm in thickness between the *crosses*; the right lobe is thicker (2.2 cm between the *crosses*) and contains a nodule measuring 1.8 cm in long axis (transverse scan)

References

Abdelmoumene N, Schlumberger M, Gardet P, et al (1994) Selective venous sampling catheterisation for localization of persisting medullary thyroid carcinoma. Br J Cancer 69:1141–1144

Adams H, Jones MC (1990) Correspondence. Clin Radiol 42:217–218

Adams H, Jones MC, Othman S, et al (1992) The sonographic appearances in postpartum thyroiditis. Clin Radiol 45:311–315

Aghini-Lombardi F, Antonangeli L, Pinchera A, et al (1997) Effect of iodized salt on thyroid volume of children living in an area previously characterized by moderate iodine deficiency. J Clin Endocrinol Metab 82:1136–1139

Ahuja A, Chick W, King W, Metreweli C (1996) Clinical significance of the comet-tail artifact in thyroid ultrasound. J Clin Ultrasound 24:129–133

Ahuja A, Ng CF, King W, Metreweli C (1998) Solitary cystic nodal metastasis from occult papillary carcinoma of the thyroid mimicking a branchial cyst: a potential pitfall. Clin Radiol 53:61–63

Ahuja AT, King W, Metreweli C (1994) Role of ultrasonography in thyroid metastases. Clin Radiol 49:627–629

Ahuja AT, Chow L, Chick W, et al (1995) Metastatic cervical nodes in papillary carcinoma of the thyroid: ultrasound and histological correlation. Clin Radiol 50:229–231

Albert SG, Alves LE, Rose EP (1987) Thyroid dysfunction during chronic amiodarone therapy J Am Coll Cardiol 9 175–183

Alonso O, Lago G, Mut F, et al (1996) Thyroid imaging with Tc-99m MIBI in patients with solitary cold nodules on pertechnetate imaging Clin Nucl Med 21 363–367

Andersen-Ranberg K, Jeune B, Hoier-Madsen M, Hegedus L (1999) Thyroid function, morphology and prevalence of thyroid disease in a population-based study of Danish centenarians. J Am Geriatr Soc 47.1238–1243

Antonelli A, Miccoli P, Ferdeghini M et al. (1995) Role of neck ultrasonography in the follow-up of patients operated on for thyroid cancer. Thyroid 5 25–28

Argalia G, D'Ambrosio F, Lucarelli F et al (1995) L'eco Doppler nella caratterizzazione della patologia nodulare tiroidea. Radiol Med 89.651–657

Arslan H, Unal O, Algun E, Harman M, Sakarya ME (2000) Power Doppler sonography in the diagnosis of Graves' disease. Eur J Ultrasound 11:117–122

Auffermann W, Clark OH, Thurnher S, Galante M, Higgings CB (1988) Recurrent thyroid carcinoma characteristics on MRI. Radiology 168.753–757

Avetis'ian IL, Iarovoi AO, Gul'Chii NV (1999) Guided fine-needle biopsy of thyroid nodular formations in the early diagnosis of thyroid carcinoma. Lik Sprava 1 106–110

Baeza A (1999) Thyroid cancer. Analysis of the diagnosis, treatment and follow-up in 151 cases. Rev Med Chil 127.581–588

Baldini M, Castagnone D, Rivolta R, Meroni L, Pappalettera M, Cantalamessa L (1997) Thyroid vascularization by color Doppler ultrasonography in Graves' disease. Changes related to different phases and to the long-term outcome of the disease. Thyroid 7.823–828

Barczynski M, Barcsynski M, Cichon S, Sulowicz W, Sydor A, Walatek B (1998) Metastasis of kidney clear cell carcinomas to the thyroid cell in patients on renal replacement therapy. Przegl Lek 55.623–625

Barraclough BM, Barraclough BH (2000) Ultrasound of the thyroid and parathyroid glands. World J Surg 24.158–165

Bartos M, Pomorski L, Narebski J (1999) The treatment of solitary thyroid nodules in non-toxic goiter with 96% ethanol injections. Wiad Lek 52.432–440

Becker D, Bair HJ, Becker W, et al (1997) Thyroid autonomy with color-coded image-directed Doppler sonography internal hypervascularization for the recognition of autonomous adenomas J Clin Ultrasound 25.63–69

Benker G, Reinwein D, Kahaly G, et al (1998) Is there a methimazole dose effect on remission rate in Graves' disease? Results from a long-term prospective study. The European Multicentre Trial Group of the treatment of hyperthyroidism with antithyroid drugs. Clin Endocrinol 49.451–457

Bennedbaek FN, Hegedus L (1997) The value of ultrasonography in the diagnosis and follow-up of subacute thryoiditis. Thyroid 7.45–50

Bennedbaek FN, Nielsen LK, Hegedus L (1998) Effect of percutaneous ethanol injection therapy versus suppressive doses of L-thyroxine on benign solitary solid cold thyroid nodules: a randomized trial. J Clin Endocrinol Metab 83:830–835

Benson DM, Rifkin MD, Rose JL, et al (1983) Characterization of benign and malignant tissues of the thyroid gland. An ultrasonic approach using RF waveform analysis and pattern recognition. Invest Radiol 18.459–462

Berghout A, Wiersinga WM, Smits NJ, Touber JL (1987) Determinants of thyroid volume as measured by ultrasonography in healthy adults in a non-iodine-deficient area. Clin Endocrinol 26.273–280

Berglund J, Aspelin P, Bondeson AG, et al (1998) Rapid increase in volume of the remnant after hemithyroidectomy does not correlate with serum concentration of thyroid stimulatory hormone. Eur J Surg 164.257–262

Birchall IWJ, Chow CC, Metreweli C (1990) Ultrasound appearance of De Quervain's thyroiditis. Clin Radiol 41.57–59

Bittman O, Bruneton JN, Fenart D, et al (1992) Imagerie des cancers anaplasiques de la thyroide. J Radiol 73:35–38

Bogazzi F, Bartalena L, Vitti P, Rago T, Brogioni S, Martino E (1996) Color flow Doppler sonography in thyrotoxicosis factitia. J Endocrinol Invest 19:603–606

Bogazzi F, Bartalena L, Brogioni S et al (1997) Color flow Doppler sonography rapidly differentiates type I and type II amiodarone-induced thyrotoxicosis. Thyroid 7:541–545

Bogazzi F, Bartalena L, Brogioni S, et al (1999) Thyroid vascularity and blood flow are not dependent on serum thyroid hormone levels: studies in vivo by color flow Doppler sonography. Eur J Endocrinol 140:452–456

Bolland GW, Lee MJ, Mueller PR, Mayo-Smith W, Dawson SL, Simenone JF (1993) Efficacy of sonographically-guided biopsy of thyroid masses and cervical lymph nodes. AJR 161.1053–1056

Bourguignat E, Marcy PY, Bobin S, Bruneton JN (1997) Cancers de la thyroide. In: Lavayssiere R, Vannetzel JM, Cabee AE (eds) TDM et IRM en carcinologie de l'adulte. Vigot, Paris, pp 140–156

Brander A, Viikinkoski P, Nickels J, Kivisaari L (1989) Thyroid gland: US screening in middle-aged women with no previous thyroid disease. Radiology 173:507–510

Brander A, Viikinkoski P, Tuuhea J, Voutilainen L, Kivisaari L (1992) Clinical versus ultrasound examination of the thyroid gland in common clinical practice. J Clin Ultrasound 20:37–42

Braun B, Blank W (1994) Color Doppler sonography-guided percutaneous alcohol instillation in the therapy of functionally autonomous thyroid nodules. Dtsch Med Wochenschr 119:1607–1612

Brkljacic B, Cuk V, Tomic-Brzac H, Bence-Zigman Z, Delic-Brkljacic D, Drinkovic I (1994) Ultrasonic evaluation of benign and malignant nodules in echographically multinodular thyroids. J Clin Ultrasound 22.71–76

Bruneton JN, Santini N, Santini J (1987) Medical ultrasound equipment, examination techniques, and ultrasonography of the normal neck. In: Bruneton JN (ed) Ultrasonography of the neck. Springer, Berlin Heidelberg New York, pp 1–21

Bruneton JN, Balu-Maestro C, Marcy PY, Melia P, Mourou MY (1994a) Very high frequency (13 Mhz) ultrasonographic examination of the normal neck. detection of normal lymph nodes and thyroid nodules. J Ultrasound Med 13: 87–90

Bruneton JN, Maestro C, Marcy PY, Padovani B (1994b) Echographie des ganglions superficiels. J Radiol 75.373–381

Bruneton JN, Marcy PY, Maestro C, Raffaelli C (1996) Echographie des nodules thyroidiens. In: Bruneton JN, Padovani B (eds) Imagerie en endocrinologie. Masson, Paris, pp 48–54

Bruneton JN, Livraghi T, Marcy PY, Tramalloni J, Tranquart F (1998) Thyroid gland. In. Bruneton JN (ed) Radiological imaging of endocrine diseases. Springer, Berlin Heidelberg New York, pp 145–180

Burch HB (1995) Evaluation and management of the solid thyroid nodule. Endocrinol Metab Clin North Am 24:663–710

Burke JS, Burke JJ, Fuller LM (1977) Malignant lymphoma of the thyroid: a clinical pathologic study of 35 patients including ultrastructural observations. Cancer 39:1587–1602

Cannoni M, Demard F (1995) Les nodules thyroïdiens du diagnostic à la chirurgie. Arnette, Paris

Cantalamessa L, Baldini M, Orsatti A, Meroni L, Amodei V, Castagnone D (1999) Thyroid nodules in Graves' disease and the risk of thyroid carcinoma. Arch Intern Med 159:1705–1708

Caraccio N, Goletti O, Lippolos PV et al (1997) Is percutaneous ethanol injection a useful alternative for the treatment of the cold benign thyroid nodule? Five years' experience. Thyroid 7:699–704

Carmeci C, Jeffrey RB, McDougall IR, Nowels KW, Weigel RJ (1998) Ultrasound guided fine-needle aspiration biopsy of thyroid masses. Thyroid 8:283–289

Carrol BA (1982) Asymptomatic thyroid nodules: incidental sonographic detection. AJR 133:499–501

Casara D, Rubello D, Saladini G et al. (1999) Clinical approach in patients with metastatic differentiated thyroid carcinoma and negative 131-I whole body scintigraphy: importance of 99m Tc MIBI scan combined with high resolution neck ultrasonography Tumori 85:122–127

Castagnone D, Rivolta R, Rescalli S, Baldini MI, Tozzi R, Cantalamessa L (1996) Color Doppler sonography in Graves' disease: value in assessing activity of disease and predicting outcome. AJR 166:203–207

Castro MR, Gharib H (2000) Thyroid nodules and cancer. When to wait and watch, when refer. Postgrad Med J 107:113–116, 119–120, 123–124

Cavalieri RR (1996) Nuclear imaging in the management of thyroid carcinoma. Thyroid 6:485–492

Cavalieri RR (1997) Iodine metabolism and thyroid physiology: current concepts. Thyroid 7:177–181

Chan ST, Brook F, Ahuja A, Brown O, Metreweli C (1999) Relationship of thyroid blood flow to reproductive events in normal Chinese females. Ultrasound Med Biol 25:223–240

Chang TC, Hong CT, Chang SL, Hsieh HC, Liaw KY, How SW (1990) Correlation between sonography and pathology in thyroid diseases. J Formos Med Assoc 89:777–783

Cheug NW, Boyages SC (1997) The thyroid gland in acromegaly: an ultrasonographic study. Clin Endocrinol (Oxf) 46:545–549

Chiu WY, Chia NH, Wan SK, Yuen CH, Cheung MT (1998) The investigation and management of thyroid nodules. A retrospective review of 183 cases. Ann Acad Med Singapore J 27:196–199

Cho YS, Lee HK, Ahn IM et al (2000) Sonographically guided ethanol sclerotherapy for benign thyroid cysts: results in 22 cases. AJR 174:213–216

Chopra S, Wastie ML, Chan S et al (1996) Assessment of completeness of thyroid ablation by estimation of neck uptake of ^{131}I on whole-body scans: comparison of quantification and visual assessment of thyroid bed uptake. Nucl Med Commun 17:687–691

Clark KJ, Cronan JJ, Scola FH (1995) Color Doppler sonography: anatomic and physiologic assessments of the thyroid. J Clin Ultrasound 23:215–223

Cochan-Priollet B, Guillausseau PJ, Chagnon S, et al (1994) The diagnostic value of fine-needle aspiration biopsy under ultrasonography in nonfunctional thyroid nodules: a prospective study comparing cytologic and histologic findings. Am J Med 97:152–157

Cohen JH, Ingbar SH, Braverman LE (1989) Thyrotoxicosis due to ingestion of excess thyroid hormone. Endocr Rev 10:113–124

Conti PS, Durski JM, Singer PA (1997) Incidence of thryoid gland uptake of F-18 FDG in cancer patients. Radiology 205 (P):220

Crescenzi A, Papini E, Pacella CM, et al (1996) Morphological changes in a hyperfunctioning thyroid adenoma after percutaneous ethanol injection: histological, enzymatic and submicroscopical alterations. J Endocrinol Invest 19:371–376

Crom DB, Kaste SC, Tubergen DG, Greenwald CA, Sharp GB, Hudson MM (1997) Ultrasonography for thyroid screening after head and neck irradiation in childhood cancer survivors. Med Pediatr Oncol 28:15–21

Cyna-Gorse F, Toubert ME, Zagdanski AM et al (1996) Récidives cervico-médiastinales des cancers thyroïdiens différenciés: valeur de l'IRM. J Radiol 77:1195–1200

Danese D, Schiacchitano S (1993) Il nodulo tiroideo. Considerazioni diagnostiche. Minerva Endocrinol 18:129–137

Danese D, Sciacchitano S, Farsetti A, Andreoli M, Pontecorvi A (1998) Diagnostic accuracy of conventional versus sonography-guided fine-needle aspiration biopsy of thyroid nodules. Thyroid 8:15–21

Degnan BM, McClellan DR, Francis GL (1996) An analysis of fine-needle aspiration biopsy of the thyroid in children and adolescents. J Pediatr Surg 31:903–907

De Lellis RA (1989) The endocrine system. In: Cotram R, Kumar V, Robbins SL (eds) Robbins pathologic basis of disease, 4th edn. Saunders, Philadelphia, pp 1214–1242

Delorme S, Weisser G, Zuna I, Fein M, Lorenz A, Van Kaick G (1995) Quantitative characterization of color Doppler images: reproducibility, accuracy, and limitations. J Clin Ultrasound 23:537–550

Derebek E, Biberoglu S, Kut O, et al (1996) Early and delayed thallium-201 scintigraphy in thyroid nodules: the relationship between early thallium-201 uptake and perfusion. Eur J Nucl Med 23:504–520

Diez O, Anorbe E, Aisa P, Saez de Ormijana J, Aguirre X, Paraiso M (1998) Acute suppurative thyroiditis secondary to piriform sinus fistula: a case report. Eur J Radiol 29:25–27

Dimai HP, Ramschak-Schwarzer S, Lax S, Lipp RW, Leb G (1999) Hyperthyroidism of Graves' disease: evidence for only unilateral involvement of the thyroid gland in a 31-year-old female patient. J Endocrinol Invest 22:215–219

Dorr V, Wurstlin S, Franck-Raue K, et al (1993) Somatostatin receptor scintigraphy (SRS) and MRI in recurrent medullary thyroid carcinoma: a comparative study. Horm Metab Res 27:48–55

Duquenne M, Rohmer V, Guyetant S et al (1997) Nodule thyroïdien isolé. Intérêt de la cytoponction et de la scintigraphie. Presse Méd 26:507–511

Eeckhoudt L, Hermans J, Merlo P, et al (1993) Analyse économique des approches diagnostiques et thérapeutiques du nodule froid de la thyroïde. Ann Endocrinol 54:293–296

Ezzat S, Sarti DA, Cain DR, Braunstein GD (1994) Thyroid incidentalomas. Prevalence by palpation and ultrasonography. Arch Intern Med 154:1838–1840

Farwell AP, Braverman LE (1996) Inflammatory thyroid disorders. Otolaryngol Clin North Am 29:541–557

Feldkamp J, Horstser FA (1995) Rationelle Diagnostik von Schilddrusenfunktionsstörungen. Z Arztl Fortbild 89:21–25

Ferrari C, Reschini E, Paracchi A (1997) Treatment of the autonomous thyroid nodule: a review. Eur J Endocrinol 135:383–390

Ferrozzi F, Bova D, Campodonico F, De Chiara F, Conti GM, Bassi P (1998) US and CT findings of secondary neoplasms of the thyroid. A pictorial essay. Clin Imaging 22:157–161

Fon LJ, Deans GT, Lioe TF, Lawson JT, Briggs K, Spence RA (1996) An audit of thyroid surgery in a general surgical unit. Ann R Coll Surg Engl 78:192–196

Fontan FJP, Carballido FC, Felipe FP, Oses JM, Martin CV (1993) Riedel thyroiditis: US, CT, and MR evaluation. J Comput Assist Tomogr 17:324–325

Franceschi M, Kujic Z, Franceschi D, Lukinac L, Roncevic S (1996) Thyroglobulin determination, neck ultrasonography and iodine-131 whole-body scintigraphy in differentiated thyroid carcinoma. J Nucl Med 37:446–451

Frasoldati A, Toschi E, Zini M, et al (1999) Role of thyroglobulin measurement in fine-needle aspiration biopsies of cervical lymph nodes in patients with differentiated thyroid cancer. Thyroid 9:105–111

Freitas JE, Freitas AE (1994) Thyroid and parathyroid imaging. Semin Nucl Med 24:234–245

Fridrich L, Messa C, Landoni C, et al (1997) Whole-body scintigraphy with 99 Tcm-MIBI, 18 F-FDG and 131-I in patients with metastatic thyroid carcinoma. Nucl Med Commun 18:3–9

Funari M, Campos Z, Gooding GA, Higgins CG (1992) MRI and ultrasound detection of asymptomatic thyroid nodules in hyperparathyroidism. J Comput Assist Tomogr 16:615–619

Galloway RJ, Smallridge RC (1996) Imaging in thyroid cancer. Endocrinol Metab Clin North Am 25:93–113

Gallowitsch HJ, Mikosch P, Kresnik E, Starlinger M, Lind P (1999) Lymphoscintigraphy and gamma probe-guided surgery in papillary thyroid carcinoma: the sentinel lymph node concept in thyroid carcinoma. Clin Nucl Med 24:744–746

Gandon J, Ledoux-Robert J (1995) Les cancers du corps thyroïde. Actualités en cancerologie cervicofaciale. Masson, Paris

Garcia-Mayor RV, Perez Mendez LF, Paramo C, et al (1997) Fine-needle aspiration biopsy of thyroid nodules: impact on clinical practice. J Endocrinol Invest 20:482–487

Garretti L, Cassinis MC, Cesarini F, Drogo M, Papotti M, Ragona R (1994) Attendibilita della diagnosi ecotomografica nella valutazione delle lesioni della tiroide. Confronto con la citologia e l'istologia. Radiol Med 88:598–605

Gemma R, Nakamura H, Mori T, Andoh S, Suzuki Y, Yoshimi T (1996) The change in 123-I uptake between 3 and 24 hours is useful in predicting early response to methimazole in patients with Graves' disease. Endocr J 43:61–66

Gharib H (1994) Fine-needle aspiration biopsy of thyroid nodules: advantages, limitations and effect. Mayo Clin Proc 69:44–49

Gharib H (1997) Changing concepts in the diagnosis and management of thyroid nodules. Endocrinol Metab Clin North Am 26:777–800

Gharib H, Goellner JR (1993) Fine-needle aspiration biopsy of the thyroid: an appraisal. Ann Intern Med 118:282–289

Gharib H, Goellner JR, Johnston DA (1993) Fine-needle aspiration cytology of the thyroid: a 12-year experience with 11,000 biopsies. Clin Lab Med 13:669–709

Gimondo P, Messina G, Caratozzolo M, Tomei A (1994) Analisi del ruelo della citologia agoaspirativa ecoguidata quale criterio di selezione nella terapia chirurgica delle malattie tiroidee. Studio retrospettivo multicentrico su 5109 pazienti. Radiol Med 87:648–652

Gimondo P, Messina G, Gimondo S (1996) Raro caso di tiroidite acuta suppurativa. Minerva Med 87:475–478

Gimondo P, Pizzi C, Gimondo S, Messina G (1998) Ultrasonography, with Doppler color, and cytologic correlations in Plummer's disease. Radiol Med (Torino) 95:193–198

Giovagnoli MR, Pisani T, Drusco A, Scardella L, Antonaci A, Vecchione A (1998) Fine-needle aspiration biopsy in the preoperative management of patients with thyroid nodules. Anticancer Res 18:3741–3745

Giuffrida D, Gharib H (1995) Controversies in the management of cold, hot, and occult thyroid nodules. Am J Med 99:642–650

Giusti M, Foppiani L, Fazzuoli L, et al (1999) An increased prevalence of thyroid echographic and auto-immune changes in hyperprolactinemic women on therapy with dopaminergic drugs. Recenti Prog Med 90:147–151

Goletti O, Lenziardi M, Lippolis PV, et al (1993) Alcolizzazione percutanea ecoguidata dei noduli tirodei freddi non neoplastici. Radiol Med 85:827–830

Gonczi J, Szabolcs I, Kovacs Z, Kakosy T, Goth M, Szilagyi G (1994) Ultrasonography of the thyroid gland in hospitalized, clinically ill geriatric patients: thyroid volume, its relationship to age and disease, and the prevalence of diffuse and nodular goiter. J Clin Ultrasound 22:257–261

Gonsorcikova V, Trebjbal D, Tajtakova M, et al. (1996) Treatment of autonomous thyroid gland nodules using percutaneaous injections of ethanol under ultrasonography control. Initial experience. Vnitr Lek 42:166–170

Gooding GA (1993) Sonography of the thyroid and parathyroid. Radiol Clin North Am 31:967–989

Gordon DL, Flisak M, Fischer SG (1999) Changes in thyroid nodule volume caused by fine-needle aspiration: a factor complicating the interpretation of the effect of thyrotropin suppression on nodule size. J Clin Endocrinol Metab 84:4566–4569

Gorman B, Charboneau JW, James EM, et al (1987) Medullary thyroid carcinoma: role of high-resolution US. Radiology 162:147–150

Greening WP, Sarker JK, Osborne MP (1980) Hemiagenesis of the thyroid gland. Br J Surg 67:446–448

Guerra U, Pizzocaro C, Terzi A, et al (1988) The use of 99m Tc (V) DMSA as imaging for the medullary thyroid carcinoma (MCT). J Nucl Med Allied Sci 32:242–247

Hamburger JI (1987) Consistency of sequential needle biopsy findings for thyroid nodules. Arch Intern Med 147:97–99

Hamburger JI (1994) Diagnosis of thyroid nodules by fine-needle biopsy: use and abuse. J Clin Endocrinol Metab 79:335–339

Hamburger JI, Miller JM, Kini SR (1983) Lymphoma of the thyroid. Ann Intern Med 99:685–693

Hancock SL, McDougall IR, Constine LS (1995) Thyroid abnormalities after therapeutic external radiation. Int J Radiat Oncol Biol Phys 31:1165–1170

Hardoff R, Baron E, Sheinfeld M, Luboshitsky R (1995) Localized manifestations of subacute thyroiditis presenting as solitary transient cold thyroid nodules. A report of 11 cases. Clin Nucl Med 20:981–984

Hatabu H, Kasagi K, Yamamoto K, et al (1991) Cystic papillary carcinoma of the thyroid gland: a new sonographic sign. Clin Radiol 43:121–124

Hatada T, Okada K, Ishii H, Utsunomiya J (1998) Evaluation of ultrasound-guided fine-needle aspiration biopsy for thyroid nodules. Am J Surg 175:133–136
Hayashi N, Tamaki N, Konishi J, et al. (1986) Sonography of Hashimoto's thyroiditis. J Clin Ultrasound 14:123–126
Hazard JB (1960). Small papillary carcinoma of the thyroid: a study with special reference to so-called non-encapsulated sclerosing tumor. Lab Invest 9:86–97
Healy JC, Shafford EA, Reznek RH, et al (1996) Sonographic abnormalities of the thyroid gland following radiotherapy in survivors of childhood Hodgkin's disease. Br J Radiol 69:671–623
Hegedus L (1990) Thyroid size determined by ultrasound. Influence of physiological factors and non-thyroidal disease. Dan Med Bull 37:249–263
Hegedus L, Kastrup S, Rasmussen N (1986) Evidence of cyclic alterations of thyroid size during the menstrual cycle in healthy women. Am J Obstet Gynecol 155:142–145
Hermann M, Roka R, Richter B, Koriska K, Gobl S, Freissmuth M (1999) Reoperation as treatment after subtotal thyroidectomy in Graves' disease. Surgery 125:522–528
Hermans R, Bouillon R, Laga K, et al (1997) Estimation of thyroid gland volume by spiral computed tomography. Eur Radiol 7:214–216
Hiromatsu Y, Ishibashi M, Miyake I, Nonaka K (1998) Technetium-99m tetrafosmin imaging in patients with subacute thyroiditis. Eur J Nucl Med 25:1448–1452
Hiromatsu Y, Ishibashi M, Miyake I, et al (1999) Color Doppler ultrasonography in patients with subacute thyroiditis. Thyroid 12:1189–1193
Hiromura T (1994) Ultrasonography of cystic thyroid nodules: sonographic-pathologic correlation. Nippon Igaku Hoshasen Gakkai Zasshi 54:500–509
Ho C, Lin JD, Huang YY, Huang HS, Huang BY, Hsueh C (1996) Clinical experience of medullary thyroid carcinoma in Chang Gung Memorial Hospital. Chang Keng I Hsueh 19:142–148
Hodgson KJ, Lazarus JH, Wheeler MH et al (1988) Duplex scan-derived thyroid blood flow in euthyroid and hyperthyroid patients. World J Surg 12:470–475
Holden A (1995) The role of colour and duplex Doppler ultrasound in the assessment of thyroid nodules. Australas Radiol 39:343–349
Hopkins CR, Reading CC (1995) Thyroid and parathyroid imaging. Semin Ultrasound CT MR 16:279–295
Hopkins CR, Reading CC (1998) Thyroid, parathyroid and other glands. In: McGahan JP, Goldberg BB (eds) Diagnostic ultrasound: a logical approach. Lippincott-Raven, Philadelphia, pp 1087–1114
Horlocker TT, Hay JE, James EM, Reading CC, Charboneau JW (1986) Prevalence of incidental nodular thyroid diseases detected during high-resolution parathyroid ultrasonography. In: Medeiros-Neto A, Gaitan E (eds) Frontiers of thyroidology, vol 2. Plenum, New York, pp 1309–1312
Horvath E, Majilis S, Yanez P, et al (1997) Thyroidite de de Quervain: diagnostic en échographie. J Radiol 78:897
Horvath F, Capuano LG, Lippolis G, et al (1993) In tema di diagnosi di natura preoperatoria del nodulo tiroideo. Minerva Chir 48:1279–1281
Hurley DL, Gharib H (1996) Evaluation and management of multinodular goiter. Otolaryngol Clin North Am 29:527–540
Huysmans D, Hermus A, Edelbroeck M, Barentsz J, Corstens F, Kloppenborg P (1997) Radioiodine for nontoxic multinodulair goiter thyroid 7:235–239
Huysmans DA, De Haas MM, Van Den Broerk WJ, et al (1994) Magnetic resonance imaging for volume estimation of large multinodular goitres: a comparison with scintigraphy. Br J Radiol 67:519–523
Ito M, Yamashita S, Ashizawa S, et al (1995) Childhood thyroid diseases around Chernobyl evaluated by ultrasound examination and fine-needle aspiration cytology. Thyroid 5:365–368
James C, Starks M, MacGillivray DC, White J (1999) The use of imaging studies in the diagnosis and management of thyroid cancer and hyperparathyroidism. Surg Oncol Clin N Am 8:145–169
James EM, Charboneau JW, Hay ID (1991) The thyroid. In: Rumack CM (ed) Diagnostic ultrasound, vol 1. Mosby, St Louis, pp 507–523
Jarlov AE, Hegedus L, Gjorup T, Hansen JEM (1991) Accuracy of the clinical assessment of thyroid size. Dan Med Bull 38:87–89
Jarlov AE, Nygard B, Hegedus L, Kastrup S, Hansen JM (1993) Observer variation in ultrasound assessment of the thyroid gland. Br J Radiol 66:625–627
Kamijo K (1994) Clinical studies on thyroid CT number in chronic thryoiditis. Endocr J 41:19–23
Kasagi K, Hatabu H, Tokuda Y, et al (1991) Lymphoproliferative disorders of the thyroid gland: radiological appearances. Br J Radiol 64:569–575
Katagiri M, Harada T, Kiyono T (1994) Diagnosis of thyroid carcinoma by ultrasonic examination: comparison with diagnosis by fine-needle aspiration cytology. Thyroidology 6:21–26
Kato A, Yamada H, Yamada T, Ishinaga H (1997) Fine-needle aspiration cytology under ultrasonographic imaging for diagnosis of thyroid tumor. Nippon Jibiinkoka Gakkai Kaiho 100:45–50
Kerr L (1994) High-resolution thyroid ultrasound: the value of color Doppler. Ultrasound Q 12:21–43
Khurana KK, Richards VI, Chopra PS, Izquierdo R, Rubens D, Mesonero C (1998) The role of ultrasonography-guided fine-needle aspiration biopsy in the management of nonpalpable and palpable thyroid nodules. Thyroid 8:511–515
Kim JK, Lee HK, Ahn IM, Lee MJ, Choi CG, Suh DC (1997) Treatment of benign cold thyroid nodules: efficacy and safety of sonographically guided percutaneous ethanol injection. Radiology 205 (P):531
Kimoto T, Suemitsu K, Eda I, Shimizu T, Ohtani M, Nabika T (1999) The efficiency of performing ultrasound-guided fine-needle aspiration biopsy following mass screening for thyroid tumors to ovoid unnecessary surgery. Surg Today 29:880–883
King AD, Ahuja AT, King W, Metreweli C (1997) The role of ultrasound in the diagnosis of a large, rapidly growing, thryroid mass. Postgrad Med J 73:412–414
King AD, Ahuja AT, To EW, Tse GM, Metreweli C (2000) Staging papillary carcinoma of the thyroid: magnetic resonance imaging vs ultrasound of the neck. Clin Radiol 55:222–226
Kirillov IUB, Stroev EA, Arijtarkhov VG, et al (1997) The dynamic observation of patients with diffuse toxic goiter in the postoperative period by means of echography. Vestn Khir Im I I Grek 156:80–82
Kobayashi M, Mogami T, Uchiyama M, et al (1997) Usefulness of 99mTc-MIBI SPECT in the metastatic lesions of thyroid cancer. Nippon Igaku Hoshasen Gakkai Zasshi 57:127–132

Komatsu M, Kobayashi S, Ito N, Sugenoya A, Ida F (1994) Ultrasonography in the diagnosis of malignant lymphoma of the thyroid. Nippon Geka Gakkai Zasshi 95:187–191

Komorowski J, Kuzdak K, Pomorski L, Bartos M, Stepien H (1998) Percutaneous ethanol injection in treatment of benign nonfunctional and hyperfunctional thyroid nodules. Cytobios 95:143–150

Kraimps JL (1999) Place des investigations complémentaires avant une thyroidectomie. Quels examens demander avant une reintervention? Ann Chir 53:78–80

Kraimps JL, Barbier J (1993) Apport de l'échographie peropératoire. Ann Endocrinol 54:235–236

Kraimps JL, Bouin-Pineau MH, Marechaud R, Barbier J (1998) Basedow's disease and thyroid nodules. A common association. Ann Chir 52:449–451

Kresnik E, Gallowitsch HJ, Mikosch P, Gomez I, Lind P (1997) Technetium-99m-MIBI scintigraphy of thyroid nodules in an endemic goiter area. J Nucl Med 38:62–65

Kuma K, Matzsuzuka F, Yokozawa T, Miyauchi A, Sugawara M (1994) Fate of untreated benign thyroid nodules: results of long-term follow-up. World J Surg 18:495–498

Kumar A, Aggarwal S, Pham DH (1994) Pharyngoesophageal (Zenker's) diverticulum mimicking thyroid nodule on ultrasonography: report of two cases. J Ultrasound Med 13:31322

Kume N, Suga K, Nishigauchi K, Kawamura M, Matsunaga N (1996) Relationship between thallium-201 uptake and tumour proliferative ability in thyroid nodules. Eur J Nucl Med 23:376–382

Kumpusalo L, Kumpusalo E, Soimakallio S, et al (1996) Thyroid ultrasound findings 7 years after the Chernobyl accident. A comparative epidemiological study in the Bryansk region of Russia. Acta Radiol 37:904–909

Kusunoki T, Murata K, Nishida S, Tomura T, Inoue M (1994) Histopathological findings of human thyroid tumors and signal intensities of MRI. Nippon Jibiinkoka Gakkai Kaiho 97:1406–1411

Lagalla R, Caruso G, Finazzo M (1998) Monitoring treatment response with color and power Doppler. Eur J Radiol 27 [Suppl 2]: S149–S159

Laitt RD, Hoh B, Wakeley C, et al. (1994) The value of the short tau inversion recovery sequence in magnetic resonance imaging of thyroid eye disease. Br J Radiol 67:244–247

Langer P (1999) Minireview: discussion about the limit between normal and thyroid goiter. Endocr Regul 33:39–45

Leclere J, Sidibe S, Lassau N, et al (1996) Aspects échographiques des métastases hépatiques des cancers médullaires de la thyroïde. J Radiol 77:99–103

Lee MJ, Ross DS, Mueller PR, Daniels G, Dawson SL, Simeone JF (1993) Fine-needle aspiration biopsy of cervical lymph nodes in patients with thyroid cancer: a prospective comparison of cytopathologic and tissue marker analysis. Radiology 187:851–854

Leenhardt L, Hejblum G, Franc B, et al (1999) Indications and limits of ultrasound-guided cytology in the management of nonpalpable thyroid nodules. J Clin Endocrinol Metab 84:24–28

Lima N, Knobel M, Cavaliere H, Sztejnsznajd E, Tomimori E, Medeiros-Neto G (1997) Levothyroxine suppressive therapy is partially effective in treating patients with benign, solid thyroid nodules and multinodular goiters. Thyroid 7:691–697

Lin JD, Huang BY (1998) Comparison of the results of diagnosis and treatment between solid and cystic well-differentiated thyroid carcinomas. Thyroid 8:661–666

Lin JD, Hsueh C, Chao TC, Weng HF, Huang BY (1997a) Thyroid follicular neoplasms diagnosed by high-resolution ultrasonography with fine-needle aspiration cytology. Acta Cytol 41:687–691

Lin JD, Huang BY, Weng HF, Jeng LB, Hsueh C (1997b) Thyroid ultrasonography with fine-needle aspiration cytology for the diagnosis of thyroid cancer. J Clin Ultrasound 25:111–118

Lin JD, Weng HF, Ho YS (1998) Clinical and pathological characteristics of secondary thyroid cancer. Thyroid 8:149–153

Lind P, Gallowitsch HJ, Langsteger W, Kresnik E, Mikosch P, Gomez I (1997) Technetium-99m-tetrofosmin whole-body scintigraphy in the follow-up of differentiated thyroid carcinoma. J Nucl Med 38:348–352

Lippi F, Ferrari C, Manetti L, et al (1996) Treatment of solitary autonomous thyroid nodules by percutaneous ethanol injection: results of an Italian multicenter study. The Multicenter Study Group. J Clin Endocrinol Metab 81:3261–3264

Livraghi T, Paracchi A, Ferrari C, Reschini E, Macchi RM, Bonifacino A (1994) Treatment of autonomous thyroid nodules with percutaneous ethanol injection: 4-year experience. Radiology 190:529–533

Loevner LA (1996) Imaging of the thyroid gland. Semin Ultrasound CT MRI 17:539–562

Loughran CF (1991). Case report: cystic lymph node metastasis from occult thyroid carcinoma: a sonographic mimic of a branchial cleft cyst. Clin Radiol 43:213–214

Lu C, Chang TC, Hsiao YL, Kuo MS (1994) Ultrasonographic findings of papillary thyroid carcinoma and their relation to pathologic changes. J Formos Med Assoc 93:933–938

Lucas A, Llatjos M, Salinas I, et al (1995) Fine-needle aspiration cytology of benign nodular thyroid disease. Value of re-aspiration. Eur J Endocrinol 132:677–680

Lucas KJ (2000) Use of thyroid ultrasound volume in calculating radioactive iodine dose in hyperthyroidism. Thyroid 10:151–155

Lugo-Vicente H, Ortiz VN, Irizarky H, Camps JI, Pagan V (1998) Pediatric thyroid nodules: management in the era of fine-needle aspiration. J Pediatr Surg 33:1302–1305

Lukomskii GI, Shulutko AM, Semikov VI (1999) Clinical and morphological characteristics and peculiarities of differentiated thyroid gland cancer course. Khirurgiia 7:4–8

Lupi A, Cerisara D, Orsolon P, De Antoni G, Vianello Dri A (1999) Thyroid nodules and Doppler ultrasonography. A new element for an old puzzle? Minerva Endocrinol 24:7–10

Lupoli G, Lombardi G, Panza N, et al (1991) MIBG scintigraphy and selective venous catheterization after thyroidectomy for MTC. Med Oncol Tumor Pharmacother 13:8101–8107

Malotte MS, Chonkich GD, Zuppan CW (1991) Riedel's thyroiditis. Arch Otolaryngol Head Neck Surg 117:214–217

Mann B, Schmale P, Stremmel W (1996) Thyroid morphology and function after surgical treatment of thyroid diseases. Exp Clin Endocrinol Diabetes 104:271–277

Massol J, Pazart L, Aho S, Strauch G, Leclere J, Durieux P (1993) Prise en charge de nodule thyroïdien. Résultats préliminaires d'une enquête de pratiques auprès de 685 médecins généralistes et spécialistes. Ann Endocrinol 54:220–225

Mayr B, Brabant G, von zur Muhlen A (1999) Incidental detection of familial medullary thyroid carcinoma by calcitonin screening for nodular thyroid disease. Eur J Endocrinol 141:286–289

Merceron RE, Cordray JP, Nys PM, et al (1997) Results of ultrasonographic and cytologic follow-up of 311 initially nonsuspicious thyroid nodules. Ann Endocrinol 58:463–468
Messina G (1999) Echography and cytologic exam by needle aspirate in the diagnosis of chronic thyroiditis. Recenti Prog Med 90:258–263
Messina G, Viceconti N, Trinti B (1998a) Ecotomografia e color-Doppler nella diagnosi di carcinoma teroideo. Ann Ital Med Int 11:263–267
Messina G, Viceconti N, Trinti B (1998b) Diagnostic items and treatment of Plummer's disease: a study on 180 patients. Clin Ter 149:191–195
Meyer D (1991) Bewertung der Schilddrusenszintigraphie sowie der Schilddrusensonographie aus chirurgischer sicht. Zentralbl Chir 116:935–942
Miccoli P, Antonelli A, Iacconi P, Alberti B, Gambuzza C, Baschieri L (1993) Prospective, randomized, double-blind study about effectiveness of Levothyroxine suppressive therapy in prevention of recurrence after operation: result at the third year of follow-up. Surgery 114:1097–1101
Miki H, Oshimo K, Inoue H, et al (1993) Incidence of ultrasonographically detected nodules in healthy adults. Tokushima J Exp Med 40:43–46
Mikosch P, Gallowitsch HJ, Kresnik E, et al (2000) Value of ultrasound-guided fine-needle aspiration biopsy of thyroid nodules in an endemic goiter area. Eur J Nucl Med 27:62–69
Mirk P, Rufini V, Summaria V, Salvatori M (1999) Diagnostic imaging of the thyroid: methodology and normal patterns. Rays 24:215–228
Mitteldorf CA, Misiara AC, De Carvalho IE (1999) Multicystic autoimmune thyroiditis-like disease associated with HIV infection. A case report. Acta Cytol 43:862–866
Morosini PP, Mancini V, Filipponi S, et al (1996a) Cytological diagnosis of thyroid nodules. Comparison of results obtained with guided echography with those from a blind biopsy. Minerva Endocrinol 21:18–25
Morosini PP, Filipponi S, Mancini V, et al (1996b) Evaluation of the role of repeat needle biopsy in the diagnosis and follow-up of thyroid nodules. Minerva Endocrinol 21:59–62
Morosini PP, Simonella G, Mancini V, et al (1998c) Color Doppler sonography patterns related to histological findings in Graves' disease. Thyroid 8:577–582
Mortensen JD, Wollner LB, Bennett WA (1955) Gross and microscopic findings in clinically normal thyroid glands. J Clin Endocrinol Metab 15:1270–1280
Muller NW, Schroder S, Schneider C, Seifert G (1985) Sonographic tissue characterization in thyroid gland diagnosis. Klin Wochenschr 63:706–710
Muller-Leisse C, Troger J, Khabirpour F, Pockler C (1988) Normal values of thyroid gland volume. Ultrasound measurements in school children 7 to 20 years of age. Dtsch Med Wochenschr 113:1872–1875
Multanen M, Haapiainen R, Leppaniemi A, Voutilainen P, Sivula A (1999) The value of ultrasound-guided fine-needle aspiration biopsy (FNAB) and frozen section examination (FS) in the diagnosis of thyroid cancer. Ann Chir Gynaecol 88:132–135
Naik KS, Bury RF (1998) Imaging the thyroid. Clin Radiol 53:630–639
Nakahara H, Noguchi S, Murakami N, et al (1997) Gadolinium-enhanced MR imaging of thyroid and parathyroid masses. Radiology 202:765–772
Naruo K, Miyamoto Y, Tada S (1999) Diagnosis of thyroid nodules by Doppler ultrasonography: a comparison between color Doppler and power Doppler ultrasonography. Nippon Igaku Hoshasen Gakkai Zasshi 59:3–11
Ng EH, Tan Sk, Nambiar R (1990) Impact of fine-needle aspiration cytology on the management of solitary thyroid nodules. Aust N Z J Surg 60:463–466
Nicolosi A, Addis E, Calo PG, Tarquini A (1994) Ipertiroidismo e cancro della tiroide. Minerva Chir 49:491–495
Nordmeyer JP, Simons M, Wenzel C, Scholten T (1997) How accurate is the assessment of thyroid volume by palpation? A prospective study of 316 patients. Exp Clin Endocrinol Diabetes 105:366–371
Nygaard B, Farber J, Veje A, Hansen JE (1997) Thyroid volume and function after 131-I treatment of diffuse non-toxic goitre. Clin Endocrinol (Oxf) 46:493–496
Okamoto T, Yamashita T, Harasawa A, et al (1994) Test performances of three diagnostic procedures in evaluating thyroid nodules: physical examination, ultrasonography and fine-needle aspiration cytology. Endocr J 41:243–247
Onishi T, Noguchi S, Murakami N, et al (1994) Extraocular muscles in Graves' ophthalmopathy: usefulness of T2 relaxation time measurements. Radiology 190:857–862
Otsuka N, Nagai K, Morita K, et al. (1994) MRI of subacute thyroiditis. Radiat Med 12:273–276
Ozdemir H, Iigit ET, Yucel C, et al. (1994) Treatment of autonomous thyroid nodules: safety and efficacy of sonographically guided percutaneous injection of ethanol. AJR 163:929–932
Pacella CM, Guglielmi R, Fabbrini R, et al (1998) Papillary carninoma in small hypoechoic thyroid nodules: prediction value of echo color Doppler evaluation. Preliminary results. J Exp Clin Cancer Ris 17:127–128
Pachucki K, Burmeister LA (1997) Evaluation and treatment of persistent thyroglobulinemia in patients with well-differentiated thyroid cancer. Eur J Endocrinol 137:254–261
Papini E, Petrucci L, Guglielmi R, et al (1998) Long-term changes in nodular goiter: a 5-year prospective randomized trial of levothyroxine suppressive therapy for benign cold thyroid nodules. J Clin Endocrinol Metab 83:780–783
Parkes AB, Adams H, Othman S, Hall R, John R, Lazarus JH (1996) The role of complement in the pathogenesis of postpartum thyroiditis: ultrasound echogenicity and the degree of complement-induced thyroid damage. Thyroid 6:177–182
Pelizzo MR, Toniato A, Grigoletto R, Bernardi C, Pagetta C (1998) Papillary carcinoma of the thyroid. A uni- and multivariate analysis of the factors affecting the prognosis inclusive of surgical treatment. Minerva Chir 53:471–482
Pisani T, Giovagnoli MR, Intrieri FS, Vecchione A (1999a) Tall cell variant of papillary carcinoma coexisting with chronic lymphocytic thyroiditis. A case report. Acta Cytol 43:435–438
Pisani T, Vecchione A, Sinopoli NT, Drusco A, Valli C, Giovagnoli MR (1999b) Cytological and immunocytochemical analysis of laterocervical lymph nodes in patients with previous thyroid carcinoma. Anticancer Res 19:3527–3530
Podoloff DA (1996) Is there a place for routine surveillance using sonography, CT, or MR imaging for early detection (notably lymphoma) of patients affected by Hashimoto's thyroiditis? Questions and answers. AJR 167:1337–1338
Premawardhana LD, Parkes DB, Ammari F, et al (2000) Postpartum thyroiditis and long-term thyroid status: prognos-

tic influence of thyroid peroxidase antibodies and ultrasound echogenicity. J Clin Endocrinol Metab 85:71–75
Price DC (1993) Radioisotopic evaluation of the thyroid and parathyroids. Radiol Clin North Amer 31:991–1015
Price R, Horvath K, Moore FD jr (1993) Surgery for solitary thyroid nodules: assessment of methods to select patients at low risk for unsuspected malignancy in the unaffected lobe and the possible utility of preoperative thyroid ultrasound. Thyroid 3:87–92
Proye C (1993) Prise en charge du nodule thyroïdien isolé. Conclusion. Ann Endocrinol (Paris) 54:297–300
Raab SS, Silverman JF, Elsheikh TM, et al (1995) Pediatric thyroid nodules: disease demographics and clinical management as determined by fine-needle aspiration biopsy. Pediatrics 95:46–49
Rago T, Vitti P, Chiovato L, et al (1998) Role of conventional ultrasonography and color flow-Doppler sonography in predicting malignancy in "cold" thyroid nodules. Eur J Endocrinol 138:41–46
Rajkovaca Z, Biukovic M, Mikac G, Skrobic M (1999) Correlation of ultrasound and radio-isotopic studies in subacute de Quervain thyroiditis. Med Pregl 52:141–145
Ralls PW, Mayekawa DS, Lee KP, et al (1988) Color-flow Doppler sonography in Graves' disease: "thyroid inferno". AJR 150:781–784
Reading CC, Gorman CA (1993) Thyroid imaging techniques (review). Clin Lab Med 13:711–724
Reinhardt MJ, Moser E (1996) An update on diagnostic methods in the investigation of diseases of the thyroid (review). Eur J Nucl Med 23:587–594
Renard E, Jaffiol C, Rouanet JP, Lamarque JL (1991) Nodules thyroidiens et goitres non fonctionnels. Apport diagnostique de l'imagerie par résonance magnétique. Presse Méd 20:214–298
Reynolds JC, Robbins J (1997) The changing role of radioiodine in the management of differentiated thyroid cancer. Semin Nucl Med 27:152–164
Rifat SF, Ruffin MT IV (1994) Management of thyroid nodules. Am Fam Physician 50:785–790
Rodriguez JM, Hernandez Q, Pinero A, et al (1999) Substernal goiter: clinical experience of 72 cases. Ann Otol Rhinol Laryngol 108:501–504
Rodriguez JM, Reus M, Moreno A, et al (1997) High-resolution ultrasound associated with aspiration biopsy in the follow-up of patients with differentiated thyroid cancer. Otolaryngol Head Neck Surg 117:694–697
Romaldini JH, Biancalana MM, Figueiredo DI, Farah CS, Mathias PC (1996) Effect of L-thyroxine administration on antithyroid antibody levels, lipid profile, and thyroid volume in patients with Hashimoto's thyroiditis. Thyroid 6:183–188
Ronga G, Fiorentino A, Paserio E et al (1990) Can iodine 131 whole-body scan be replaced by thyroglobulin measurement in the postsurgical follow-up of differentiated thyroid carcinoma? J Nucl Med 31:1766–1771
Rosen IB, Azadian A, Walfish PG, Salem S, Lansdown E, Bedard YC (1993) Ultrasound-guided fine-needle aspiration biopsy in the management of thyroid disease. Am J Surg 1766:346–349
Ross DS (1991) Evaluation of the thyroid nodule. J Nucl Med 32:2181–2192
Rubello D, Gasparoni P, Roth G et al. (1996) Functional meaning of scintigraphic and echographic patterns, and of circulating anti-peroxidase antibodies in asymptomatic chronic thyroiditis. Q J Nucl Med 40:359–364
Sadoul JL (1995) Génèse des nodules thyroïdiens. Mécanismes physiologiques et pathologiques, implications cliniques. Ann Endocrinol 56:5–22
Sakaguchi T, Arakawa A, Takahashi M (2000) Appropriate use of ultrasonography in the neck . Semin Roentgenol 35:54–62
Sashi R, Tomura N, Hashimoto M, Kobayashi M, Watarai J (1997) Growth patterns of benign and malignant thyroid tumors estimated by CT. Radiat Med 15:7–11
Sato K, Okamura K, Hirata T, et al (1996) Immunological and chemical types of reversible hypothyroidism; clinical characteristics and long-term prognosis. Clin Endocrinol 45:519–528
Schlumberger M, Archangioli O, Peirarski JD, Tubiana M, Parmentier C (1988) Detection and treatment of lung metastases of differentiated thyroid carcinoma in patients with normal chest X-rays. J Nucl Med 29:1790–1794
Schumm-Draeger PM (1998) Ultrasound-guided percutaneous thyroid nodules. A review. Exp Clin Endocrinol Diabetes 106 [Suppl 4]:S59–S62
Schweiger U, Hosten N, Cordes M, et al (1996) Die Duplexsonographie in der Schilddrusenfunktionsdiagnostik. Rofo Fortschr Geb Rontgenstr Neuen Bildgeb Verfahr 164:114–118
Scott AM, Macapinlac H, Zhang J, et al (1995) Image registration of SPECT and CT images using an external fiduciary band and three-dimensional surface fitting in metastatic thyroid cancer. J Nucl Med 36:100–103
Seabold JE, Lawson MA, Gurll NJ, et al (1997) F-18 FDG PET Scans in thyroid cancer patients with negative total body diagnostic I-131 scans. Radiology 205:(P)399
Set PA, Oleszczuk-Raschke K, von Lengerke JH, Bramswig J (1996) Sonographic features of Hashimoto thyroidis in childhood. Clin Radiol 51:167–169
Seya A, Oeda T, Terano T, et al (1990) Comparative studies in fine-needle aspiration cytology with ultrasound scanning in the assessment of thyroid nodule. Jpn J Med 29:478–480
Shafford EA, Kingston JE, Healy JL, Webb JA, Plowman PN, Reznek RH (1999) Thyroid nodular disease after radiotherapy to the neck for childhood Hodgkin's disease. Br J Cancer 80:808–814
Shah DH, Samuel AM (1996) Metastasis to the liver in well-differentiated carcinoma of the thyroid. Thyroid 6:607–611
Shamma FN, Abrahams JJ (1992) Imaging in endocrine disorders. J Reprod Med 37:39–45
Shimamoto K, Satake H, Sawaki A, Ishigaki T, Funahashi H, Imai T (1998) Preoperative staging of thyroid papillary carcinoma with ultrasonography. Eur J Radiol 29:4–10
Shimaoka K, Sokal IE, Pickren JW (1962) Metastatic neoplasms in the thyroid gland: pathological and clinical findings. Cancer 15:557–565
Shimamoo K, Endo T, Ishigaki T, Sakuma S, Makino N (1993) Thyroid nodules: evaluation with color Doppler ultrasonography. J Ultrasound Med 12:673–678
Simeone JF, Daniels GH, Hall DA, et al (1987). Sonography in the follow-up of 100 patients with thyroid carcinoma AJR 14:45–49
Simon D, Goretzki PE, Witte J, Roher HD (1996) Incidence of regional recurrence guiding radicality in differentiated thyroid carcinoma. World J Surg 20:860–866
Singer PA (1996) Evaluation and management of the solitary thyroid nodule. Otolaryngol Clin North Am 29:577–591
Singer PA, Cooper DS, Daniels GH, et al (1996) Treatment guidelines for patients with thyroid nodules and well-dif-

ferentiated thyroid cancer. American Thyroid Association Arch Intern Med 156 2165–2172

Sironi M, Cozzi L, Pareschi R, Spreafico GL, Assi A (1999) Occult sporadic medullary microcarcinoma with lymph node metastases. Diagn Cytopathol 21.203–206

Smyth PP, Hetherton AM, Smith DF, Radcliff M, O'Herlihy C (1997) Maternal iodine status and thyroid volume during pregnancy correlation with neonatal iodine intake. J Clin Endocrinol Metab 82.2840–2843

Solbiati L, Cioffi V, Ballarati E (1992) Ultrasonography of the neck. Radiol Clin North Am 30.951–954

Solbiati L, Livraghi T, Ballarati E, Ierace T, Crespi L (1995) Thyroid gland. In. Solbiati L, Rizzatto G (eds) Ultrasound of superficial structures. High frequencies, Doppler and interventional procedures. Churchill Livingstone, Edinburgh, pp 49–85

Solbiati L, Ierace T, Cova L, Dellanoce M, Marelli P (1999) Percutaneous ethanol injection of autonomously functioning thyroid nodule. Rays 24.348–357

Solivetti FM, Nasrollah N, Paganelli C, De Majo A (1998) Lyphadenopathy as specific ultrasonography index of subacute thyroiditis. Preliminary data. Radiol Med (Torino) 96:596–598

Som P (1992) Detection of metastasis in cervical lymph nodes: CT and MR criteria and differential diagnosis. AJR 158:961–969

Som PM, Brandwein M, Lidov M, Lawson W, Biller HF (1994) The varied presentations of papillary thyroid carcinoma cervical nodal disease. CT and MR findings. AJNR 15.1123–1128

Sophocleous S, Ehrenheim C, Fischer J, Hundeshagen H (1997) Low-risk thyroid carcinoma. Therapy, follow-up and prognosis. Nuklearmedizin 36:93–102

Sostre J, Reyes MM (1991) Sonographic diagnosis and grading of Hashimoto' thyroiditis. J Endocrinol Invest 14.115–121

Spiezia S, Cerbone G, Assanti AP, Colao A, Siciliani M, Lombardi G (2000) Power Doppler ultrasonographic assistance in percutaneous ethanol injection of autonomously functioning nodules. J Ultrasound Med 19:39–46

Sponza M, Fabris B, Bertoletto M, Ricci C, Armini L (1997) Role of Doppler color ultrasonography and of flowmetric analysis in the diagnosis and follow-up of Graves' disease. Radiol Med (Torino) 93.405–409

Stern WD, Laniado M, Vogl W, et al (1994) Farbkodierte duplexsonographie und konstrastverstarkte Magnetresonanztomographie szintigraphisch kalter Schilddrusenknoten. Rofo Fortschr Geb Rontgenstr Neuen Bildgeb Verfahr 160:3–10

Strauss S (1999) Cricoid cartilage masquerading as a tumor on thyroid ultrasound. Br J Radiol 72.644–647

Sugino K, Ito K Jr, Ozaki O, Mimura T, Iwasaki U, Ito K (1998) Papillary microcarcinoma of the thyroid. J Endocrinol Invest 21:445–448

Sweeney DC, Johnston GS (1995) Radioiodine therapy for thyroid cancer. Endocrinol Metab Clin North Am 24.803–809

Szabolcs I, Podoba J, Feldkamp J, et al (1997) Comparative screening for thyroid disorders in old age in areas of iodine deficiency, long-term iodine prophylaxis and abundant iodine intake. Clin Endocrinol (Oxf) 47:87–92

Takamatsu J, Yoshida S, Yokozawa T, et al (1998) Correlation of antithyroglobulin and antithyroid-peroxidase antibody profiles with clinical and ultrasound characteristics of chronic thyroiditis. Thyroid 8:1101–1106

Takashima S, Fukuda H, Kobayashi T (1984) Thyroid nodules: clinical effects of ultrasound-guided fine-needle aspiration biopsy. J Clin Ultrasound 22.535–542

Takashima S, Matsuzuka F, Nagareda T, Tomiyama N, Kozuka T (1992) Thyroid nodules associated with Hashimoto thyroiditis. assessment with US. Radiology 185.125–130

Takashima S, Fukuda H, Nomura N, Kishimoto H, Kim T, Kobayashi T (1995a) Thyroid nodules: re-evaluation with ultrasound. J Clin Ultrasound 23:179–184

Takashima S, Fukuda H, Tomiyama N, Fujita N, Iwatani Y, Nakamura H (1995b) Hashimoto thyroiditis. correlation of MR imaging signal intensity with histopathologic findings and thyroid function test results. Radiology 197:213–219

Takashima S, Nomura N, Noguchi Y, Matsuzuka F, Inoue T (1995c) Primary thyroid lymphomas. evaluation with US, CT, and MRI. J Comput Assist Tomogr 19.282–288

Takashima S, Nomura N, Tanaka H, Itoh Y, Miki K, Harada T (1995d) Congenital hypothyroidism. assessment with ultrasound. AJNR 16:1117–1123

Takashima S, Sone S, Takayama F, Maruyama Y, Hasegawa M, Wang Q (1997) Differentiated thyroid carcinomas: prediction of tumor invasion into surrounding structures with MR imaging. Radiology 205 (P).604

Taki S, Kakuda K, Kakuma K et al (1997) Thyroid nodules: evaluation with US-guided core biopsy with an automated biopsy gun. Radiology 202:874–877

Tambouret R, Szyfelbein WM, Pitman MB (1999) Ultrasound-guided fine-needle aspiration biopsy of the thyroid. Cancer 87:299–305

Tan GH, Gharib H (1997) Thyroid incidentalomas: management approaches to nonpalpable nodules discovered incidentally on thyroid imaging. Ann Intern Med 126:226–231

Tan GH, Gharib H, Reading CC (1995) Solitary thyroid nodule. Comparison between palpation and ultrasonograhy. Arch Intern Med 155.2418–2423

Tarantino L, Giorgio A, Perotta A, Aloisio V, Forestieri MC (1997) Percutaneous ethanol injection (PEI) of large autonomous hyperfunctioning thyroid adenoma. Radiology 205 (P): 531

Tarantino L, Giorgio A, Mariniello N, et al (2000) Percutaneous ethanol injection of large autonomous hyperfunctioning thyroid nodules Radiology 214:143–148

Tatsuno S, Miyamoto Y, Ishihara K, Irie T, Kobori K, Tada S (1994) Ultrasonography in primary malignant lymphoma of the thyroid. Nippon Igaku Hoshasen Gakkai Zasshi 54.853–859

Tennvall J, Palmer J, Cederquist E, et al (1981) Scintigraphic evaluation and dynamic studies with thallium-201 in thyroid lesions with suspected cancer. Eur J Nucl Med 6: 295–300

Tessler FN, Tublin ME (1999) Thyroid sonography. current applications and future directions. AJR 173:437–443

Tollin SR, Mery GM, Jelveh N, et al (2000) The use of fine-needle aspiration biopsy under ultrasound guidance to assess the risk of malignancy in patients with a multinodular goiter. Thyroid 10:235–241

Tourniaire J, Nicolas MH, Paulin C, et al (1997) Nodules thyroidiens: dosage d'hormone thyréotrope sérique et cytoponction versus scintigraphie comme examens de premiere intention. Etude prospective de 150 dissections. Presse Med 26:752–755

Tramalloni J, Swagier-Uzan C, Moreau JF (1997) Etude de l'efficacite de la cytoponction echoguidee des nodules thyroidiens en fonction de leur taille. J Radiol 78.897

Tranquart F, Girard JJ, Baulieu JL, Pourcelot L (1996) Echographie de la pathologie inflammatoire et fonctionnelle de la thyroïde. In: Bruneton JN, Padovani B (eds) Imagerie en endocrinologie. Masson, Paris, pp 60–63

Ugur O, Kostakglu L, Guler N, et al (1996) Comparison of 99mTc (V)-DMSA, 201-TI and 99m-Tc-MIBI imaging in the follow-up of patients with medullary carcinoma of the thyroid. Eur J Nucl Med 23:1367–1371

Van den Breckel MWM, Stel HV, Castelijns J, et al (1990) Cervical lymph node metastasis: assessment of radiologic criteria. Radiology 177:373–384

Van Espen MB, Hermans J, Bodart F, Schmitz A, François D, Beauduin M (1997) Autonomous thyroid adenoma. Value of thallium scintigraphy and pathology. Ann Endocrinol 58:482–493

Verde G, Papini E, Pacella CM, et al (1994) Ultrasound-guided percutaneous ethanol injection in the treatment of cystic thyroid nodules. Clin Endocrinol 41:719–724

Versamidis K, Varsamidou E, Mavropoulos G (2000) Doppler ultrasonography in predicting relapse of hyperthyroidism in Graves' disease. Acta Radiol 41:45–48

Viateau-Poncin J (1992) Echographie de la thyroïde, 2nd edn. Vigot, Paris

Vidone RA, Silverberg SG (1966) Carcinoma of the thyroid in surgical and post-mortem material. Ann Surg 164:291–299

Visset J (1999) Quels examens demander devant un nodule thyroidien. Ann Chir 53:71–74

Vitti P, Lampis M, Piga M, et al (1994) Diagnostic usefulness of thyroid ultrasonography in atrophic thyroiditis. J Clin Ultrasound 22:375–379

Vitti P, Rago T, Mazzeo S, et al (1995) Thyroid blood flow evaluation by color-flow Doppler sonography distinguishes Graves' disease from Hashimoto's thyroiditis. J Endocrinol Invest 18:857–861

Wanet PM, Sand A, Abramovici J (1996) Physical and clinical evaluation of high-resolution thyroid pinhole tomography. J Nucl Med 37:2017–2020

Wang Q, Takashima S, Sone S, Takayama F, Maruyama Y, Hasegawa M (1997) MR imaging of medullary thyroid carcinoma: correlation with pathologic findings. Radiology 205 (P): 604

Wernecke K, Diederich P (1994) Sonographic features of mediastinal tumors. AJR 163:1357–1364

Wesche MFT, Tiel-v.Buul MM, Smits NJ, Wiersinga WM (1998) Ultrasonographic versus scintigraphic measurement of thyroid volume in patients referred for 131-I therapy. Nucl Med Com 19:341–346

Wiest PW, Hartshorne MF, Inskip PD, et al (1998)Thyroid palpation versus high-resolution thyroid ultrasonography in the detection of nodules. J Ultrasound Med 17:487–496

Witterick IJ, Abel SM, Noyek AM, et al (1993) Nonpalpable occult and metastatic papillary thyroid carcinoma. Laryngoscope 103:149–155

Woeber KA (1995) Cost-effective evaluation of the patient with a thyroid nodule. Surg Clin North Am 75:357–363

Yarman S, Mudun A, Alagol F, et al (1997) Scintigraphic varieties in Hashimoto's thyroiditis and comparison with ultrasonography. Nucl Med Commun 18:951–956

Yasuda S, Shohtsu A, Ide M, et al (1998) Chronic thyroiditis: diffuse uptake of FDG at PET. Radiology 207:775–778

Yeh HC, Futterweit W, Gilbert P (1996) Micronodulation: ultrasonographic sign of Hashimoto thyroiditis. J Ultrasound Med 12:813–819

Ying M, Brook F, Ahuja A, Metreweli C (1998) The value of thyroid parenchymal echogenicity as an indicator of pathology using the sternomastoid muscle for comparison. Ultrasound Med Biol 24:1097–1105

Yokoyama N, Nagayama Y, Kakezono F, et al (1988) Determination of the volume of the thyroid gland by a high-resolution ultrasonic scanner. J Nucl Med 27:1475–1479

Yokozawa T, Fukata S, Kuma K, et al (1996) Thyroid cancer detected by ultrasound-guided fine-needle aspiration biopsy. World J Surg 20:848–853

Yoshimura R, Kodama S, Nakamura H (1995) Classification of congenital hyperthyroidism based on scintigraphy, ultrasonography and the serum thyroglobulin level. Kobe J Med Sci 41:71–82

Zaidi H (1996) Comparative methods for quantifying thyroid volume using planar imaging and SPECT. J Nucl Med 37:1421–1426

Zardo F, Soldo P, Altissimi G, Parnasi E, Bertin S (1999) Hashimoto's thyroiditis and thyroid cancer: a report of a clinical case and a review of the literature. G Chir 20:174–176

Zingrillo M, D'Aloiso L, Ghiggi MR, et al (1996a) Thyroid hypoechogenicity after methimazole withdrawal in Graves' disease: a useful index for predicting recurrence? Clin Endocrinol 45:201–206

Zingrillo M, Torlontano M, Ghiggi MR, et al (1996b) Percutaneous ethanol injection of large thyroid cystic nodules. Thyroid 6:403–408

Zingrillo M, Collura D, Ghiggi MR, Nirchio V, Trischitta V (1998) Treatment of large cold benign thyroid nodules not eligible for surgery with percutaneous ethanol injection. J Clin Endocrinol Metab 83:3905–3907

Zohar Y, Strauss M (1994) Occult distant metastases of well-differentiated thyroid carcinoma. Head Neck 16:438–442

2 Parathyroid Glands

Jean Noël Bruneton, Tito Livraghi, Robin Lecesne, Francesca Meloni

CONTENTS

J.N. Bruneton, MD
Service de Radiologie, Hôpital de l'Archet, 151, route de St.-Antoine Ginestière, B.P. 3079, F-06202 Nice Cedex 3, France
T. Livraghi, MD
Unita Raiologia, Ospedale Civile, Via C. Battisti, 23, I-20059 Vimercate (MI), Italy
R. Lecesne, MD
Service de Radiodiagnostic, Hôpital du Haut Lévêque, F-33604 Pessac, France
F. Meloni, MD
Unita Raiologia, Ospedale Civile, Via C. Battisti, 23, I-20059 Vimercate (MI), Italy

The parathyroid glands secrete parathyroid hormone (PTH, the main endocrine regulator of calcium and phosphorus), which is down-regulated by serum ionized calcium. Parathyroid disorders are dominated by primary hyperparathyroidism, for which the role of imaging remains controversial.

2.1 Definitions

2.1.1 Primary Hyperparathyroidism

Primary hyperparathyroidism (PHPT) is a common endocrine disorder diagnosed today essentially in women over the age of 60 years following a long, insidious course. This explains why, in the past, this disorder often went unrecognized until complications (bone, renal) or exacerbation of hypercalcemia occurred. Today, PHPT is nearly always discovered during routine serum calcium assays. Conclusive diagnosis is based on demonstration of hypercalcemia with hypophosphatemia, associated with an inappropriate (normal or elevated) plasma intact PTH level.

Diagnostic difficulties are encountered in three situations (SADOUL 1996):

- Severe hypercalcemia, which is suggestive of malignant tumoral hypercalcemia
- PHPT with normocalcemia, which must be distinguished from idiopathic hypercalciuria
- PHPT with a normal PTH concentration

In each case, the clinical setting and laboratory values should provide the correct diagnosis; imaging should not be used to make a positive diagnosis.

Parathyroid adenomas, the most frequent cause of PHPT, are usually solitary. Parathyroid hyperplasia, which affects all four glands, is much less frequent (fewer than 20% of patients), but asymmetrical enlargement of two or three parathyroid glands may be confused with multiple parathyroid adenomas (less than 3% of patients). One third of all patients with primary hyperplasia have familial hyperparathyroidism or a multiple endocrine neoplasia (MEN) syndrome (LIVOLSI and HAMILTON 1994). Parathyroid carcinoma is a rare cause of PHPT.

2.1.2
Secondary and Tertiary Hyperparathyroidism

In patients with chronic renal failure, hyperplasia of the parathyroid glands causes secondary hyperparathyroidism (SHPT). Chronic oversecretion of PTH secondary to hypocalcemia results in enlargement of all four parathyroid glands. The presence of supernumerary glands, sometimes in unusual locations, appears more frequent in this population, and has been attributed to overstimulation of embryonic rests disseminated throughout the cervical and mediastinal fat (LOSSEF et al. 1993). In these patients, renal phosphate retention and reduced intestinal calcium absorption lead to hypocalcemia. Oversecretion of PTH causes the radiologically and histologically demonstrable lesions of osteitis fibrosa cystica. SHPT is one of the most frequent complications of chronic renal failure.

Tertiary hyperparathyroidism (THPT) corresponds to autonomous growth of an enlarged parathyroid gland (LOSSEF et al. 1993).

2.2
Anatomy

2.2.1
General Features

Most individuals (84%) have four parathyroid glands, located behind the thyroid lobes, between the common carotid artery and the internal jugular vein laterally, the laryngopharynx medially, and the longus colli muscle posteriorly (AKERSTROM et al. 1984).

Average gland weight ranges from 20 to 40 mg, and normal parathyroids usually measure 3–6 mm in length, 2–4 mm in width, and 1–3 mm in thickness. Although anatomic structures with these dimensions are usually visible on imaging studies, this is unfortunately not the case for normal parathyroid glands, because neither their echotexture (sonography), density (CT), or signal intensity (MRI) allows differentiation from adjacent tissues.

Topographically, the parathyroid glands are grouped around the terminal branches of the inferior thyroid artery. The superior parathyroid glands, located above this artery, are posterolateral to the esophagus. The inferior parathyroid glands usually lie just below the point of entry of the thyroid artery into the thyroid space (BISMUTH et al. 1975).

2.2.2
Variations in Location

The embryology of the parathyroid glands explains the possible variations in number and location.

2.2.2.1
Inferior Parathyroid Glands

The parathyroid glands, recognizable in the embryo of 8–9 mm, arise from the third and fourth branchial pouches. When the third branchial pouch separates from the pharynx, the inferior parathyroid glands (P3), which derive from the third pouch, form a bilobate complex with the thymic lobe (thymus 3). Embryonic descent of the heart into the thorax is accompanied by descent of thymus 3 and P3. In the 18-mm embryo, the P3 glands usually come to rest at the lower pole of the thyroid, where they remain after dissociation of the thyroid from the thymus. The two inferior parathyroid glands occasionally fail to dissociate from the thymus and migrate more caudally than usual into the lower part of the neck, the anterior mediastinum, or even the pericardium. In other instances, premature separation of the thymus and P3 results in unusually high-lying P3 glands, above the thyroid and the P4 parathyroids.

In an anatomic study, WANG (1976) demonstrated that fewer than half (42%) of all P3 glands were located at the lower thyroid pole; 41% were intrathymic (39% in the lower neck, within the thymic tongue, and 2% in the mediastinum). Ectopic parathyroids represented only 2%, and corresponded to undescended glands in the superior lateral neck, above the upper pole of the thyroid, or behind the middle third of the thyroid; the remaining 15% were juxtathyroidal.

2.2.2.2 *Superior Parathyroid Glands*

The superior parathyroid glands (P4) form a bilobate complex with the lateral lobes of the thyroid. When the thyroid lobes unite, the P4 glands separate from the thyroid tissue and acquire their definitive position immediately above the point at which the inferior thyroid artery crosses the recurrent nerve. Owing to their midline location, the P4 glands are associated with the midline structures of the neck. These glands migrate less than the P3 glands, and their positions are thus fairly constant, at least in height. Wang (1976) found that the P4 glands were located at the cricothyroid junction in over 75% of cases and behind the upper pole of the thyroid in 22%; only 1% were retropharyngeal or retroesophageal. Other authors have confirmed this distribution of ectopic glands. In particular, Zeze et al. (1995) reported a frequency of 35.1% for ectopic parathyroids in patients with renal hyperparathyroidism; the majority were found in a cervical location.

2.2.2.3 *Influence of Parathyroid Pathologies*

The incidence of ectopic superior parathyroid glands can reach 10% in pathological conditions; this is due to the risk of migration, under the effect of gravity, between the posterior margin of the esophagus and the posterosuperior mediastinum. In contrast, a pathological condition does not increase the risk of migration for the inferior parathyroids (THOMPSON et al. 1982).

2.2.2.4 *Intrathyroidal Parathyroid Glands*

Subcapsular and intraparenchymal intrathyroid locations are uncommon (AKERSTROM et al. 1984; ANDRÉ et al. 1999; PROYE et al. 1994); the incidence is higher for pathological parathyroid tissue (less than 5% of cases) than for normal parathyroid tissue (only 0.2%). LIBUTTI et al. (1997) found the incidence of intrathyroid parathyroid glands to be only 7%. Although the P4 glands are usually considered at greatest risk of occurring in an intrathyroid location, most intrathyroid parathyroids are actually P3 glands (44 of 47 cases seen by PROYE et al. 1994).

2.2.3 Variations in Number

While nearly 95% of individuals have four parathyroid glands (AKERSTROM et al. 1984), numerous anatomic studies have shown that the number actually varies from 2 to 8. The incidence of supernumerary glands ranges from 2% to 13%; this anomaly is due to multiple divisions of one or more glands or to parathyroid rests during embryonic descent (rudimentary glands). Less often (3%), only three parathyroid glands are present. Regardless of the cause, the existence of supplementary sites of parathyroid tissue can create major diagnostic and therapeutic difficulties.

2.2.4 Vascularity

Each parathyroid gland receives a terminal arteriole arising essentially from the branches of the inferior thyroid artery and, accessorily, from the superior thyroid artery. Ectopic glands, which are generally supplied by the inferior thyroid artery, may receive a mediastinal artery (internal mammary artery or thymic artery) (BISMUTH et al. 1975).

Venous return is ensured by three pairs of veins originating from an anastomotic plexus. The inferior thyroid veins drain separately, or after anastomosis, into the innominate venous trunk, while the superior and middle thyroid veins drain into the internal jugular vein. Numerous anatomic variations are possible, regardless of whether there are any ectopic glands (the latter may drain into the inferior thyroid veins or at the level of the internal mammary, thymic or azygos veins). Awareness of these anatomic variants is essential before performing venous sampling for PTH assays.

2.2.5 Histological Types

2.2.5.1 *Adenoma*

Adenoma is the most frequent cause of PHPT. Although dimensions are variable, mean diameter is 15 mm and average weight 1 g. Lesions smaller than 8 mm are referred to as microadenomas. Histologically, over 90% are composed of chief cells; less than 10% are composed of oncocytes (DUBOST et al. 1984).

Multiple adenomas occur in less than 5% of cases. Unless necrosis has occurred, tumor size is correlated with the serum PTH level (DUBOST et al. 1984). Giant, often necrotic, adenomas have been described on rare occasion; when located deep within the prevertebral space, such lesions can reach huge dimensions (PALESTINI et al. 1997).

Adenomas can undergo cystic degeneration, either as a nonfunctional true cyst or as a lesion with a cystic component (microcystic adenomas are more common than macroscopic forms). Lipoadenomas (hamartomas) are a clinicopathological entity corresponding to an admixture of glandular and fatty tissue (OBARA et al. 1989).

2.2.5.2 *Hyperplasia*

Hyperplasia is much more common than adenoma in SHPT. Hyperplastic glands tend to be smaller than adenomas, but gland enlargement is often asymmetrical and differential diagnosis from adenoma can thus be difficult. This justifies an intraoperative search for a normal homolateral gland that confirms the diagnosis of adenoma (VOGEL et al. 1998). Intraoperative PTH assays are another means of avoiding misdiagnosing hyperplasia: If a solitary adenoma is at cause, the serum PTH drops after tumor ablation (MOORE et al. 1999).

2.2.5.3 *Carcinoma*

An infrequent cause of PHPT (2% of cases), parathyroid carcinoma typically corresponds to a cervical mass that invades adjacent anatomic structures. Although difficulties may exist for gross differentiation from adenoma, local invasion is usually detectable, at least histologically. Twenty percent of patients already have metastatic disease at diagnosis, and the prognosis at 5 years is 50% (SCHANTZ and CASTELMAN 1973; SPINELLI et al. 1994).

2.3 Ultrasonography

Several observations concerning sonography in particular, and imaging studies in general, warrant mention:

- No currently available imaging modality can identify a normal parathyroid gland.
- Imaging studies provide merely topographical data; parathyroid hyperfunction is diagnosed biochemically.
- The number and location of parathyroid glands vary considerably; this limits the value of US, which cannot satisfactorily explore the entire cervical region and is unsuitable for examination of the mediastinum.
- Influence of the histopathological type of lesion; adenomas are generally three times larger than hyperplastic glands (1.8±0.4 g for adenomas vs 0.6±0.1 g for hyperplastic glands) (KANEGAE et al. 1994).
- Interventional sonography can be used for diagnostic (US-guided FNA) and especially therapeutic procedures (US-guided percutaneous ethanol ablation).

2.3.1 Ultrasound (US) Technique

Examination is performed with the patient supine and the neck hyperextended, if necessary with the aid of a pad placed under the shoulders. Transducers must be adapted to patient morphology. High-frequency (up to 13 MHz) probes are preferable, but patients with a thick neck or multinodular goiter and obese individuals are best examined with a lower frequency transducer in order to achieve adequate depth of penetration.

Sonograms are obtained in the sagittal and axial planes, following localization of the longus colli muscle and the neurovascular bundle (inferior thyroid artery and recurrent laryngeal nerve). Owing to the possibility of anatomic variations, scanning should be performed from the angle of the mandible down to the superior mediastinum (Hopkins and Reading 1995).

Detection of ectopic glands requires particular techniques:

- A search for paratracheal or paraesophageal glands necessitates examination of the lateral neck by rotation of the patient's head to the contralateral side. This maneuver is of limited help, however, because even a large lesion may remain inaccessible to the sonographic beam (Reading 1991).
- The search for glands within the cervical thymus requires that scanning be performed during swallowing in order to raise the mediastinal structures upwards.
- Attempts to demonstrate mediastinal glands should be performed via a suprasternal approach, using a low-frequency probe (5 MHz), angled caudally for maximum penetration (Fugazzola et al. 1995).

Other, more recent techniques do not always provide decisive information, but may help to solve certain diagnostic dilemmas:

- Color Doppler (CD) and power Doppler (PD) can easily visualize the thyroid veins and arteries, and in particular the inferior thyroid arteries (Calliada et al. 1993; Gooding and Clark 1992).
- Harmonic imaging and US contrast agents have not proven truly useful for investigation of hyperparathyroidism.
- US guidance is helpful for diagnostic and therapeutic procedures (Du et al. 1994; Sacks et al. 1994).
- Esophageal endosonography may be indicated if doubt persists after examination of the mediastinum by scintigraphy or MRI (Palestini et al. 1997); intraoperative US is used only occasionally (Trombetta et al. 1996).

2.3.2 Gray-Scale Imaging

Lesion size (adenomas are easier to diagnose than hyperplasia) and topographic variations can both create difficulties for sonographic examination. No new sonographic findings have been described recently, and all currently recognized features were described prior to 1990. Despite the introduction of CD and PD and the increasing use of US guidance for FNA and percutaneous ethanol ablation (PEA) (Chen et al. 1999), initial evaluation by sonography has not undergone any major changes. Furthermore, the relatively high frequency of diagnostic pitfalls makes examination by a well-trained operator essential (Figs. 2.1–2.3).

2.3.2.1 Echotexture

The typical sonographic features of adenoma and hyperplasia were described in the late 1980s (Graif et al. 1987; Randel et al. 1987). These solid oval masses characteristically show low echogenicity, owing to their uniform hypercellularity that creates few acoustic interfaces (Kinoshita et al. 1985). Dynamic study reveals lesion mobility during swallowing, a feature that should be sought systematically. Other sonographic features are observed in 15%–20% of cases (Fugazzola et al. 1995):

- A mass isoechoic to the thyroid gland
- A hyperechoic mass (relative to the thyroid), owing to fibrosis or microcystic degeneration or a complex mass (partly solid, partly anechoic) due to necrotic or hemorrhagic degeneration. An infrequent finding, hyperechogenicity was attributed by Kinoshita et al. (1985) to the presence of numerous fibrous trabeculae, which are more common in parathyroid carcinoma than in adenoma. A hyperechoic parathyroid nodule should thus suggest this rare etiology, especially if there are signs of local invasion.
- Internal cystic spaces (3.8%)
- Calcifications (2.5%). A rare phenomenon, calcifications are encountered in patients with longstanding hyperplasia, SHPT, or carcinoma (Graif et al. 1987; Randel et al. 1987). Calcifications are very rare in adenomas.
- Lipoadenomas (Obara et al. 1989) with a predominant fatty component appear hyperechoic.

2.3.2.2 Shape

Parathyroid adenoma and hyperplasia typically manifest as an oval or lobular mass oriented in a craniocaudal direction. When an echogenic line is seen separating the mass from the thyroid, and when the mass is mobile during swallowing, the diagnosis of a parathyroid adenoma is highly probable. Rounded glands (less common than oval lesions), tubular masses on longitudinal scans, and bilobate or triangular shapes have also been described (Fugazzola et al. 1995).

2.3.2.3 Diameter

Along with location, lesion diameter is another important criterion for sonographic diagnosis. A

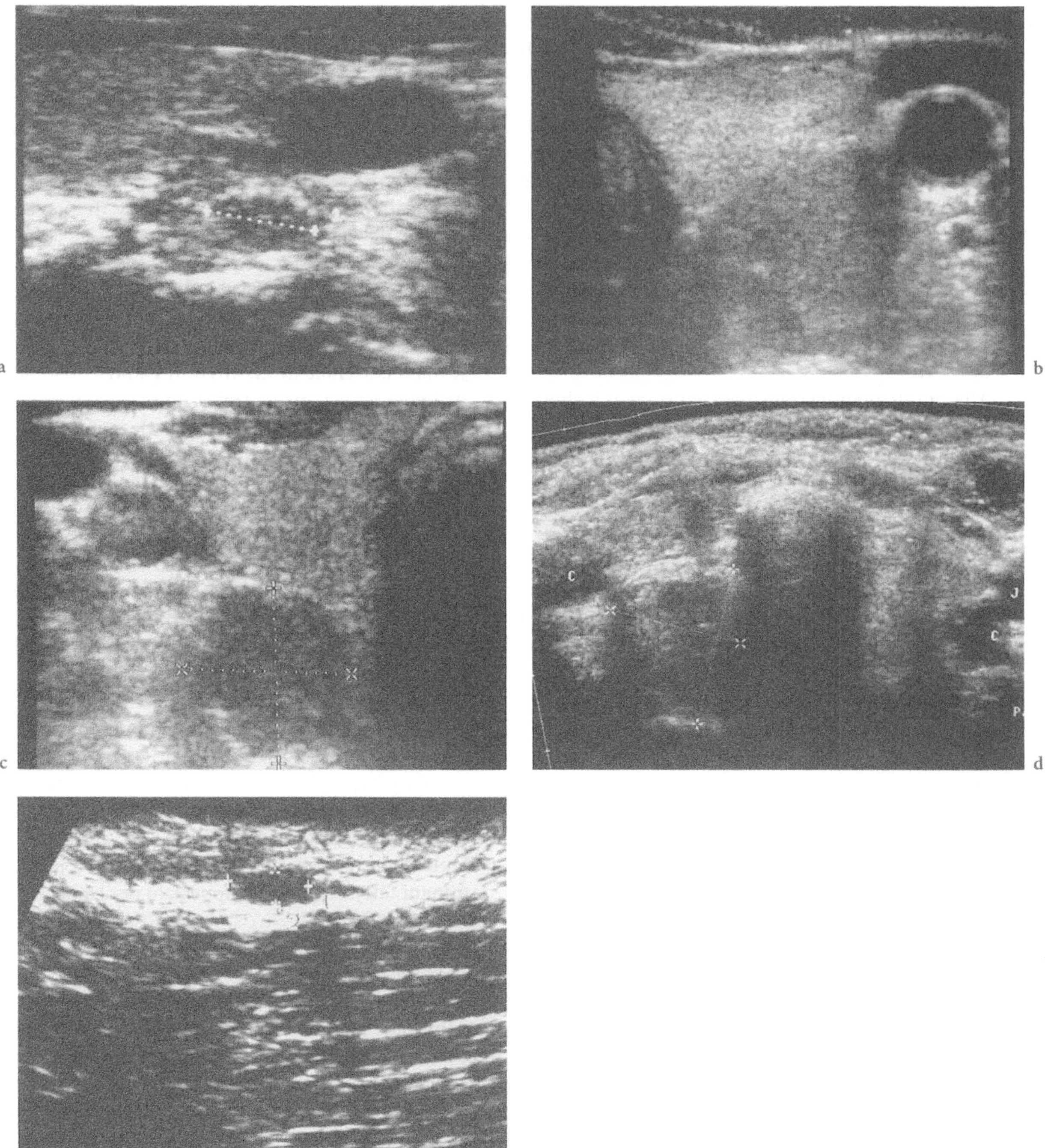

Fig. 2.1a–e. Parathyroid adenoma. **a** Retrothyroid parathyroid adenoma located below the inferior tip of the thyroid; the adenoma is hypoechoic to the thyroid, from which it is separated by an echoic interface. **b** Parathyroid adenoma hypoechoic to the thyroid, without any clear interface (axial scan). **c** Parathyroid adenoma hypoechoic to the thyroid, measuring 1.4 cm in diameter (axial scan). **d** SieScape study of a parathyroid adenoma (2.1/1.8 cm between the *two crosses*) hypoechoic to the thyroid, from which it is separated by an echoic interface (*C* common carotid artery; *J* internal jugular vein). **e** Small parathyroid adenoma that developed in the forearm of a patient with chronic renal failure who had undergone total parathyroidectomy with brachial grafting of a gland; easily detected owing to the cutaneous scar, the adenoma measures 0.5/0.2 cm between the *two crosses*

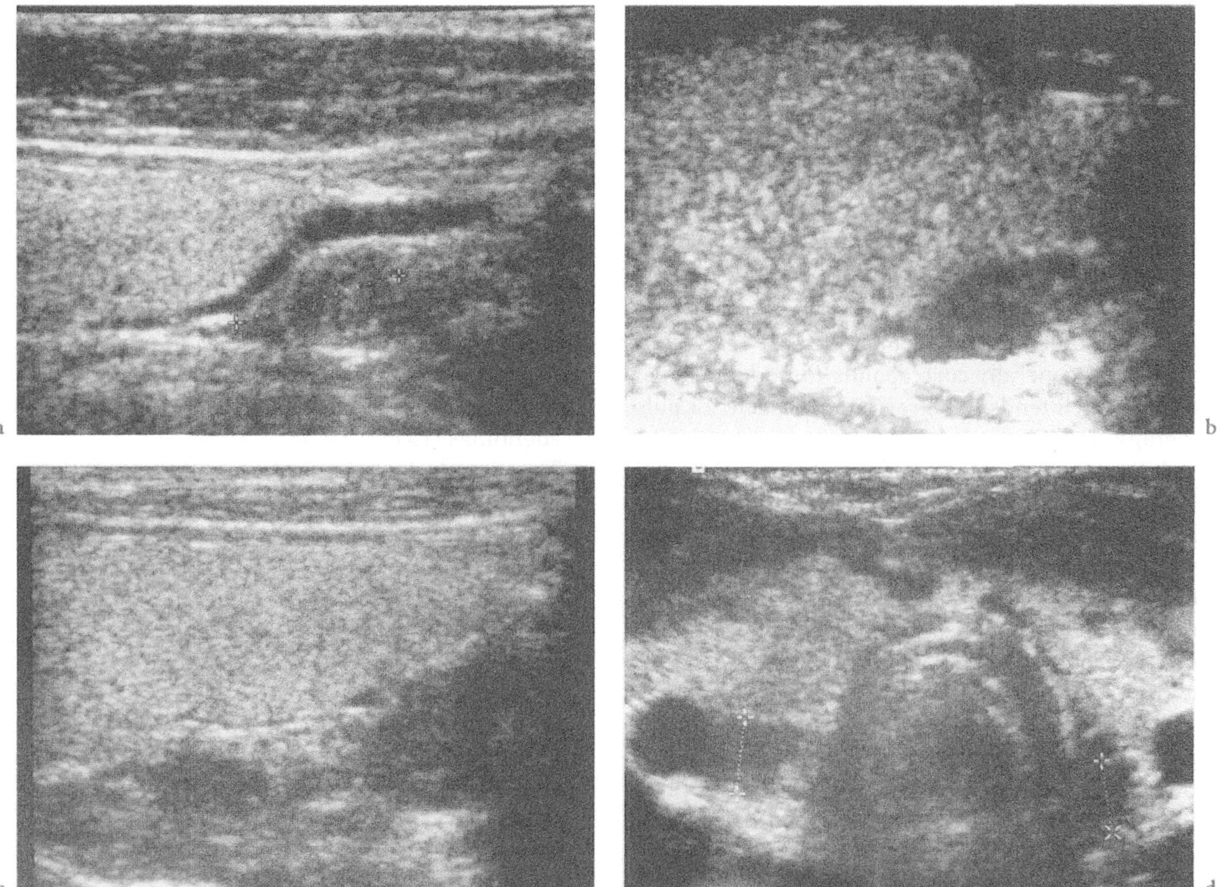

Fig. 2.2a–d. Parathyroid hyperplasia. **a** Hyperplastic left inferior parathyroid gland (1.1 cm between the *two crosses*) separated from the thyroid by a weakly echoic zone. **b** Small hyperplastic right inferior parathyroid gland detected by its marked hypoechogenicity compared with the thyroid, despite the absence of a line of separation. **c** Hyperplastic retrothyroid right superior and inferior parathyroid glands (sagittal scan). **d** Axial scan of the cervical region showing the thyroid lobes posteriorly and the internal carotid arteries medially; the two 6 mm hypoechoic areas correspond to two hyperplastic parathyroid glands in a patient with renal failure

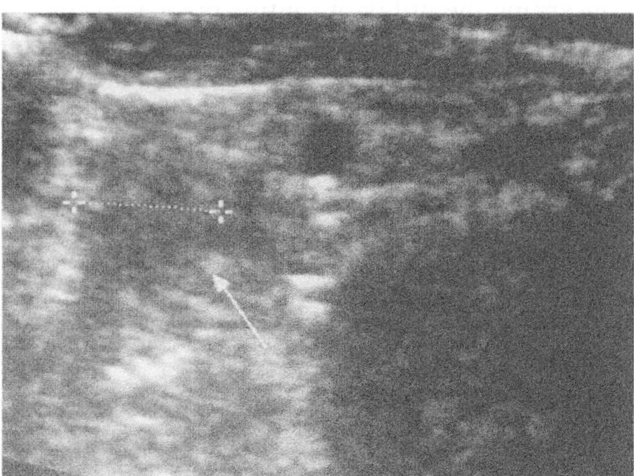

Fig. 2.3. Sonogram of the lateral neck revealing a hypoechoic and especially ill-defined nodule (15 mm between the *two crosses*). No preoperative diagnosis was made; a small parathyroid carcinoma was found at surgery

diameter of 1 cm corresponds roughly to 0.5 cm^3 or 0.5 g (Fukagawa et al. 1997). The size of the smallest detectable parathyroid lesion varies in the literature, depending on whether diameter, volume, or weight is considered: 0.5+0.8 cm for Schwerk et al. (1985), 0.36 g for Lloyd et al. (1990), and 0.5 cm^3 for Fukagawa et al. (1996). For Reading et al. (1982), sonography has a sensitivity of less than 29% for adenomas weighing under 0.1 g.

Accurate measurement of lesion size may be helpful for therapeutic management. In SHPT, a volume of 0.5 cm^3 generally corresponds to nodular hyperplasia, which tends to be resistant to calcitriol pulse therapy (Fukagawa et al. 1997).

Interestingly, certain parathyroid adenomas escape US detection even though there is no topographic problem and they are large enough for sonographic visualization. Lerner (1996) considered such cases to be the result of massive infiltration by fatty tissue, responsible for underestimation of size or even failure to recognize the lesion owing to the low contrast with the surrounding fat. However, this histological explanation was refuted by Sacks et al. (1994). The giant adenomas that account for 4.6% of cases would involve difficulties for etiological diagnosis rather than for localization, were it not for the biological context (Randel et al. 1987).

Volumetric data are currently used to monitor patients with SHPT treated by calcitriol because the severity of SHPT is correlated with the diameter of the enlarged glands (Gladziwa et al. 1992). Surveillance of lesion size is thus recommended (Huraib et al. 1997; Malberti et al. 1996). For Katoh et al. (2000), parathyroid gland size has a prognostic role, because it can predict the therapeutic potential of calcitriol in SHPT. Patients without any sonographically visible enlarged parathyroid glands tend to respond to calcitriol more often than individuals with larger, sonographically detectable hyperplastic glands.

2.3.2.4 Localization

As emphasized in the section on parathyroid anatomy (Sect. 2.2), at least for typical forms, sonography permits detection of an enlarged parathyroid mass or masses posterior or lateral to the thyroid. Superior pathological glands are more difficult to detect than those in lower locations (Torregrosa et al. 1998). Accurate search for ectopic glands requires a skilled operator:

- An ectopic gland in the lateral neck, along the common carotid artery, may suggest an enlarged and perhaps inflammatory node, but there is no echogenic hilum and, above all, the lesion is usually solitary. Furthermore, CD fails to demonstrate the typical nodal vascular pattern. An ectopic parathyroid within the carotid artery sheath may be overlooked by the surgeon. Accurate description of all sonographically visualized lesions in a written report is essential to help reduce the number of unproductive cervicotomies.
- Retroesophageal and retrotracheal cervical parathyroid glands are responsible for numerous false-negative errors, even when US is performed by skilled operators, the only exception being giant adenomas (Palestini et al. 1997).
- The search for a thymic parathyroid requires hyperextension of the neck, scanning during swallowing, and examination of the entire cervicomediastinal region, if necessary using an endovaginal probe permitting analysis of a wide sector.
- In patients who have had a forearm autograft, hypertrophy of even only a few millimeters in diameter (as encountered in SHPT) can usually be readily detected opposite the scar, because the gland's echotexture relative to the adjacent structures changes as soon as pathological hyperfunction occurs.
- Intrathyroid parathyroid glands are discussed in Sect. 2.3.2.6.

2.3.2.5 Number of Lesions Detected

The potential variation in the number of glands and the topographic limitations of sonography explain the false-negative findings with the technique, and hence the reservations expressed by certain authors concerning the utility of routine preoperative localization studies. The limitations of US related to lesion size must also be taken into account, not only for hyperplasia but also, for some authors, for diagnosis of adenoma, owing to the low but real possibility of a double adenoma. The reticence expressed by most authors in the literature concerns primarily SHPT (Heller et al. 1993; Hewin et al. 1997; Koong et al. 1998; Pons et al. 1997) (see Sect. 2.5.1).

2.3.2.6 Relations with the Thyroid Gland

A retrothyroid oval mass that appears hypoechoic to the thyroid and is mobile during swallowing is highly suggestive of a parathyroid adenoma. An additional sonographic feature should also be sought: an echogenic line separating the mass from the thyroid. This diagnostic feature is inconstant, however, and CD does not always provide the solution.

An enlarged intrathyroid parathyroid gland may manifest as an oval mass without the typical appearance of thyroid nodules: The mass is homogeneously hypoechoic and often superficial. Parathyroids deep within the thyroid parenchyma are rare, having been estimated at less than 20% of all intrathyroid parathyroid glands by Proye et al. (1994). Regardless of whether sonography shows one or more enlarged parathyroid glands, detection of one or more thyroid nodules should always be indicated in the sonographic report.

Sonographic search for parathyroid enlargement is often difficult in patients with multinodular goiter. Owing to the frequency of thyroid nodules, coexisting thyroid lesions are common, occurring in 29%–57.6% of cases in the literature (Chen et al. 1999; Gooding and Clark 1992; Lane et al. 1998; Marcocci et al. 1998). Coexisting multinodular goiter reduces the value of sonography for the detection of small parathyroid lesions by nearly 10% (Mazzeo et al. 1996).

Serial US studies (performed in particular for thyroid nodules) and technological improvements have lead to the detection of parathyroid "incidentalomas" (Frasoldati et al. 1999). This diagnosis should be considered whenever a lesion with the typical sonographic features of adenoma is imaged, especially if located in a typically retrothyroid position, whether laboratory values are abnormal or not. Frasoldati et al. (1999) observed sonographic incidentalomas in 2.3% of studies performed for the workup of thyroid disease. However, only nine of their 38 patients actually had a parathyroid lesion corresponding to a true anatomic incidentaloma; the real frequency is thus closer to 0.5% (Figs. 2.4 and 2.5).

2.3.3 Color Doppler (CD) and Power Doppler (PD)

Although the complementary information obtained with CD and PD is not yet considered decisive, several features should be sought systematically at the end of a conventional sonographic examination:

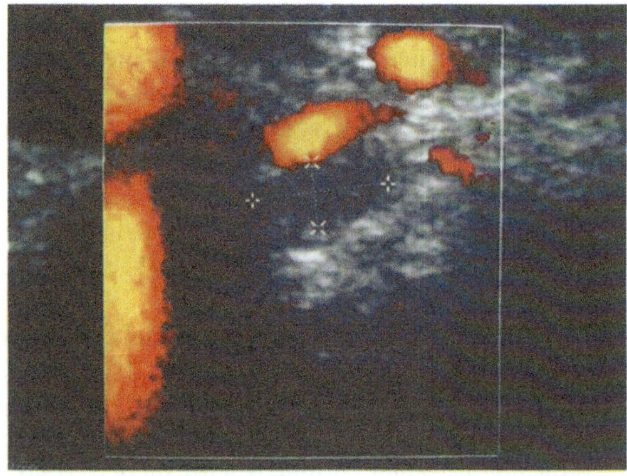

Fig. 2.4. Parathyroid incidentaloma (5.3/2.5 mm hypoechoic lesion)

a

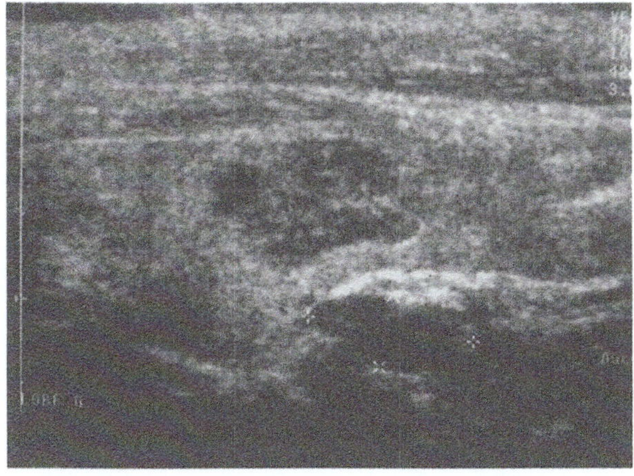

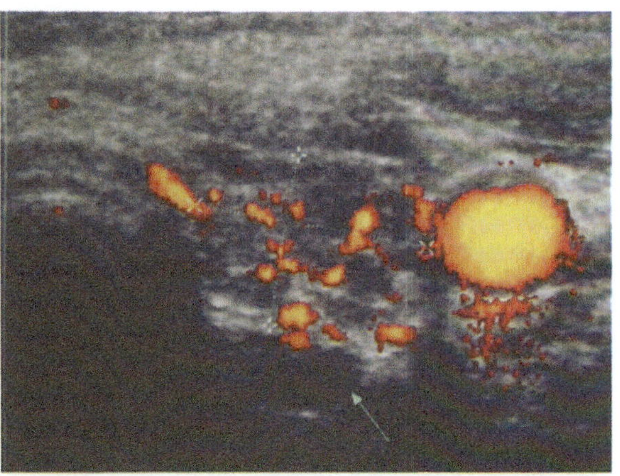

b

Fig. 2.5a,b. Parathyroid incidentaloma discovered during workup of a patient with Hashimoto's disease. **a** Inhomogeneous, pseudonodular thyroid; a less echoic nodule (4.2/9.9 mm between the *two crosses*) is visible deep within the parenchyma (sagittal scan). **b** Power Doppler study of the right lateral neck revealing the vascularity in Hashimoto's disease; diminished thyroid lobe volume (9.4/13.2 mm); a weakly echoic parathyroid nodule (*arrow*) is visible, separated from the thyroid by an echogenic line. US-guided FNA resulted in diagnosis of a parathyroid adenoma, despite the absence of any biochemical anomaly

- An increase in the peak systolic velocity in the thyroid artery (superior or inferior) supplying the parathyroid adenoma. Asymmetry in peak velocity has a sensitivity of 96.5% and a specificity of 83.1% for localization of both the side and the level of an adenoma (Varsamidis et al. 1999).
- For Lane et al. (1998), an extrathyroid feeding artery leading to an adenoma was visible in 35 of 42 lesions as a vascular pedicle enveloped in fat that typically arose from the inferior thyroid artery.

A prominent feeding vessel can serve as a road map to the lesion; this finding increases the sensitivity of sonography from 73% to 83% and aids in differentiation from the esophagus, a normal lymph node, or an adenopathy. The vascular arc sometimes formed by the vessel feeding the parathyroid adenoma distinguishes it from the contralateral side, where this feature is absent (Fig. 2.6). This road-map approach appears more sensitive for an adenoma than for multiglandular disease (Lane et al. 1998).

- Parathyroid lesions show little or no tumor vascularity (Chen et al. 1999); Doppler signals had low sensitivity (33%) but high specificity (93%) for De Feo et al. (2000) (Fig. 2.7).
- CD or PD may contribute to differential diagnosis from nodular thyroid disease (Meola et al. 1999). Whereas thyroid nodules at least 1 cm in diameter tend to be vascular, parathyroid lesions are typically avascular, although with increased size they may demonstrate vascularity (Gooding and Clark 1992).

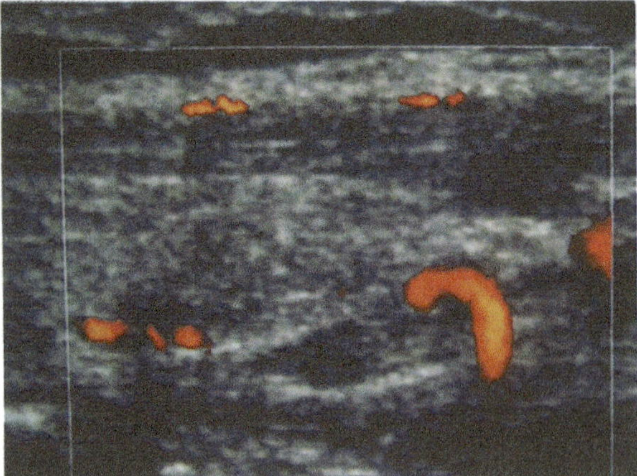

Fig. 2.6. Power Doppler analysis of the lower cervical region (sagittal scan): The vascular arc formed by a periadenomatous arteriole permitted detection of a small (<5 mm) parathyroid lesion (sagittal scan)

- CD and PD are helpful for monitoring response to calcitriol therapy for SHPT (Pretolesi et al. 1997). A positive response is associated with a reduction in intraglandular flow (scored from 0 to 2, where 0 is avascular, 2 is vascular signals covering over 50% of the lesion), and this modification in vascularity parallels the changes in serum PTH. For patients with parathyroid hyperplasia treated by PEA, volumetric data must be supplemented by a search for a reduction in blood flow; this is readily assessed, and any revascularization is generally associated with relapse (Fukagawa et al. 1996, 1997; Lemmi et al. 1994).

Overall, CD can serve as a diagnostic aid by improving the sensitivity of sonography, especially in patients with associated thyroid disease (Meola et al. 1999) (Fig. 2.8).

2.3.4 Differential Diagnosis

Differential diagnosis is usually not complicated, owing to the elevated specificity of sonography (over 90% for Fugazzola et al. 1995).

Vascular structures do not present any problem for differential diagnosis, thanks to CD. In contrast, diagnosis of thyroid lesions (see Sect. 2.3.2.6) can be troublesome, and FNA is not always sufficient, in particular for follicular tumors and less often for papillary carcinomas (Mincione et al. 1986). Differentiation from a normal lymph node with the typical oval shape and an echogenic hilum is usually easy. CD generally permits analysis of nodal vascularity, aided if necessary by the injection of contrast material to increase the visibility of intranodal vascular structures. If a doubt persists, US-guided FNA is indicated. The sonography report should mention this mass, which usually lies lateral to the carotid artery. Other, less common, etiologies include congenital cystic disease and sarcoid granulomata (Nabriski et al. 1992).

2.3.5 US-guided Diagnostic Procedures

Cytological examination of fine-needle aspirates using routine staining techniques (Papanicolaou, May-Grünwald-Giemsa) permits only limited morphological analysis. The Grimelius silver stain cytochemical technique can be a helpful complement but is time con-

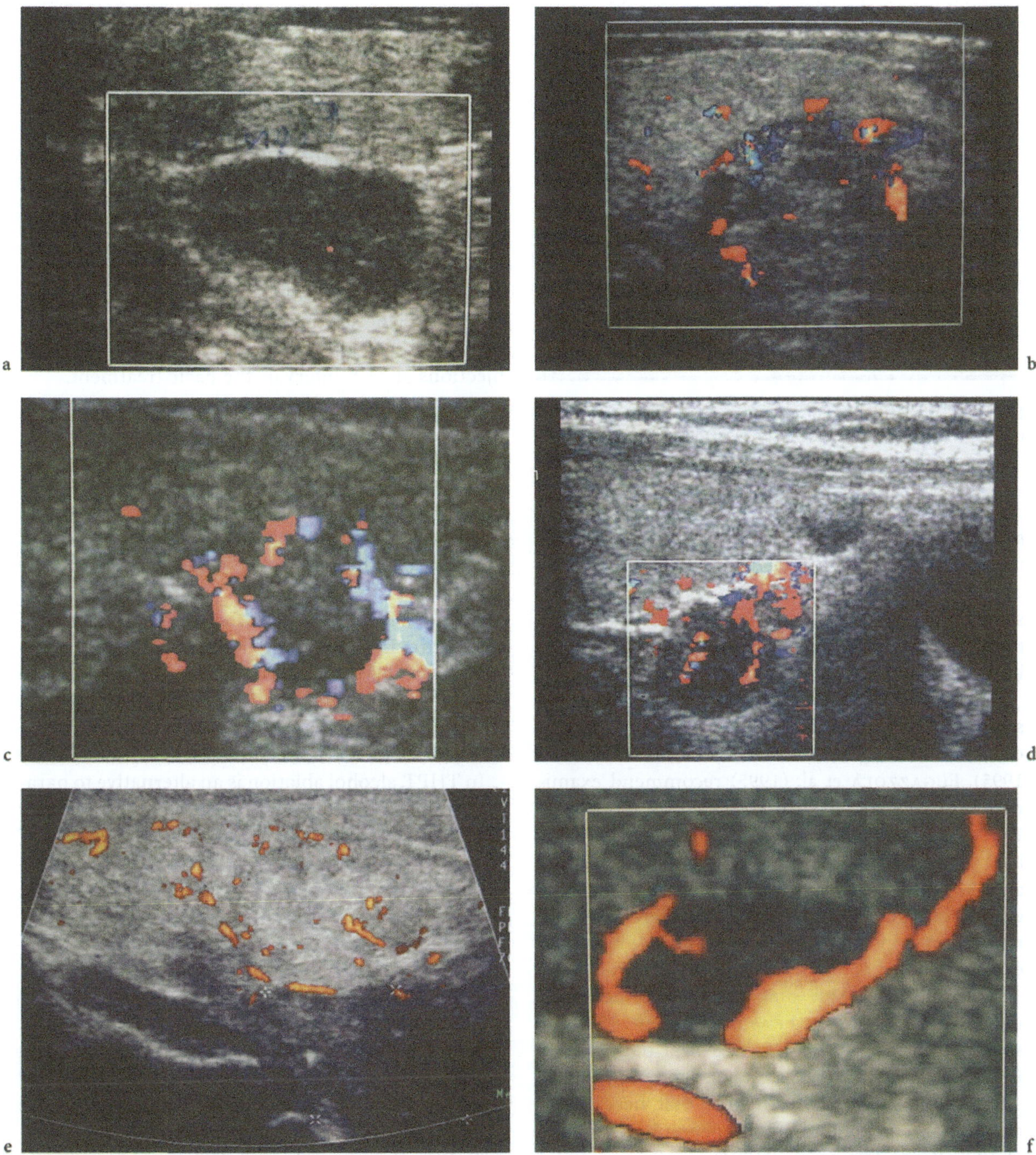

Fig. 2.7a–f. Vascular patterns of parathyroid lesions. **a** Hypoechoic nodule with punctate vascularity. **b** Large (3 cm) nodule of parathyroid origin with essentially peripheral vascularity. **c** Centimeter-sized parathyroid nodule with extensive peripheral vascularity. **d** Vascularity (veins and arteries) of an inferior parathyroid adenoma. **e** Multinodular goiter descending into the mediastinum ("diving goiter"); presence of a hypoechoic mass posteriorly (2.6/1.7 cm between the *two crosses*) without any detectable vascularity. **f** Essentially peripheral arterial vascularity of a hyperplastic right inferior parathyroid gland; this vascular pattern has no specificity for diagnosis of adenoma or hyperplasia

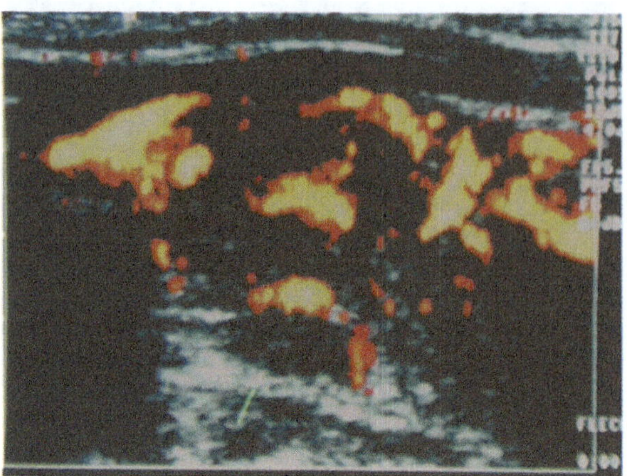

Fig. 2.8. Differentiation of the thyroid and a parathyroid nodule was improved by use of power Doppler

suming (Fugazzola et al. 1995). Cytological examination is hampered by inadequate material in 17% of cases (Halbauer et al. 1991), but it had a mean sensitivity of 86.9% in the literature review of Fugazzola et al. (1995). Most false-negative errors are related to insufficient cellularity (Abati et al. 1995).

Radioimmunologic PTH assays in venous blood samples have a specificity of 100% and a sensitivity of 72.2%–96% (Fugazzola et al. 1995; Mazzeo et al. 1995). Fugazzola et al. (1995) recommend examination of two aspirates from each suspicious lesion. PTH radioimmunologic assays are generally associated with measurement of thyroglobulin (Chang et al. 1998; Mazzeo et al. 1995). Finally, immunoperoxidase staining of PTH contributes to differential diagnosis from a thyroid lesion (Chang et al. 1998; Sardi et al. 1992).

The indications for diagnostic US-guided FNA include incidentalomas (Frasoldati et al. 1999), any sonographically suspicious mass in a patient with PHPT (Mazzeo et al. 1995), and discovery after failed parathyroid surgery of a nodule that necessitates tissue characterization before reoperation (Abati et al. 1995; Kairaluoma et al. 1994).

2.3.6 US-guided Therapeutic Procedures

Although percutaneous calcitriol therapy has been used to treat parathyroid nodules (Fukagawa et al. 1996), percutaneous ethanol ablation (PEA) by injecting lesions with 95% ethanol is currently the most frequently used approach (Figs. 2.9–2.11).

2.3.6.1 Technique

Solbiati et al. (1985) were the first to propose PEA, performed under US guidance using 21- or 22-gauge needles. Slow injection produces echogenic images corresponding to the ethanol and microbubbles of air. The amount of ethanol injected corresponds to 70%–100% of the pretreatment volume of the lesion. Response to therapy is apparent as a drop in PTH after 1–2 weeks. The frequency of injection sessions depends on the serum PTH concentration, although Karstrup et al. (1993) consider a maximum of three injections at 24-h intervals the basic treatment.

2.3.6.2 Indications

- In PHPT, the indications for PEA include high surgical risk (in particular due to age), patient refusal of surgery, and severe intercurrent disease (Lemmi et al. 1994).
- In SPHT, PEA is an attractive therapeutic alternative, provided there are no more than two enlarged parathyroid glands. In patients refractory to calcitriol pulse therapy, PEA of the largest glands may restore the response to calcitriol (Fukagawa et al. 1996; Kitaoka et al. 1994).
- In THPT, alcohol ablation is an alternative to parathyroidectomy (Cintin et al. 1994), in particular following subtotal parathyroidectomy with symptomatic hyperparathyroidism due to hypertrophy of the remaining tissue (Fletcher et al. 1998).

2.3.6.3 Results

The majority of studies to date concern SHPT, in which PEA nearly always obviates the need for surgery (Kakuta et al. 1999). Fugazzola et al. (1995) report that complete remission is achieved in 35%–40% of cases at 2 years, and a partial response (30%–50% reduction in PTH) is achieved in 60% of cases. While results are not as good with PEA as with surgery, this is probably attributable to the failure of imaging studies to detect areas of hyperplasia that go untreated (Fugazzola et al. 1995). Results are also less satisfactory for THPT: response to PEA is unpredictable and results are poor compared with those of surgical parathyroidectomy (Fletcher et al. 1998). Cintin et al. (1994) reported failure with ethanol injection in 33% of patients with THPT.

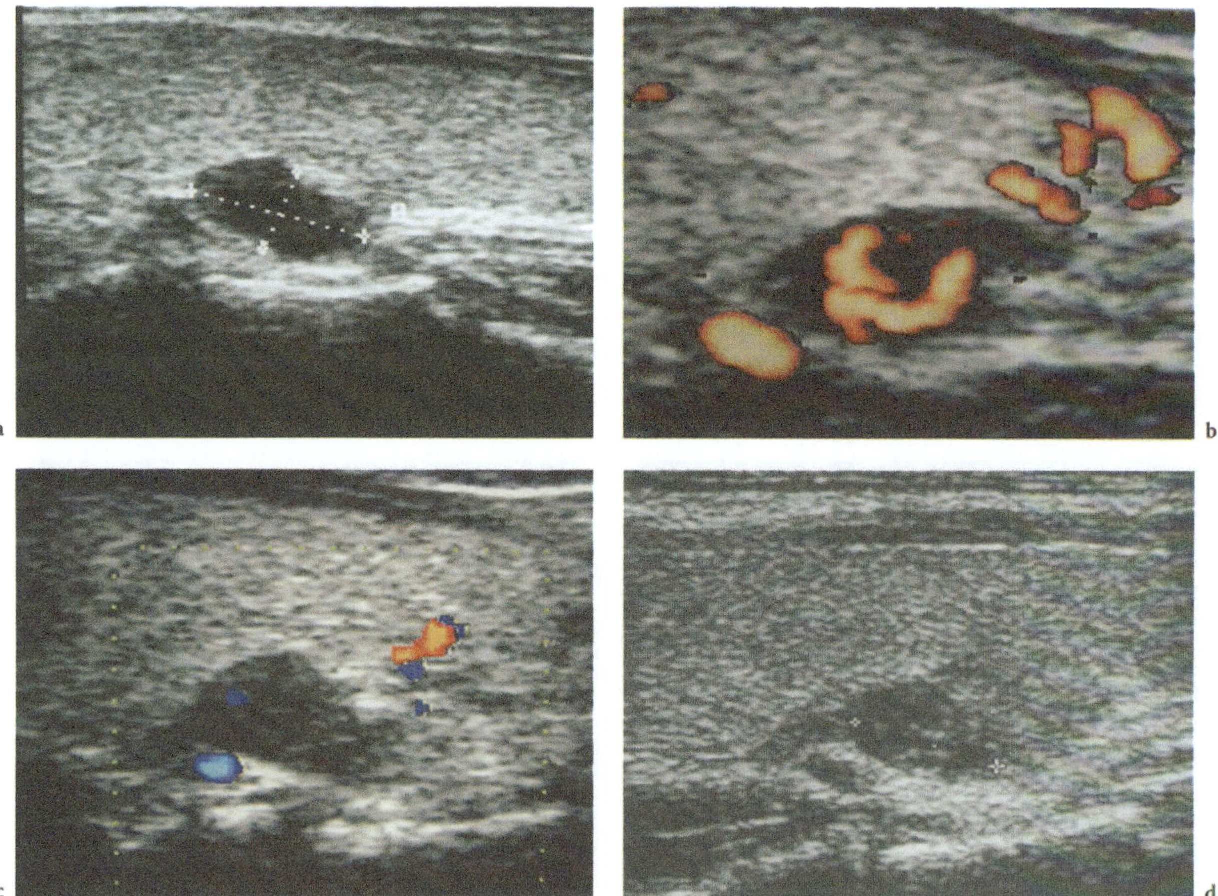

Fig. 2.9a–d. Parathyroid adenoma treated by percutaneous alcohol ablation (PEA). **a** Parathyroid adenoma (12/6 mm between the *two crosses*). **b** Power Doppler study revealing extensive lesion vascularity. **c** Disappearance of the tumor vascularity on a follow-up sonogram taken 4 months after PEA was accompanied by normalization of the PTH level. **d** Sonographic follow-up of the lesion 14 months after PEA, appearance of small echoic zones within the lesion, which appears less well defined and has decreased slightly in size (9 mm between the *two crosses*)

2.3.6.4 Incidents and Accidents

Along with the fibrotic sequelae due to ethanol injection that can impede future exploratory surgery, the most common adverse effect is recurrent nerve palsy. This rare but usually reversible complication occurred in two of 32 patients for Kitaoka et al. (1994) and one of 46 patients for Kakuta et al. (1999). However, permanent involvement has also been reported: two cases of laryngeal nerve palsy in 39 patients for Fletcher et al. (1998) and one case of vocal cord paralysis for Karstrup et al. (1993). To avoid this complication, the procedure should be stopped immediately whenever ethanol leakage is suspected during injection. For the same reason, use of less traumatic needles with a closed conical tip and three small side holes is recommended (Solbiati et al. 1985).

2.3.6.5 US and Follow-up

Sonography is particularly suitable for the surveillance of treated patients (Lemmi et al. 1994) as it can depict a reduction in gland size, hyperechogenicity, or, occasionally, a calcification. CD, which can demonstrate a reduction in vascularity (Fukagawa et al. 1997), merits use before and after PEA: Before the procedure it visualizes areas of vascularity that should be targeted in priority; after injection, CD documents the tissue destruction associated with the decrease in blood flow. In addition to serum PTH assays, patient monitoring may benefit from CD for detection of recurrence manifesting as the reappearance of intranodular vessels.

Any increase in lesion size detected by sonography, any increase in vascularity, and especially any

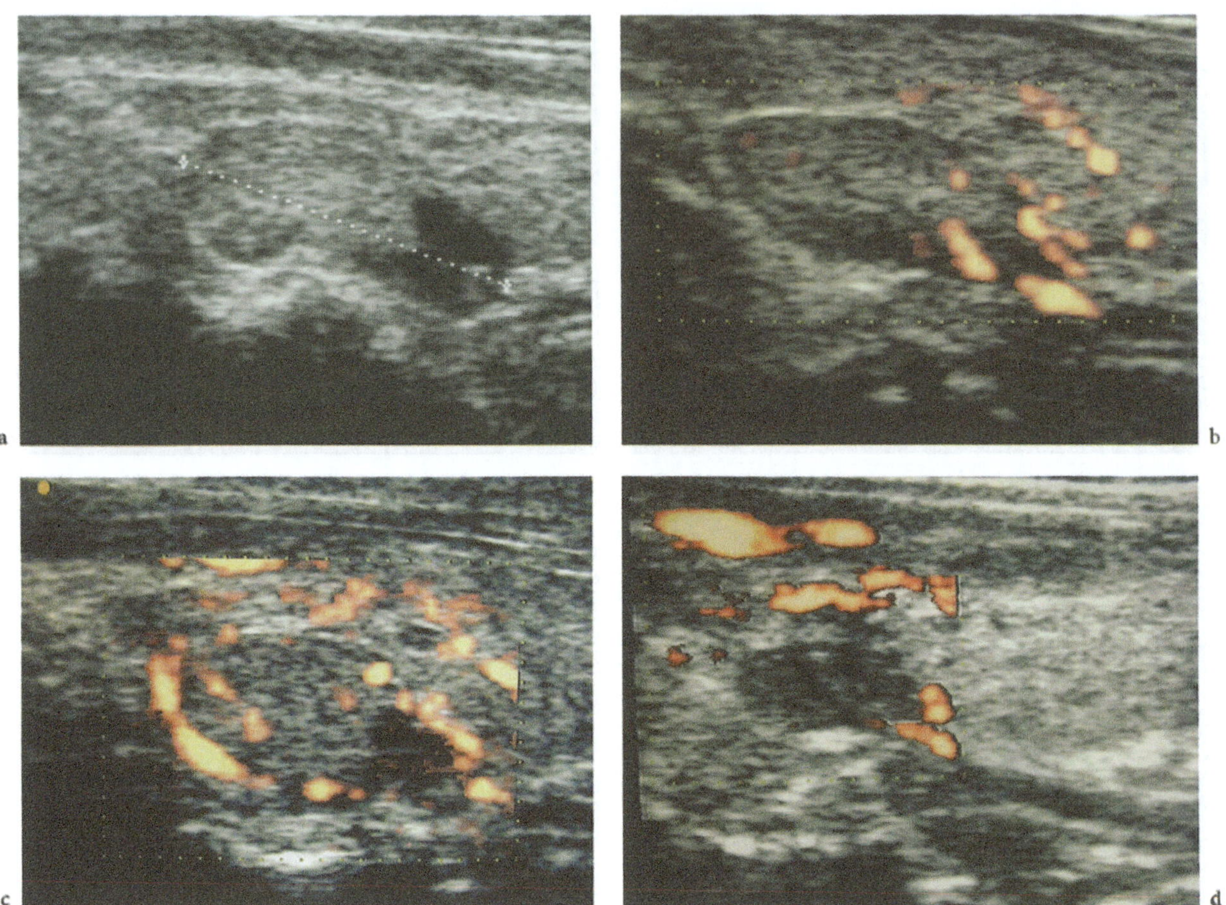

Fig. 2.10a–d. Parathyroid adenoma treated by PEA. a Complex echotexture of the parathyroid lesion (2.1 cm in greatest dimension). b Power Doppler analysis revealed the essentially lower pole vascularity of the adenoma. c Contrast administration improved visualization of lesion vascularity. d Power Doppler follow-up study 1 year after PEA demonstrated greater than 50% reduction in size and disappearance of the intralesional vascularity. These sonographically visible changes were associated with normalization of the PTH level

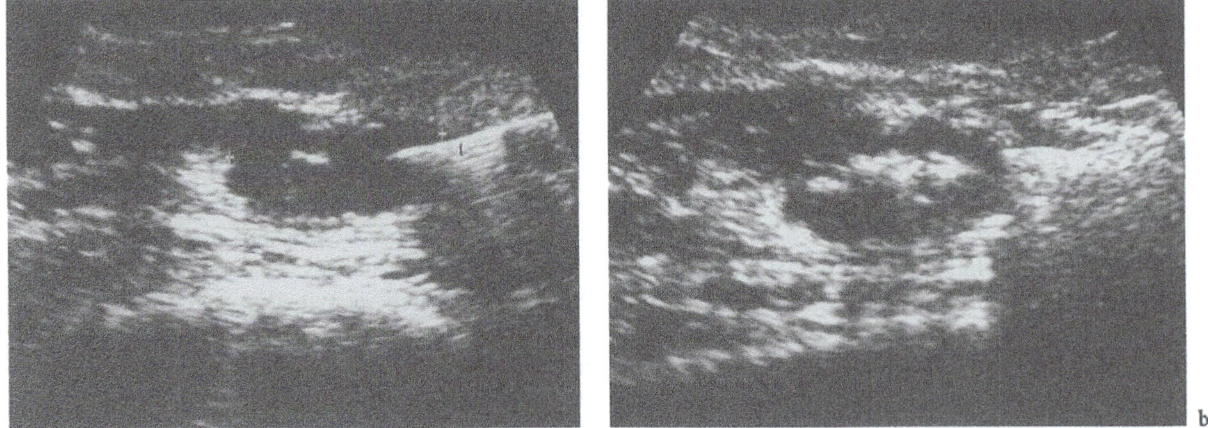

Fig. 2.11a,b. Brachial parathyroid adenoma treated by PEA. a Percutaneous puncture of the lesion. b US examination immediately following PEA: internal echoes corresponding to ethanol within the lesion

elevation in circulating PTH should prompt a new PEA session.

2.3.7 Accuracy of US

2.3.7.1 *Primary Hyperparathyroidism*

The sensitivity and specificity of sonography for preoperative localization of parathyroid glands in literature reports from 1995 to 1999 are listed in Table 2.1. Only CHOU et al. (1997), HEWIN et al. (1997), KOONG et al. (1998) and PURCELL et al. (1999) report a low specificity. All other investigators confirmed the values reported in the earlier literature, underscoring the notion that the technological progress in US and new techniques such as CD are not fundamental for the diagnosis of PHPT (BRUNETON et al. 1996). Recent data confirm the high specificity of sonography. The results obtained with US are similar to those reported for other imaging modalities, in particular scintigraphy.

Table 2.2 presents the sensitivity of US as a function of histology; the better results for adenoma are logical, because these lesions are usually larger than hyperplastic glands.

2.3.7.2 *Secondary Hyperparathyroidism*

Table 2.3 lists data from the recent literature concerning the sensitivity and specificity of sonography for SHPT. Although the specificity of US remains satisfactory for diagnostic localization, its sensitivity is lower for SHPT than for PHPT. Scintigraphy and probably MIBI appear to be a more valuable diagnostic approach to SHPT.

Table 2.2. Sensitivity of sonography as a function of histology (adenoma, hyperplasia), regardless of the type (primary or secondary) of hyperparathyroidism (1990–1998)

	Adenoma (%)	Hyperplasia (%)
SAKAMOTO et al. (1990)	88	20
STEIN and WEXLER (1990)	78	36
HASSELGREN and FIDLER (1992)	58	28
CASAS et al. (1993)	69	80
BILLY et al. (1995)	50	25
MUSLUMANOGLU et al. (1995)	100	66
LIGHT et al. (1996)	57	24
Ishibashi et al. (1998)	78	78

2.3.7.3 *Persistent and Recurrent Hyperparathyroidism*

Persistent hyperparathyroidism corresponds to the failure of hypercalcemia to disappear after surgery. The main cause is one or more lesions that are overlooked during surgery (lesions in unusual sites, a second adenoma, undiagnosed primary hyperplasia).

Recurrent hyperparathyroidism is less common, and may be due to a parathyroid carcinoma or parathyroidomatosis (FUGAZZOLA et al. 1995).

Table 2.4 lists the frequency of sonographic and scintigraphic diagnoses and the types of lesions that

Table 2.1. Sensitivity (*Se*) and specificity (*Sp*) of Doppler ultrasound (*US*) and radionuclide studies (*MIBI, thallium*) in the literature (1995–1999) for preoperative localization of parathyroid glands in primary hyperparathyroidism

	US (%)		MIBI (%)		Thallium (%)	
	Se	Sp	Se	Sp	Se	Sp
CAIXAS et al. (1995)	75		95.2		57.1	
MUSLUMANOGLU et al. (1995)	77.8				63.8	
LIOU et al. (1996)	75	95.8			87.5	100
MAZZEO et al. (1996)	85		82		62	
CHOU et al. (1997)	55	100			70	100
FRIEDRICH et al. (1997)	69.4					
HEWIN et al. (1997)	38				60	
KOSLIN et al. (1997)	84					
OKADA et al. (1997)	76.7				61.3	
HUANG et al. (1998)	71				49	
ISHIBASHI et al. (1998)	78	40	83	83		
KOONG et al. (1998)	18.2		40			
LANE et al. (1998)	83	98	62	99		
TORREGROSA et al. (1998)	68	97			94	100
Purcell et al. (1999)	57	98	54	99		

Table 2.3. Sensitivity (*Se*) and specificity (*Sp*) of ultrasound (*US*) and radionuclide studies (*MIBI, thallium*) reported in the literature (1996–1998) for diagnostic localization of secondary hyperparathyroidism

	US (%)		MIBI (%)		Thallium (%)	
	Se	Sp	Se	Sp	Se	Sp
Liou et al. (1996)	32.4	87.7			32.4	100
Fletcher et al. (1997)	64	100				
Jeanguillaume et al. (1998)	54		82			
Torregrosa et al. (1998)	41	89	54	89		

Table 2.4. Reoperation: preoperative diagnosis (US, MIBI, thallium) and histology (adenoma, hyperplasia) in the literature (1984–1999)

	Imaging (sensitivity, %)			Histology (%)	
	US	MIBI	Thallium	Adenoma	Hyperplasia
Krudy et al. (1984)	32				
Clark et al. (1985)	50		36		
Levin et al. (1987)	56		49		
Aufferman et al. (1988)	57		68		
Fraker et al. (1990)				72.4	27.6
Casas et al. (1993)	69				
Weber et al. (1994)				48.5	51.5
Numerow et al. (1995)	77	80		78.3	11.7
Tezelman et al. (1995)				56.8	43.2
Fayet et al. (1997)		83			
Mariette et al. (1998)a		69		50	38
Thompson et al. (1999)	75	82			

[a]"Normal" but overweight gland in 9.5%, carcinoma in 2.5%.

go undetected. Sonography has only moderate sensitivity for persistent and recurrent hyperparathyroidism, but during the past few years it has been no lower than that observed during the initial diagnostic workup of hyperparathyroidism. This may be attributable to the fact that these patients are generally managed by specialized teams, as concerns both surgery and sonography.

Histological studies reveal that hyperplasia involves more preoperative diagnostic problems than adenoma. The majority of problems with adenoma are related to an ectopic location or to the existence of a double adenoma, the essential cause of initial therapeutic failure in nearly all studies.

According to Mariette et al. (1998), McIntyre et al. (1994), and Rodriguez et al. (1994), the reasons for failure of initial parathyroid operations include a gland in a normal location (25%–44%), reflecting inexperience with this type of surgery); a mediastinal location (22%–55%); a deep cervical location (0%–19%); an intrathyroidal location (0%–12.5%); a location level with or above the common carotid bifurcation (0%–2.5%); and the presence of supernumerary glands (12.7%–39.5%).

Even when performed by highly trained operators, sonographic examination is of lower quality in patients with cervical fibrosis due to previous surgery. Diagnosis of even a small nodule in such patients should prompt US-guided FNA and a PTH assay.

2.3.7.4 Value of US Combined with Other Imaging Modalities

The limitations of sonography and the widespread availability of other imaging techniques have led numerous authors to propose exploration strategies combining US and one or more other modalities:

- Combination with thallium scintigraphy has a sensitivity of 61%–86% for localization of adenomas in patients with PHPT (Arkles et al. 1996; Summers 1996).
- Combination with MIBI scintigraphy has a sensitivity of 86% for adenomas (Prager et al. 1999)

and 78%–96% for the diagnosis of PHPT (De Feo et al. 2000; Purcell et al. 1999).
- Combination with CT has a sensitivity of 87%, regardless of the type of hyperparathyroidism (Lemmi et al. 1994)
- A combination of three imaging modalities (sonography, CT, thallium subtraction scintigraphy) reportedly has a positive predictive value of 96% for preoperative detection of hyperplasia and adenomas (Okada et al. 1997)

2.4 Nonsonographic Imaging Modalities

2.4.1 MIBI

MIBI scintiscanning is currently considered the most accurate localization technique, in particular for SHPT and persistent and recurrent HPT. Introduced during the past decade (Taillefer et al. 1992), this dual-phase method is based on the difference in the rate of ^{99m}Tc-MIBI washout from the thyroid and parathyroid tissues; scans obtained after 2–3 h reveal a contrast between the thyroid and the pathological parathyroid tissue.

In the literature review by Darcourt et al. (1998), MIBI scintiscanning had a mean sensitivity of 91.8% for adenoma (304 cases), 61.7% for hyperplasia (188 cases), and 92.6% for ectopic adenoma (27 cases). Comparison with thallium studies in the literature reveals the consistent superiority of MIBI (Tables 2.1, 2.3, and 2.4).

Technical adaptations have been proposed to improve diagnostic accuracy, in particular single photon-emission computed tomography (SPECT) with analysis of early images (Chen et al. 1997) and simultaneous iodine-123/^{99m}Tc-sestamibi SPECT subtraction imaging (Neumann et al. 1997).

De Feo et al. (2000) advocate increased use of ^{99m}Tc-MIBI scintigraphy and sonography. Beginning the examination sequence with scintigraphy allows optimization of sonography to characterize the parathyroid nodules demonstrated by MIBI. When scintigraphy is normal, a sonographic search can be made for subcentimeter lesions or lesions with necrotic areas or weak metabolic activity. When cervical MIBI scintiscanning is positive, cervical US is useful to correct false-positive findings, in particular by accurate characterization of thyroid nodules and lymph nodes.

2.4.2 Other Imaging Modalities

2.4.2.1 *Computed Tomography*

Cervicomediastinal CT, a second-line technique, is performed with contiguous, 5-mm-thick scans between the hyoid bone and the tracheal bifurcation after administration of intravenous iodinated contrast medium.

Regardless of the etiology, CT usually demonstrates a homogeneous or an inhomogeneous solid lesion showing variable enhancement after contrast injection. Enlarged retrothyroid parathyroid glands are usually separated from the thyroid gland by a thin line of fat. Intratumor variations in density have the same significance as the variations in echotexture observed at sonography, and reflect changes in internal architecture: calcifications, necrotic or hemorrhagic degeneration, lipoadenoma. The sensitivity of CT is essentially equivalent to that of sonography (50%–87% in the review of Higgins and Auffermann 1988).

The main limitations of CT concern lesion size, particularly in cases of hyperplasia. In addition to the need for iodinated contrast injection, which may be a problem in patients with chronic renal failure, the quality of cervicomediastinal CT scans (except for the most recent CT units) can be altered by artifacts of respiration or swallowing and by the position of the shoulders. Generally speaking, the presence of surgical clips, postoperative fibrosis or an intrathyroid adenoma create diagnostic difficulties.

2.4.2.2 *Magnetic Resonance Imaging*

Like CT, MRI is reserved as a second-line modality. Axial and coronal scans are obtained at the cervical and mediastinal levels. T_1-weighted spin-echo sequences and STIR sequences are usually used. These sequences are actually complementary, because T_1-weighted images provide excellent spatial resolution, while STIR sequences increase the contrast between the abnormal parathyroid gland and adjacent structures, despite their lower spatial resolution. T_2-weighted sequences and gadolinium enhancement of T_1-weighted images are unnecessary because the contrast between the parathyroid gland and the adjacent structures is not optimal. Nevertheless, in the absence of STIR sequences, a T_2-weighted sequence with fat saturation is recommended.

Regardless of the sequence, MRI, like other imaging modalities, can reveal only gland enlargement. The most common finding is a mass of intermediate signal intensity that is isointense to muscle and the thyroid on T_1-weighted images and isointense or hyperintense to fat on T_2-weighted sequences. On STIR sequences, an abnormal parathyroid gland is easily detectable as an extremely hyperintense structure within the suppressed fat. This contrast phenomenon is also observed on T_2-weighted images with fat saturation, although contrast is not as good because fat saturation is not homogeneous.

MRI is a sensitive technique that has similar efficacy for preoperative evaluation of PHPT and etiological workup of recurrent HPT. In the literature, its sensitivity has been evaluated at between 65% and 80% (Bruneton et al. 1996; Hewin et al. 1997; Ishibashi et al. 1998; McDermott et al. 1996). False-positive findings are attributable to nodular thyroid disease or lymphadenopathy. False-negative errors are related to small gland size, the existence of multiple lesions, or an atypical signal (isointense on T_2-weighted sequences). As adenomas tend to be larger than hyperplastic glands, they are easier to detect. Size is not the only factor affecting detection, however, because atypical signals are more frequent with hyperplasia than with adenomas (McDermott et al. 1996).

2.4.2.3
Thallium-Technetium Subtraction Scintigraphy

The indications for this scintigraphic technique have declined markedly since the introduction of MIBI. This dual-isotope subtraction technique has a sensitivity of 49%–94% (Table 2.1) in PHPT and 32.4%, according to Liou et al. (1996), in SHPT. Sensitivity ranges from 36%–68% for recurrent and persistent hyperparathyroidism (Table 2.4).

2.4.2.4
Invasive Imaging Procedures

Invasive imaging techniques must be performed in highly specialized units by radiologists familiar with their use for patients who have often already undergone multiple surgical procedures.

Arteriography requires selective catheterization of the arteries feeding the parathyroid glands. The superior and inferior thyroid arteries must be catheterized at the cervical level. Search for an ectopic thoracic adenoma requires selective catheterization of the internal thoracic arteries, in particular the internal mammary artery. The normal parathyroid glands are not visible, but presence of an adenoma or hyperplasia creates an arteriographic blush. Arteriography had a sensitivity of 60% for Brennan et al. (1982).

Venous blood sampling requires selective catheterization of the thyroid veins (superior, middle, and inferior) and the thymic, vertebral, and internal thoracic veins. It may be performed alone or as a complement to arteriography. Staged venous sampling allows identification of a PTH gradient, permitting localization of an adenoma or hyperplasia. A gradient is considered significant if the PTH peak is twice the baseline value. Indication of all sampling sites on a map of the relevant venous system can guide the surgical procedure. Performed essentially after the failure of one or more parathyroid operations, catheterization is often difficult, owing to the presence of ligations and anastomoses. The sensitivity of venous sampling, which requires operator expertise, is close to 80% for Miller et al. (1987).

2.5
Indications for Ultrasound and Other Imaging Modalities

2.5.1
Value of Preoperative Localization Studies in the Literature

The many literature reports in the 1990s on the potential value of preoperative localization studies were followed by a series of publications claiming that such studies were of no true benefit. However, during the past 2 years, a number of authors have emphasized the value of preoperative localization studies, essentially as a means of decreasing operative dissection.

2.5.1.1
Arguments Against Preoperative Localization Studies

The main arguments against such studies are as follows:

- Inaccuracy of imaging techniques in general (Hewin et al. 1997; Koong et al. 1998; Light et al. 1996; Walgenbach et al. 1999), in particular for SHPT (Heller et al. 1993; Pons et al. 1997).
- Failure of imaging studies to detect multiple lesions (Heller et al. 1993; Moore et al. 1999; Zmora et al. 1995)

- Efficacy of surgery even without imaging studies (Chou et al. 1997; Koong et al. 1998), although results are unquestionably best when the operative procedure is performed by an experienced parathyroid surgeon (Summers 1996).

2.5.1.2 Arguments in Favor of Preoperative Localization Studies

The purpose of preoperative imaging is to improve surgical management and, if possible, limit the procedure to unilateral neck exploration.

Preoperative imaging is often considered sufficient, even when only a single accurate localization modality is used, be it sonography (Friedrich et al. 1997; Koslin et al. 1997; Vogel et al. 1998) or MIBI (Moka et al. 1997; Wei and Burke 1995). Various combinations of two sensitive imaging techniques have been advocated to improve diagnostic accuracy prior to unilateral neck exploration: sonography and MIBI (Profanter et al. 1999; Purcell et al. 1999), sonography and thallium scintigraphy (Huang et al. 1998), sonography and CT (Okada et al. 1997)

Certain authors set additional conditions, such as use of extemporaneous histopathological examination (Friedrich et al. 1997), identification of a normal parathyroid gland on the initial operative side (Vogel et al. 1998), or intraoperative PTH assays that should reveal a marked decrease after ablation of the lesion (Moore et al. 1999).

The advantages achieved with improved pretherapy localization include decreased operative time (Friedrich et al. 1997; Koslin et al. 1997; Song et al. 1999; Wei and Burke 1995), a reduction in postoperative complications such as laryngeal nerve injury or hypoparathyroidism (Thompson et al. 1999; Vogel et al. 1998), and lower operative costs (Koslin et al. 1997).

2.5.2 Primary Hyperparathyroidism

Despite current controversy concerning the role of preoperative localization, such studies remain extremely important for patients with malignant hypercalcemia who respond poorly to medical therapy and for whom unsuccessful surgery may have dire consequences.

When the patient's general condition contraindicates a prolonged surgical procedure, when treatment must be performed under local anesthesia, or when PEA is envisaged, the pretherapy workup must be as accurate as possible. Sonography should be the initial imaging technique in such situations, taking care to keep the its limitations in mind. It thus currently appears realistic to supplement US with MIBI scintigraphy.

When PEA is planned, CD provides complementary information that improves analysis of the vascular areas of the lesion that should be treated with priority. Post-therapy surveillance, if necessary after several sessions of ethanol injection, is performed using sonography and CD or PD, along with serum PTH assays.

Persistent and recurrent postoperative hyperparathyroidism present problems for sonographic identification of postoperative fibrosis, in particular following a radical procedure. The same is true for CT and MRI. The slightest doubt after sonography should prompt FNA plus PTH assay, but MIBI appears to be the most effective technique as it is less impeded by fibrosis. Angiographic procedures are reserved for cases where noninvasive imaging is negative or inconclusive.

2.5.3 Secondary Hyperparathyroidism

A correlation exists between the elevation in PTH and serum alkaline phosphatase concentrations and the presence of sonographically visible parathyroid anomalies. A third of all hemodialysis patients have sonographic evidence of enlargement of one or more parathyroid glands (Bruneton et al. 1996). Sonographic findings for SHPT are similar to those described for PHPT, and the lesions are generally hypoechoic. Gladziwa et al. (1992) found that patients in whom sonography demonstrated parathyroid enlargement had disease of greater clinical or biochemical severity than patients with a negative sonographic study. US has no indications for screening, however, because the PTH level predicts or excludes the existence of parathyroid anomalies.

Recently, sonography has been used to evaluate changes in parathyroid volume in patients on calcitriol therapy; the reduction in gland size after 1 year of treatment reflects biochemical and clinical improvement (Huraib et al. 1997). Malberti et al. (1996) attributed a prognostic role to parathyroid volume for patient management.

The excellent sensitivity of sonography should be emphasized for follow-up of patients who have undergone parathyroid autografting, especially into the forearm. Sonography can detect millimeter-sized lesions opposite the cutaneous scar corresponding to graft-dependent HPT. Sonographic localization also facilitates therapeutic PEA.

Outside of these cases, whenever a surgical indication exists owing to the inefficacy of medical treatment, the search for parathyroid enlargement can benefit from imaging studies. While sonography should be the initial modality of choice, the frequency of hyperplastic processes, sometimes in unusual localizations, warrants use of a second exploration technique (MIBI scintigraphy). PEA appears indicated for persistent and recurrent HPT owing to the encouraging results achieved in these fragile patients (Solbiati et al. 1985).

Parathyroid imaging remains controversial, and no recent improvements have been made in sonography owing to the limitations of the technique related to lesion size and topography. Even when enhanced with contrast agents, CD provides no decisive information and requires additional investigations by specialized teams. The most important change appears to be the increasingly frequent use of PEA. Patient management using this approach is difficult to quantitate, but it is unquestionably in progression, particularly in Italy. Owing to the results achieved with PEA, the indications for parathyroid surgery merit re-evaluation for all types of hyperparathyroidism.

References

Abati A, Skarnlis MC, Shawker T, Solomon D (1995) Ultrasound-guided fine-needle aspiration of parathyroid lesions: morphological and immunocytochemical approach. Hum Pathol 26:338–343

Akerström G, Malmaeus J, Bergström R (1984) Surgical anatomy of human parathyroid glands. Surgery 95:14–21

André V, Andre M, Le Dreff P, Granier H, Forlodou P, Garcia JF (1999) Adénome parathyroidien intrathyroidien. J Radiol 80:591–592

Arkles LB, Jones T, Hicks RJ, De Luise MA, Chou ST (1996) Impact of complementary parathyroid scintigraphy and ultrasonography on the surgical management of hyperparathyroidism. Surgery 120:845–851

Auffermann N, Gooding GA, Okerlund MD, et al (1988) Diagnosis of recurrent hyperparathyroidism: comparison of MR imaging and other imaging techniques. AJR 150:1027–1033

Billy HT, Rimkus DR, Hartzman S, Latimer RG (1995) Technetium-99m-sestamibi single agent localization versus high-resolution ultrasonography for the preoperative localization of parathyroid glands in patients with primary hyperparathyroidism. Am Surg 61:882–888

Bismuth V, Fendler JP, Grellet J, et al (1975) Le diagnostic artériographique des adénomes parathyroidiens. A propos de 45 cas. J Radiol 56:235–244

Brennan MF, Doppman JL, Kurdy AG, Marx SJ, Spiegel AM, Auerbach GD (1982) Assessment of techniques for preoperative parathyroid gland localization in patients undergoing preoperation for hyperparathyroidism. Surgery 91:6–11

Bruneton JN, Laurent F, Chevallier P, Drouillard J (1996) Imagerie non isotopique des parathyroides. In: Bruneton JN, Padovani B (eds) Imagerie en endocrinologie. Masson, Paris, pp 84–94

Caixas A, Berna L, Piera J, et al (1995) Utility of 99m Tc-sestamibi scintigraphy as a first-line imaging procedure in the preoperative evaluation of hyperparathyroidism. Clin Endocrinol (Oxford) 43:525–530

Calliada F, Sala G, Conti MP, et al (1993) Applicazioni cliniche del color-Doppler: le ghiandole paratiroidi. Radiol Med 85:114–119

Casas AT, Burke GJ, Sathyanarayana, Mansberger AR jr, Wei JP (1993) Prospective comparaison of technetium-99m-sestamibi/iodine-123 radionuclide scan versus high-resolution ultrasonography for the preoperative localization of abnormal parathyroid glands in patients with previously unoperated primary hyperparathyroidism. Am J Surg 166:369–373

Chang TC, Tung CC, Hsiao YL, Chen MH (1998) Immunoperoxidase staining in the differential diagnosis of parathyroid from thyroid origin in fine needle aspirates of suspected parathyroid lesions. Acta Cytol 42:619–624

Chen CC, Holder LE, Scovill WA, Chan AM, Gann DS (1997) Comparison of parathyroid imaging with technetium-99m-pertechnetate/sestamibi and technetium-99m-sestamibi SPECT. J Nucl Med 38:834–839

Chen MH, Chang TC, Hsiao Yl, Chang TH, Huang SH (1999) Combination of color Doppler ultrasonography and ultrasound-guided fine-needle aspiration cytology for localization of parathyroid lesions. J Formos Med Assoc 98:506–511

Chou FF, Wang PW, Sheen-Chen SM (1997) Preoperative localisation of parathyroid glands in primary hyperparathyroidism. Eur J Surg 163:889–895

Cintin C, Karstrup S, Ladefoged SD, Joffe P (1994) Tertiary hyperparathyroidism treated by ultrasonically guided percutaneous fine-needle ethanol injection. Nephron 68:127–220

Clark OH, Okerlund MD, Moss AA, et al (1985) Localization studies in patients with persistent or recurrent hyperparathyroidism. Surgery 98:1083–1094

Darcourt J, Gray M, Bussiere F (1998) Parathyroid glands. Scintigraphy. In: Bruneton JN (ed) Radiology of endocrine diseases. Springer, Berlin Heidelberg New York, pp 192–199

De Feo ML, Colagrande V, Biagini C, et al (2000) Parathyroid glands: combination of 99mTc MIBI scintigraphy and US for demonstration of parathyroid glands and nodules. Radiology 214:393–402

Du SD, Chang TC, Chen YL, et al (1994) Ultrasonography and needle aspiration cytology in the diagnosis and management of parathyroid lesions. J Formos Med Assoc 93:153–159

Dubost C, Lecharpentier Y, Bouteloup PY (1984) Chirurgie des glandes parathyroïdes. Traitement de l'hyperparathyroïdie. Encycl Med Chir Techniques Chirurgicales, Thorax. Editions Techniques, Paris, 42070, 40.10.06

Fayet P, Hoeffel C, Fulla Y (1997) Technetium-99m sestamibi scintigraphy, magnetic resonance imaging and venous blood sampling in persistent and recurrent hyperparathyroidism. Br J Radiol 70:459–464

Fletcher S, Jones RG, Rayner HC et al (1997) Assessment of renal osteodystrophy in dialysis patients: use of bone alkaline phosphatase, bone mineral density and parathyroid ultrasound in comparison with bone histology. Nephron 75:412–419

Fletcher S, Kanagasundaram NS, Rayner HC, et al (1998) Assessment of ultrasound-guided percutaneous ethanol injection and parathyroidectomy in patients with tertiary hyperparathyroidsm. Nephrol Dial Transplant 13:3111–3117

Fraker Kl, Doppman JL, Shawker TH, Marx SJ, Spiegel AM, Norton JA (1990) Undescended parathyroid adenoma: an important etiology for failed operations for primary hyperparathyroidism. World J Surg 14:342–348

Frasoldati A, Pesenti M, Toschi E, Azzarito C, Zini M, Valcavi R (1999) Detection and diagnosis of parathyroid incidentalomas during thyroid sonography. J Clin Ultrasound 27:492–498

Friedrich J, Krause U, Saller B, Eigler FW (1997) Unilateral neck exploration in primary hyperparathyroidism. Langenbecks Arch Chir [Suppl Kongressbd] 114:1157–1160

Fugazzola C, Bermamo-Andreis I, Solbiati L (1995) Parathyroid glands. In: Solbiati L, Rizzato G (eds) Ultrasound of superficial structures: high frequencies, Doppler and interventional procedures. Churchill Livingstone, Edinburgh, pp 87–113

Fukagawa M, Kitaoka M, Kurokawa K (1996) Ultrasonographic intervention of parathyroid hyperplasia in chronic dialysis patients: a theoretical approach. Nephrol Dial Transplant 11 [Suppl 3]:125–129

Fukagawa M, Kitaoka M, Kurokawa K (1997) Ultrasonographic evaluation of parathyroid hyperplasia. Nephrol Dial Transplant 12:2461–2468

Gladziwa U, Ittel TH, Dakshinamurty KV, Schacht B, Riehl J, Sieberth HG (1992) Secondary hyperparathyroidism and sonographic evaluation of parathyroid gland hyperplasia in dialysis patients. Clin Nephrol 38:162–166

Gooding GA, Clark OH (1992) Use of color-Doppler imaging in the distinction between thyroid and parathyroid lesions. Am J Surg 164:51–56

Graif M, Itzchak Y, Strauss S, Dolev E, Mohr R, Wolfstein I (1987) Parathyroid sonography: diagnostic accuracy related to shape, location and texture of the gland. Br J Radiol 60:439–443

Halbauer M, Crepinko I, Tomc Brzac H, Simonivic I (1991) Fine-needle aspiration cytology in the preoperative diagnosis of ultrasonically enlarged parathyroid glands. Acta Cytol 35:728–735

Hasselgren PO, Fidler JP (1992) Further evidence against the routine use of parathyroid ultrasonography prior to initial neck exploration for hyperparathyroidism. Am J Surg 164:337–340

Heller KS, Attie JN, Dubner S (1993) Parathyroid localization: inability to predict multiple gland involvement. Am J Surg 166:367–359

Hewin DF, Brammar TJ, Kabala J, Farndon JR (1997) Role of preoperative localization in the management of primary hyperparathyroidism. Am J Surg 84:1377–1380

Higgins CB, Auffermann W (1988) MR imaging of thyroid and parathyroid glands: a review of current status. AJR 151:1095–1106

Hopkins CR, Reading CC (1995) Thyroid and parathyroid imaging. Semin Ultrasound CT MR 16: 279–295

Huang SH, Lai IR, Liaw KY, Cheng YC, Hsiao YL, Chang TC (1998) Preoperative localization procedures for initial surgery in primary hyperparathyroidism. J Formos Med Assoc 97:679–683

Huraib S, Abu-Aisha H, Abed J, Al Wakeel J, Al Desouki M, Memon N (1997) Long-term effect of intravenous calcitriol on the treatment of severe hyperparathyroidism, parathyroid gland mass and bone mineral density in haemodialysis patients. Am J Nephrol 17:118–129

Ishibashi M, Nishida H, Hiromatsu Y, Kojima K, Tabuchi E, Hayabuchi N (1998) Comparison of technetium-99m-MIBI, technetium-99m-tetrofosmin, ultrasound and MRI for localization of abnormal parathyroid glands. J Nucl Med 39:320–324

Jeanguillaume C, Urena P, Hindie E, et al (1998) Secondary hyperparathyroidism: detection with I-123-Tc-99m-sestamibi subtraction scintigraphy versus US. Radiology 207:207–213

Kairaluoma MV, Kellosalo J, Makarainen H, Haukipuro K, Kairaluoma MI (1994) Parathyroid re-exploration in patients with primary hyperparathyroidism. Ann Chir Gynaecol 83:202–206

Kakuta T, Fukagawa M, Fujisaki T, et al (1999) Prognosis of parathyroid function after successful percutaneous ethanol injection therapy guided by color Doppler flow mapping in chronic dialysis patients. Am J Kidney Dis 33:1091–1099

Kanegae K, Itoh K, Kato C, et al (1994) Detection and localization of parathyroid adenomas and hyperplasias in patients with hyperparathyroidism using thallium-201/technetium-99m parathyroid subtraction scintigraphy. Kaku Igaku 31:441–449

Karstrup S, Hegedus L, Holm HH (1993) Acute change in parathyroid function in primary hyperparathyroidism following ultrasonically guided ethanol injection into solitary parathyroid adenomas. Acta Endocrinol (Copenh) 129:377–380

Katoh N, Nakayama M, Shigematsu T, et al (2000) Presence of sonographically detectable parathyroid glands can predict resistance to oral pulsed-dose calcitriol treatment of secondary hyperparathyroidism. Am J Kidney Dis 35:465–468

Kinoshita Y, Fukase M, Uchihashi M, et al (1985) Significance of preoperative use of ultrasonography in parathyroid neoplasms: comparison of sonographic textures with histologic findings. J Clin Ultrasound 13:457–460

Kitaoka M, Fukagawa M, Ogata E, et al (1994) Reduction of functioning parathyroid cell mass by ethanol injection in chronic dialysis patients. Kidney Int 46:1110–1117

Koong HN, Choong LH, Soo KC (1998) The role for preoperative localization techniques in surgery for hyperparathyroidism. Ann Acad Med Singapore 27:192–195

Koslin DB, Adams J, Andersen P, Everts E, Cohen J (1997) Preoperative evaluation of patients with primary hyperparathyroidism: role of triple-resolution ultrasound. Laryngoscope 107:1249–1253

Krudy AG, Shawker TH, Doppman JL, et al (1984) Ultrasonic parathyroid localization in previously operated patients. Clin Radiol 35:113–118

Lane MJ, Desser JS, Weigel RJ, Jeffrey RB jr (1998) Use of color and power Doppler sonography to identify feeding arteries associated with parathyroid adenomas. AJR 171:819–823

Lemmi A, Baroni M, Malaspina C, et al (1994) Percutaneous alcohol injection in hyperparathyroidism. Experience in 11 cases with an 18-month follow-up. Radiol Med (Torino) 88:840–843

Lerner RM (1996) Underdiagnosis of parathyroid adenomas by sonography. AJR 167:814–815

Levin KE, Gooding GA, Okerlund M, et al (1987) Localizing studies in patients with persistent or recurrent hyperparathyroidism. Surgery 102:917–925

Libutti SK, Bartlett DL, Jaskowiak NT, et al (1997) The role of thyroid resection during reoperation for persistent or recurrent hyperparathyroidism. Surgery 122:1883–1187

Light VL, Mettenry CR, Jayoura D, Sodee DB, Miron SD (1996) Prospective comparison of dual-phase technetium-99m-sestamibi scintigraphy and high-resolution ultrasonography in the evaluation of abnormal parathyroid glands. Am Surg 62:562–567

Liou MJ, Huang HS, Lin JD, et al (1996) The accuracy of ultrasonography and 201Tl-99m Tc subtraction scan in localization of parathyroid lesions. Chang Keng I Hsueh 19:121–128

Livolsi VA, Hamilton R (1994) Intraoperative assessment of parathyroid gland pathology. A common view from the surgeon and the pathologist. Am J Clin Pathol 102:365–373

Lloyd MN, Lees WR, Milroy EJ (1990) Pre-operative localisation in primary hyperparathyroidism. Clin Radiol 41:239–243

Lossef SV, Ziessman HA, Alijani MR, Gomes MN, Barth KH (1993) Multiple hyperfunctioning mediastinal parathyroid glands in a patient with tertiary hyperparathyroidism. AJR 161:285–286

Malberti F, Corradi B, Cosci P, Calliada F, Marcelli D, Imbasciati E (1996) Long-term effects of intravenous calcitriol therapy on the control of secondary hyperparathyroidism. Am J Kidney Dis 28:704–712

Marcocci C, Mazzeo S, Bruno-Bossio G, et al (1998) Preoperative localization of suspicious parathyroid adenomas by assay of parathyroid hormone in needle aspirates. Eur J Endocrinol 139:72–77

Mariette C, Pellissier L, Combemale F, Quievreux JL, Carnaille B, Proye C (1998) Reoperation for persistent or recurrent primary hyperparathyroidism. Langenbecks Arch Surg 383:174–179

Mazzeo S, Caramella D, Lencioni R, et al (1995) Preoperative imaging in the detection of parathyroid tumefaction in patients with primary hyperparathyroidism. The author's own experience. Radiol Med (Torino)90:747–755

Mazzeo S, Caramella D, Lencioni R, et al (1996) Comparison among sonography, double-tracer subtraction scintigraphy, and double-phase scintigraphy in the detection of parathyroid lesions. AJR 166:1465–1470

McDermott VG, Mendez Fernandez RJ, Meakem TJ III, Stolpen AH, Spritzer CE, Gefter WB (1996) Preoperative MR imaging in hyperparathyroidism: results and factors affecting parathyroid detection. AJR 166:705–710

McIntyre RC Jr, Kumpe DA, Liechty RD (1994) Reexploration and angiographic ablation for hyperparathyroidism. Arch Surg 129:499–503

Meola M, Barsotti M, Lenti C, Luperini M, Cavanna L, Barsotti G (1999) Color Doppler in the imaging workup of primary hyperparathyroidism. J Nephrol 12:270–274

Miller DL, Doppmann JL, Krudy AG, et al (1987) Localization of parathyroid adenomas in patients who have undergone surgery II. Invasive procedures. Radiology 161:138–141

Mincione GP, Borrelli D, Cicchi P, Ipponi PL, Fiorini A (1986) Fine-needle aspiration cytology of parathyroid adenoma. A review of seven cases. Acta Cytol 30:65–69

Moka D, Voth E, Larena-Avellaneda A, Schicha H (1997) 99m-Tc-MIBI SPECT parathyroid gland scintigraphy for the preoperative localization of small parathyroid gland adenomas. Nuklearmedizin 36:240–244

Moore FD jr, Mannting F, Tanasijevic M (1999) Intrinsic limitations to unilateral parathyroid exploration. Ann Surg 230:382–391

Muslumanoglu M, Terzioglu T, Ozarmagan S, Tezelman S, Guloglu R (1995) Comparison of preoperative imaging techniques (thallium technetium scan and ultrasonography) and intraoperative staining (with methylene blue) in localizing the parathyroid glands. Radiol Med (Torino) 90:444–447

Nabriski D, Bendahan J, Shapiro MS, Freund U, Lidor C (1992) Sarcoidosis masquerading as a parathyroid adenoma. Head Neck 14:384–386

Neumann DR, Esselstyn CG jr, Go RT, Wong Co, Rice TW, Obuchowski NA (1997) Comparison of double-phase 99m Tc-sestamibi with 123 I-99m Tc-sestamibi subtraction SPECT in hyperparathyroidism. AJR 169:1671–1674

Numerow LM, Morita ET, Clark OH, Higgins CB (1995) Persistent/recurrent hyperparathyroidism: a comparison of sestamibi scintigraphy, MRI, and ultrasonography. J Magn Reson Imaging 5:702–708

Obara T, Fujimoto Y, Ito Y, et al (1989) Functioning parathyroid lipoadenoma. Report of four cases: clinicopathological and ultrasonographic features. Endocrinol Jpn 36:135–145

Okada Y, Mizutani Y, Takeuchi H, Shigeno C, Konishi J, Yoshida O (1997) Preoperative imaging for parathyroid localization in primary hyperparathyroidism. Int J Urol 4:338–342

Palestini N, Quaglino F, Abbona GC, Durando R, Robecchi A (1997) Primary hyperparathyroidism sustained by a giant adenoma of the parathyroid gland. Ann Ital Chir 68: 697–700

Pons F, Torregrosa JV, Vidal-Sicart S, et al (1997) Preoperative parathyroid gland localization with technetium-99m sestamibi in secondary hyperparathyroidism. Eur J Nucl Med 24:1494–1498.

Prager G, Czemy C, Kurtaran A, Passler C, Scheuba C, Niederle B (1999) The value of preoperative localization studies in primary hyperparathyroidism. Chirurg 70:1082–1088

Pretolesi F, Silvestri E, Di Maio G (1997) US imaging and color Doppler in patients undergoing inhibitory therapy with calcitriol for secondary hyperparathyroidism. Eur Radiol 7:721–725

Profanter C, Klingler A, Strolz S, et al (1999) Surgical therapy for primary hyperparathyroidism in patients with previous thyroid surgery. Am J Surg 178:374–376

Proye C, Bizard JP, Carnaille B, Quievreux JL (1994) Hyperparathyroidism and intrathyroid parathyroid gland. 43 cases. Ann Chir 48:501–506

Purcell GP, Dirbas FM, Jeffrey RB, et al (1999) Parathyroid localization with high-resolution ultrasound and technetium Tc 99m sestamibi. Arch Surg 134:824–828

Randel SB, Gooding GAW, Clark OH, Stein RM, Winkler B (1987) Parathyroid variants: US evaluation. Radiology 165:191–194

Reading CC (1991) The parathyroid. In: Rumack CM, Wilson SR, Charboneau JW (eds) Diagnostic ultrasound. Mosby, St Louis, pp 524–539

Reading CC, Charboneau WJ, James EM, et al (1982) High-resolution parathyroid sonography. AJR 139:539–546

Rodriguez JM, Tezelman S, Siperstein AE, et al (1994) Localization procedures in patients with persistent or recurrent hyperparathyroidism. Arch Surg 129:870–875

Sacks BA, Pallotta JA, Cole A, et al (1994) Diagnosis of parathyroid adenomas: efficacy of measuring parathormone levels in needle aspirates of cervical masses. AJR 163:1223–1226

Sadoul JL (1996) Parathyroides. Introduction clinique. In: Bruneton JN, Padovani B (eds) Imagerie en endocrinologie. Masson, Paris, pp 81–83

Sakamoto W, Kishimoto T, Nishisaka M, et al (1990) Clinical study on 32 patients who underwent parathyroidectomy at Osalla City University Hospital. Nippon Hingokika Gakkai Zasshi 81:230–235

Sardi A, Bolton JS, Mitchell WT jr, Merritt CR (1992) Immunoperoxidase confirmation of ultrasonographically guided fine-needle aspirates in patients with recurrent hyperparathyroidism. Surg Gynecol Obstet 175:563–568

Schantz A, Castelman B (1973) Parathyroid carcinoma: a study of 70 cases. Cancer 31:600–605

Schwerk WB, Grun R, Wahl R (1985) High-resolution realtime sonography of parathyroid tumors. Ultraschall Med 6:13–18

Solbiati L, Giangrande A, De Pra L, Bellotti E, Cantu P, Ravetto C (1985) Percutaneous ethanol injection of parathyroid tumors under US guidance: treatment for secondary hyperparathyroidism. Radiology 155:607–610

Song AU, Phillips TE, Edmond CV, Moore DW, Clark SK (1999) Success of preoperative imaging and unilateral neck exploration for primary hyperparathyroidism. Otolaryngol Head Neck Surg 121:393–397

Spinelli C, Berti P, Miccoli P (1994) Carcinoma of the parathyroids. Surgical experience in 3 cases. Minerva Chir 49:1342–1347

Stein BL, Wexler MJ (1990) Preoperative parathyroid localization: a prospective evaluation of ultrasonography and thallium-scintigraphy in hyperparathyroidism. Can J Surg 33:175–180

Summers GW (1996) Parathyroid update: a review of 220 cases. Ear Nose Throat J 75:434–439

Taillefer R, Boucher Y, Potvin C, et al (1992) Detection and localization of parathyroid adenomas in patients with hyperparathyroidism using a simple radionuclide imaging procedure with technetium-99m-sestamibi (double-phase study). J Nucl Med 33:1801–1807

Tezelman S, Shen W, Siperstein AE, Duh QY, Clark OH (1995) Persistent or recurrent hyperparathyroidism in patients with double adenomas. Surgery 118:1115–1122

Thompson GB, Grant CS, Perrier ND, et al (1999) Reoperative parathyroid surgery in the era of sestamibi scanning and intraoperative parathyroid hormone monitoring. Arch Surg 134:699–704

Thompson NW, Eckhauser FE, Harness JK (1982) The anatomy of primary hyperparathyroidism. Surgery 92:814–821

Torregrosa JV, Palomar MR, Pons F, et al (1998) Has double-phase MIBI scintigraphy usefulness in the diagnosis of hyperparathyroidism? Nephrol Dial Transplant 13 [Suppl 3]:37–40

Trombetta C, Lissiani A, Moro U, Belgrano E (1996) Infrequent application of intraoperative ultrasonography in urology. Arch Ital Urol Androl 68 [Suppl 5]:31–36

Varsamidis K, Varsamidou E, Mavropoulos G (1999) Color Doppler sonography in the detection of parathyroid adenomas. Head Neck 21:648–651

Vogel LM, Lucas R, Czako P (1998) Unilateral parathyroid exploration. Am Surg 64:693–697

Walgenbach S, Dutkowski P, Andreas J, Gorges R, Bockisch A, Juginger T (1999) 99m Tc-MIBI-scintigraphy before parathyroid surgery? Zentralbl Chir 124:214–219

Wang CA (1976) The anatomic basis of parathyroid surgery. Ann Surg 183:271–275

Weber CJ, Sewell CW, McGarity WC (1994) Persistent and recurrent sporadic primary hyperparathyroidism: histopathology, complications, and results of reoperation. Surgery 116:991–998

Wei JP, Burke GJ (1995) Analysis of savings in operative time for primary hyperparathyroidism using localization with technetium 99m sestamibi scan. Am J Surg 170:488–491

Zeze F, Ikoh H, Ohsato K (1995) Hyperplasia and adenoma of the ectopic parathyroid gland. Nippon Rinsho 53:920–924

Zmora O, Schachter PP, Heyman Z, Shabtay M, Avigad I, Ayalon A (1995) Correct preoperative localization: does it permit a change in operative strategy for primary hyperparathyroidism?

3 Salivary Glands

Charles Raffaelli, Nicolas Amoretti, Bruno Carlotti

CONTENTS

The salivary glands form a distinct anatomic and functional system. The spectrum of salivary gland disease varies greatly; although sometimes quite specific, salivary pathologies are often rare or of uncertain pathogenesis. Infection and inflammatory lesions predominate, but a wide variety of tumors are also encountered. Technological progress in sonography has made this noninvasive procedure with multiple operating modes the initial imaging technique of choice for the salivary glands. Owing to the superficial location of these glands, high-frequency ultrasound (US) transducers provide markedly better spatial resolution than other imaging modalities. US can also effectively guide and improve the safety of aspiration biopsy of inflammatory and tumoral lesions. Color Doppler allows assessment of salivary gland function and accurate analysis

C. Raffaelli, MD
Service de Radiodiagnostic, Hôpital Pasteur, 30, avenue Voie Romaine, BP 69, F-06002 Nice Cedex 1, France
N. Amoretti, MD
Service de Radiodiagnostic, Hôpital Pasteur, 30, avenue Voie Romaine, BP 69, F-06002 Nice Cedex 1, France
B. Carlotti, MD
Otorhinolaryngologiste, 88, boulevard de Cimiez, F-06000 Nice, France

of tumor vascularity. A valuable technique in constant progression, sonography is necessary and sufficient in many circumstances. However, achievement of optimum results requires both familiarity with multiplanar anatomy and technical expertise.

3.1 Anatomy

The first components of the digestive tract with a secretory function, the salivary glands are divided into major glands (parotid, submandibular, and sublingual glands, all paired and symmetrical) and accessory glands, ubiquitous structures of variable distribution. All of the salivary glands are exocrine glands; the glandular tissue is composed of acinar or tubuloacinar cells that produce a mucous, serous-mucous or mixed secretion whose composition varies with the excretory phase.

The major salivary glands are lobular structures with long, highly branched excretory ducts (intralobular ducts, interlobular ducts, and collector or interlobar ducts). Secretion is ensured by acini that are surrounded by myoepithelial cells. The lobules of the parotid contain only serous-secreting cells, whereas the submandibular gland contains both serous- and mucous-secreting cells; the sublingual gland has a predominantly mucous secretion.

The saliva contains mucin and several enzymes (essentially amylases). Saliva has numerous functions: lubrification of the oral tissues; moistening and softening of the food, which facilitates mastication and swallowing; mediation of taste sensations by solubilization of aliment; facilitation of speech; enzymatic digestion of starches (Hermann and Cier 1979).

3.1.1 Parotid Gland

The largest of the main salivary glands, the parotid occupies most of the retromandibular space; it extends anteriorly onto the ascending ramus of the mandible.

The pathogenesis of inflammatory, tumoral, and lymphoepithelial parotid lesions can be explained by the specificity of parotid embryogenesis. Development of the ductal epithelium (ductal canalization) precedes differentiation of the glandular acini. The capsule encasing the parotid gland forms later than that of the other salivary glands, after emergence of the lymphatic ducts; the parenchyma thus contains both lymph nodes and ducts. During the terminal phase of gland encapsulation, salivary epithelial cells may be included within the intraparotid and periparotid lymph nodes (Silvers and Som 1998).

The parotid space is bounded as follows (Bouchet and Cuilleret 1991a) (Fig. 3.1):

- Laterally, by the superficial cervical fascia and the subcutaneous plane
- Anteromedially, by the paratonsillar region (anterior subparotid space)
- Posteromedially, by the retrostyloid space (posterior subparotid space), which contains the internal carotid artery, the internal jugular vein, and cranial nerves IX, X, and XI
- Anteriorly, by the infratemporal and masseter regions
- Superiorly, by the temporal region
- Inferiorly, by the bicarotid region and the posterior pole of the submandibular space

Enclosed within a well-defined fibrous capsule, the parotid is intimately connected to the walls of the parotid space. Irregularly shaped, like an inverted pyramid with a subcutaneous base, the parotid presents three surfaces (anterior, posterior, and lateral) and an internal pharyngeal border. The parotid gland has a variable number of extensions that often extend beyond the limits of the parotid space; the size of

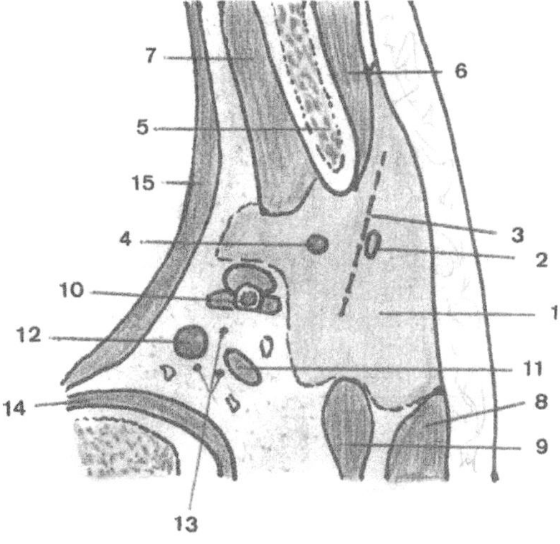

Fig. 3.1. Parotid space: transverse scan. *1* Parotid gland, *2* venous plane, *3* facial nerve, *4* external carotid artery, *5* ramus of mandible, *6* masseter muscle, *7* medial pterygoid muscle, *8* sternocleidomastoid muscle, *9* digastric muscle, *10* styloid apophysis, *11* internal jugular vein, *12* internal carotid artery, *13* cranial nerves IX, X, XI, *14* prevertebral muscles, *15* wall of the pharynx

these extensions varies greatly from one individual to another (Fig. 3.2):

- Anteriorly, there is often a superficial and sometimes voluminous masseter extension that may image as a true accessory parotid.
- Posteriorly, a pharyngeal extension may project between the stylomandibular and sphenomaxillary ligaments. Over 50% of individuals have a pharyngeal parotid extension that is closely connected to the lateral pharyngeal wall (Bruneton et al. 1987).
- Inferiorly, the parotid extends an average of 1 cm below the angle of the mandible. Some individuals have a true parotid extension that may extend up to 4 cm, separated from the submandibular gland by a fascial extension.
- Other, smaller extensions are encountered inconsistently (posterior extension towards the styloid diaphragm, superior extension into the pretragal region, inferior extension towards the carotid region).

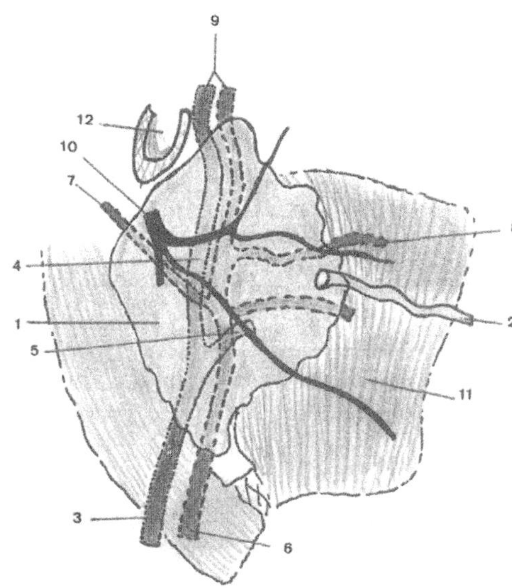

Fig. 3.2. Right parotid gland: lateral view. *1* Parotid gland, *2* Stensen's duct, *3* external jugular vein, *4* venous plane of the parotid, *5* retromandibular vein, *6* external carotid artery, *7* posterior auricular artery, *8* internal maxillary artery, *9* superficial temporal artery and vein, *10* trunk of the facial nerve, *11* masseter muscle, *12* external acoustic meatus

The parotid excretory duct (Stensen's duct) has a mean diameter of 3 mm and averages 4 cm in length. Emerging from the anterior border of the superficial lobe, at the level of the masseter extension, this duct runs forwards, lateral to the masseter, together with the transverse facial artery. After running deeply towards the buccal surface of the cheek, the duct pierces the buccinator muscle and drains via a prominent papilla into the oral cavity, opposite the second upper molar. In approximately 20% of individuals, Stensen's duct receives the duct of an accessory parotid gland as it crosses the masseter muscle (Silvers and Som 1998).

Awareness of the neurovascular relationships of the parotid is essential. The facial nerve emerges from the skull base through the stylomastoid foramen and penetrates the parotid posteriorly. After running anteriorly through the gland, the facial nerve divides into major trunks (zygomatic, buccal, mandibular, and cervical branches) lateral to the mandible and the external carotid artery. Arising from the confluence of the internal maxillary vein and the superficial temporal vein, the venous plane lies deep to the deep aspect of the facial nerve trunk. Venous drainage is primarily into the external jugular vein, and sometimes to the facial vein via the intraparotid communicant vein or retromandibular vein (Gaillard et al. 1981).

The external carotid artery penetrates the posteromedial surface of the parotid. The deepest vascular element of the parotid, the external carotid artery passes upwards through the gland, ending 4 cm above the angle of the mandible where it divides into two terminal branches (superficial temporal artery and maxillary artery).

An important lymphatic junction, the parotid space contains supra- and subfascial extraglandular lymph nodes as well as nodes within the gland parenchyma itself. These nodes receive lymph from a vast anatomic territory including, in addition to the parotid, the eyeball and ocular adnexa, the deep regions of the face, and the temporal region of the scalp (Gaillard et al. 1981).

By convention, the parotid is divided into two major lobes (superficial or lateral and deep or medial), based on their position with respect to the facial nerve and its branches. This division is actually of little value, however, because there is no actual anatomic plane of separation. Nevertheless, the parotid gland can be conveniently divided into three portions: superficial (exofacial), deep (endofacial), and inferior (infrafacial).

3.1.2 Submandibular Gland

Located in the lateral portion of the suprahyoid region, the submandibular gland fills most of the submandibular area bounded by the internal aspect of the mandible, the suprahyoid muscles, and the internal aspects of the base of the tongue and the pharynx.

On anteroposterior views, the submandibular area appears triangular, bounded laterally by the superficial cervical fascia and medially by the suprahyoid muscles and the lateral pharyngeal wall. In the internal wall of the submandibular space course the hypoglossal nerve, the lingual artery and vein, and the facial artery (Fig. 3.3).

Posteriorly, the submandibular area occupies the inferior part of the paratonsillar space, separated from the parotid by a fibrous septum.

The almond-shaped submandibular gland is intimately related to the submandibular space. Inferiorly, the gland extends beyond the horizontal body of the mandible to enter in contact with the subcutaneous plane (Bouchet and Cuilleret 1991b). Its lower aspect may extend inferiorly beyond the greater horn of the hyoid bone; its superior aspect is intimately related to the mylohyoid muscle.

Near the posterosuperior border of the mylohyoid muscle, a small, deep part of the gland is closely related to the posteromedial aspect of the homolateral sublingual gland. This small, deep extension runs forward in the gutter between the mylohyoid and hyoglossal muscles (intermuscular hiatus) and thus communicates with the floor of the mouth (Bouchet and Cuilleret 1991b).

The main excretory duct of the submandibular gland (Wharton's duct) has a mean length of 4 cm and a mean diameter of 3 mm. It exits the deep portion of the gland and runs obliquely, following an anteromedial course, in contact with the anterior extension and the internal borders of the mylohyoid muscle, medial to the sublingual gland. After passing through the intermuscular hiatus, Wharton's duct ends in the anterior floor of the mouth on the sublingual papilla, at the inferior extremity of the frenulum of the tongue; it thus presents a close and potentially dangerous relationship with the lingual nerve.

The arterial supply to the submandibular gland is via branches of the facial artery; venous drainage is to the facial vein. These vessels cross the superoexternal aspect of the gland. In contrast to the parotid, the submandibular gland contains no lymph nodes. However, the walls of the submandibular space contain a rich lymphatic network that drains the floor of the mouth, half of the tongue, the nose, the cheek, and the eyelid. The submandibular lymph nodes are classed in four groups according to their position with respect to the facial vein (pre- or retroglandular and pre- or retrovascular). The most constant node lies at the superior border of the gland, near the lingual nerve.

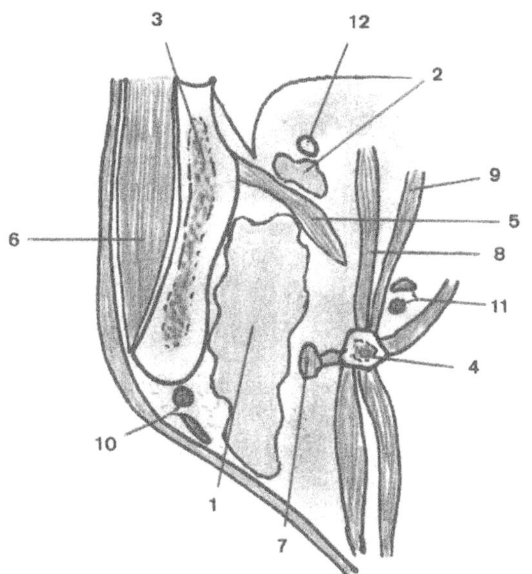

Fig. 3.3. Submandibular space: anteroposterior view. *1* Submandibular gland, *2* anterior extension of the submandibular gland, *3* mandible, *4* hyoid bone, *5* mylohyoid muscle, *6* masseter muscle, *7* digastric muscle, *8* hyoglossal muscle, *9* styloglossus muscle, *10* facial artery and vein, *11* lingual artery and vein, *12* Wharton's duct

3.1.3 Sublingual Gland

A part of the floor of the mouth, the sublingual space is bounded by the inner surface of the mandibular gingiva and the hyoglossal and mylohyoid muscles forming the sublingual floor (Fig. 3.4). This compartment of the oral cavity contains the sublingual gland, the deep anterior portion of the submandibular gland, Wharton's duct, the excretory ducts of the sublingual gland, the lingual and hypoglossal nerves, and the sublingual blood vessels and lymphatics (Yasumoto et al. 1993).

The almond-shaped sublingual gland lies on the mylohyoid muscle, between the mandible and the genioglossus muscle; it is in contact with the contralateral sublingual gland. Posteriorly, the sublingual gland is in direct contact with the anterior part of the submandibular gland, located posteromedially in the floor of the mouth (Yasumoto et al. 1993).

The sublingual gland is drained by numerous small ducts (ducts of Walther), some of which unite to form the major sublingual duct (Bartholin's duct); Bartholin's duct may empty into Wharton's duct or open directly into the floor of the mouth (BOURJAT and KAHN 1995).

The sublingual gland is supplied by the sublingual artery, which arises from the lingual artery, and by branches of the submental artery that pierce the mylohyoid muscle to reach it (YASUMOTO et al. 1993).

Lymphatic drainage from the sublingual area is into the homolateral submental and submandibular group of suprahyoid lymph nodes.

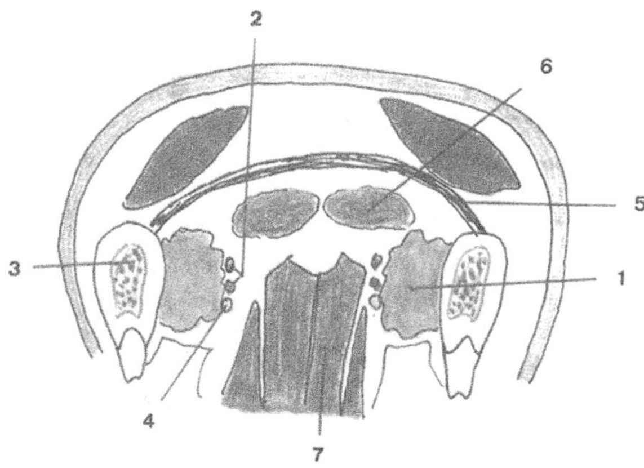

Fig. 3.4. Floor of the mouth: longitudinal scan. *1* Sublingual gland, *2* lingual vessels, *3* mandible, *4* Wharton's duct, *5* mylohyoid muscle, *6* geniohyoid muscle, *7* genioglossus muscle

3.1.4 Accessory Salivary Glands

The minor salivary glands are small glandular islets disseminated throughout the cervicofacial region, including the oral cavity, the tongue, the palate, the paranasal sinuses, the pharynx, and the larynx; they are also found in the trachea and bronchi. These accessory glands have a mixed seromucous structure, except for those on the hard palate, which contain only mucous-secreting cells. The number of accessory salivary glands has been estimated at over 750 (SILVERS and SOM 1998).

3.2 Sonographic Anatomy

3.2.1 Technical Modalities

High-frequency sonography (7.5–13 MHz) is usually performed with a linear probe (STEINER 1994c). A lower frequency (2–4 MHz) sector probe facilitates examination of the parotid in individuals with a thick neck, because the depth of beam penetration compensates for the loss of spatial resolution. The B-mode settings must be carefully adjusted. Use of a water bath improves evaluation of very superficial structures. Color Doppler requires use of a low pulse repetition frequency (PRF) (approx. 15 cm/s), with a low band pass filter and elevated persistence for parenchymal analysis (RAFFAELLI et al. 1995). A color Doppler unit capable of demonstrating very slow flow (less than 5 cm/s) may prove useful owing to the small diameter of the normal vascular structures. The pressure exerted by the probe must be minimal to avoid obliteration of color signals (MARTINOLI et al. 1994). The patient is examined in the supine position, with the neck hyperextended; bilateral scanning of all of the salivary glands and the cervical node-bearing areas is obligatory and permits comparative analysis. Measurement of the peak systolic velocity (PSV) by pulsed Doppler requires angle correction, and thus awareness of the direction of the vessel being analyzed. For tortuous intraparenchymal vessels, measurement is easier with power Doppler.

3.2.2 Parotid Gland

The parotid is imaged using both transverse scans at a right angle to the ascending ramus of the mandible and longitudinal scans (RAFFAELLI et al. 1995). On transverse views (Fig. 3.5), the gland is surrounded by the acoustic shadows created by the ascending ramus of the mandible anteriorly and the mastoid posteriorly. These adjacent bony structures form a true acoustic window for exploration of the parotid. The greater the distance between the mastoid and the mandible, the better the quality of parotid examination (BRUNETON et al. 1987). The superficial planes are limited medially by a thin, strongly echoic line corresponding to the superficial cervical fascia (BRUNETON et al. 1987).

The normal parotid parenchyma is sonographically homogeneous (Fig. 3.6); its echogenicity is usually similar to that of the thyroid gland but markedly lower than that of the adjacent masseter muscle. Gland echogenicity varies considerably, depending on the fat content; the presence of overabundant fat may create a strongly hyperechoic pattern, with strong posterior attenuation.

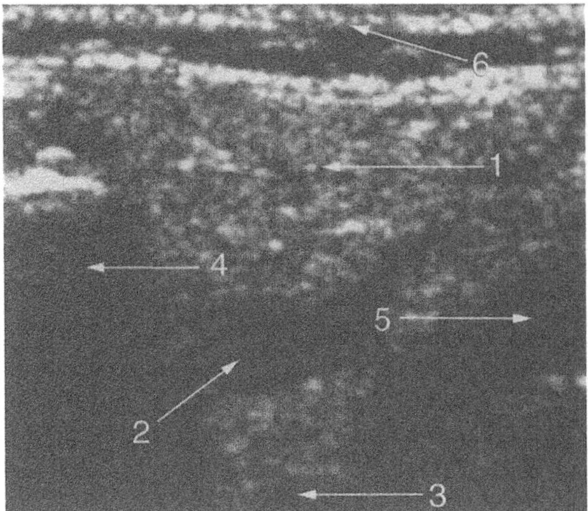

Fig. 3.5. Transverse scan of a parotid gland: *1* parotid parenchyma, *2* venous plane, *3* external carotid artery, *4* ramus of mandible, *5* acoustic shadow of the mastoid, *6* superficial cervical fascia

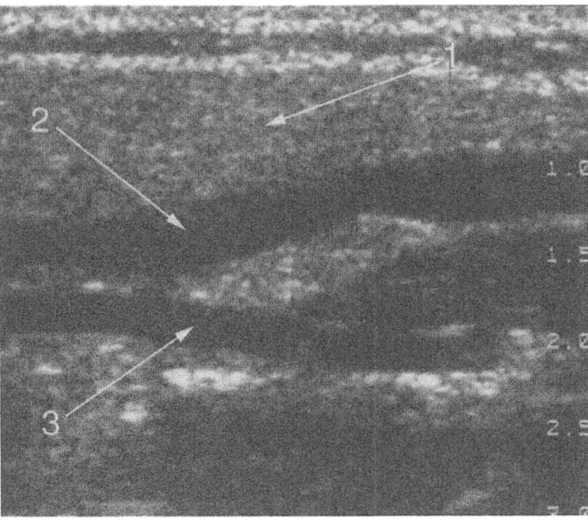

Fig. 3.6. Longitudinal scan of a parotid gland: *1* parotid parenchyma, *2* venous plane, *3* external carotid artery

The normal parotid gland averages 46.3±7.7 mm in length; the retromandibular portion measures 22.8±3.6 mm (Dost and Kaiser 1997). The entire infrafacial part of the parotid gland is visible sonographically, as is the superficial part; the endofacial portion is only partially accessible to sonography. The portion of the parotid gland between the venous plane and the external carotid artery is usually well visualized, if necessary by using a low-frequency transducer. The pharyngeal parotid extension is usually not visible (Gritzmann 1989) but the masseter extension is consistently accessible to US study (Fig. 3.7). Examination of the retrostyloid space and its relations with the parotid is usually not possible. In favorable cases, the muscles and the stylomandibular ligament separating the parotid space from the posterior subparotid area can be identified as a slightly irregular hypoechoic zone (Bruneton et al. 1987). Although the facial nerve is not directly visible by US, its position can be deduced by locating the venous plane of the parotid that lies against the superficial aspect of the nerve trunk (Bruneton et al. 1987). This venous plane can be accurately located by B-mode imaging in 70% of normal subjects, if necessary with the aid of a Valsalva maneuver (Fig. 3.8). Color Doppler and especially power Doppler are more effective, permitting visualization of the venous plane in 93% of patients (Thoron et al. 1996) (Fig. 3.9). Scanning is optimal in the longitudinal oblique plane, after localization of the external jugular vein at the lower pole of the gland.

The external carotid artery and the inconstant external carotid vein may be visualized within the deep portion of the parotid gland by color Doppler using longitudinal scans. The external carotid artery gives off five or six branches to the parotid parenchyma; these vessels usually run parallel to the drainage veins of the gland that empty into the venous confluence (Martinoli et al. 1994).

The normal intraglandular ductal system is not visible sonographically. Stensen's duct is inconstantly visible; it should be sought systematically on transverse scans parallel to the horizontal body of the mandible, anterior to the masseter, at the extremity of the masseter parotid extension, using a water bath if needed (Fig. 3.10). When dilated, Stensen's duct may be followed as it runs within the buccal surface of the cheek to its ostium. The initial, intraparotid segment

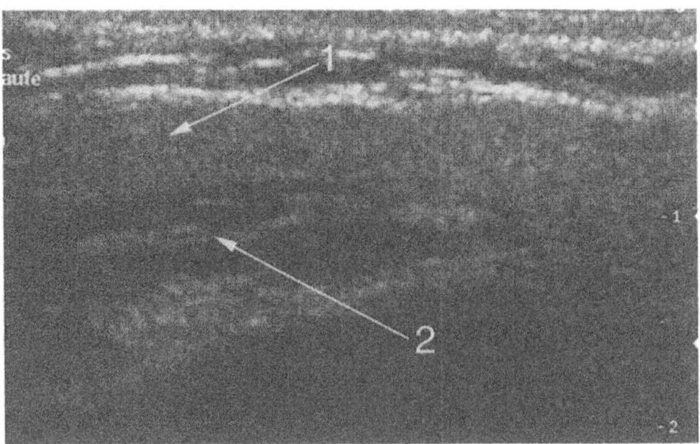

Fig. 3.7. Transverse scan: masseter extension of the parotid. *1* Masseter extension, *2* masseter

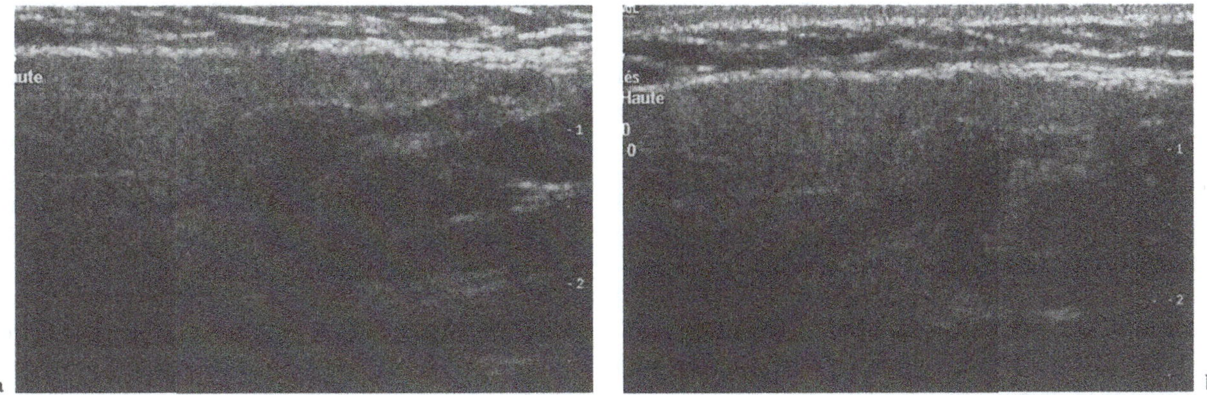

Fig. 3.8 a Oblique longitudinal scan of the parotid gland: The venous plane of the parotid is difficult to identify during uncontrolled breathing. b Same patient as in a: The venous plane of the parotid is visible on this oblique longitudinal scan obtained during a Valsalva maneuver

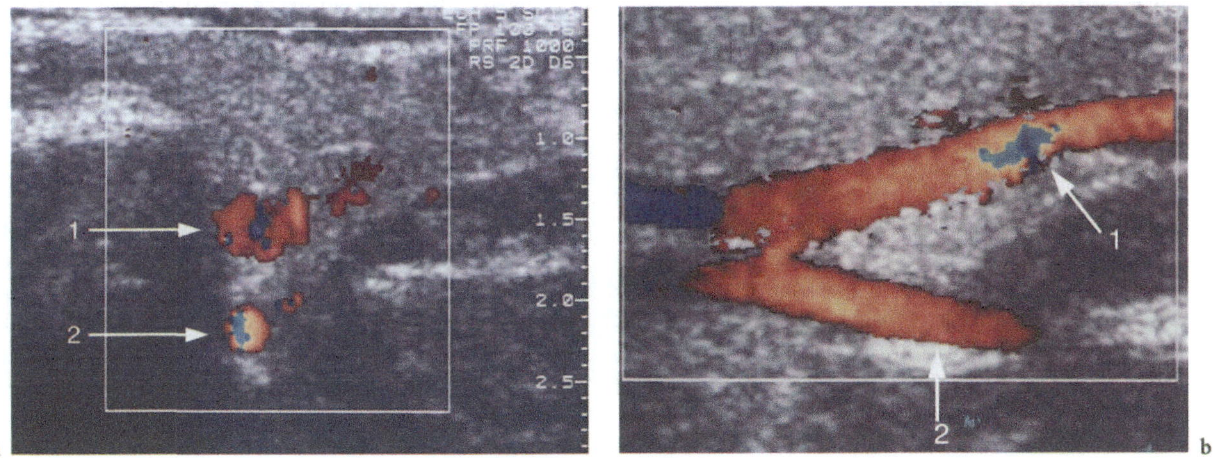

Fig. 3.9a,b. Color Doppler: a transverse scan, b oblique longitudinal scan. *1* venous plane of the parotid, *2* external carotid artery

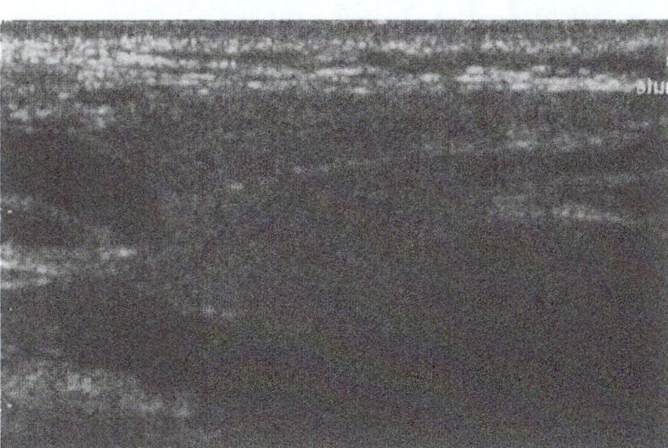

Fig. 3.10. Longitudinal scan of the parotid: note the hyperechoic line delimiting the intraparotid portion of Stensen's duct

of Stensen's duct is sometimes visible as two hyperechoic lines at the level of the anterior segment of the gland; this provides an indication of the position of the nearby intraglandular facial nerve (Marsot-Dupuch et al. 1992).

Currently, small intra- or periparotid nodal structures are visualized sonographically in the normal parotid (Katz 1991). These well-delimited, hypoechoic oval nodes smaller than 1 cm in diameter have a central hyperechoic structure corresponding to the nodal hilum (Raffaelli et al. 1995) (Fig. 3.11). Color Doppler allowing detection of slow flows (PRF less than 10 cm/s) may demonstrate the hilar-type vascular pattern of these nodes. A pretragal node is nearly always visible.

3.2.3 Submandibular Gland

The entire submandibular gland can be visualized sonographically (Bartlett and Pon 1984) using recurrent oblique scans and a high-frequency transducer (Figs. 3.12, 3.13). Use of a small probe facilitates access to the gland, as it can easily be inserted under the external border of the mandible.

The body of the gland can be accurately examined using oblique transverse and longitudinal scans (Raffaelli et al. 1995). Gland echogenicity is comparable to that of the parotid, and is less variable. The normal submandibular gland has a mean length of 35±5.7 mm (Dost and Kaiser 1997).

The mylohyoid muscle is readily visualized, allowing localization of the anterior extension of the submandibular gland that lies against the deep aspect of the mylohyoid.

The facial artery arises from the external carotid artery, sometimes in common with the lingual artery. The facial artery loops laterally around the submandibular gland, where it is readily localized by color Doppler (Fig. 3.14). Like the facial vein, the facial artery gives off several branches to the deep parenchyma of the submandibular gland that are detectable by color Doppler; the arrangement of these branches reflects the lobar architecture of the submandibular gland parenchyma (Martinoli et al. 1994).

A tubular structure with thick, echogenic walls is often visualized within the gland on color-Doppler sonograms. This longitudinal vessel is an intraparenchymal branch of the facial vein and must not be confused with a dilated excretory duct (Martinoli et al. 1994) (Fig. 3.15).

The sublingual vessels are identified by color Doppler on the internal aspect of the submandibular gland. These tubular structures give off branches to the lingual muscles and to the sublingual gland (Yasumoto et al. 1993).

The normal intraglandular ductal structures cannot be seen by sonography. On oblique anterior transverse scans of the floor of the mouth and median longitudinal scans obtained with the probe in a submental position, Wharton's duct is visible in 53% of subjects as it courses through the sublingual space (Yasumoto et al. 1993) (Fig. 3.16). On longitudinal scans, the duct

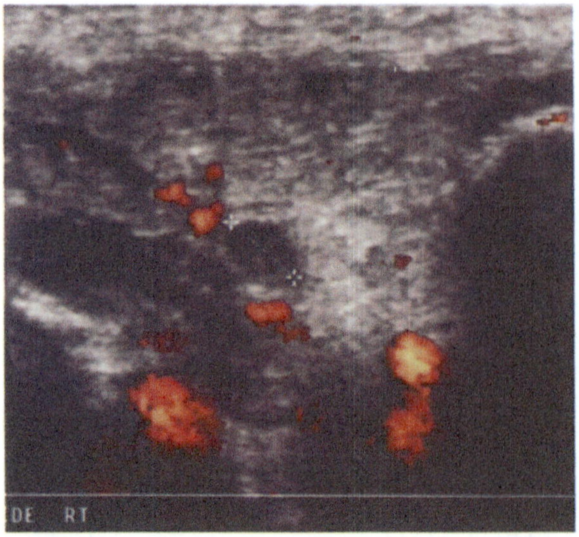

Fig. 3.11. Transverse scan of a normal parotid in an asymptomatic patient: intraparotid node

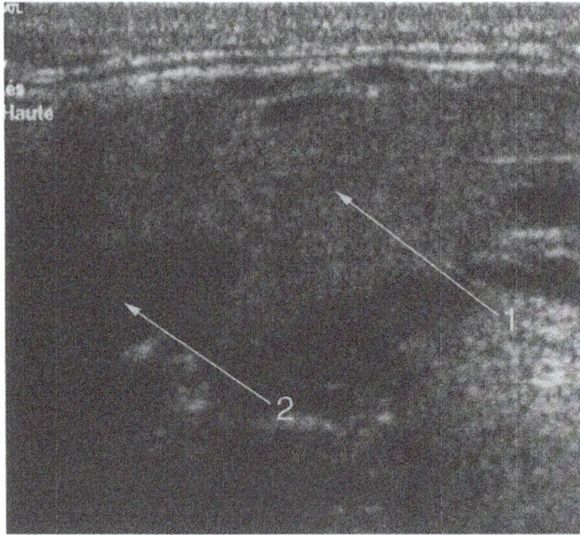

Fig. 3.12. Recurrent transverse scan of a submandibular gland. *1* submandibular gland, *2* mylohyoid muscle

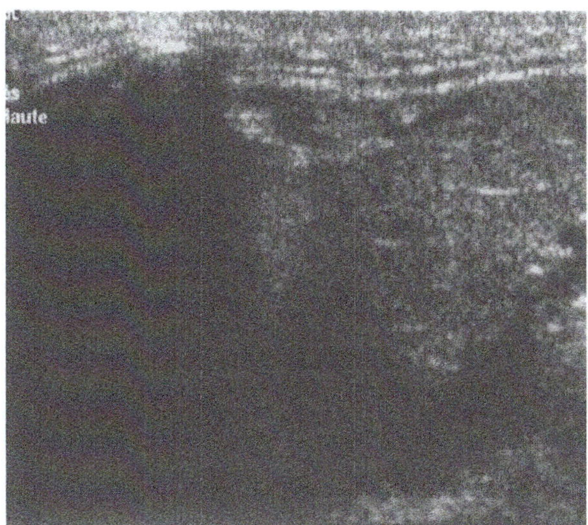

a

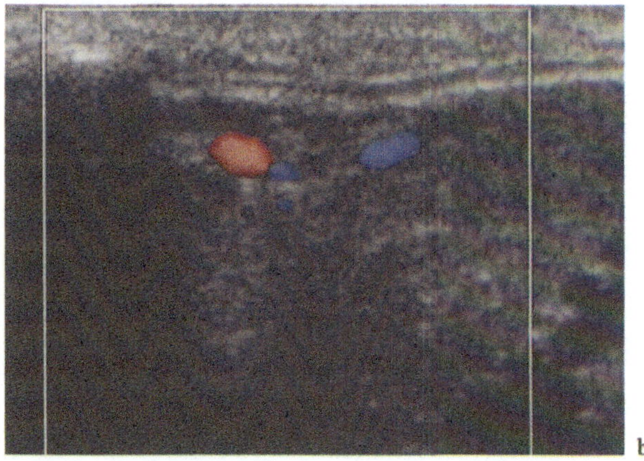

b

Fig. 3.13a,b. Longitudinal scan of a submandibular gland in B-mode (**a**) and color Doppler (**b**)

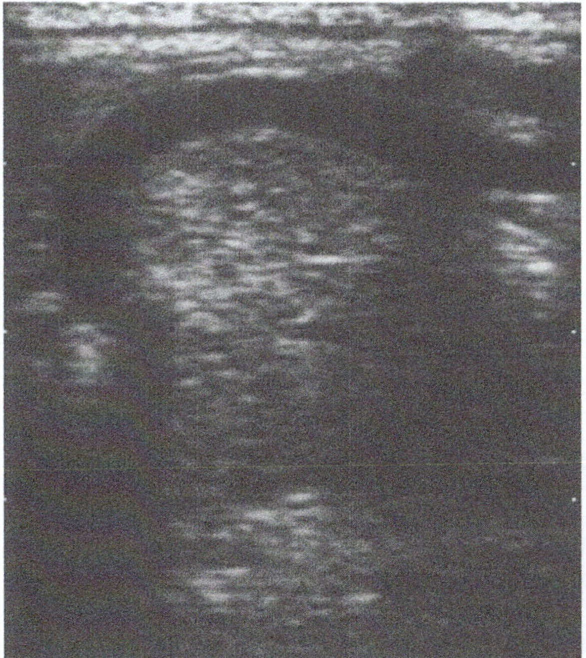

Fig. 3.14. Submandibular gland: loop of the facial artery

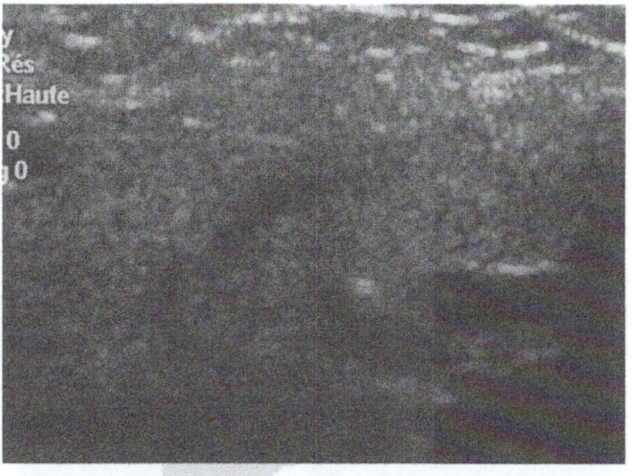

a

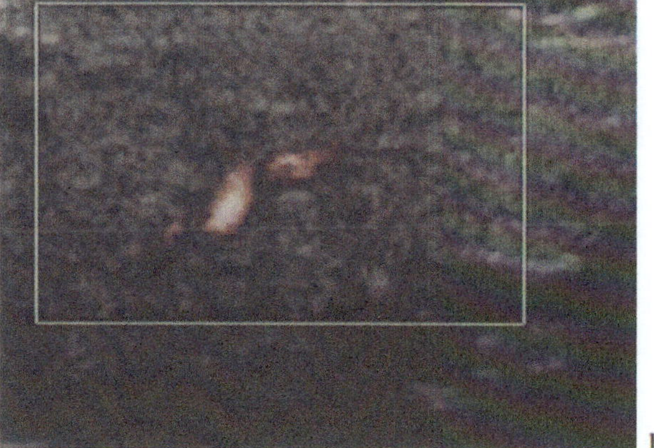

b

Fig. 3.15a,b. Recurrent transverse scan of the submandibular gland: **a** The anechoic tubular structure in the center of the gland parenchyma suggests ductal dilatation, but power Doppler (**b**) reveals its vascular origin

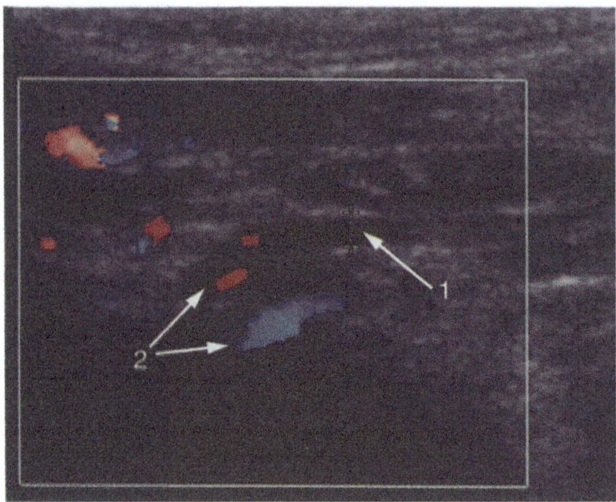

Fig. 3.16. Oblique transverse scan of the floor of the mouth: color Doppler. *1* Wharton's duct, *2* sublingual vessels

images as an anechoic structure with a mean diameter of less than 3 mm running in contact with the superointernal border of the sublingual gland. The submandibular duct cannot be formally distinguished by B-mode imaging from the usually adjacent, though slightly anterior, sublingual vessels. Color Doppler allows identification of the submandibular duct because it is the only structure without any signal (YASUMOTO et al. 1993). When dilated, all of Wharton's duct can be assessed on 45° oblique transverse scans.

In the normal subject, nodal structures are visible sonographically in the submandibular space. They are easy to distinguish from the gland because they typically have a hyperechoic hilum.

3.2.4 Sublingual Gland

The small size of the sublingual space and its superficial location make it particularly accessible to high-frequency sonography (NEUHOLD et al. 1986) (Figs. 3.17, 3.18).

Longitudinal and transverse scans are obtained from a submental position; a water bath is often very helpful. The sublingual gland is best imaged in the transverse plane. Although the gland is nearly always visible (93% of subjects), precise delineation can be difficult, and good images are obtained in only 36% of cases (YASUMOTO et al. 1993).

The echogenicity of the sublingual gland is similar to that of the other major salivary glands. Mean length on oblique transverse scans is 32 mm, while mean width is 12 mm; sonographic data are well-correlated with anatomic findings (YASUMOTO et al. 1993).

a

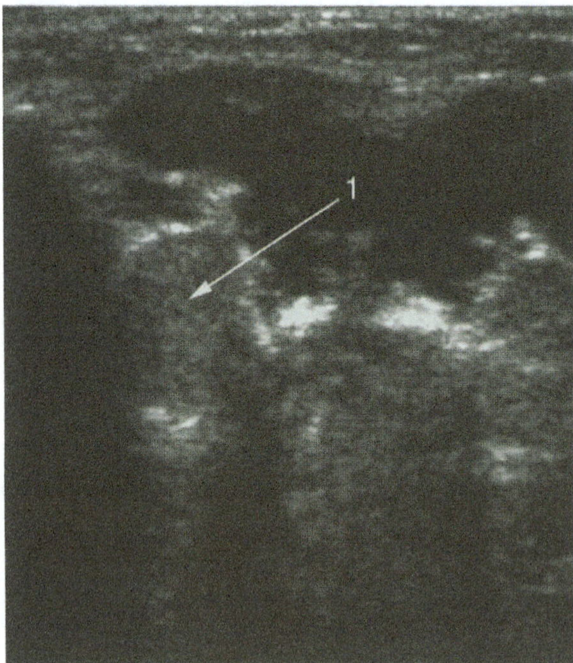

b

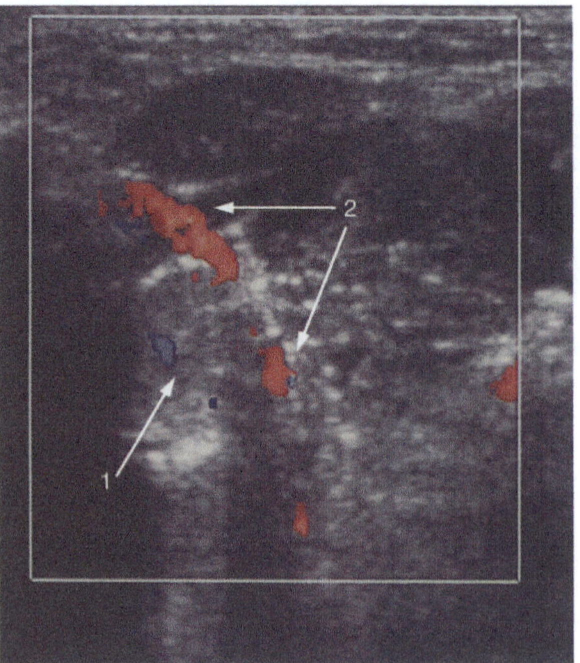

Fig. 3.17a,b. Sublingual gland: longitudinal scan, B-mode (**a**) and color Doppler (**b**). *1* sublingual gland, *2* sublingual vessels

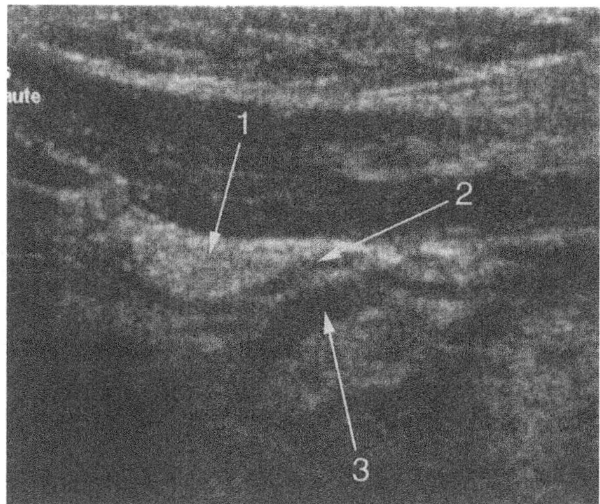

Fig. 3.18. Sublingual gland: oblique transverse scan. *1* sublingual gland, *2* sublingual artery, *3* Wharton's duct

The sublingual gland is related to the mandible (which creates an acoustic shadow that hampers exploration of the anterior part of the gland) and to the mylohyoid and genioglossus muscles, both of which are readily identified by US.

Color Doppler demonstrates the lingual vessels coursing beneath the deep margin of the submandibular gland and the anterior submental artery that pierces the mylohyoid muscle to supply the tongue (Martinoli et al. 1994).

The normal intraglandular ductal system and the excretory ducts are not visible by sonography.

3.2.5 Accessory Salivary Glands

The normal accessory salivary glands cannot be visualized by US. High-frequency intraoral sonography may prove helpful for the diagnosis of salivary masses or cysts involving the accessory glands, and in particular palatal lesions (Ishii et al. 1999).

3.2.6 Specific Techniques

3.2.6.1 Ultrasonic Tracking Systems and Three-dimensional Imaging

The ultrasonic tracking systems developed by certain manufacturers, such as the Siemens SieScape (Fig. 3.19), permit continuous freehand acquisition of an anatomic structure that extends considerably beyond the field of the transducer. This allows visualization, on a single scan, of the entire parotid in the coronal plane or of the base of the tongue and both sublingual and submandibular glands.

Such acquisitions have limited diagnostic value, and are useful primarily for biometric studies or comparative analyses. However, because the documents obtained resemble the images obtained with other radiological techniques, they help to improve the credibility of sonography.

B-mode imaging today can be completed by color Doppler or power Doppler. Use of three-dimensional B-mode surface imaging for salivary gland US has not been reported to date. Three-dimensional reconstructions with power Doppler appear more interesting, particularly for evaluation of the vascular relations of tumors and their overall vascularity (Fig. 3.20).

3.2.6.2 Stimulation of Saliva Secretion

Secretion of saliva is controlled by the parasympathetic fibers via the cranial nerves (chorda tympani,

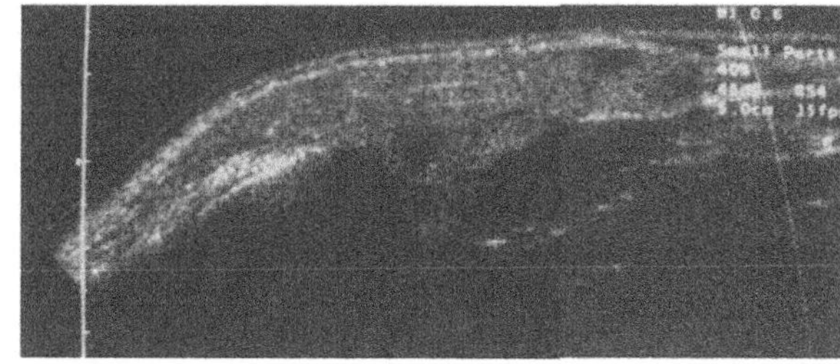

Fig. 3.19. SieScape B-mode study: longitudinal scan of a parotid

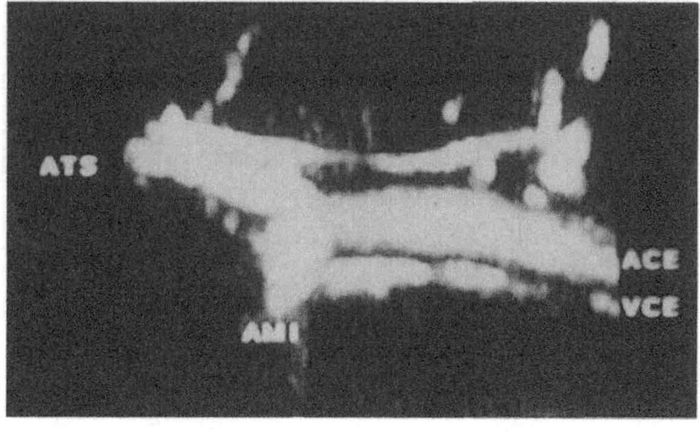

Fig. 3.20. Three-dimensional imaging with power Doppler: external carotid artery and its parotid branches

trigeminal nerve, glossopharyngeal nerve). Salivary secretion is accompanied by intense hyperemia with a drop in arterial resistance (KOHLER and WINTER 1985). Daily saliva production in the adult ranges from 1000 to 1500 cc. The parotid and submandibular glands have an equivalent secretion that represents 90% of the total salivary secretion; 5% is produced by the sublingual glands and 5% by the accessory salivary glands.

Several clinical tests of salivary function allowing qualitative assessment have been described (KOHLER and WINTER 1985). Salivary scintigraphy allows quantitative evaluation, but this costly procedure is rarely used. Doppler sonography permits both qualitative and quantitative analysis of salivary stimulation. The examination is performed before and after intraoral lemon juice stimulation. The patient is instructed to keep the lemon juice under the tongue because saliva secretion ceases rapidly as soon as the lemon juice is swallowed. Salivary gland vascularity can be assessed by color Doppler US or power Doppler (MARTINOLI et al. 1994) (Fig. 3.21). Arterial PSVs and the resistive indices (RIs) of the parenchymal arteries can be measured before and after lemon stimulation, but measurements are often artifacted by buccal movements (MARTINOLI et al. 1994).

Color Doppler US of pre- and post-stimulation arterial blood flow reveals significant changes for the submandibular glands, namely a constant increase in the arterial PSV and a decrease in the RI (ARIJI et al. 1998). In the study of MARTINOLI et al. (1994), the mean PSV during stimulation rose from 8.48±2.84 cm/s to 24.03±10.72 cm/s and the RI dropped from 0.70±0.04 to 0.58±0.04.

3.2.6.3
US-guided Aspiration Biopsy

Fine-needle (22-gauge) aspiration biopsy (FNAB) of salivary gland masses (especially parotid masses) remains controversial. Procedure safety is improved by US and color Doppler guidance, allowing avoidance of necrotic zones and major vessels (MARTINOLI et al. 1994).

Certain investigators consider FNAB sufficiently accurate (specificity 72%) to warrant systematic use (FELD et al. 1999; KATE et al. 1998); others consider the procedure unjustified, owing to the risk of tumor seeding (especially for pleomorphic adenomas), the high rate of false-negative errors, and the fact that surgical excision is usually proposed anyway for all parotid and submandibular gland masses (SILVERS and SOM 1998).

Despite this debate, salivary gland FNAB is useful in a number of situations: lesions where surgery is not absolutely indicated from the outset (elderly subject or poor surgical candidate), suspected pseudotumoral inflammatory pathology, context or history of non-Hodgkin's lymphoma or disseminated neoplasia, submandibular location.

Aspiration biopsy of fluid masses in the parotid or floor of the mouth is routine practice and allows diagnosis of an abscess or sialocele (MAGARAM and GOODING 1981).

a 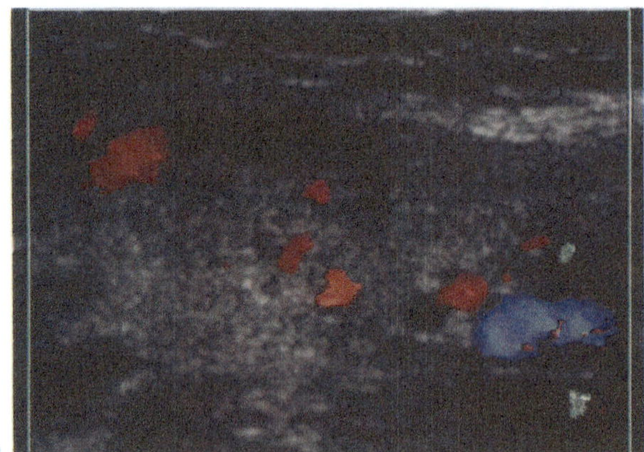

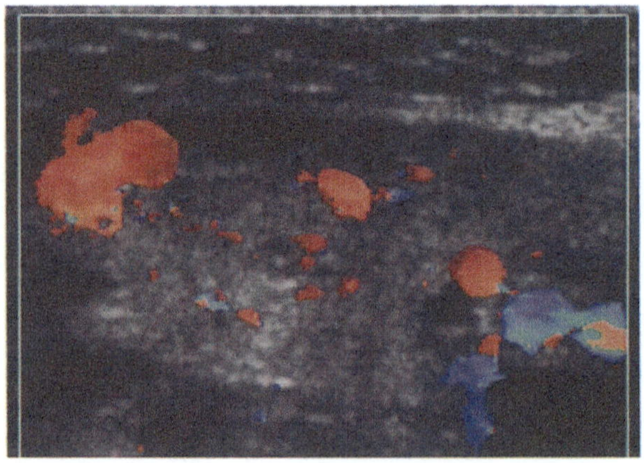 b

Fig. 3.21a,b. Submandibular gland: color Doppler before (**a**) and after (**b**) stimulation of saliva secretion with lemon juice. Multiplication of the number of signals reflects gland hyperemia

3.3 Other Imaging Modalities

While sonography is often the first technique for salivary gland imaging, other modalities are also frequently used during initial workup or as complementary procedures. No consensus has been reached concerning the role of and the indications for the various techniques. Technical progress, particularly in MRI, explains the continuous changes in salivary gland examination protocols. Although MRI has become the gold standard for salivary gland tumors, CT remains indicated for lesions of infectious origin and salivary gland pathologies in children.

3.3.1 Sialography

Following a series of plain films centered on the salivary gland under investigation, cannulation of the ostium of Stensen's duct or Wharton's duct permits opacification of the parotid or submandibular gland duct system with a water-soluble contrast agent. Sialograms are obtained during filling with the contrast material and then during evacuation, after removal of the catheter.

This difficult-to-perform technique requires an experienced operator. Accidents are not uncommon, and failed duct cannulation has been reported in up to 20% of all submandibular sialographies (Laudenbach and Moreau 1974).

Sialography permits detailed analysis of the salivary ducts, and in particular the search for a developmental anomaly or salivary calculi. Detailed radiological findings can be obtained for inflammatory processes involving the gland parenchyma, including the secondary ducts, and the glandular acini are sometimes opacified, but sialograms are often difficult to interpret. Sialography is increasingly being replaced by other imaging techniques for inflammatory processes, and has been completely abandoned for salivary gland tumors.

3.3.2 Scintigraphy

Like the thyroid, the parotid and submandibular glands take up the radioactive tracer technetium pertechnetate (Tc 99m); the sublingual glands and accessory glands do not. Following intravenous tracer injection, digitized scans are taken at regular short intervals; delayed films are also obtained. Curves of tracer uptake and elimination are plotted; administration of lemon juice allows assessment of tracer evacuation. Radionuclide scanning does not permit anatomic study; it merely allows assessment of gland function. Salivary gland tumors are characterized as a function of tracer uptake (Reinhardt and Dross 1984).

^{99m}Tc scintigraphy can usefully confirm decreased salivary function and is indicated in particular for the diagnosis of certain tumors with increased activity, such as cystadenolymphoma and oncocytoma (Higashi et al. 1987).

Gallium scintigraphy and positron emission tomography have also been used, but results to date have been disappointing (Higashi et al. 1989; Keyes et al. 1994).

3.3.3 CT

CT studies of salivary gland disease must cover the entire cervicofacial region in order to evaluate all of the salivary glands and the node-bearing areas. Contiguous 2-mm-thick CT scans obtained in the axial projection before and after of injection contrast medium are sometimes supplemented by longitudinal scans for analysis of the parotid glands.

The major salivary glands (including the sublingual glands) are readily visualized by CT. The density of the normal parotid is often lower than that of the other salivary glands, owing to its fat content (Bernier et al. 1994).

CT can accurately define the various glands, the fat-containing spaces, and the vascular structures; the pharyngeal parotid extension and the adjacent parapharyngeal space are also clearly visualized (Bryan et al. 1982). The facial nerve itself is not visible as it courses through the parotid. High-resolution CT scans permit optimum analysis of the mandible but are rarely useful in practice. The spatial resolution of CT is lower that of high-frequency sonography, and the submandibular duct can be visualized in only 60% of normal subjects, in the space between the mylohyoid and hyoglossal muscles (Aasen and Kolbenstvedt 1992).

3.3.4 MRI

All of the salivary glands can be evaluated by MRI using a head coil; use of surface coils has proven unsatisfactory (Bourjat and Kahn 1995). Axial and coronal views (3-mm-thick sections) are obtained; transverse scans are occasionally helpful for evaluation of the masseter extension of the parotid (Marsot-Dupuch et al. 1992).

Both T_1- and T_2-weighted sequences are performed. Gadolinium injection is not routinely recommended. Examination of the parotid requires T_1-weighted sequences with fat suppression (Vogl et al. 1990).

MRI permits detailed analysis of the superficial planes; the superficial cervical fascia in particular is well-visualized. Owing to its fat content, the parotid has a high T_1-weighted signal intensity. The facial nerve is visible as it exits the stylomastoid foramen, behind the parotid (Teresi et al. 1987a). Visibility of the intraparotid portion of the facial nerve remains controversial; only the adjacent ductal structures can be formally identified (Thibault et al. 1993).

The submandibular gland has a signal intensity intermediate between that of muscle and fat. MRI permits optimum analysis of the floor of the mouth and the sublingual glands, which are hyperintense to the adjacent muscles on T_1-weighted sequences (Bernier et al. 1994).

MR sialography has recently been described for examination of the parotid and the submandibular glands. Contiguous 3-mm-thick sections are obtained using T_2-weighted sequences (RT: 9000; ET: 270) with a circular coil (Lomas et al. 1996). The major salivary ducts and their first-order branches are well-analyzed. Although less accurate than conventional sialography, MR sialography will undoubtedly progressively replace it, namely for inflammatory pathologies (Varghese et al. 1999).

3.4 Cysts and Malformations

3.4.1 Cystic Lesions

Cystic lesions of the salivary glands are rare, accounting for less than 5% of all sonographically detected salivary gland masses (Rice 1984). The majority of true cysts occur in the parotid gland.

3.4.1.1 HIV-related Lymphoepithelial Cysts

Currently the most common type of parotid cyst, lymphoepithelial cysts occur in up to 83% of HIV-positive individuals. The complex pathophysiology of these lesions has been attributed to a combination of diffuse intraparotid lymphoid infiltration and dilatation of gland excretory ducts secondary to partial obstruction (Tunkel et al. 1989; Vona et al. 1994). The trophism for the parotid can be explained by the developmental particularities of this gland; lymphoepithelial cysts of the submandibular glands are much less common (Gottesman et al. 1996).

Cyst formation can be an early manifestation of HIV infection, occurring in patients who are still asymptomatic; they are thus not correlated with the stage of the disease (Holliday et al. 1988). In particular, patients usually do not have any opportunistic infections or symptoms of overt AIDS at initial diagnosis of the cysts (Shugar et al. 1988). Clinically, the cysts manifest as bilateral and sometimes painful parotid enlargement. Cervical lymphadenopathy is observed in 20%–80% of patients (Martinoli et al. 1994; Vona et al. 1994).

Sonography usually suffices for diagnosis of these predominantly superficial, multicystic parotid masses (Fig. 3.22). The highly echogenic septa may contain vessels demonstrable by color Doppler US (Fig. 3.23). The cysts often have an echoic, pseudotissular echotexture (the precipitation of calcium oxalate crystals creates high-level echoes in suspension). The surrounding gland parenchyma appears normal in the adult, but in children it may be inhomogeneous and indicative of associated parotitis. Certain lymphoepithelial cysts have a hyperechoic, vascularized solid component corresponding to lymphoid tissue. Such mixed-type cysts always have a hilar-type vascular pattern on color Doppler studies; on spectral analysis the mean PSV is less than 20 cm/s and the RI is relatively low RI (mean 0.57). US-guided FNAB of these cysts often reveals a mucinous content. Bacterial superinfection has been reported in 30% of cases and an association with cytomegalovirus in 50% (Martinoli et al. 1994; Vona et al. 1994).

Other imaging techniques are usually not required for diagnosis; they are reserved for preoperative workup of atypical mixed lesions with a predominance of solid components or involvement of the deep portion of the parotid. CT and MRI can confirm the fluid nature of the lesion (Gooding et al. 1992). Parotid cysts have an extremely high intensity signal on T_2-weighted sequences; on T_1-weighted images the signal intensity may be difficult to interpret because of the thickness of cyst contents.

The features and the pathogenesis of HIV-related lymphoepithelial cysts are similar to those of the bilateral cystic parotid lesions encountered in Sjögren's

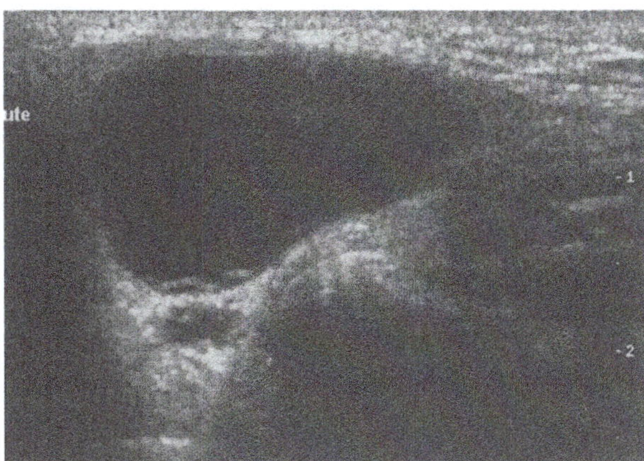

Fig. 3.22. HIV-positive patient. Large cystic parotid mass containing echoic sediment. Small associated posterior cystic mass. Lymphoepithelial cysts

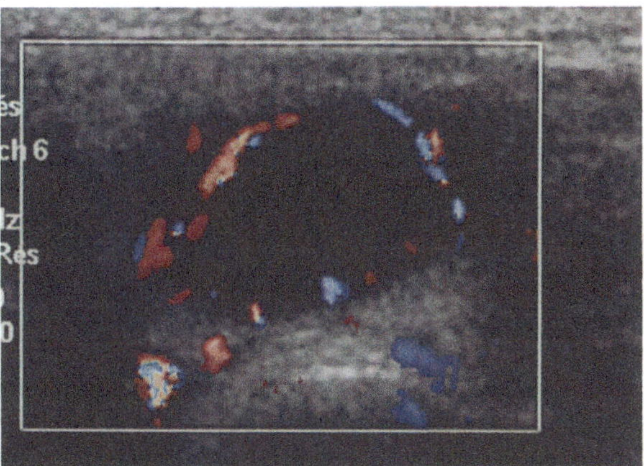

Fig. 3.23. Lymphoepithelial cyst in an HIV-positive patient; the parietal hypervascularity on color Doppler is related to a lymphoid tissue component

syndrome and Warthin's tumor, which are the main differential diagnoses. Sjögren's syndrome occurs in a different clinical context, however, and the cysts are usually much smaller and more numerous. In the absence of cervical lymphadenopathy, lymphoepithelial cysts may mimic Warthin's tumor on imaging studies. HIV serological tests, US-guided FNAB (which may demonstrate the presence of oncocytes, a characteristic of Warthin's tumor), and radionuclide scans showing intense tracer uptake are required to correct the diagnosis. The natural history of these cysts includes episodes of pain and multiple infections that may necessitate surgical drainage. Cysts often regress spontaneously in the terminal phase of AIDS, paralleling the aggravation of the immune deficiency (Vona et al.1994).

3.4.1.2
Auriculobranchial Fistulas and Cysts

These congenital anomalies are related to defective coalescence of the edges of the first branchial arch, on either side of the first branchial cleft. Mean age at diagnosis is 7 years. Parotid lesions may not manifest until a late stage as a cystic mass syndrome (often superinfected) or a retromandibular fistula. These cysts extend into the triangle of Poncet, formed by the union of the external acoustic meatus, the inferior margin of the mandible, and the homolateral greater horn of the hyoid bone. The external acoustic meatus and the drum must be examined systematically to search for the superior orifice of the fistula at the level of the plane of the meatus (Gaillard et al. 1981).

These solitary, well-delimited cysts are readily demonstrated by US. Features are pathognomonic; they are frequently homogeneously echogenic owing to their high content of cholesterol crystals (Gritzmann 1989). Color Doppler confirms their avascular nature (Fig. 3.24).

Fistulography of the inferior tract is rarely possible owing to inflammatory changes; when feasible, it shows the tract's ascending course towards the external acoustic meatus.

The existence of associated signs is indispensable for diagnosis of an intraparotid branchial cleft cyst, which is most likely a solitary lymphoepithelial cyst (Fig. 3.25) that can develop in response to any chronic inflammatory disease, with or without any relationship to an immune disorder (Silvers and Som 1998). CT or MRI is sometimes useful to confirm the cystic

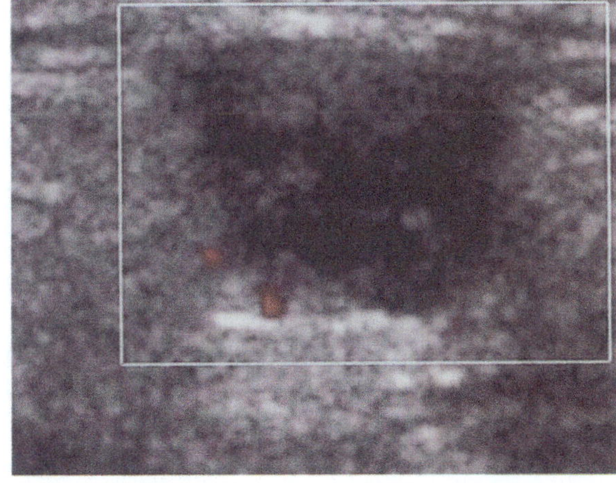

Fig. 3.24. Hypoechoic mass in the upper pole of a parotid gland. No vascularity detectable by power Doppler. First branchial cleft cyst

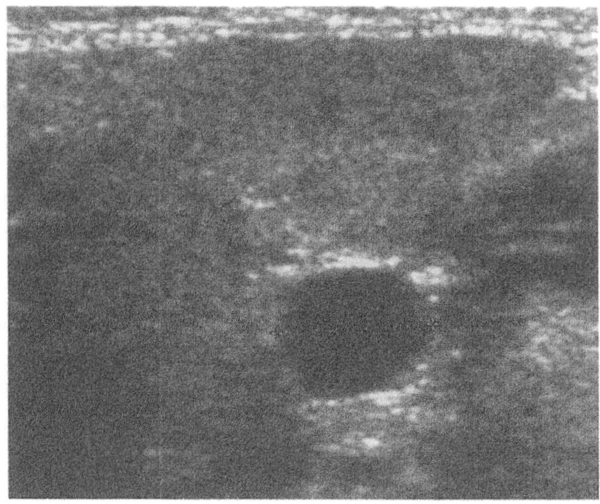

Fig. 3.25. Thin-walled echolucent cyst deep within the parotid. No associated signs. Solitary lymphoepithelial cyst

nature of the lesion, to rule out the presence of a tissue component, or to obtain precise topographical information for preoperative planning.

Diagnosis of second branchial cleft cysts and fistulas is rarely a problem in salivary pathologies owing to their infrahyoid location. Other lesions occurring in the same locations may mimic branchial cleft cysts. Dermoid cysts are subcutaneous or infralobular superficial parotid masses connected by a fibrous tract to the cartilage of the auricle. Fibrochondromas manifest as pedunculate subcutaneous lesions of the parotid region associated with auricular malformations (Gaillard et al. 1981).

3.4.1.3 Salivary Cysts

Salivary cysts (sialoceles) are secondary to retention of saliva accumulation following obstruction of the ductal system; traumatic section of the excretory ducts can also result in development of a cystic salivary lesion (Fig. 3.26). Intermittent ductal obstruction and postinflammatory stricture are the usual causes; complete ductal obstruction usually leads to acinar and glandular atrophy (Peel and Gnepp 1985). Such cysts may be very large.

Retention cysts (also referred to as mucoceles) have a propensity for the buccolingual accessory salivary glands and the sublingual glands (mucous retention cysts of the sublingual gland are called ranulas). Retention cysts of the submandibular gland are less common (Meseguer et al. 1996). Imaging demonstrates a strictly fluid mass in the floor of the mouth; sonography reveals a solitary, well-delimited, echo-free mass (Gritzmann 1989). Located along the mylohyoid muscle, retention cysts usually include a thin anterior extension. Simple ranulas are true cysts with an epithelial lining; rupture of the wall of a simple ranula below the level of the mylohyoid muscle creates a usually painful pseudocyst (plunging ranula). Evaluation of these cysts in the floor of the mouth often requires a complementary imaging modality (usually MRI) to search for a tissue component. The differential diagnosis includes a number of other cystic lesions: epidermoid cyst, dermoid cyst, thyroglossal duct cyst, cystic hygroma. Diagnosis often requires histological examination (Coit et al. 1987). Diagnosis of a parotid cyst may be suggested by a clinical context of trauma or colic, in which case sonography may demonstrate a sialolith.

Sialography may be useful after trauma or when a suspected sialolith is not visible sonographically (Reinhardt and Dross 1984).

3.4.1.4 Polycystic Disease of the Parotid

This rare inherited disorder with a marked female predominance manifests as bilateral parotid enlargement; the recurrent episodes of swelling often begin in childhood. The parotid glands contain multiple cystic areas (Brown et al. 1993). Few studies have investigated the sonographic features of these rare lesions, but US may suggest the diagnosis when HIV serological tests are negative.

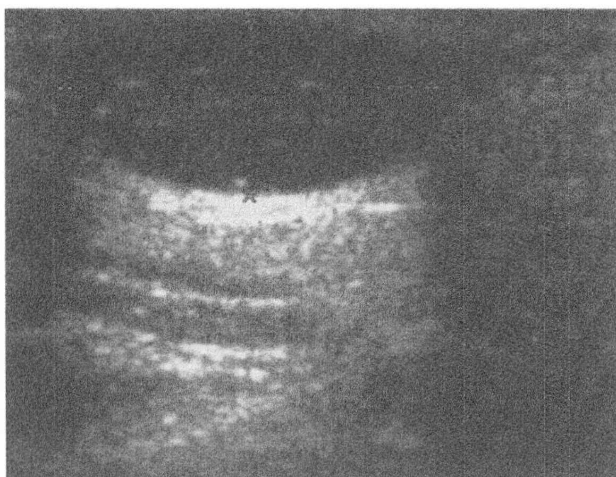

Fig. 3.26. Cystic mass with thick contents following facial trauma, with a penetrating injury of the parotid region. Superinfected parotid cyst

3.4.2 Malformations

Developmental anomalies of the salivary glands are rare. Glandular aplasia essentially affects the parotid, and may be unilateral (ALMADORI et al. 1997).

Anomalies can also exist in the position of the submandibular glands; enlargement of an accessory salivary gland may suggest a tumor. When accessible to sonography, these masses are readily diagnosed, owing to the echogenicity of the gland, the absence of a submandibular gland in the normal position, and positive results on color Doppler following saliva stimulation with lemon juice (CARNEY et al. 1996).

3.5 Salivary Gland Tumors

Although uncommon, tumors of the salivary glands have highly diverse origins. Occurring at an incidence of less than 3 per 100,000 population, salivary lesions account for less than 3% of all cervicofacial tumors and less than 0.1% of all deaths from cancer.

Parotid tumors are by far the most frequent; sublingual tumors are exceedingly rare. It has been estimated that for every 100 parotid tumors there are ten submandibular tumors, ten tumors arising in the accessory salivary glands, and only one sublingual tumor (THACKRAY and LUCAS 1974). Certain extremely rare benign or malignant lesions such as angiomyolipomas, sebaceous adenomas, various sarcomas, and primary parotid melanomas have no specific imaging features and require histological examination for diagnosis.

3.5.1 Benign Tumors

3.5.1.1 Pleomorphic Adenoma

Pleomorphic adenoma (benign mixed tumor) represents 70%–80% of all benign major salivary gland tumors; 84% occur in the parotid glands, 8% in the submandibular glands, 6.5% in the accessory salivary glands, and only 0.5% in the sublingual glands (SILVERS and SOM 1998). These multitissue lesions have a predominant epithelial component and varying amounts of myxoid, chondroid, myoepithelial, or osteoid tissue. Chondromyxoid lesions predominate (95% of cases). Female predominance has been observed for these slow-growing epithelial tumors. According to THACKRAY and LUCAS (1974), 90% of parotid tumors are well-delimited, firm and mobile nodules arising on the superficial part of the parotid, lateral to the plane of the facial nerve.

On US examination, the solid, encapsulated superficial mass appears well-demarcated and hypoechoic, with discrete posterior enhancement (Fig. 3.27) (BRUNETON et al. 1980). One or more extracapsular satellite nodules are present in 25% of cases and can cause recurrence if left untreated (Fig. 3.28) (BYRNE et al. 1989). Large tumors tend to be lobular, with an inhomogeneous echotexture related to necrosis, or to cystic or hemorrhagic changes (SOM et al. 1988); massive calcifications are sometimes present (Fig. 3.29).

Color Doppler US usually reveals a basket-like pattern of peripheral flow signals that is uncommon with other types of parotid tumors (Fig. 3.30) (MARTINOLI et al. 1994). There are no statistically significant differences in the RI or pulsatility index (PI) between pleomorphic adenoma and cystadenolymphoma (BENZEL et al. 1995).

For typical lesions, sonography is sufficient to suggest the diagnosis and indicate surgical excision (Fig. 3.31). Complementary imaging studies, usually MRI, are indicated for large (more than 3 cm) or atypical lesions and whenever spread to the pharyngeal parotid extension is suspected. MRI findings are highly variable. Small pleomorphic adenomas usually have a lower signal intensity than the surrounding tissue on T_1-weighted images and a high intensity signal on T_2-weighted views; they typically show homogeneous contrast enhancement after gadolin-

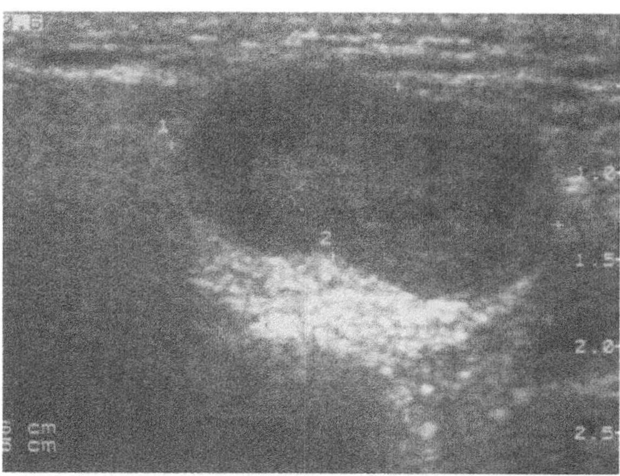

Fig. 3.27. Superficial, solid and well-delimited, homogeneously hypoechoic parotid nodule with posterior enhancement. Pleomorphic adenoma

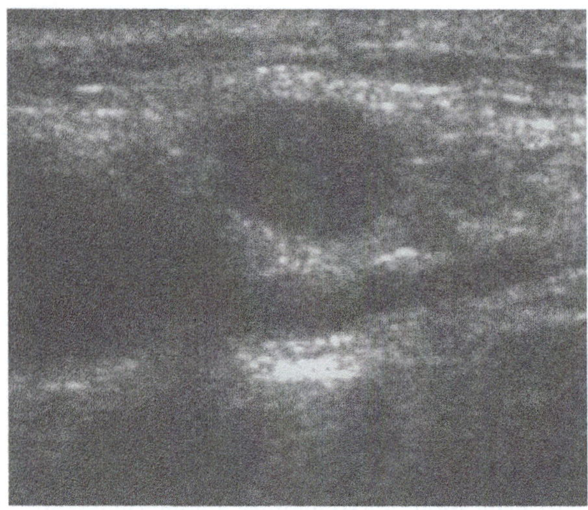

a

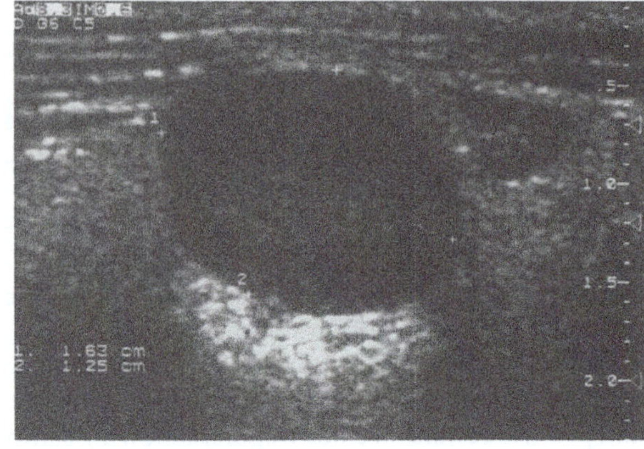

b

Fig. 3.28a,b. Satellite nodules of a pleomorphic adenoma

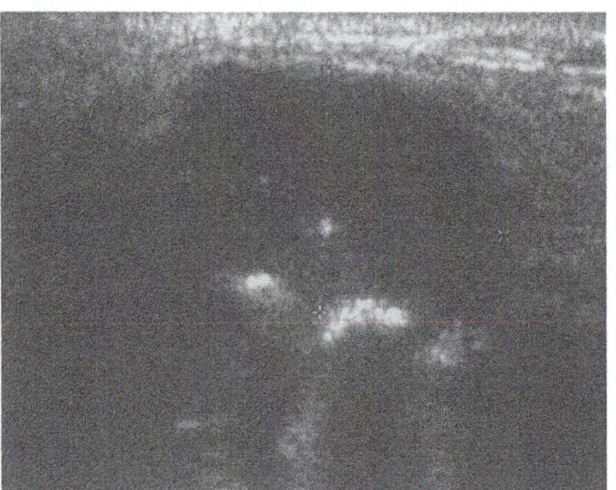

Fig. 3.29. Partially calcified pleomorphic parotid adenoma

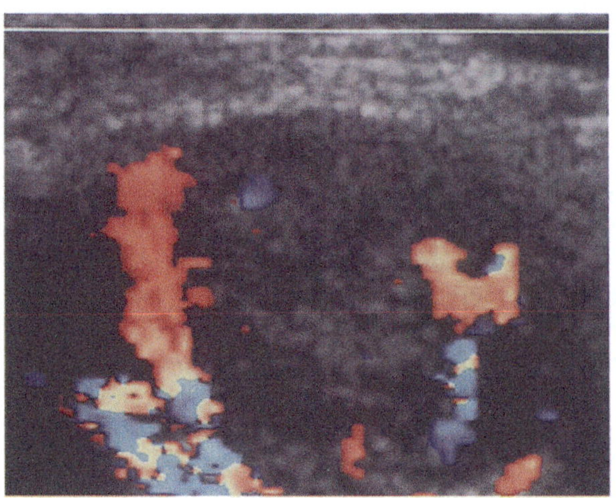

Fig. 3.30. Pleomorphic adenoma: peripheral hypervascularity on color Doppler

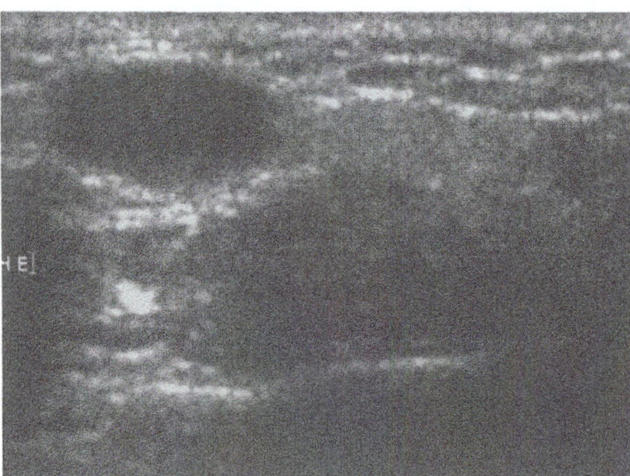

Fig. 3.31. Small, slow-growing hypoechoic parotid nodule involving the masseter extension. Pleomorphic adenoma

ium injection (Sigal 1996). Large tumors often contain sites of necrosis; their mucoid content may produce a high signal intensity on T_2-weighted sequences; zones of myxoid degeneration are also common.

Surgical excision must be followed by attentive sonographic or MRI surveillance; recurrence is seen in 3%–13% of cases 5–10 years after surgery and is related to the surgical technique; tumor enucleation is insufficient, and care must be taken to remove an intact capsule to avoid seeding the operative field (Fig. 3.32). An estimated 25% of all untreated pleomorphic adenomas undergo malignant transformation (carcinoma ex pleomorphic adenoma, which has a poor prognosis). This possibility should be entertained whenever imaging reveals focal irregularities in tumor contours.

Even in the absence of malignant transformation, pleomorphic adenoma is one of the rare histologically benign tumors with a metastatic potential (Gaillard et al. 1981).

3.5.1.2
Basal Cell Adenoma

This rare tumor represents only 2% of all salivary gland adenomas; it has a propensity for the labial accessory glands, but the parotid and other accessory glands may also be affected. Occurring essentially in elderly individuals as a small, solitary, solid encapsulated tumor, basal cell adenoma has a benign course. However, these tumors can easily be confused with adenoid cystic carcinoma (cylindroma), which may result in untimely and mutilating therapy (Gaillard et al. 1981).

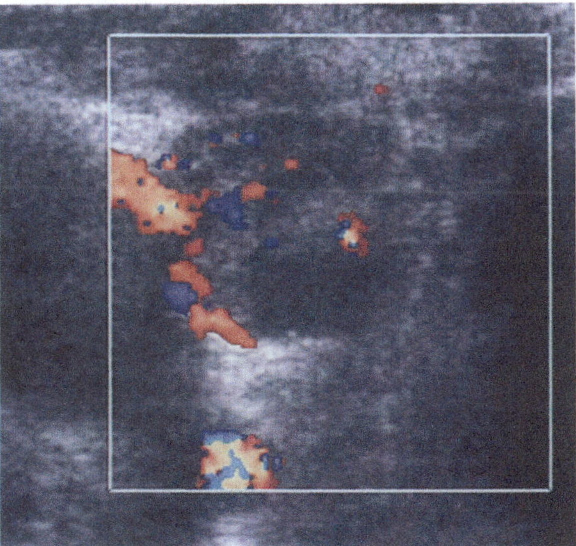

Fig. 3.32. Recurrence of a pleomorphic adenoma in the parotidectomy bed

3.5.1.3
Oncocytoma

Also referred to as oxyphilic granular cell adenoma or oncocytic adenoma, this rare salivary gland tumor is composed of acidophilic granular cells (oncocytes) grouped together in strands in a thin connective-tissue stroma. Although usually benign, there have been several reports of malignant oncocytoma (Nakada et al. 1998).

Sonography may suggest the diagnosis by demonstrating small, well-delimited, and often multifocal parotid or submandibular nodules of low echogenicity (Fig. 3.33). There are no associated cervical adenopathies (Bruneton et al. 1987).

Oncocytomas show strong tracer uptake on scintigraphy (Higashi et al. 1987). US-guided FNAB permits histological diagnosis. Therapeutic abstention is the rule.

3.5.1.4
Papillary Cystadenolymphoma

Also referred to as adenolymphoma or Warthin's tumor, papillary cystadenolymphoma Is the result of proliferation of the intraglandular ducts within the preexistent intraparotid lymph nodes (Cabanne and Bonenfant 1980). These lesions accounts for 6%–10% of all parotid tumors (Bruneton et al. 1987). Submandibular gland involvement is very rare. Male predominance has been observed; age at diagnosis is generally more than 40 years.

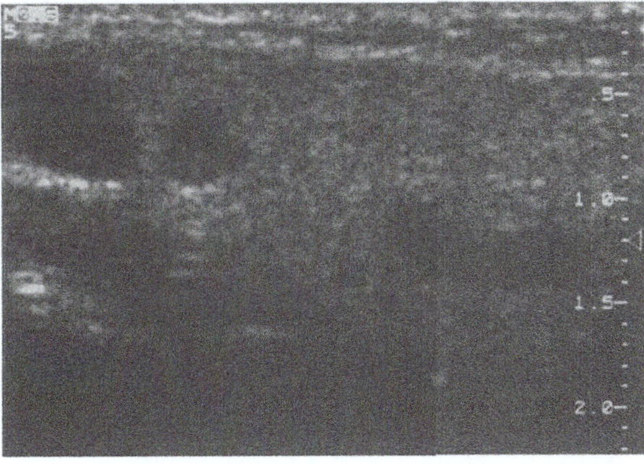

Fig. 3.33. Multiple hypoechoic parietal nodules in a patient with oncocytosis

The encapsulated tumor may contain one or more cystic masses, and hemorrhagic changes are common; only 5%–15% of cases are bilateral. The most typical clinical presentation is a swelling on the lower aspect of the parotid in an elderly Caucasian man (Fig. 3.34).

Sonography depicts a well-delimited, often small posteroinferior lesion in the infrafacial portion of the parotid. An echo-free cystic component with posterior enhancement coexists with tissue contingents (Shimizu et al. 1999). The larger the lesion, the more predominant the cystic portion; only the presence of parietal nodules permits differentiation of the tumor from a simple cyst. Other possible US findings include fine posterior echoes, multiple septa, layering internal echoes (Fig. 3.35), and an inhomogeneous echotexture suggestive of pleomorphic adenoma (Bruneton et al. 1987).

Color Doppler reveals the hilar disposition of flow signals with centrifugal distribution, but this feature is not specific (Fig. 3.36) (Martinoli et al. 1994) On color Doppler and power Doppler, use of a low PRF (<5 cm/s) and an appropriate color gain may reveal small avascular intratumoral zones corresponding to cysts that may be initially overlooked by B-mode imaging (Fig. 3.37) (Benzel et al. 1995).

Technetium scintigraphy can confirm the diagnosis by demonstrating intense tracer uptake (Higashi et al. 1987). MRI is reserved for atypical or large lesions and for preoperative staging. The MR signal is heterogeneous, but the cystic portions usually have a high intensity signal on T_2-weighted sequences. Signal intensity on T_1-weighted images is highly variable, owing to the frequent presence of a hemorrhagic component. Exoparotid development of a large tumor may lead to confusion with a necrotic laterocervical nodal mass or a second branchial cleft cyst.

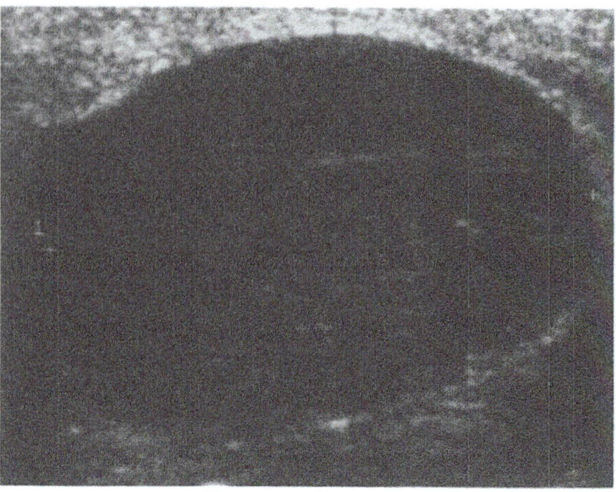

Fig. 3.35. Essentially cystic Warthin's tumor containing hemorrhagic sediment

Sonography suffices for the surveillance of papillary cystadenolymphoma; surgical excision is indicated only if the tumor causes discomfort (Bruneton et al. 1987).

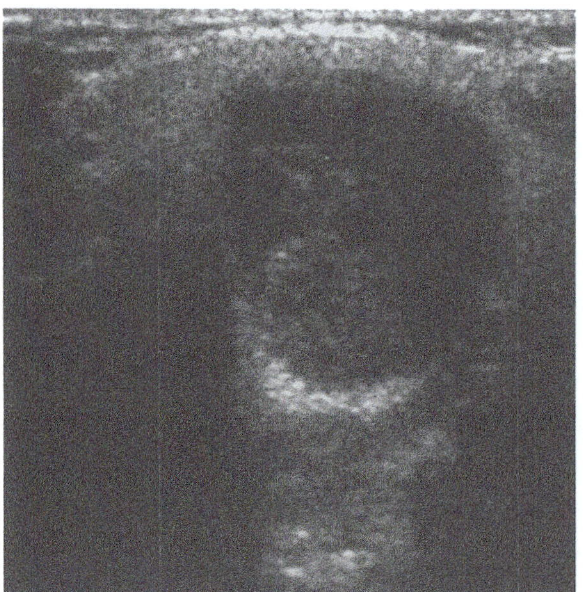

Fig. 3.34. Transverse scan of the parotid: small superficial nodule in the lower pole in an elderly individual. Presence of cystic cavities. Warthin's tumor

3.5.1.5 Hemangioma and Lymphangioma

These lesions of vascular origin represent less than 5% of all salivary gland neoplasms (Silvers and Som 1988). The majority arise in the parotid; involvement

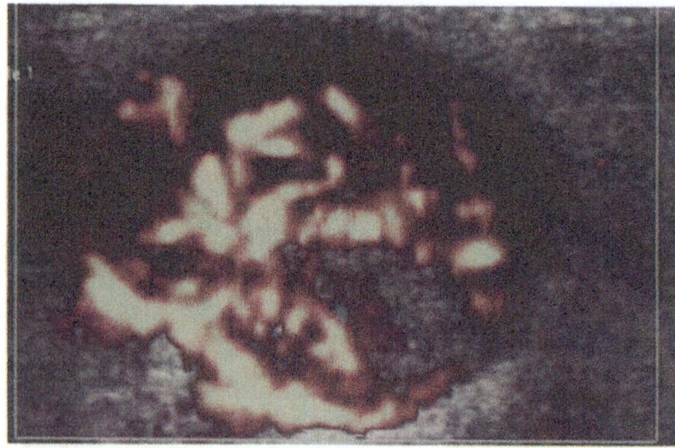

Fig. 3.36. Warthin's tumor: power Doppler reveals hilar-type central vascularity. Avascular layering internal echoes of hemorrhagic origin

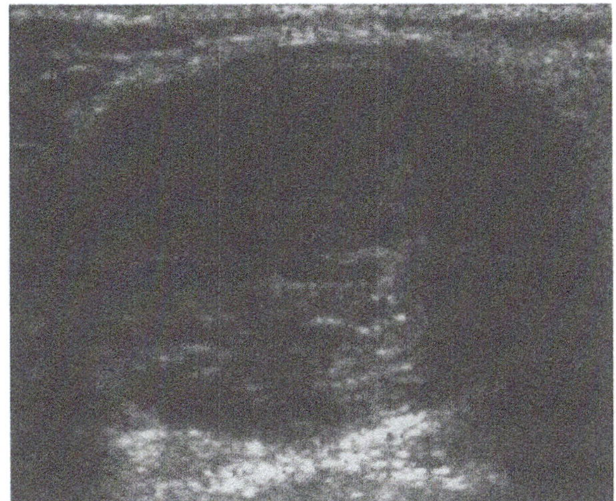

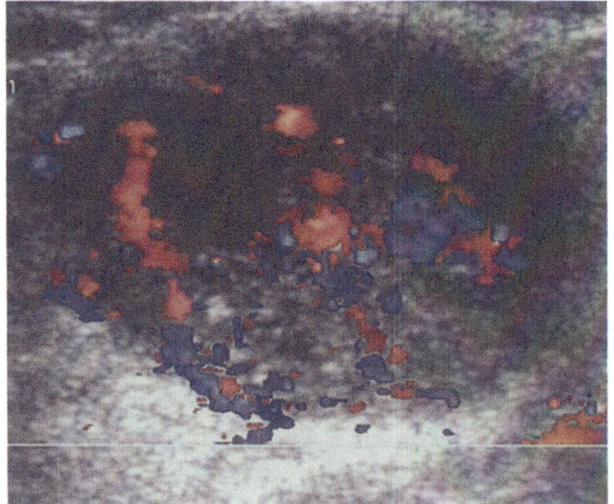

a b

Fig. 3.37a,b. Warthin's tumor: color Doppler demonstrates avascular zones corresponding to the cystic components

of the submandibular glands is rare. Differential diagnosis of these nonepithelial tumors can be difficult.

Capillary hemangioma of the parotid gland is the most frequent salivary gland neoplasm in children. Congenital capillary hemangioma accounts for 90% of all parotid tumors in the first 12 months of life. Following a period of rapid enlargement, spontaneous regression is common.

Lymphangiomas may be diagnosed at any age, although 80%–90% are seen in young children (SILVERS and SOM 1988). Several pathological types have been described: strictly vascular lesions (cavernous lymphangioma), tumors with an extensive cystic component (cystic lymphangioma), and intermediate lesions in which no one pathological type predominates (hemangioendothelioma). These unilateral cervical masses may spread to the parotid or submandibular glands or invade the vascular structures. Infection or hemorrhage can cause sudden enlargement, prompting diagnosis in the adult. Facial nerve paralysis is possible.

These sonographically homogeneous or septated cystic lesions have a soft or semi-firm consistency (Fig. 3.38). Cyst contents tend to be echoic but may contain a hemorrhagic sediment. Repeated infections result in thickening of the cyst wall and increase the

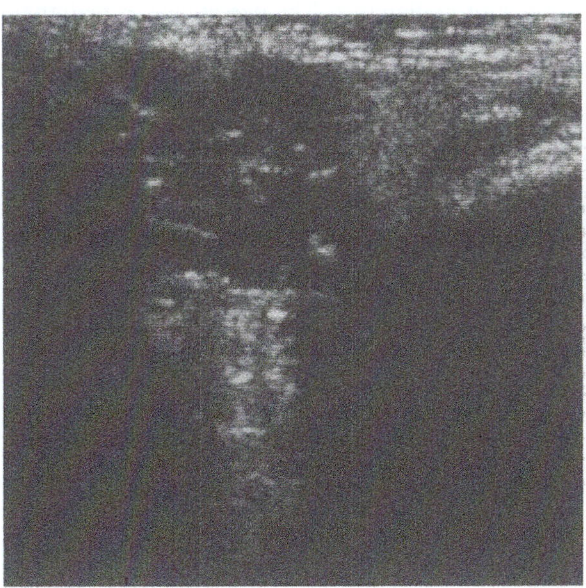

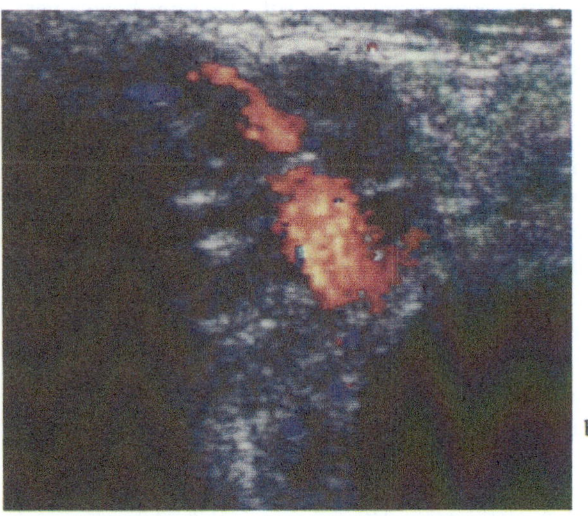

a b

Fig. 3.38a,b. Cystic lymphangioma of the parotid bed: multicystic mass. Color Doppler demonstrates vessels in the septa

echogenicity of cyst contents (RAFFAELLI et al. 1995). Arciform calcifications corresponding to phleboliths are possible.

Color Doppler analysis of tumor vascularity reveals numerous vessels in the septa (Fig. 3.39). Pulsed Doppler often demonstrates the existence of venous signals related to ectatic veins.

MRI is often necessary for a complete topographic workup of large or atypical lesions. Cystic lesions have a low signal intensity on T_1-weighted sequences and a high-intensity signal on T_2-weighted images; the septa appear hypointense on both T_1- and T_2-weighted sequences. Gadolinium injection enhances the vascular structures. Treatment of these cystic masses consists in either conventional surgery or percutaneous sclerotherapy by injection of Ethibloc under US guidance. Injection of the sclerosing agent often causes an inflammatory reaction, sometimes intense, that resolves under medical therapy. Results are excellent, with either disappearance of the lesions or marked regression allowing excision under satisfactory conditions (BERNIER et al. 1994).

3.5.1.6 Lipoma

This benign soft tissue neoplasm can develop within the parotid or in the submandibular space, close to the parotid. Approximately 90% of cases are ordinary lipomas; fibrolipomas (infiltrating lipomas with a fibrous component) and those rare parotid lipomas occurring as part of a lipomatosis syndrome account for the remainder (BOURJAT and KAHN 1994; SILVERS and SOM 1998).

Often superficial, these soft swellings have a very slow growth pattern. The well-defined lesions tend to be echogenic and compressible by the US transducer (BRUNETON et al. 1987); their echogenicity is usually similar to that of the subcutaneous fat, although hypoechoic forms have been described (Fig. 3.40) (CHIKUI et al. 1997). CT is indicated whenever doubt persists concerning diagnosis, and for evaluation of highly advanced lesions. CT can affirm the diagnosis by demonstrating the lesion's typical fat density (density between -65 and -125 HU). Differential diagnosis from extensive, ill-defined fibrotic changes or hemorrhage by CT can be difficult because the increased attenuation of lipomas is similar to that of muscle. Color Doppler or CT demonstration of intratumoral vessels must be interpreted with caution, because well-differentiated liposarcomas, though exceptional, can mimic an ordinary lipoma. Intratumoral vascularity is thus an indication for surgical excision.

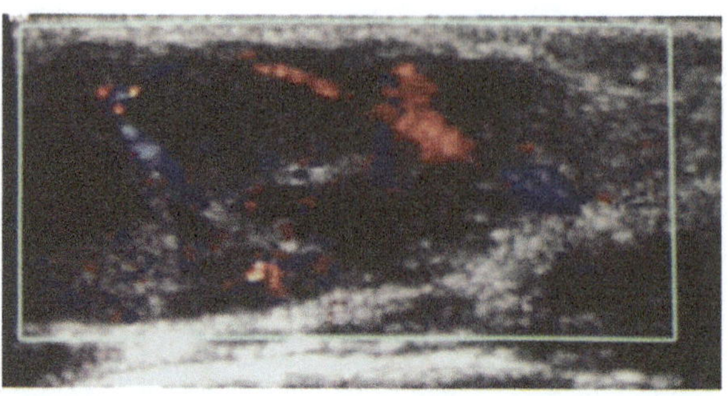

Fig. 3.39. Parotid hemolymphangioma: tissue and cystic components with hypervascularity on color Doppler

3.5.1.7 Neurogenic Tumors

Both schwannomas and neurofibromas occur in the parotid gland. These well-circumscribed, frequently cystic lesions arise primarily from the facial nerve trunk or its branches. The multiple neurofibromas seen in neurofibromatosis type I show a low fat attenuation that may mimic a lipoma (SILVERS and SOM 1998). Diagnosis often requires histological examination.

3.5.2 Malignant Tumors

The incidence of malignant tumors is apparently higher in certain populations, such as the Inuit or previously irradiated patients (SILVERS and SOM 1998). The smaller the affected salivary gland, the higher the risk of malignancy. The percentage of malignant lesions is 20% for the parotid, 60% for the submandibular gland, and 80% for the sublingual glands and accessory salivary glands (SILVERS and SOM 1998).

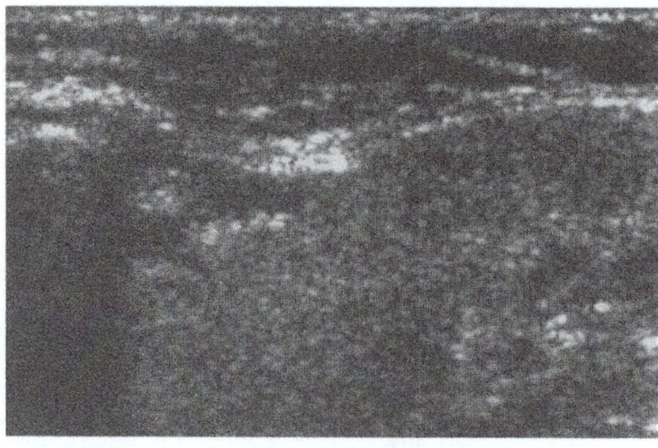

Fig. 3.40. Lipoma of the submandibular space

The risk of malignancy is also very high in children. Although salivary gland tumors are uncommon in the pediatric population, 30%–35% of such neoplasms are malignant (Silvers and Som 1998).

Imaging features may suggest malignancy, but such studies are used especially for disease staging. The TNM classification for malignant parotid tumors is based on tumor size, the presence of extraparenchymal spread, facial nerve involvement, and the existence of nodal or visceral metastases. Regional nodal metastasis is associated with a poor prognosis (Andersen et al. 1991). Facial nerve invasion corresponds to stage-IV disease from the outset and is predictive of nodal involvement in 66%–77% of cases; the 5-year survival for such patients is only 9%–14%. Approximately 20% of all malignant parotid tumors metastasize to the viscera (Silvers and Som 1998). The metastatic potential of these lesions varies considerably as a function of the histological type. While the 5-year survival rate is often high, it is not very significant, because certain tumors such as adenoid cystic carcinomas are very slow-growing.

Surgical resection remains the rule whenever feasible, and is increasingly supplemented by radiotherapy or chemotherapy for high-grade malignant tumors.

Parotid TNM staging system

Primary tumor (T)

TX: Primary tumor cannot be assessed
T0: No evidence of primary tumor
T1: Tumor 2 cm or less in greatest dimension without extraparenchymal extension
T2: Tumor greater than 2 cm but not more than 4 cm in greatest dimension without extraparenchymal extension
T3: Tumor more than 4 cm but not more than 6 cm in greatest dimension, or tumor having extraparenchymal extension without seventh nerve involvement
T4: Tumor more than 6 cm in greatest dimension, or tumor invades the skull base or seventh nerve

Regional lymph nodes (N)

NX: Regional lymph nodes cannot be assessed
N0: No regional lymph node metastasis
N1: Metastasis in a single ipsilateral lymph node, 3 cm or less in greatest dimension
N2: Metastasis in a single ipsilateral lymph node more than 3 cm but not more than 6 cm in greatest dimension; or multiple ipsilateral lymph nodes, none more than 6 cm in greatest dimension; or bilateral or contralateral lymph nodes, none more than 6 cm in greatest dimension
N3: Metastasis in a lymph node more than 6 cm in greatest dimension

Distant metastasis (M)

MX: Distant metastasis cannot be assessed
M0: No distant metastasis
M1: Distant metastasis

Stage grouping

Stage I: T1 or T2, N0, M0
Stage II: T3, N0, M0
Stage III: T1 or T2, N1, M0
Stage IV: T4, N0, M0 or T3 or T4, N1, M0 or any T, N2 or N3, M0 or any T, any N, M1

3.5.2.1 Mucoepidermoid Carcinoma

Erroneously termed carcinomas, these tumors represent approximately 30% of all salivary gland malignancies. Fifty percent affect the parotid glands while 45% develop from the accessory salivary glands, especially those in the palate and buccal mucosa (Lack and Upton 1988). Children and young adults are often affected, there being a slight female predominance. For many years the malignancy of these tumors was overestimated, and the proportion of aggressive malignant forms is actually only approximately 5% (Gaillard et al. 1981). Mucoepidermoid tumors contain both mucous and squamous cells (Gaillard et al. 1981; Silvers and Som 1998).

Histologically, mucoepidermoid tumors are classed in three grades that are correlated with their course and prognosis (Healey et al. 1970). Low-grade tumors are well-delimited lesions with regular contours and may include cystic areas or focal calcification. Their appearance is often similar to that of pleomorphic adenoma (Fig. 3.41). In contrast, infiltrating high-grade tumors have indistinct margins (Fig. 3.42).

The frequency of recurrence after resection is comparable to that of pleomorphic adenoma.

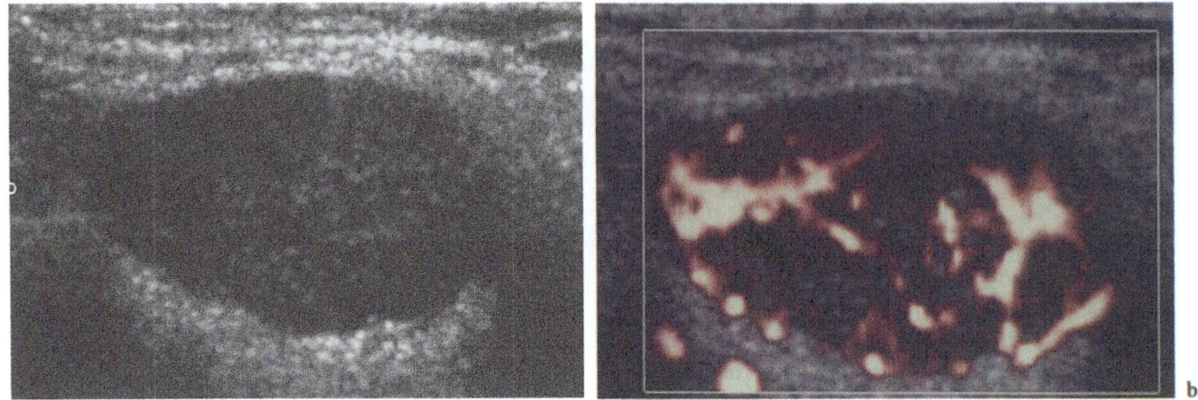

Fig. 3.41. a Low-grade mucoepidermoid parotid tumor. Well-delimited, homogeneously hypoechoic lesion with posterior enhancement. **b** Power Doppler reveals diffuse hypervascularity

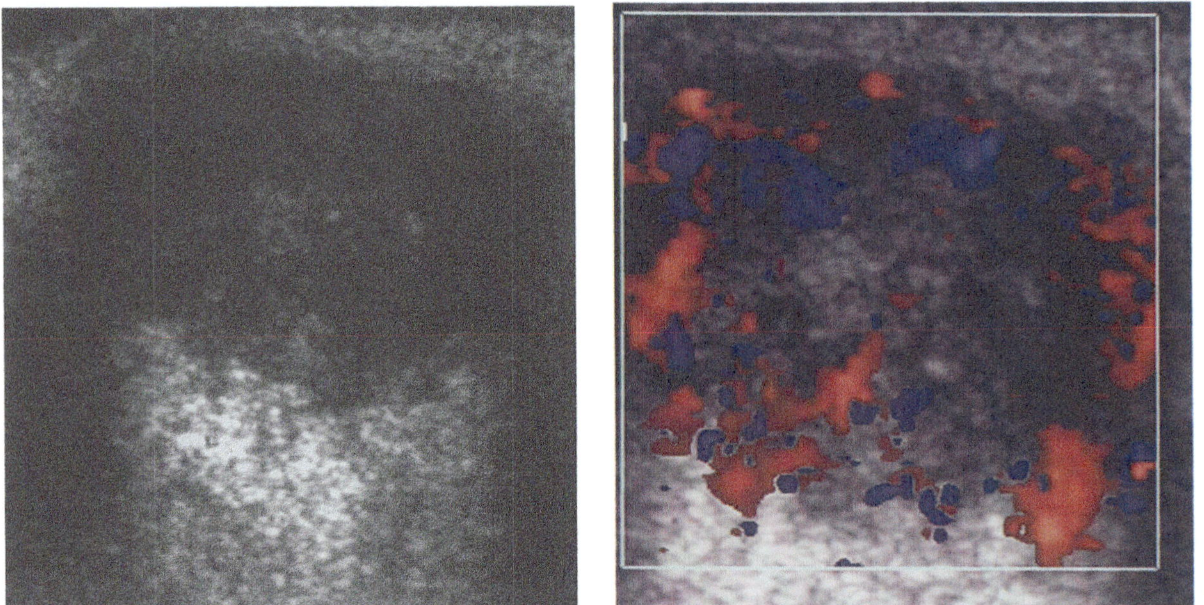

Fig. 3.42. a Inhomogeneously hypoechoic parotid tumor with posterior enhancement and irregular margins. **b** Color Doppler reveals peripheral hypervascularity suggesting a central zone of necrosis. High-grade mucoepidermoid tumor

3.5.2.2
Acinic Cell Tumor

Also referred to as acinic cell carcinoma despite its low malignant potential, this tumor occurs at all ages. It represents 2%–4% of all major salivary gland tumors and 15%–17% of all parotid malignancies. Parotid sites predominate (80% of cases), but the accessory salivary glands of the buccal mucosa or lips are involved in 10% of cases. Submandibular gland involvement is rare (4%); 3% of parotid acinic cell tumors are bilateral (Gaillard et al. 1981; Peel and Gnepp 1985; Silvers and Som 1998). In children, acinic cell tumors are the second most frequent parotid malignancy after mucoepidermoid carcinoma.

Two histological types coexist: a form composed of highly differentiated granular cells similar to normal salivary tissue, and a clear cell form that may be mistaken for a parotid metastasis of renal cancer (Gaillard 1981).

Acinic cell tumors have no specific imaging features and often manifest as a well-delimited lesion with a benign appearance. Regional nodal metastases occur in 10%–19% of cases, distant visceral metastases (mainly lung and bone) in 15% (Silvers and Som 1998). The rate of growth is very slow and the course may be marked by multiple recurrences (GAILLARD et al. 1981).

The 5-year survival rate is high (80%–90%), but survival drops to 56% at 20 years (THACKRAY and LUCAS 1974; SILVERS and SOM 1998).

3.5.2.3 Adenoid Cystic Carcinoma

Adenoid cystic carcinomas account for 4%–15% of all salivary gland tumors, 2%–6% of parotid tumors, 15% of submandibular gland tumors, 15% of sublingual gland tumors, and 25%–31% of accessory salivary gland tumors (SIGAL et al. 1992).

The typical patient is a woman over 40 years of age. These ubiquitous solitary lesions can invade all of the facial structures, including the palatal region. Facial nerve paralysis may be observed in cases of parotid involvement.

These slow-growing invasive tumors spread both locally and by intracranial infiltration, in particular along the nerve sheaths; they also have a non-negligible potential for metastasis to the lung (BYRNE and SPECTOR 1988). Contiguous spread to the mandible may eventually result in bone erosion (GAILLARD et al. 1981). Imaging features are nonspecific. Small tumors often have a benign US appearance. Large lesions have irregular contours (Fig. 3.43), particularly when they involve the accessory salivary glands. Palatal lesions can be evaluated by intraoral sonography. MRI is helpful for tumor staging. In particular, gadolinium-enhanced, T_1-weighted sequences with fat suppression readily demonstrate perineural infiltration (facial, trigeminal, mandibular nerves, etc.), especially at the base of the skull following retrograde tumor extension (SIGAL et al. 1992).

Prolonged survival is common, even among patients with lung metastases. Treatment consists in surgical excision and often requires more extensive tissue and nerve sacrifice than initially predicted by preoperative imaging studies (BRUNETON et al. 1987).

3.5.2.4 Carcinoma

The general term "carcinoma" covers several histological types (CABANNE and BONENFANT 1980; GAILLARD et al. 1981):

- Adenocarcinoma and certain extremely aggressive malignancies (salivary duct carcinomas) resemble breast carcinoma histologically.
- Undifferentiated carcinoma
- Squamous cell carcinoma
- Carcinoma ex pleomorphic adenoma

Carcinomas represent only 3% of all parotid tumors and generally occur after the age of 50 years; there is a marked male predominance. Primary squamous cell carcinomas of salivary gland origin are rare. Care must be taken not to confuse them with a periparotid nodal metastasis from a regional squamous cell carcinoma (often a skin cancer of the face or scalp or, less frequently, a pharyngeal carcinoma). Clinical signs are suggestive: firm, fixed, painful mass,

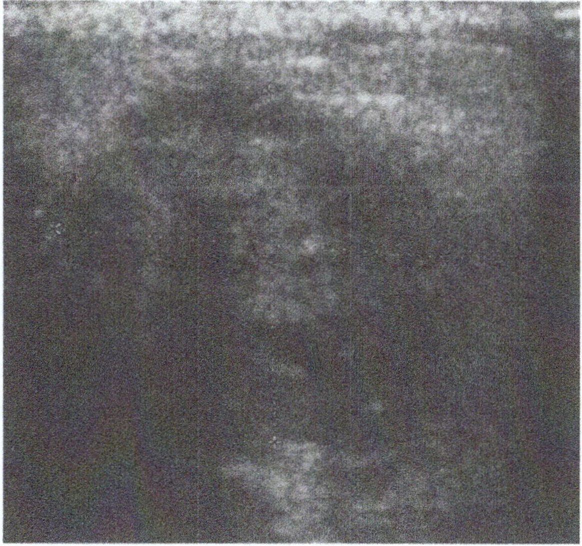
a

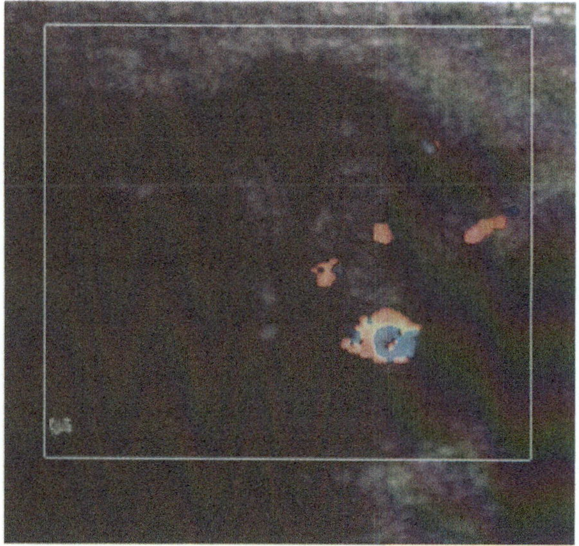
b

Fig. 3.43a,b. Ill-defined, inhomogeneous parotid tumor with weak vascularity, a slow growth pattern, and associated facial paralysis. Adenoid cystic carcinoma

sometimes ulcerated, with facial nerve paralysis and satellite adenopathies.

Sonography generally does not reveal any features suggestive of malignancy for lesions smaller than 2 cm, and the usual diagnosis is pleomorphic adenoma (Raffaelli et al. 1995). The irregular contours of larger tumors reflect their invasive nature (Fig. 3.44). Late-stage lesions appear heterogeneous, owing to necrosis and hemorrhagic changes; tumor limits are indistinct (Fig. 3.45). Sonography is the best technique for assessment and quantification of spread to the cervical nodes (Fig. 3.46, 3.47) (Bruneton et al. 1987). Color Doppler US can help to demonstrate the marked hilar-type hypervascularization (PSV over 60 cm/s) of malignant parotid tumors that distinguishes them from pleomorphic adenomas, which typically show a peripheral vascular pattern or total absence of vascularity (Fig. 3.48) (Aluffi et al. 1997; Martinoli et al. 1994; Schade et al. 1998).

Disease staging often requires a second imaging technique (CT or MRI) to examine the pharyngeal parotid extension and the parapharyngeal and retrostyloid spaces and to search for parapharyngeal or retromandibular adenopathies that cannot be detected by US (Bourjat and Kahn 1995).

Total parotidectomy with sacrifice of the facial nerve and cervical node resection is systematic, but the overall prognosis remains poor. The 5-year survival is only approximately 30% for adenocarcinoma (Byrne et al. 1989).

3.5.2.5 Lymphoma

Primary non-Hodgkin's lymphoma (NHL) of the parotid gland is rare; only 100 cases have been reported in the literature. Diagnosis of this malignancy that develops from the intraparotid lymphoid tissue is based on histological demonstration of intraglandular lymphomatous tissue, without any intra- or extraglandular nodal involvement.

Secondary lymphomatous involvement of the salivary glands by systemic disease is more common, as is salivary NHL in Sjögren's syndrome (Bruneton et al. 1982). Secondary salivary gland involvement occurs in 1%–8% of all lymphomas, with parotid lesions accounting for 80% of cases. The enlarged parotid contains multinodular lesions of low echogenicity with posterior enhancement (Fig. 3.49). Sonography permits analysis of the other salivary glands and the cervical node-bearing areas in search of lymphomatous nodes, which frequently have typical features:

- These well-delimited nodal masses are often homogeneous and hypoechoic or even echolucent, with posterior enhancement (Fig. 3.50). Color Doppler demonstrates their tissue character.
- Often compressive, these masses do not cause jugular vein thrombosis until a late stage, and even then much more rarely than the metastatic nodes of head and neck cancers.

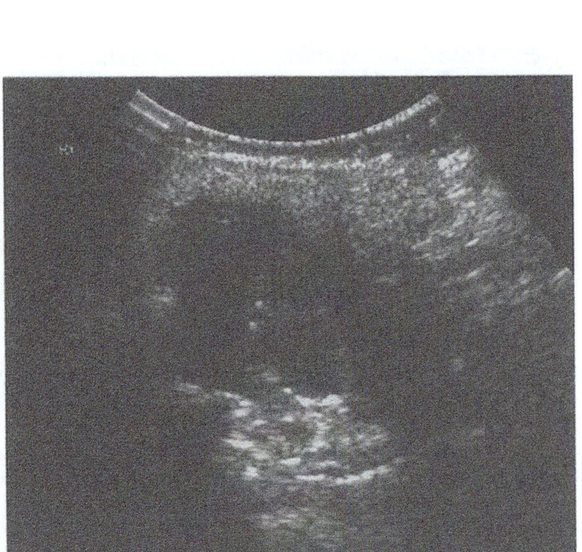

Fig. 3.44. Large, aggressive, inhomogeneous parotid tumor with associated facial paralysis. Undifferentiated carcinoma

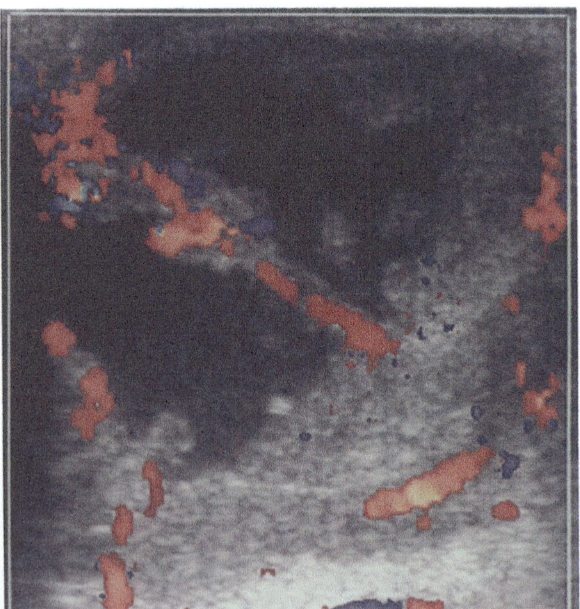

Fig. 3.45. Necrotic parotid carcinoma

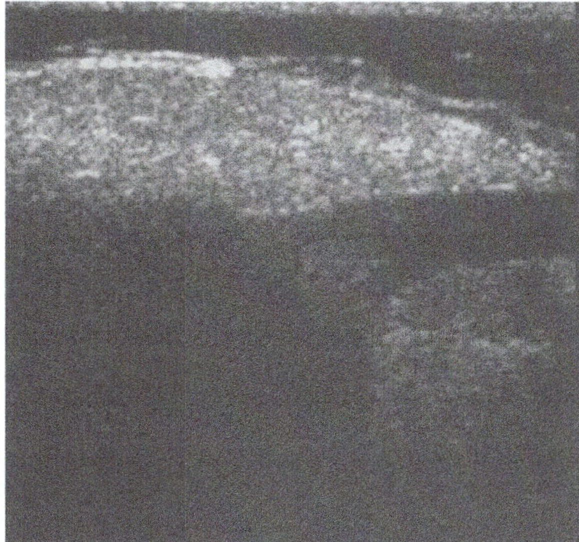

a

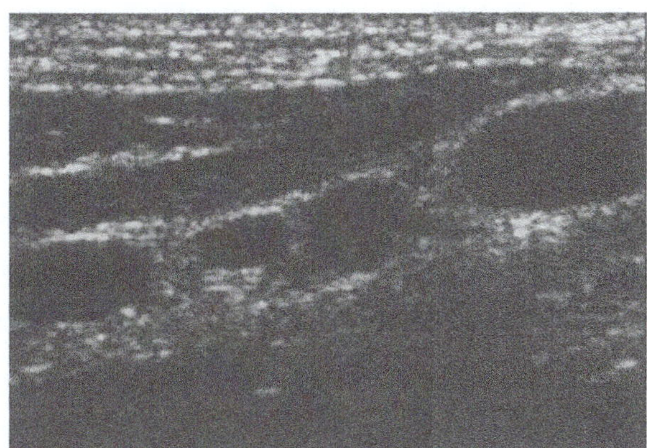

b

Fig. 3.46a,b. Parotid carcinoma ex pleomorphic carcinoma. Cervical nodal metastases

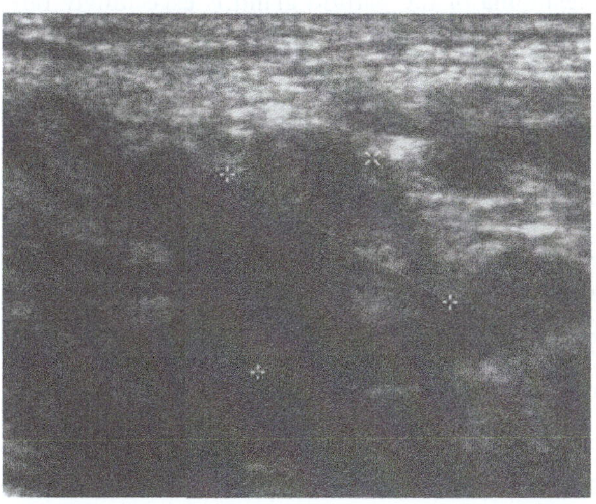

Fig. 3.47. Carcinoma of the submandibular gland

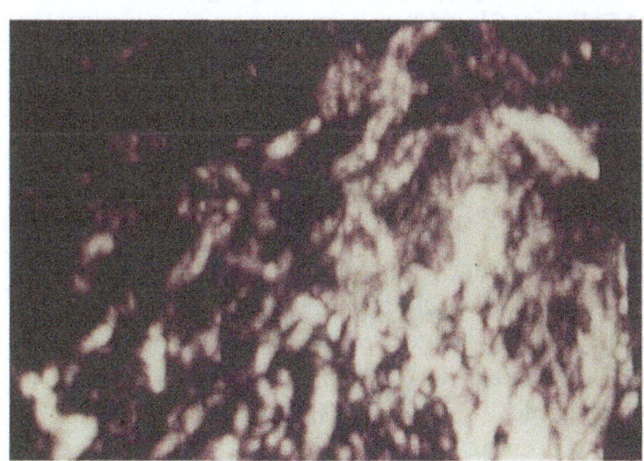

a

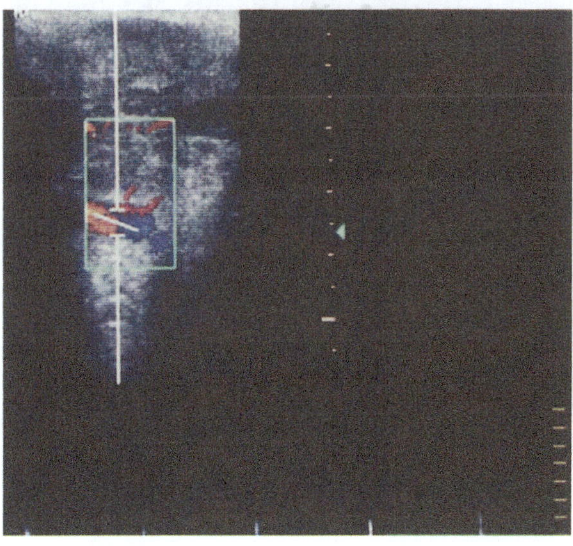

b

Fig. 3.48a,b. Parotid carcinoma. a 3-D power Doppler demonstrates irregular hypervascularity; b spectral analysis reveals systolic velocities higher than 60 cm/s

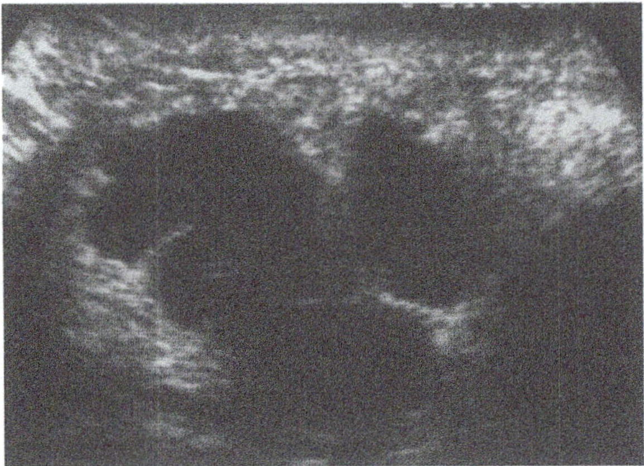

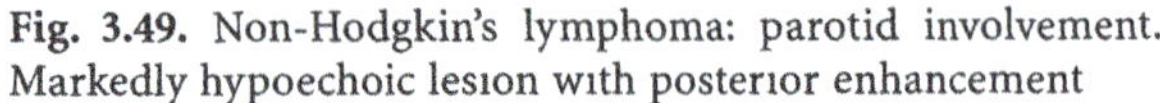

Fig. 3.49. Non-Hodgkin's lymphoma: parotid involvement. Markedly hypoechoic lesion with posterior enhancement

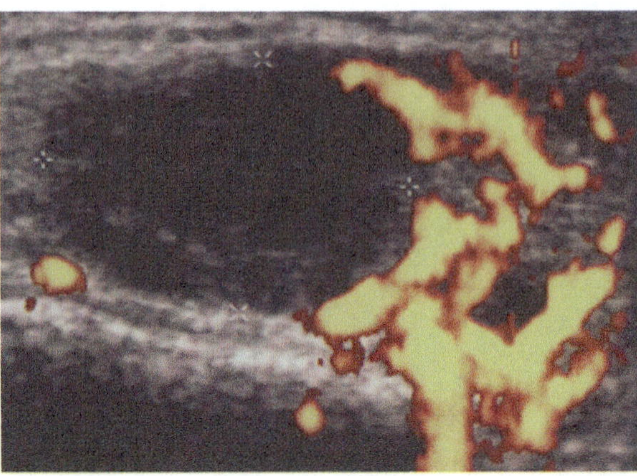

Fig. 3.50. Parotid lymphoma: hypovascular hypoechoic mass

CT and MRI are contributory, and the nodal lesions usually remain homogeneous after contrast administration. In the absence of nodal involvement, a cystadenolymphoma is sometimes suspected, and histological examination is required to correct the diagnosis (Bruneton et al. 1982).

3.5.2.6
Metastases

Being a drainage site for head and neck cancers, and especially cancers of the face and scalp, the parotid space is a frequent site of intraparotid and periparotid nodal metastases. Malignant melanoma of the temporal scalp metastasizes to the periparotid lymph nodes in 80% of cases (Fig. 3.51); primary malignant melanoma of the parotid gland is exceedingly rare (Silvers and Som 1998). These solitary or multiple nodal metastases can be differentiated from normal or inflammatory intraparotid nodes by the absence of a central hilum (Raffaelli et al. 1995).

Salivary metastases secondary to hematogenous spread have also been described, particularly in the parotid. Malignant melanoma is the predominant etiology, followed by cancers of the lung, kidney, breast, and digestive tract. Although imaging studies do not provide any etiological information, the clinical context and rapid growth of the nodule suggest the diagnosis of metastasis (Bruneton et al. 1982).

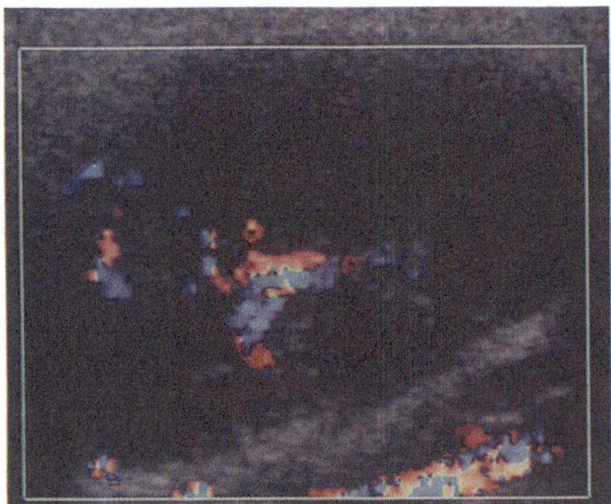

Fig. 3.51. Intraparotid nodal metastasis of a malignant melanoma of the scalp

3.5.3
Role of Sonography in the Staging of Salivary Gland Tumors

The sensitivity of sonography for the detection of salivary gland tumors varies from 87.2% to 100% (Akin et al. 1991; Gozzi et al. 1990; Kress et al. 1993; Rinast et al. 1990; Wagner et al. 1987). US is much more accurate than sialography for diagnosis of salivary gland tumors and cysts (Akin et al. 1991). The specificity of sonography for salivary gland tumors ranges from 74% to 100% (Gozzi et al. 1990; Kress et al. 1993; Rinast et al. 1990). In a series of 121 patients (Grazioli et al. 1994), US had an accuracy of only 77.6%, versus 86.1% for CT and 94.4% for MRI. In another series of 18 patients, aspiration cytology provided the correct diagnosis in 72% of cases (Feld et al. 1999).

3.5.3.1 Presumptive Determination of Origin

Sonography has a specificity of 98% for positive diagnosis of the parotid or submandibular origin of a tumor, i.e., differentiation of its peri- or intraglandular origin (HAUSEGGER et al. 1993). US can also rule out masseter hyperplasia, often seen in bruxism, particularly in young women (RAFFAELLI et al. 1995). Invasion of the parotid by a masseter rhabdomyosarcoma is rare, but it is difficult to differentiate from a malignant parotid tumor by imaging.

3.5.3.2 Diagnosis of Malignancy

Differentiation of benign and malignant salivary lesions is based on clinical information and morphological criteria. Combined use of such data allows prediction of malignancy in 90% of cases (BRYAN et al. 1982; SOM and BILLER 1989; SOM et al. 1988; TRAPPE et al. 1991). Sonography can accurately identify 74%–83% of benign lesions (BRUNETON and MOUROU 1993; GOZZI et al. 1990; KLEIN et al. 1989).

Clinically, most benign salivary tumors are painless, slow-growing masses that are firm and mobile at palpation. Cystic lesions, lymphoepithelial cysts, and lymphangiomas, however, tend to be more symptomatic, including painful inflammatory episodes; the recurrent nature of inflammation is the only suggestive feature.

Malignant tumors tend to be very firm and fixed in position; these rapidly growing lesions also tend to be painful. Malignant parotid tumors, for example, are responsible for 12%–14% of all cases of facial nerve paralysis. Although pain is not always synonymous with malignancy, pain in a patient with a recognized malignant tumor is frequently the result of neural invasion, and thus a predictor of a poor prognosis. The 5-year survival rate among patients with pain is only 35%, versus 68% in asymptomatic patients (SILVERS and SOM 1998).

Benign salivary tumors are usually encapsulated, and manifest on US as well-delimited lesions with regular contours (Fig. 3.52). However, the most frequent low-grade malignant salivary tumors (mucoepidermoid carcinomas and certain acinic cell tumors), some adenoid cystic carcinomas, and, generally speaking, most malignant tumors smaller than 2 cm in diameter also appear smoothly outlined (SILVERS and SOM 1998).

High-grade malignancies (high-grade mucoepidermoid carcinomas, adenocarcinomas, squamous cell carcinomas) are infiltrating masses with indistinct margins (Fig. 3.53). Benign tumors rarely have irregular margins, except as the result of inflammatory or hemorrhagic changes, as may occur after a biopsy.

While diagnosis of a high-grade malignant tumor is thus fairly easy, differentiation of low-grade malignant tumors and benign tumors is usually not possible with imaging studies. Submandibular, sublingual, and palatal tumors have a poor prognosis, as do salivary gland tumors in children.

Several sonographic criteria of malignancy have been defined; although not pathognomonic, their

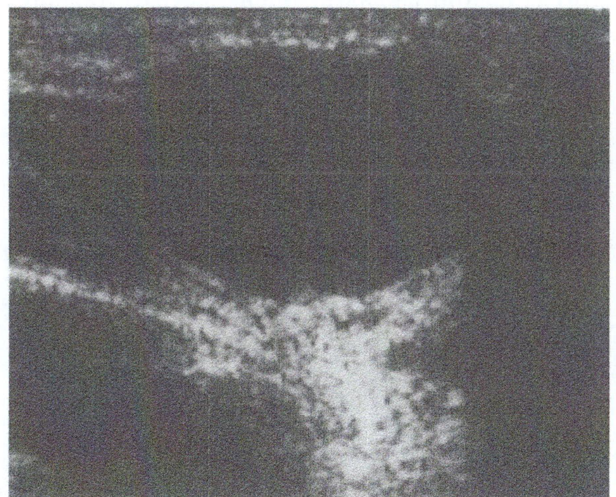

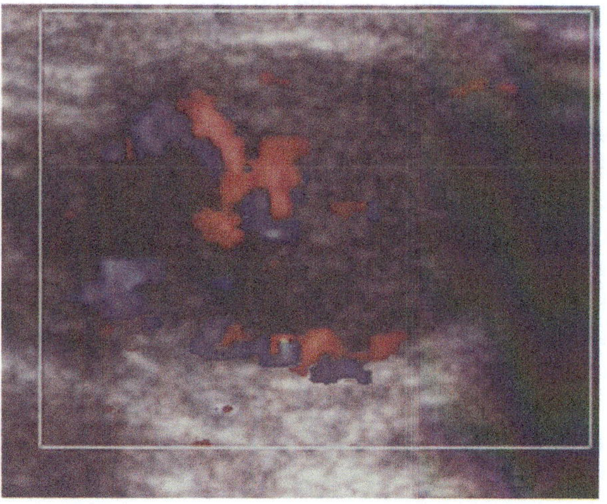

Fig. 3.52a,b. Parotid tumor (2.5 cm) with sonographic features of benignity: well-defined margins, posterior enhancement, superficial location, regular vascular pattern on color Doppler

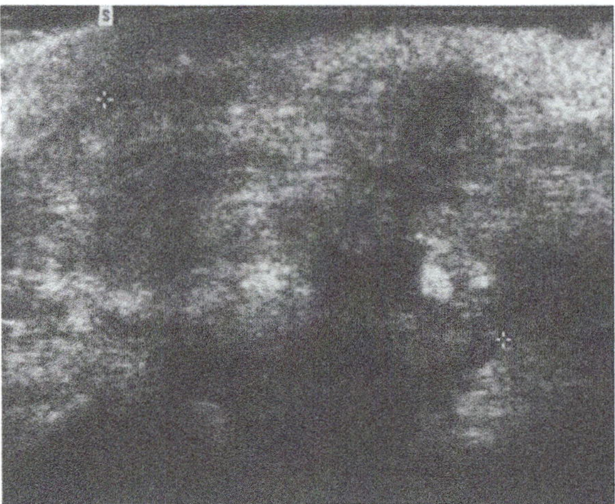

Fig. 3.53. Inhomogeneous, poorly-defined carcinoma of the submandibular gland

value increases when they are combined (Raffaelli et al. 1995):

- Contour irregularities
- Hypervascularity on color Doppler (PSV greater than 60 cm/s)
- Invasion localized to a muscle in contact with the tumor
- Presence of cervical adenopathies

CT is not very effective for differentiation of malignant and benign masses, owing to the similarity of their attenuation. Analysis of the MRI tumor signal is more interesting (Freling et al. 1992; Teresi et al. 1978b). Benign lesions and low-grade malignant tumors often contain variable quantities of watery secretions (serous and mucoid materials) that produce low T_1-weighted signal intensities and high T_2-weighted signal intensities. In contrast, high-grade tumors contain little serous and mucoid material, which explains their low signal intensities on all sequences (especially T_2-weighted images) (Som and Biller 1989). Although areas of fibrosis and granulomatous processes also produce relatively low T_2-weighted signal intensities, any poorly defined mass with a low T_2-weighted signal intensity should raise the suspicion of a high-grade malignancy (Silvers and Som 1998).

3.5.3.3
Etiological Diagnosis

Affirmation of the salivary origin of a tumor that develops in a buccal, labial, or palatal accessory salivary gland or an accessory gland in the deep regions of the face can be difficult. With the exception of salivary cysts in the floor of the mouth, most of these lesions are malignant; adenoid cystic carcinomas predominate. Roughly speaking, the same is true for tumors of the sublingual glands.

Submandibular tumors are dominated by adenoid cystic carcinomas, the most frequent etiology, and mucoepidermoid carcinoma.

Discovery of a mass in the parotid region can involve diagnostic difficulties, although a number of disease patterns have been defined. Imaging studies sometimes suggest the etiology. US, for example, accurately diagnosed 57% of the tumors in the study of Klein et al. (1989). A combination of sonography and MRI is usually recommended; CT is of limited value (Grazioli et al. 1994; Steiner et al. 1994b). The possibility of pseudotumoral infectious masses or inflammatory disease should also be entertained (Fig. 3.54).

Salivary gland tumors represent less than 5% of all tumors in children. Diagnosis is made by clinical examination and Doppler sonography. Hemangiomas predominate (50%), but malignant tumors (especially mucoepidermoid carcinomas) are also common (35%). Adenopathies of the parotid space are fairly frequent and can be painful and rapidly growing. They are often related to acute otitis, which is responsible for 5% of all cases of peripheral facial nerve paralysis. A rapidly expanding mass of the parotid space with facial nerve paralysis may suggest a malignant tumor, and especially rhabdomyosarcoma, which is not uncommon. On sonograms, inflammatory nodes usually appear well-delimited and conserve their central hyperechoic hilum (Fig. 3.55). MRI is helpful whenever doubt persists: Adenopa-

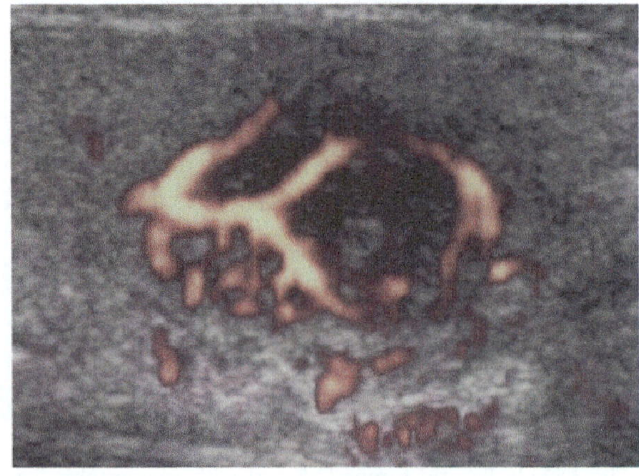

Fig. 3.54. Hypervascular, ill-defined hypoechoic parotid lesion. Infectious context. Pseudotumoral parotitis

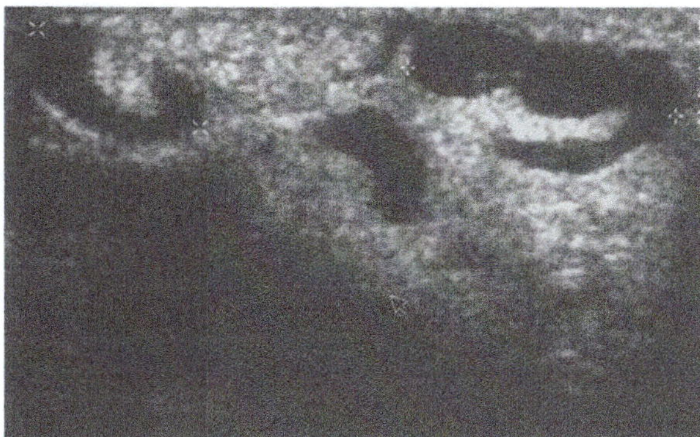

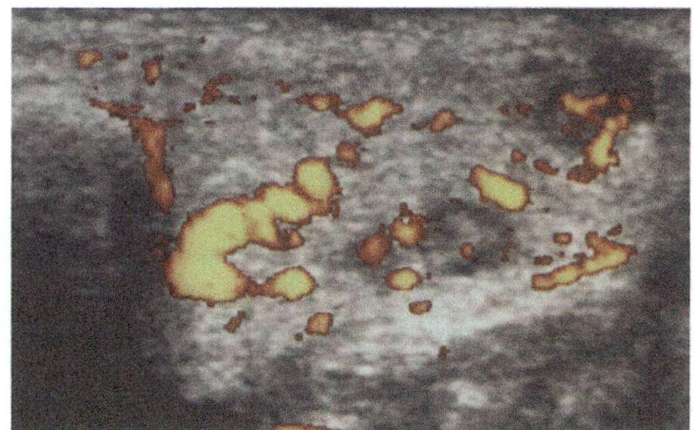

Fig. 3.55a,b. Typical inflammatory intraparotid nodes: smaller than 1 cm; preservation of a hyperechoic central hilum

thies have a very high intensity signal on T_2-weighted sequences, whereas high-grade malignant tumors tend to have a low-intensity signal.

In the adult, the differential diagnosis for a solitary, sonographically benign-appearing lesion larger than 2 cm includes, in order of decreasing frequency, pleomorphic adenoma, cystadenolymphoma, mucoepidermoid carcinoma, adenoid cystic carcinoma, and acinic cell tumor. Sudden changes in a long-standing lesion are strongly suggestive of carcinoma ex pleomorphic adenoma. Color Doppler US studies may be a useful complement for parotid tumors, as tumor hypervascularity is a predictor of malignancy (Benzel et al. 1995). A solitary lesion with the sonographic features of malignancy should suggest a high-grade mucoepidermoid carcinoma, carcinoma, or adenoid cystic carcinoma. MRI demonstration of perineural invasion along the facial nerve is suggestive of adenoid cystic carcinoma.

Detection of a solitary contralateral lesion should suggest a cystadenolymphoma or an acinic cell tumor.

Unilateral multinodular lesions are suggestive of a pleomorphic adenoma, oncocytoma, lymphoma, or nodal metastases of regional tumors (Bruneton et al. 1987). A diagnosis of lymphoma can be suggested by the history and the presence of cervical adenopathies. Scintigraphy reveals intense tracer uptake in the case of oncocytomas. Regional examination is required to search for a malignant melanoma of the temporal region or a squamous cell carcinoma (Fig. 3.56). US-guided FNAB is also an effective diagnostic procedure. Adenopathies in the posterior parotid space, close to the stylomastoid foramen have been associated with facial nerve paralysis in patients with Lyme disease (Mann et al. 1992). There have been rare reports of synchronous double benign parotid tumors of different histological types, essentially pleomorphic adenoma and Warthin's tumor (Franzen and Koegel 1996).

Bilateral multinodular lesions may suggest non-Hodgkin's lymphoma, local-regional nodal metastases, tuberculosis, sarcoidosis, or oncocytosis (Bruneton et al. 1985). Sarcoidosis has a propensity for the submandibular gland. Lingual cancers and carcinomas in the floor of the mouth can spread to the lymph nodes of both submandibular spaces, occasionally causing dilatation of Wharton's duct on the same side as the tumor (Larsson et al. 1987).

The presence of massive calcifications should suggest pleomorphic adenoma. Smaller calcifications may be related to a mucoepidermoid tumor or, in the context of hemangioma, phleboliths.

Cystic masses require a careful etiological evaluation. Examination of the external acoustic meatus and the drum may suggest a first branchial cleft cyst. HIV serological tests should be performed, as lymphoepithelial cysts are common in HIV-infected

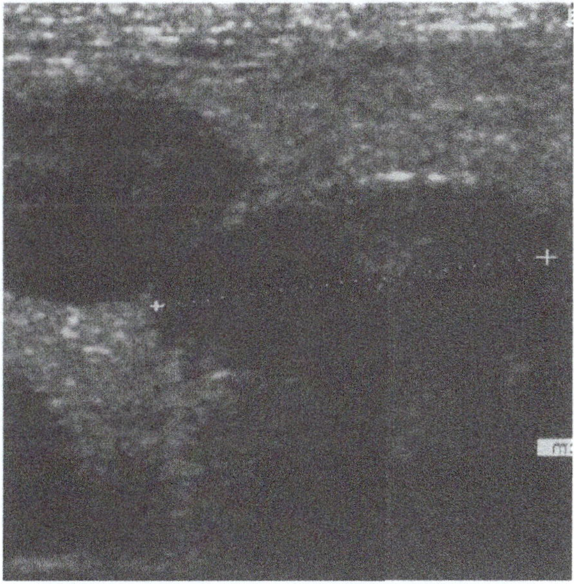

Fig. 3.56. Parotid metastases of a squamous cell carcinoma

patients. The possibility of a cystadenolymphoma can be determined by radionuclide scanning, as these lesions show high tracer uptake. Certain mucoepidermoid tumors also have a cystic component. Bilateral, diffuse cystic parotid lesions with swelling of the submandibular glands and decreased saliva flow should prompt a search for Sjögren's syndrome.

Facial nerve paralysis associated with a parotid mass should initially suggest a high-grade malignant tumor. The possibility of a granulomatous disease, Sjögren's syndrome, and Lyme disease must also be investigated (Fig. 3.57).

Inflammatory lesions can mimic a tumor. Pseudotumoral Sjögren's syndrome may image sonographically as multiple, bilateral hypoechoic lesions smaller than 5 mm; MRI may reveal a suggestive appearance on T_2-weighted sequences. Sialography remains valuable for the diagnosis of tuberculosis. A presumptive diagnosis of sarcoidosis based on the history may be confirmed by demonstration of thoracic or cervical node involvement. Kimura's disease is a benign, chronic condition seen essentially in Asians. It affects young, predominantly male subjects (80% of cases). The painless cervical swelling is often associated with eosinophilia. Sonography demonstrates one or more hypoechoic parotid or submandibular nodules, sometimes associated with regional adenopathies. US-guided FNAB may suggest the diagnosis (Ahuja et al. 1995). When steroids prove ineffective, the treatment of choice is surgery. Angiolymphoid hyperplasia with eosinophilia causes subcutaneous masses similar to those in Kimura's disease; the lesions are ubiquitous, but the majority of cases are extraglandular and occur in a preauricular location. Doppler sonography reveals a well-defined mass with high central vascularization supplied by a large artery that enters the lesion directly (Ussmuller et al. 1997). Treatment consists in surgical excision.

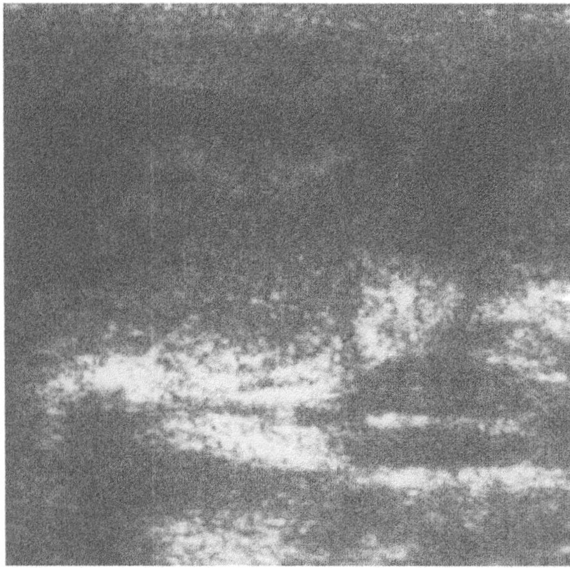

Fig. 3.57. Multiple hypoechoic intra- and retroparotid masses in a patient with peripheral facial paralysis. Lyme disease

Diagnosis occasionally requires histological examination of the surgical specimen, which may reveal a rare pathology such as necrotizing sialometaplasia or Wegener's granulomatosis, or nonspecific lesions such as chronic inflammation of the parotid or submandibular gland (Gaillard et al. 1981; Lustmann et al. 1994; Russo et al. 1998).

3.5.3.4 *Staging*

Staging is based on an association of sonography and MRI; CT is helpful for accurate demonstration of extraglandular spread, and in particular osseous infiltration of the mandible or at the level of the base of the skull (Marsot-Dupuch et al. 1992; Whyte and Byrne 1987). Sonography allows optimal staging of the local-regional lymph nodes. MRI can accurately demonstrate extension to the retrostyloid space, the pharyngeal parotid, and the deep regions of the face for accessory salivary gland tumors.

MRI offers better diagnostic accuracy than US for the detection of multifocal pleomorphic adenomas and bilateral space-occupying lesions (Grazioli et al. 1994).

Tumor spread to the facial nerve is difficult to assess, regardless of the imaging technique used. Sonography and color Doppler US can accurately localize the venous confluence of the parotid on oblique longitudinal scans; invasion of this plane suggests involvement of the facial nerve (Fig. 3.58).

3.6 Sialolithiasis

Sialolithiasis is always limited to the gland itself and is not correlated with similar biliary or renal pathologies. An estimated 1.2% of the general population is affected. Most salivary stones occur in the submandibular glands (80%–92% of sialoliths); the parotid gland is involved in only 6%–19% of cases and the sublingual glands in 1%–2% (Silvers and Som 1998).

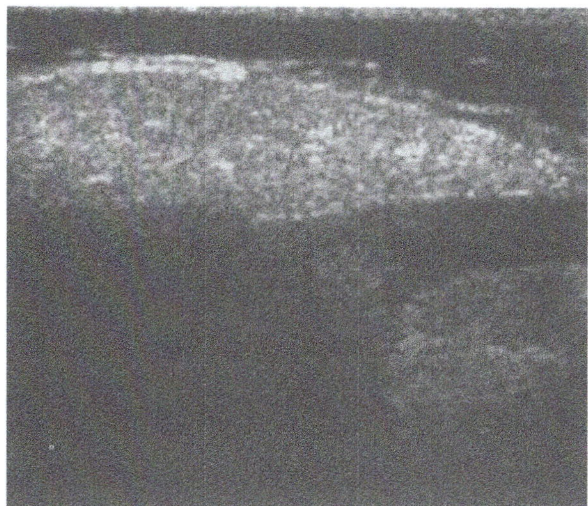

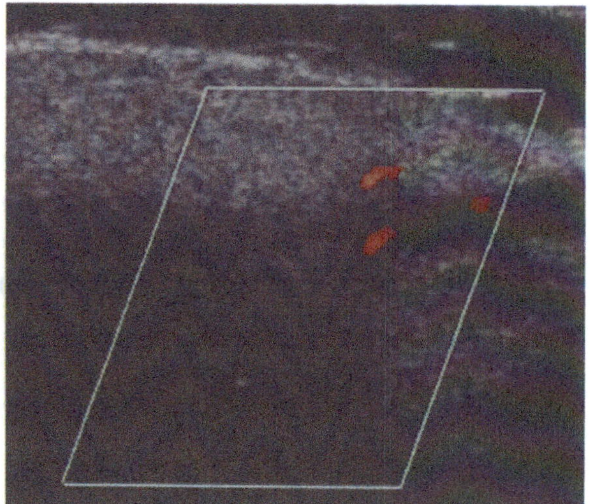

Fig. 3.58a,b. Carcinoma invading the venous plane of the parotid

Three quarters of stones are solitary, and multigland disease is rare (3%) (Bourjat and Beaujeux 1994). Two thirds of all patients with chronic sialadenitis have at least one stone. The majority of sialoliths are smaller than 1 cm, particularly those in the parotid (Gaillard 1981). Imaging studies (usually sonography or sialography) play an important role in diagnosis of these stones composed of calcium or oxalate deposits (Schurawitzki et al. 1987).

Impacted ostial stones are often managed by surgical excision. Salivary calculi can also be removed via the duct under sialographic control using a probe equipped with a Dormia basket (Kelly and Dick 1990). US-guided extracorporeal lithotripsy is an attractive and noninvasive solution for management of parotid stones (Ottaviani et al. 1996).

3.6.1 Submandibular Gland Lithiasis

Submandibular gland calculi produce suggestive clinical symptoms (episodes of salivary colic or sialadenitis). Left untreated, such stones may cause ductal lesions or chronic inflammation (Reinhardt and Dross 1984).

Submandibular gland stones are usually solitary and radiopaque. Only 15% occur in the hilum or parenchyma; 85% occur in Wharton's duct, the majority (35%) in the midportion of the duct, around the mylohyoid muscle; only 30% are ostial (Levy et al. 1962). Plain films remain helpful for diagnosis and can reveal stones composed of calcium deposits (Larsson et al. 1987)

In addition to demonstration of the stone, sonography can accurately determine its localization, evaluate the intraglandular ductal system, and even analyze Wharton's duct when this is dilated (Figs. 3.59–3.61).

Gland enlargement is an associated US feature in 94% of cases; ductal ectasia occurs in 61% (Angelelli et al. 1990). High-frequency intraoral sonography using a conventional endoscopic probe or small, dig-

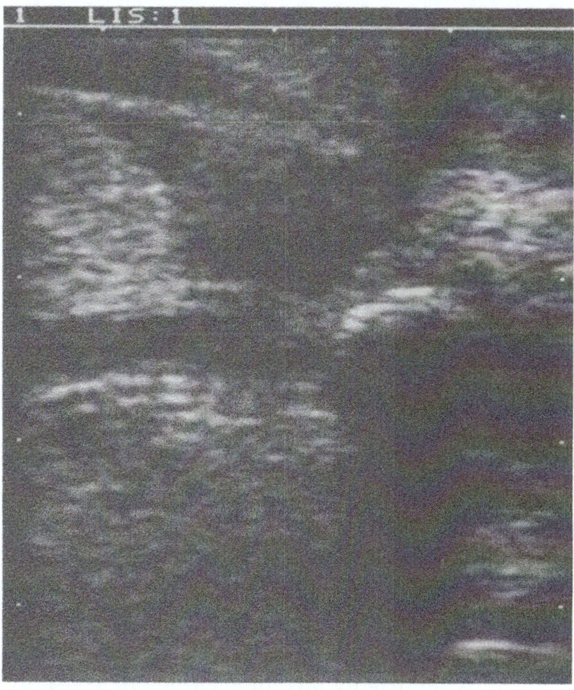

Fig. 3.59. Salivary colic. Oblique transverse scan of the floor of the mouth revealing a stone impacted in Wharton's duct

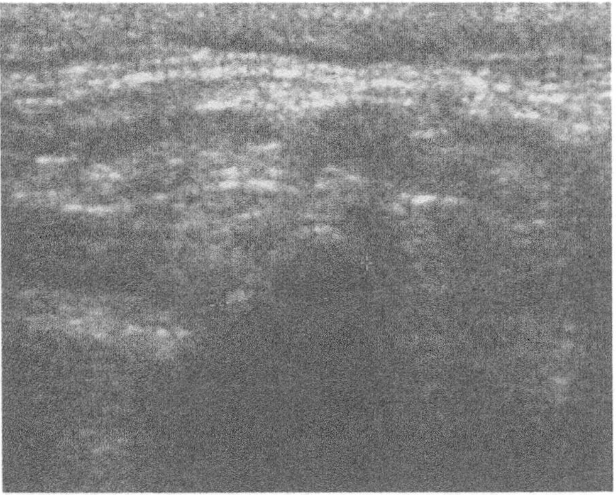

Fig. 3.60. Atrophy of a submandibular gland containing a large sialolith

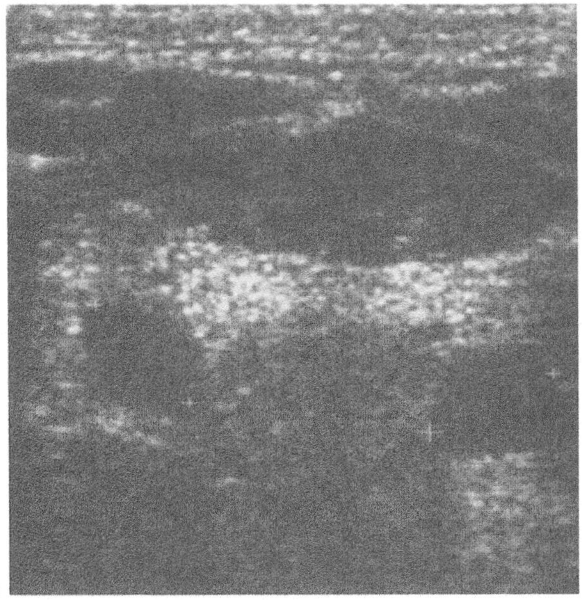

a

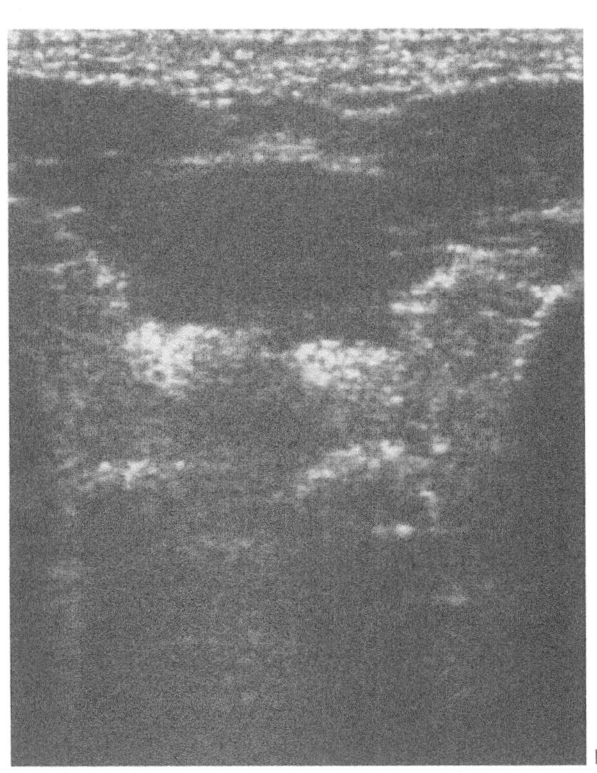

b

Fig. 3.61a,b. Severe denutrition. Longitudinal scan of the floor of the mouth. Bilateral calculi impacted in the terminal segment of both Wharton's ducts

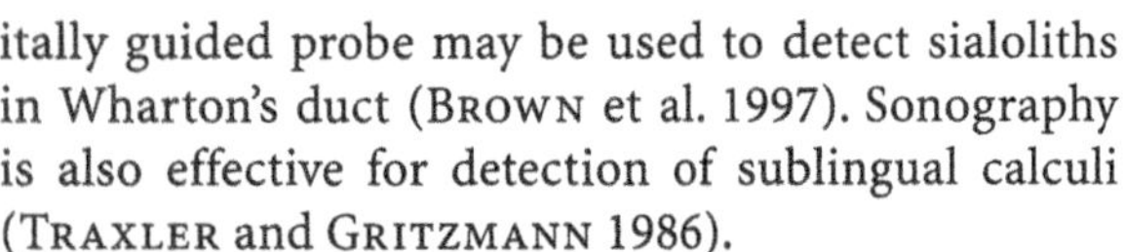

itally guided probe may be used to detect sialoliths in Wharton's duct (Brown et al. 1997). Sonography is also effective for detection of sublingual calculi (Traxler and Gritzmann 1986).

Sialography is still occasionally helpful for evaluation of ductal obstruction or to search for a radiolucent stone not visible on sonograms (Reinhardt and Dross 1984). MR sialography associated with plain films reportedly has an accuracy of 100% for the detection of submandibular gland stones (Varghese et al. 1999).

3.6.2 Parotid Lithiasis

Although symptoms are often not very suggestive, lithiasis should be sought whenever a patient presents clinically with chronic parotitis or recurrent acute parotitis. Plain films tend to be ineffective, because 40% of stones are radiolucent (Bourjat and Kahn 1995).

Sonography detects 90% of parotid stones, often in the extraglandular portion of Stensen's duct, which may be dilated (Bruneton et al. 1987). The small size and low calcium component of the calculi complicates detection within the parenchyma and necessitates attentive analysis. A posterior acoustic shadow is seen occasionally (Fig. 3.62). Demonstration of a twinkling artifact behind a hyperechoic structure is highly suggestive of a stone. The minimum size of stones demonstrable by high-frequency sonography is approximately 2+3 mm (Yoshimura et al. 1989).

The major differential diagnosis for patients who suffer painful episodes such as salivary hernia is a parotid megaduct, i.e., a permanent, global, and bilateral dilatation of Stensen's duct (Gaillard et al. 1981) (Fig. 3.63). Sonographic demonstration of bilateral, uniform dilatation without any detectable stone suggests a megaduct. Sialography may prove helpful when sonographic evaluation is noncontributory and can also rule out a stone or stenosis of the terminal segment of Stensen's duct.

3.6.3 Extracorporeal Lithotripsy

Like renal stones, salivary stones can be fragmented under sonographic guidance using electromagnetic or piezoelectric shockwaves (Hessling et al. 1993; Iro et al. 1990). The procedure is performed under mere sedation, without a need for anesthesia. Stones ranging from 3 to 13 mm in diameter are amenable to lithotripsy. Results are better for parotid stones (elimination of 56.3%–82%) than for submandibular stones (less than 50%). Although complete stone fragmentation is achieved in most cases, the residual fragments are larger than 3 mm for 30% of all submandibular stones. Adverse effects such as sialorrhagia, glandular or subcutaneous hematoma, and transient gland swelling occur in approximately 25% of cases. No adverse effects on the facial nerve have ever been reported (Hessling et al. 1993; Ottaviani et al. 1996).

3.7 Sialadenitis

3.7.1 Acute Sialadenitis

Acute sialadenitis is characterized by acute, painful swelling of a salivary gland (usually the parotid gland) due to recurrent infection. The submandibular gland is often spared, probably because its mucin-rich salivary secretion plays a protective role (Silvers and Som 1998).

The most common cause of parotitis is the mumps virus, but other viruses have also been implicated: influenza virus, Coxsackie A virus; echovirus, cytomegalovirus, and Epstein-Barr virus. An ascending bacterial infection, promoted by decreased saliva production, immune depression, or surgery, can also cause parotitis (Gaillard et al. 1981; McQuone 1999). The most commonly responsible organisms are *Staphylococcus aureus*, various strains of *Streptococcus*, and *Haemophilus influenzae*. Acute suppurative parotitis of toxic origin has been linked to poisoning by organophosphates (Leuwer et al. 1990). The diagnosis is made clinically. Examination may reveal redness of the ostium of Stensen's duct, with discharge of pus. Suppuration is a potential complication.

The use of sialography remains controversial (Bourjat and Kahn 1995). Difficult to perform

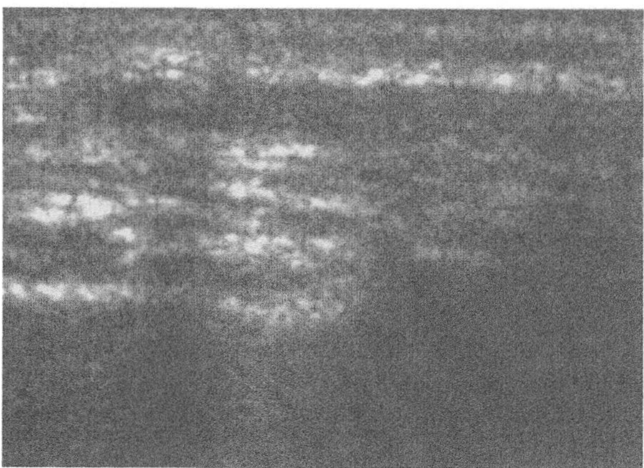

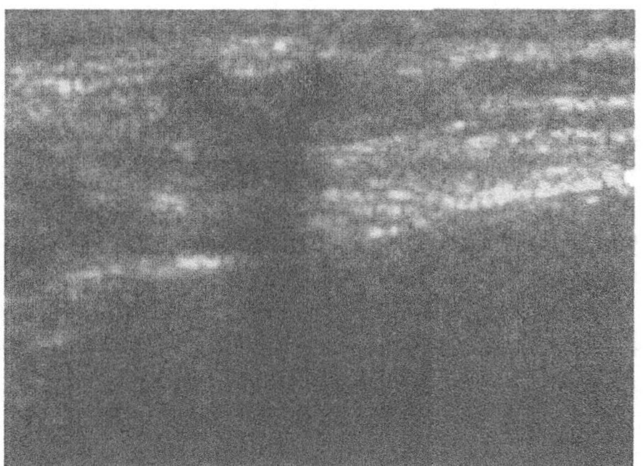

Fig. 3.62a,b. Transverse (**a**) and longitudinal (**b**) scans of the jugal region. Dilated Stensen's duct with echoic contents; the endoductal echoic mass with posterior acoustic shadowing corresponds to a calculus

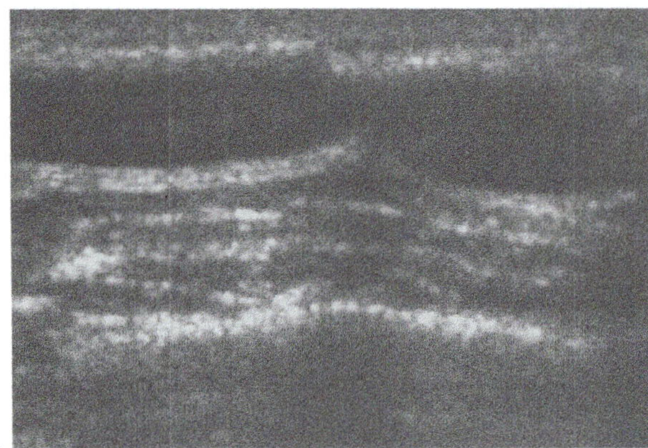
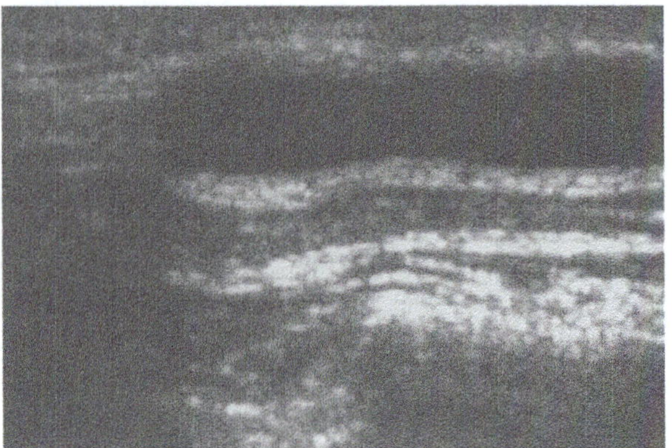

Fig. 3.63a,b. Marked bilateral dilatation of Stensen's ducts without any visible calculi: megaducts

because of the associated pain, sonography reveals diffuse, homogeneous enlargement of the affected gland. Cervical adenopathies may be associated (Bruneton et al. 1987). The gland and the course of Stensen's duct must be carefully examined to avoid overlooking a stone (Kessler et al. 1995). When an intraglandular abscess develops, sonography reveals a well-delimited anechoic or hypoechoic mass with posterior enhancement (Fig. 3.64).

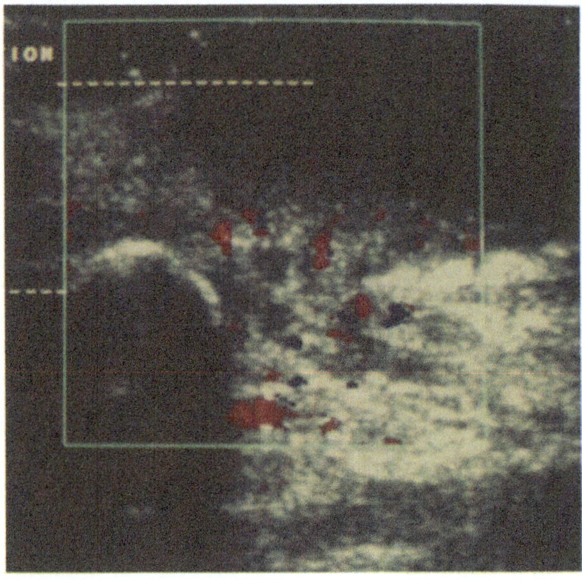

Fig. 3.64. Parotid abscess. Inhomogeneity due to the thick contents. Doppler reveals the absence of vascularity

3.7.2 Chronic Sialadenitis

3.7.2.1 Chronic Recurrent Parotitis

Manifesting clinically as recurrent acute episodes that cease in several weeks, chronic parotitis includes both an adult form and an infantile form that often regresses at puberty. There may be a history of infection or lithiasis (Reinhardt and Dross 1984); hyposialosis is common.

Chronic recurrent parotitis is characterized by periacinar lymphocytic infiltration associated with microcystic ductal dilatations (Gaillard 1981). Sialography confirms the diagnosis by demonstrating acinar ectasia and sometimes the moniliform appearance of Stensen's duct (Iko 1984).

Sonography has recently proven its excellent sensitivity for the diagnosis of sialectasia (Murray et al. 1996). On sonograms, the sometimes enlarged parotid contains multiple round hypoechoic areas ranging from 2 to 4 mm in diameter (Fig. 3.65), i.e., larger than the punctate shadows corresponding to the pools of contrast medium shown by sialography. According to Nozaki et al. (1994), these areas correspond to acinar ectasia and the surrounding lymphocytic infiltration. This suggestive appearance was observed in 62% of the glands examined by Shimizu et al. (1998). On rare occasions, US examination is strictly normal. Sonography permits reliable evaluation of disease severity and post-therapy follow-up, and US findings are well-correlated with sialographic images (Encina et al. 1996). US is recommended as the first-line technique for children with recurrent parotitis; sialography is reserved for atypical forms when sonography is noncontributory.

Certain pseudotumoral forms involve difficulties for diagnosis, and surgery may be required to confirm the benign nature of a chronic parotid nodule (Bernier et al. 1994).

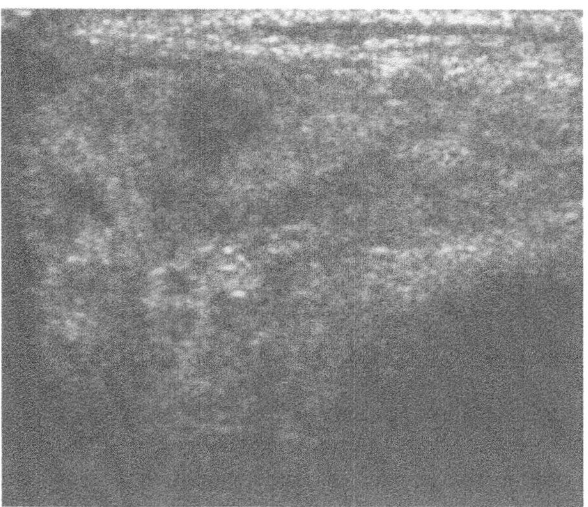

Fig. 3.65. Chronic recurrent parotitis. Heterogeneous appearance of the gland parenchyma that contains small (5 mm or less) hypoechoic masses

3.7.2.2 Granulomatous Diseases

3.7.2.2.1 Tuberculosis

Primary tuberculosis of the salivary glands is rarely seen today except in immunodepressed patients. Parotid sites predominate (70% of cases), followed by involvement of the submandibular glands (27%) and sublingual glands (3%) (SILVERS and SOM 1998). Salivary gland tuberculosis must be distinguished from nodal involvement, which is common after spread of disease through the regional lymph nodes of the submandibular space.

The highly variable clinical presentation ranges from sialadenitis with nodal involvement (acute tuberculous sialadenitis) to chronic sialitis. A pseudotumoral syndrome with facial nerve paralysis is also possible. The natural course of the adenopathies is to cutaneous fistulization. Bilateral involvement is exceptional (GAILLARD et al. 1981).

Sonography reveals an enlarged gland with a heterogeneous echostructure containing poorly delimited areas of low echogenicity and associated lymphadenopathy (DAGHFOUS et al. 1994). Sialography may suggest the diagnosis by demonstrating multiple filling defects within dense parenchymal opacification of inflammatory origin (LAUDENBACH et al. 1994). US-guided FNAB centered on the necrotic zones, followed by direct examination and culture on Lowenstein medium, may suggest the diagnosis, thereby obviating the need for exploratory surgery.

3.7.2.2.2 Sarcoidosis

The parotid glands are involved in 10%–30% of patients with sarcoidosis; solitary involvement of the parotid is infrequent but may be the first and only manifestation of the disease. Bilateral parotid gland enlargement occurs in 83% of patients (SILVERS and SOM 1998).

This systemic granulomatous disease is characterized by noncaseating granulomas (IKO et al. 1986).

Enlargement of the parotid glands is often asymmetrical. On manual palpation, the gland has a granular consistency. IKO et al. (1986) reported associated thoracic sarcoidosis in 86% of their patients and simultaneous submandibular gland enlargement in 5%.

Several clinical forms have been described (GAILLARD et al. 1981):

- Heerfordt's syndrome, a triad of parotid gland enlargement, uveitis, and facial nerve paralysis
- Pseudotumoral forms, with or without facial nerve paralysis

Imaging studies are not very contributory. Sonography may be useful for pseudotumors, particularly those involving the submandibular glands, by demonstrating the presence of multiple nodules within the gland. On sialograms, the gland parenchyma may appear intensely mottled or finely punctated by acinar or ductal ectasia. US-guided aspiration biopsy may suggest the diagnosis when salivary involvement is solitary (KELLY et al. 1994).

3.7.2.2.3 Other Granulomatous-type Diseases

Toxoplasmosis and cat-scratch disease can produce imaging features similar to those of tuberculosis and sarcoidosis, but imaging is not specific. Cervical lymphadenopathy is the predominant clinical symptom. The history and specific serological tests orient the diagnosis.

Actinomycosis due to bacteria of the genus *Actinomyces* manifests as chronic infection of the mandible, and is related to poor buccodental status. The infection may spread by contiguity to the salivary glands and the soft tissues, often leading to fistulization (GAILLARD et al. 1981). The existence of bone lesions and perimandibular infiltration (masticator space disease) suggest the diagnosis of cervicofacial actinomycosis (Sa'do et al. 1993).

3.8 Sialosis

Sialosis, a group of noninfectious, nontumoral pathologies of highly varied etiologies (often of parotid origin), is characterized by an association of gland enlargement (usually bilateral), with or without hyposialosis. Although sialography remains the imaging technique of reference, high-frequency sonography is increasing used as the first-line imaging technique and often proves sufficient (Murray et al. 1996).

3.8.1 Sjögren's Syndrome

Sjögren's syndrome is a systemic autoimmune disorder of the exocrine glands (in particular the salivary and lacrimal glands) and the second most common autoimmune disease after rheumatoid polyarthritis. In addition to the primary form (sicca syndrome), a secondary form of Sjögren's syndrome is associated with a connective-tissue disease (usually rheumatoid polyarthritis). Age at diagnosis is between 40 and 60 years, with a marked female predominance (90% of cases).

The pathological changes correspond to lymphocytic infiltration and myoepithelial islets that obstruct or compress the intercalated ducts, resulting in dilated pseudocystic acini (Cabanne and Bonenfant 1980). The natural history, aggravated by episodes of superinfection, is characterized by the formation of parenchymal cavities of highly variable dimensions.

Sicca syndrome is characterized by a "dry eye and mouth syndrome" associating varying degrees of hyposialosis, xerophthalmia, and nasal dryness. Parotid enlargement is classic, but all of the salivary glands are affected. Atypical pseudotumors and forms suggesting acute sialadenitis also occur. Transformation to non-Hodgkin's lymphoma has been reported in 5%–10% of cases (Bruneton et al. 1987).

Positive diagnosis is based on biopsy of the accessory salivary glands of the lips or soft palate (Bourjat and Beaujeux 1994). The primary role of imaging is morphological and functional evaluation of the affected glands. Scintigraphy reveals the decreased saliva production.

Parotid sialography is interesting, owing to the parallel between the evolution of radiologic signs and the severity of histological involvement. On sialograms, the early stage of the disorder manifests as numerous punctate pools of contrast material corresponding to sialectasia. The intermediate stage is characterized by larger, globular collections of contrast throughout the gland following parenchymal and ductal extravasation of the contrast medium. Cavitary and destructive forms of sialectasia are observed in the late stage (Laudenbach and Moreau 1974).

In the initial stage of Sjögren's syndrome, sonography reveals a homogeneous or sometimes finely heterogeneous gland parenchyma (Fig. 3.66). The submandibular glands have a heterogeneous US pattern on B-mode imaging in 88% of cases; this sonographic appearance is less common in the parotid gland (33%) (Kawamura et al. 1990). As the disease progresses, the gland parenchyma becomes heterogeneous and often hypoechoic, with multiple low echogenicity masses ranging in size from 2 to 5 mm (Fig. 3.67) (Bradus et al. 1988; Gritzmann 1989); this appearance is seen in 43% of cases (Takashima et al. 1992a). Color Doppler analysis of parotid blood flow reveals moderately or greatly increased perfusion correlated with the severity of glandular changes in 52% of patients with Sjögren's syndrome (Steiner et al. 1994a). US has a sensitivity of 76%–88% for primary Sjögren syndrome's but less than 50% for the secondary form (De Vita et al. 1992; Makula et al. 1996; Napoli et al. 1996). Quantitative texture analysis of the sono-

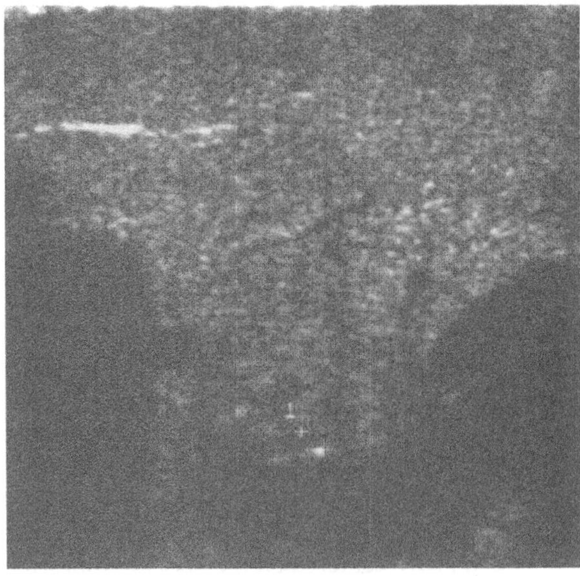

Fig. 3.66. Sjögren's syndrome: early stage with enlargement of the parotid, which appears finely heterogeneous

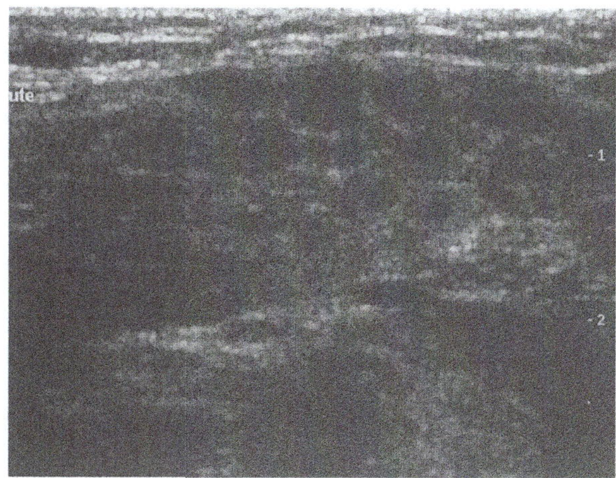

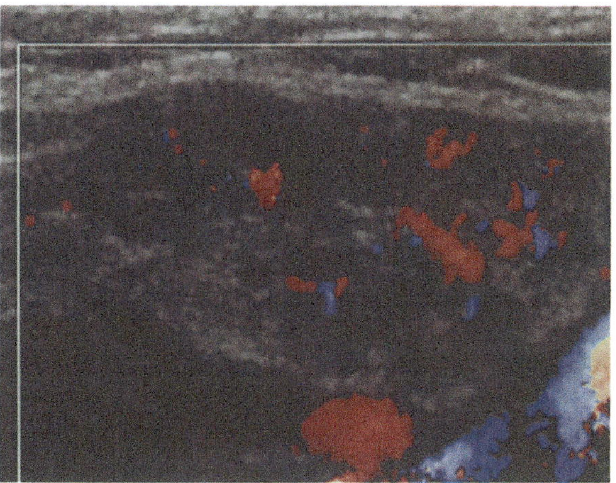

Fig. 3.67a,b. Advanced pseudotumoral Sjögren's syndrome. **a** Multiple hypoechoic intraparotid masses. **b** Hypervascularity on color Doppler

graphic features of the parotid revealed significant modifications in 96.9% of patients compared with an age-matched population of healthy volunteers (Ariji et al. 1996). Use of a sonographic scoring system (range 0–6) to describe gland inhomogeneity provides good correlation with the sialographic stage. US has a diagnostic accuracy of only 80% for diagnosis of Sjögren's syndrome, versus almost 100% for sialography (Yoshiura et al. 1997).

Multicystic masses have also been described as the sole manifestation of primary Sjögren's syndrome, similar to the multicystic disease seen in HIV-positive individuals with lymphoepithelial cysts (AIDS parotitis) (Ahmad et al. 1998).

MRI is less specific than sialography. The lymphocytic aggregates are hypointense on T_1- and T_2-weighted sequences, while the dilated ducts are hyperintense on T_2-weighted sequences. The "salt-and-pepper" sign, a characteristic mixture of hypointense and hyperintense foci, is observed on T_2-weighted images (Takashima et al. 1991). MRI is usually performed as a complement to sonography for pseudotumors in Sjögren's syndrome (Takashima et al. 1992b).

Sonographic surveillance of the cervical node-bearing areas has been recommended, owing to the risk of transformation to malignant parotid lymphoma (Bruneton et al. 1987).

3.8.2 Salivary Calcinosis

This rare but not exceptional disease, similar to Sjögren's syndrome, produces multiple small (2–3 mm) calcifications throughout the parotid parenchyma (Laudenbach et al. 1977). Ductal migration of these concretions and their associated symptoms (salivary colic) are rare. Involvement is usually bilateral. Plain films rarely demonstrate these calcifications that have a low density. Their bilateral nature and multiplicity rule out calculi or phleboliths. Sialography may reveal sialectasia. Sonography can prove helpful for diagnosis by revealing multiple bilateral intraparotid calcifications (Fig. 3.68).

3.8.3 Sialadenosis

The general term sialadenosis refers to any asymptomatic, usually bilateral and symmetrical enlarge-

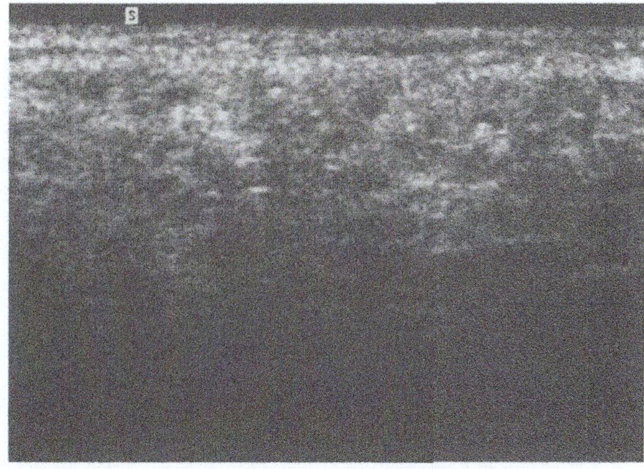

Fig. 3.68. Inhomogeneously hyperechoic parotid with posterior echo attenuation owing to multiple calcifications in the gland parenchyma. Salivary calcinosis

ment of the parotid glands that is neither inflammatory nor neoplastic in origin. Histological examination reveals acinar enlargement with fat infiltration (Cabanne and Bonenfant 1980).

The causes of sialadenosis are multiple; endocrine disorders linked to alcoholism, malnutrition, diabetes, or hyperuricemia predominate. Allergic or toxic causes are much less common. The prognosis is favorable after correction of the metabolic anomaly.

The diagnosis is made clinically. Sialography demonstrates rarefaction of the intraglandular ducts that create a typical "dead-tree" appearance. Sonography is useful when extensive gland enlargement suggests a subjacent tumor; US demonstration of homogeneous and often hyperechoic parotid enlargement related to fatty pathological changes confirms the diagnosis (Fig. 3.69).

3.9 Trauma

Most cases of salivary gland trauma concern the parotid gland, as the submandibular glands are protected by the horizontal body of the mandible.

3.9.1 Gland Fractures and Injuries

True gland fractures are frequently associated with bone involvement (mandibular or zygomatic fractures); this is particularly true for submandibular gland lesions. Injury to Stensen's duct may result in partial or complete section (Bernier et al. 1994; Bourjat and Beaujeux 1994). Extensive gland fracture manifests as a rapidly expansive mass in the parotid or submandibular space.

Ductal injuries may result in development of an internal or external salivary gland fistula or a sialocele (salivary cyst) that may or may not communicate with the duct (pseudocyst).

Sialography using water-soluble agents allows analysis of ductal lesions and opacification of fistulas and salivary cysts (Reinhardt and Dross 1984). CT is helpful for overall local-regional workup and can demonstrate the frequently associated osseous lesions. Sonography has few indications for traumatic injuries, although it may prove useful for demonstration of a sialocele or to determine the size of a hematoma (Fig. 3.70).

3.9.2 Foreign Bodies

Salivary gland trauma following penetration of a foreign body is not uncommon, particularly in children. Penetrating injuries of the floor of the mouth, the oral cavity, or the parotid region often result in impaction of the object in the submandibular gland or parotid parenchyma. If the injury is overlooked initially, the object may not be detected until complications occur (Wooley et al. 1998). The initial search for the object should be made sonographically, and US is often more effective than plain films or CT, especially for nonmetallic objects (Becelli et al. 1995).

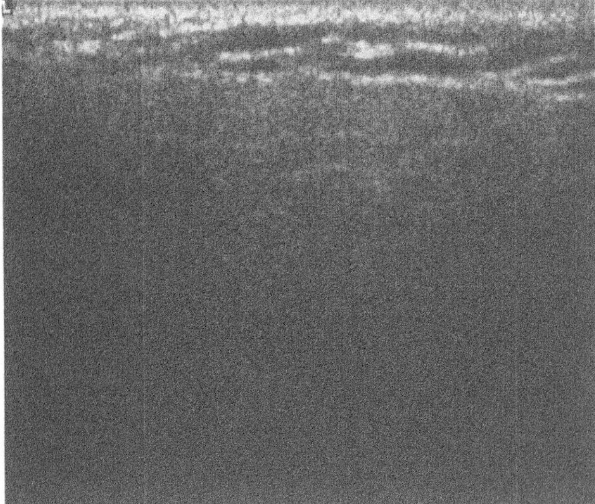

Fig. 3.69. Parotid sialadenosis

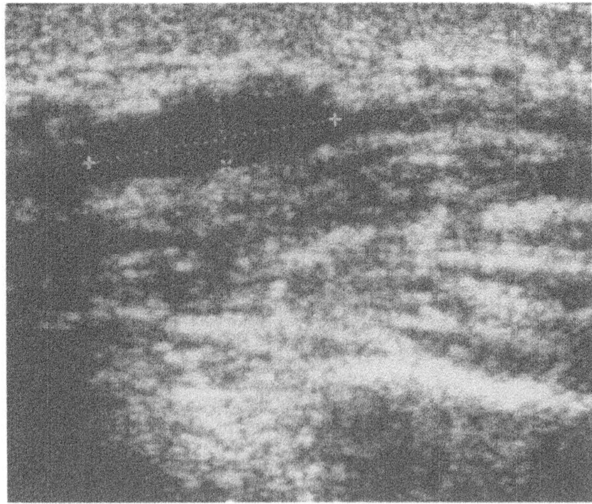

Fig. 3.70. Jugal injury with partial section of Stensen's duct. Post-traumatic formation of a sialocele

3.9.3 Pneumoparotitis

Reflux of air into the acini of the parotid via Stensen's duct is a rare cause of gland enlargement. This condition, related to an increase in intrabuccal pressure, is seen in glassblowers, players of wind instruments, and individuals with tics who puff out their cheeks. Air may diffuse to the hemiface (CURTIN et al. 1992; GAILLARD et al. 1981). Sonography or CT can demonstrate air bubbles within the parotid (Fig. 3.71).

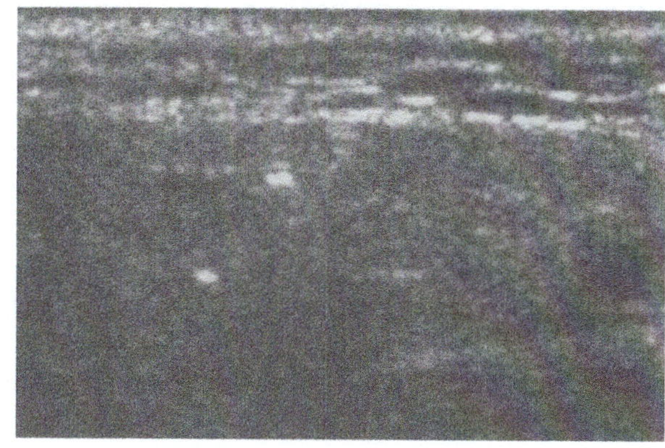

Fig. 3.71. Pneumoparotitis: the small intraglandular echoic spots without acoustic shadowing correspond to microbubbles of air in the gland ducts

3.10 Post-therapeutic Features

Sonography is increasingly used for follow-up of nontumoral salivary gland pathologies such as chronic recurrent parotitis, sarcoidosis, and Sjögren's syndrome. Parameters for surveillance include gland size, the echogenicity and degree of homogeneity of the parenchyma, and the visibility of acinar ectasia (DE VITA et al. 1992; MAKULA et al. 1996; NAPOLI et al. 1996). Abnormal findings can be ranked using a five-point rating scale (YOSHIURA et al. 1997). Sonography should thus limit recourse to sialography, which, though effective, is traumatic and exposes the patient to ionizing radiation.

Imaging is used systematically for post-therapeutic surveillance of salivary gland tumors. MRI is often indispensable, namely for carcinomas and adenoid cystic carcinomas that may spread to the deep regions of the face (Fig. 3.72, 3.73). Sonography is performed as the initial technique to search for recurrence in the parotidectomy bed, especially for pleomorphic adenomas (Fig. 3.74) (RAFFAELLI et al. 1995). US is also the imaging modality of choice for evaluation of the cervical node chains. The parotidectomy bed images as a depression that is partially filled in by hyperechoic fibrotic tissue. In such cases, the vascular axes are more superficial and well-visualized by color Doppler (Fig. 3.75). The venous plane may remain visible after superficial extrafacial parotidectomy. Sonography is particularly indicated for detection of small, highly superficial lesions of low echogenicity within the fibrotic tissue. Small hypoechoic subcutaneous masses that are tender to palpation may correspond to plexiform neuromas (GAILLARD et al. 1981) (Fig. 3.76).

Head and neck irradiation extensively modifies the appearance of the salivary glands. Postirradiation sialadenitis may be acute or chronic. The acute

a

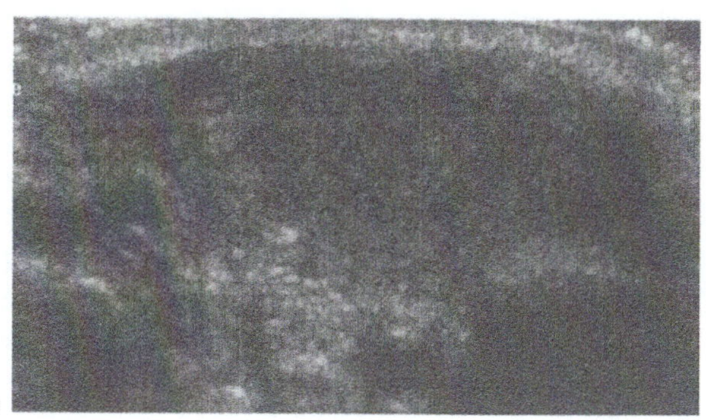

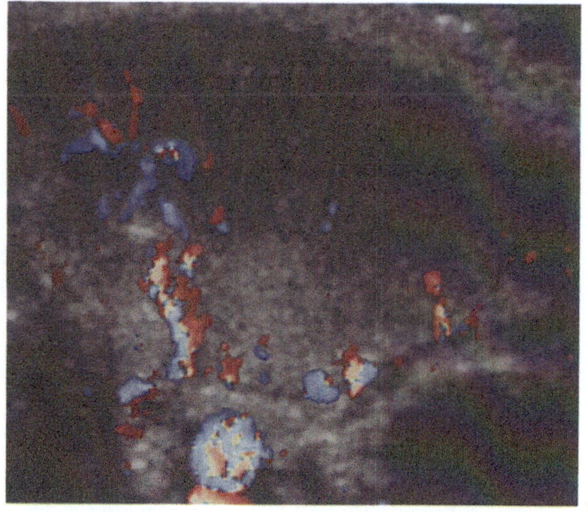

b

Fig. 3.72a,b. Recurrence of an adenoid cystic carcinoma in the parotid space after parotidectomy

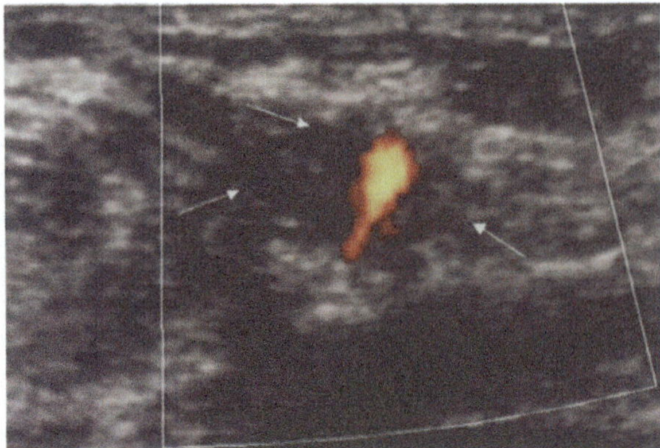

Fig. 3.73. Jugal recurrence of an adenoid cystic carcinoma

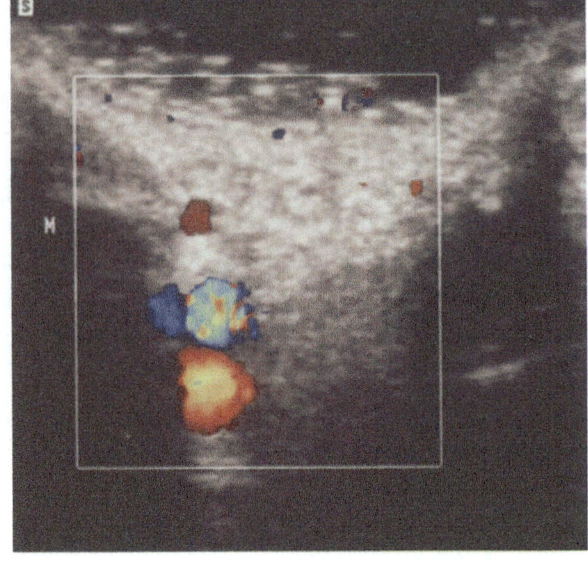

Fig. 3.75. Extrafacial parotidectomy bed. the operative cavity is partially filled in by echoic fibrous tissue. The venous plane remains visible

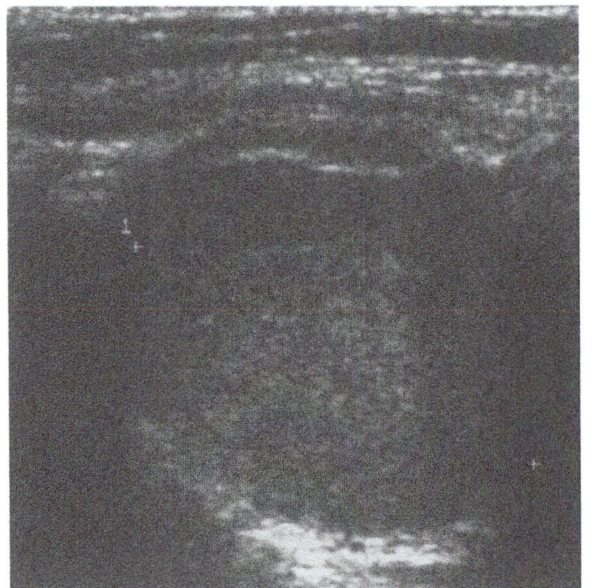

Fig. 3.74. Recurrence of a pleomorphic adenoma after parotidectomy

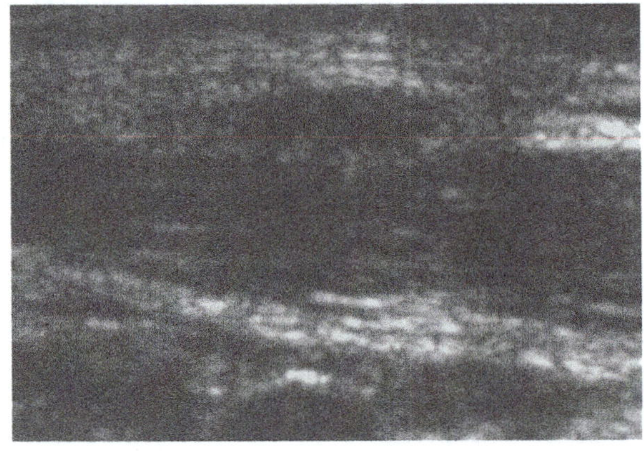

Fig. 3.76. Small, superficial and painful hypoechoic nodular mass in a total parotidectomy bed, anterior to a muscle flap. Plexiform neuroma

form develops 1–4 days after irradiation with doses of more than 10 Gy. The chronic form occurs following curative irradiation of tumors of the oral cavity or oropharynx. Hyposialosis is frequent, and usually manifests as symptoms of xerostomia (Bronstein et al. 1987). The submandibular glands are most often involved owing to the radiation fields used.

US may demonstrate atrophy and hyperechogenicity of the gland parenchyma. In the acute phase, the salivary glands have an inhomogeneous parenchymal echogenicity and irregular margins in more than 50% of cases (Fig. 3.77). Power Doppler US reveals irregular vascularization, with alternation of focal hyperemia and hypovascular or avascular zones; this confirms the elevated resistance of the smaller vessels after radiotherapy (Fig. 3.78) (Cardello et al. 1998).

External radiation therapy increases the incidence of salivary gland malignancies, especially in patients irradiated in childhood, where it is a late sequela, appearing 10–25 years after irradiation (Silvers and Som 1998).

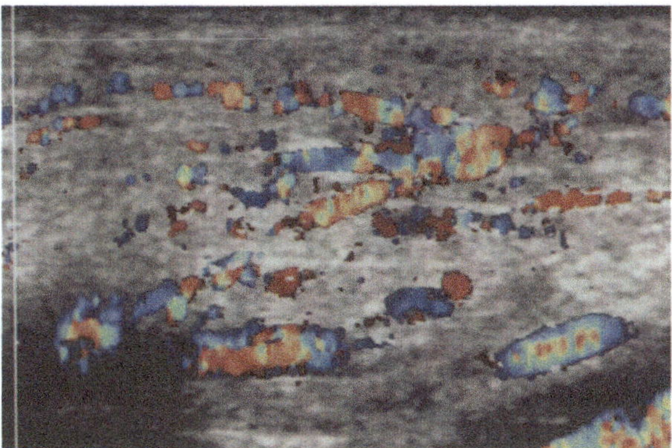

Fig. 3.77. Radiation-induced parotitis

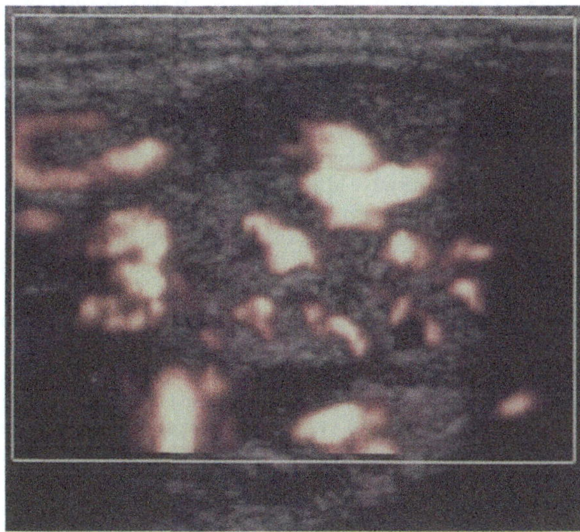

Fig. 3.78. Inhomogeneous swelling of the submandibular gland following radiotherapy for cancer of the floor of the mouth. Hypervascularity on power Doppler. Acute-stage post-radiation sialadenitis

References

Aasen S, Kolbenstvedt A (1992) CT appearances of normal and obstructed submandibular duct. Acta Radiol 33:414–419

Ahmad I, Ray J, Cullen RJ, Shortridge RT (1998) Bilateral and multicystic major salivary gland disease: a rare presentation of primary Sjögren's syndrome. J Laryngol Otol 112:1196–1198

Ahuja AT, Loke TKL, Mok CO, Chow LTC, Metreweli C (1995) Ultrasound of Kimura's disease. Clin Radiol 50:170–173

Akin I, Esmer N, Gercecker M, Aytac S, Erden I, Akan H (1991) Sialographic and ultrasonographic analyses of major salivary glands. Acta Otolaryngol 111:600–606

Almadori G, Ottaviani F, Del Ninno M, Cadoni G, De Rossi G, Paludetti G (1997) Monolateral aplasia of the parotid gland. Ann Otol Rhinol Laryngol 106:522–525

Aluffi P, Fonio N, Gandini G, Pia F (1997) Doppler color ultrasonography in the diagnosis of parotid tumors. Acta Otorhinolaryngol Ital 17:52–57

Andersen LJ, Therkildsen MH, Ockelmann HH (1991) Malignant epithelial tumors in the minor salivary glands, the submandibular glands and the sublingual glands. Cancer 68:2431–2437

Angelelli G, Favia G, Macarini L, Lacaita MG, Laforgia A (1990) Echography in the study of sialolithiasis. Radiol Med (Torino) 79:220–223

Ariji Y, Okhi M, Eguchi K, Izumi M, et al (1996) Texture analysis of sonographic features of the parotid gland in Sjögren syndrome. AJR Am J Roentgenol 166:935–941

Ariji Y, Yuasa H, Ariji E (1998) High-frequency color Doppler sonography of the submandibular gland: relationship between salivary secretion and blood flow. Oral Surg Oral Med Oral Pathol Oral Radiol Endod 86:476–481

Bartlett LJ, Pon M (1984) High-resolution real-time ultrasonography of the submandibular salivary gland. J Ultrasound Med 3:433–437

Becelli R, Belli E, Matteini C (1995) Diagnostic and surgical problems in a case of post-traumatic retention of a foreign body in the submandibular gland. Minerva Stomatol 44:539–542

Benzel W, Zenk J, Iro H (1995) Color Doppler ultrasound studies of parotid tumors. HNO 43:25–30

Bernier P, Halimi P, Trotoux J (1994) Imagerie des glandes salivaires. In: Trotoux J, Halimi P (eds) L'imagerie moderne en ORL. Arnette, Paris, pp 393–417

Bouchet A, Cuilleret J (1991a) La région sus-hyoïdienne. In: Bouchet A, Cuilleret J (eds) Anatomie topographique, descriptive et fonctionnelle. Le cou et le thorax. Simep, Paris, pp 723–737

Bouchet A, Cuilleret J (1991b) La région parotidienne. In: Bouchet A, Cuilleret J (eds) Anatomie topographique, descriptive et fonctionnelle. Le cou et le thorax. Simep, Paris, pp 767–779

Bourjat P, Beaujeux R (1994) L'imagerie des glandes salivaires. Rev Im Med 6:393–405

Bourjat P, Kahn JL (1995) Imagerie des glandes salivaires. Encycl Med Chir, Paris, France, Radiodiagnostic, 32800 A[20], 11 p

Bradus RJ, Hybarger P, Gooding GAW (1988) Parotid gland: US findings in Sjögren syndrome. Radiology 169:749–751

Bronstein AD, Nyberg DA, Schwartz AN, Shuman WP, Griffin BR (1987) Increased salivary gland density on contrast-enhanced CT after head and neck radiation. AJR Am J Roentgenol 149:1259–1263

Brown E, August M, Pich BZ, Weber A (1993) Polycystic disease of the parotid glands. AJNR Am J Neuroradiol 16:1128–1131

Brown JE, Escudier MP, Whaites EJ, Drage NA, Ng SY (1997) Intra-oral ultrasound of a submandibular duct calculus. Dentomaxillofac Radiol 26:252–255

Bruneton JN, Mourou MY (1993) Ultrasound in salivary gland diseases. J Otorhinolaryngol Relat Spec 55:284–289

Bruneton JN, Fenart D, Vallicioni J, Demard F (1980) Séméiologie échographique des tumeurs de la parotide. A propos de 40 observations. J Radiol 60:151–154

Bruneton JN, Caramella E, Boublil JL, Roux P, Abbes M, Demard F (1982) Echographic aspects of thyroid and parotid localizations in non-Hodgkin lymphomas. Rofo Fortschr Geb Roentgenstr Neuen Bildgeb Verfahr 136:530–533

Bruneton JN, Caramella E, Roux P, Fenart D, Manzino JJ (1985) Comparison of ultrasonographic findings for multinodular lesions of the salivary glands. Eur J Radiol 5:295–296

Bruneton JN, Normand F, Santini N, Balu-Maestro C (1987) Salivary glands. In: Bruneton JN (ed) Ultrasonography of the neck. Springer, Berlin Heidelberg New York, pp 64–80

Bryan RN, Miller RH, Ferreyro RI, Sessions RB (1982) Computed tomography of the major salivary glands. AJR Am J Roentgenol 139:547–554

Byrne MN, Spector JG (1988) Parotid masses: evaluation, analysis and current management. Laryngoscope 98:99–105

Byrne MN, Spector JG, Garvin CF, Gado MH (1989) Preoperative assessment of parotid masses: a comparative evaluation of radiologic techniques to histopathologic diagnosis. Laryngoscope 99:284–292

Cabanne F, Bonenfant JL (1980) Glandes salivaires. In: Cabanne F, Bonenfant JL (eds) Anatomie pathologique. Maloine, Paris, pp 754–764

Cardello P, Trinci M, Messineo D, et al (1998) Diagnostic imaging of the salivary glands in patients undergoing radiotherapy of head and neck neoplasms. Radiol Med (Torino) 95:224–231

Carney AS, Sharp JF, Cozens NJ (1996) Atypically located submandibular gland diagnosed by Doppler ultrasound. J Laryngol Otol 110:1171–1172

Chikui T, Yonetsu K, Yoshiura K, et al (1997) Imaging findings of lipomas in the orofacial region with CT, US and MRI. Oral Surg Oral Med Oral Pathol Oral Radiol Endod 84:88–95

Coit WE, Harnsberger HR, Osborn AG (1987) Ranulas and their mimics: CT evaluation. Radiology 10:211–216

Curtin JJ, Ridley NT, Cumberworth VL, Glover GW (1992) Pneumoparotitis. J Laryngol Otol 106:178–179

Daghfous MH, Nagi S, Ben Hajel H, et al (1994) Sialo-ultrasonographic approach of primary tuberculosis of the salivary glands. J Radiol 75:229–232

De Vita S, Lorezon G, Rossi G, Sabella M, Fossaluzza V (1992) Salivary gland echography in primary and secondary Sjögren's syndrome. Clin Exp Rheumatol 10:351–356

Dost P, Kaiser S (1997) Ultrasonographic biometry in salivary glands. Ultrasound Med Biol 23:1299–1303

Encina S, Ernst P, Villanueva J, Pizarro E (1996) Ultrasonography: a complement to sialography in recurrent chronic childhood parotitis. Rev Stomatol Chir Maxillofac 97:258–263

Feld R, Nazarian LN, Needleman L, et al (1999) Clinical impact of sonographically guided biopsy of salivary gland masses and surrounding lymph nodes. Ear Nose Throat J 78:908–912

Franzen A, Kogel K (1996) Synchronous double tumors of the parotid gland. Laryngorhinootologie 75:437–440

Freling NJM, Molenaar WM, Vermey A, et al (1992) Malignant parotid tumors: clinical use of MR imaging and histologic correlation. Radiology 185:691–696

Gaillard J, Gandon J, Laudenbach P, et al (1981) In: Gaillard J (ed) Pathologie médicale et chirurgicale de la région parotidienne. Arnette, Paris

Gooding GAW, Sooy CD, Hybarger CP (1992) Ultrasonography of cystic parotid lesions in HIV infection: similarity of sonographic appearance with Sjögren syndrome. J Ultrasound Med 11:35–38

Gottesman RI, Som PM, Mester J, Silvers AR (1996) Observations on two cases of apparent submandibular gland cysts in HIV-positive patients: MR and CT findings. J Comput Assist Tomogr 20:444–447

Gozzi G, Di Bonito L, Bazzocchi M, Vasciaveo A, Bassini A, Bellis GB (1990) Echography and cytology in the study of spreading pathology of the salivary glands. Radiol Med 80:273–276

Grazioli L, Olivetti L, Stanga C, et al (1994) Comparison of ultrasound, CT and MRI in the assessment of parotid masses. Eur Radiol 4:549–556

Gritzmann N (1989) Sonography of the salivary glands. AJR Am J Roentgenol 153:161–166

Hausegger KW, Krasa H, Pelzmann W, Grasser RK, Frisch C, Simon H (1993) Sonography of the salivary glands. Ultraschall Med 14:68–74

Healey WV, Perzin KH, Smith L (1970) Mucoepidermoid carcinoma of salivary gland origin. Cancer 26:366–368

Hermann H, Cier JF (1979) La sécrétion salivaire. In: Hermann H, Cier JF (eds) Précis de physiologie. Masson, Paris, pp 43–51

Hessling KH, Schlick RW, Luckey R, Gratz K, Qaiyumi SA, Allhoff EP (1993) The therapeutic value of ambulatory extracorporeal shockwave lithotripsy of salivary calculi. Results of a prospective study. Laryngorhinootologie 72:109–115

Higashi T, Murahashi H, Ikuta H, Mori Y, Watanabe Y (1987) Identification of Warthin's tumor with technetium-99m pertechnetate. Clin Nucl Med 12:796–800

Higashi T, Shindo J, Everhart FR, et al (1989) Technetium-99m pertechnetate and gallium-67 imaging in salivary gland disease. Clin Nucl Med 14:504–514

Holliday RA, Cohen WA, Schinella RA, et al (1988) Benign lymphoepithelial parotid cysts and hyperplastic cervical adenopathy in AIDS risk patients: a new CT appearance. Radiology 168:439–441

Iko BO (1984) Computed tomography and sialography of chronic pyogenic parotitis. Br J Radiol 57:1083–1090

Iko BO, Chinwuba CE, Myers EM, Teal JS (1986) Sarcoidosis of the parotid gland. Br J Radiol 59:547–552

Iro H, Schneider T, Nitsche N, Waitz G, Ell C (1990) Extracorporeal piezoelectric lithotripsy of salivary calculi. Initial clinical experiences. HNO 38:251–255

Ishii J, Nagasawa H, Wadamori T, et al (1999) Ultrasonography in the diagnosis of palatal tumors. Oral Surg Oral Med Oral Pathol Oral Radiol Endod 87:39–43

Kate MS, Kamal MM, Bobhate SK, Kher AV (1998) Evaluation of fine-needle capillary sampling in superficial and deep-seated lesions. An analysis of 670 cases. Acta Cytol 42:679–684

Katz P (1991) Intérêt de l'échographie en pathologie salivaire. J Radiol 72:271–277

Kawamura H, Taniguchi N, Itoh K, Kano S (1990) Salivary glands echography in patients with Sjögren's syndrome. Arthritis Rheum 33:505–510

Kelly IMG, Dick R (1990) Technical report: interventional sialography Dormia basket removal of Wharton's duct calculus. Clinical Radiology 43:205–206

Kelly IM, Lees WR, Watts RW (1994) Case report: grey-scale and colour Doppler ultrasound appearance of acute sarcoidosis of the parotid gland. Clin Radiol 49:425–426

Keyes JW, Harkness BA, Greven KM, Williams DW, Watson NE,

Mcguirt WF (1994) Salivary gland tumors: pretherapy evaluation with PET. Radiology 192:99–102
Kessler A, Strauss S, Eviatar E, Segal S (1995) Ultrasonography of an infected parotid gland in an elderly patient: detection of sialolithiasis during the acute attack. Ann Otol Rhinol Laryngol 104:736–737
Klein K, Turk R, Gritzmann N, Traxler M (1989) The value of sonography in salivary gland tumors. HNO 37:71–75
Kohler PF, Winter ME (1985) A quantitative test for xerostomia: the Saxon test, an oral equivalent of Schirmer test. Arthritis Rheum 28:1128–1132
Kress E, Schulz HG, Neumann T (1993) Diagnosis of diseases of the large salivary glands of the head by ultrasound, sialography and CT-sialography. A comparison of methods. HNO 41:345–351
Lack EE, Upton MP (1988) Histopathologic review of salivary gland tumors in children. Arch Otolaryngol Head Neck Surg 114:898–906
Larsson SG, Lufkin RB, Hoover LA (1987) Computed tomography of the submandibular salivary glands. Acta Radiol 28:693–696
Laudenbach P, Moreau R (1974) Sialographie. In: Fischgold H (ed) Traité de radiodiagnostic. Masson, Paris, pp 111–125
Laudenbach P, Bonneau E, Top T, Tran CP (1977) Calcinoses salivaires. J Radiol Electrol 58:413–418
Laudenbach P, Poncet JL, Carlier R, Doyon D (1994) Protocole d'exploration en imagerie de la pathologie salivaire. J Radiol 75:585–596
Leuwer A, Weisser B, Siewert B, Vetter H, Dusing R (1990) Acute purulent parotitis as a sequela of alkylophosphate (E 605) poisoning. Laryngorhinootologie 69:469–471
Levy DM, Remine WH, Devine KD (1962) Salivary gland calculi. JAMA 181:115–1119
Lomas DJ, Carroll NR, Johnson G, Antoun NM, Freer CE (1996) MR sialography (work in progress). Radiology 200:129–133
Lustmann J, Segal N, Markitziu A (1994) Salivary gland involvement in Wegener's granulomatosis. A case report and review of the literature. Oral Surg Oral Med Oral Pathol 77:254–259
Magaram D, Gooding GAW (1981) Ultrasonic guided aspiration of parotid abscess. Arch Otolaryngol 107:549–550
Makula E, Pokorny G, Rajtar M, Kiss I, Kovacs A, Kovacs L (1996) Parotid gland ultrasonography as a diagnostic tool in primary Sjögren's syndrome. Br J Rheumatol 35:972–977
Mann WJ, Amedee RG, Schreiber J (1992) Ultrasonography for the diagnosis of Lyme disease in cases of acute facial paralysis. Laryngoscope 102:525–527
Marsot-Dupuch K, Katz P, Chabolle F, Niklaus P, Firhat M (1992) Imagerie des processus expansifs parotidiens. Feuillets Radiol 32:414–427
Martinoli C, Derchi LE, Solbiati L, Rizzatto G, Silvestri E, Giannoni M (1994) Color Doppler sonography of the salivary glands. AJR Am J Roentgenol 163:933–941
McQuone SJ (1999) Acute viral and bacterial infections of the salivary glands. Otorhinolaryngol Clin North Am 32:793–811
Meseguer H, Merino Galvez E, Ruiz JA (1996) Mucocele of the submaxillary salivary gland. An Otorrinolaringol Ibero Am 23:319–327
Murray ME, Buckenham TM, Joseph AE (1996) The role of ultrasound in screening patient referred for sialography: a possible protocol. Clin Otolaryngol 21:21–23
Nakada M, Nishizaki K, Akagi H, Masuda Y, Yoshino T (1998) Oncocytic carcinoma of the submandibular gland: a case report and literature review. J Oral Pathol Med 27:225–228
Napoli V, Tozzini A, Neri E, et al (1996) The imaging diagnosis of Sjögren's syndrome: echography, sialography and scintigraphy compared in the study of the salivary glands. Minerva Stomatol 45:141–148
Neuhold A, Fruhwald F, Balogh B, Wicke L (1986) Sonography of the tongue and the floor of mouth. Part I: Anatomy. Eur J Radiol 6:103–107
Nozaki H, Harasawa A, Hara H, Kohno A, Shigeta A (1994) Ultrasonographic features of recurrent parotitis in childhood. Pediatr Radiol 24:98–100
Ottaviani F, Capaccio P, Campi M, Ottaviani A (1996) Extracorporeal electromagnetic shock-wave lithotripsy for salivary gland stones. Laryngoscope 106:761–764
Peel RZ, Gnepp DR (1985) Diseases of the salivary glands. In: Barnes L (ed) Surgical pathology of the head and neck. Marcel Dekker, New York, pp 535–552
Raffaelli CP, Iffenecker C, Sigal R, et al (1995) Imagerie des glandes salivaires. Encycl Med Chir, Paris, France, Radiodiagnostic, 33-020-A-10, 16 p
Reinhardt G, Dross J (1984) Exploration radiologique des glandes salivaires. Encycl Med Chir, Paris, France, Radiodiagnostic 33-020-A-10, 17 p
Rinast E, Gmelin E, Hollands-Thorn B (1990) Imaging diagnosis of parotid diseases: a comparison of methods. Laryngorhinootologie 69:460–463
Russo A, Dell'Aquila A, Prota V, Sica GS (1998) Necrotizing sialometaplasia of the submandibular gland. Report of a case. Minerva Stomatol 47:273–277
Sa'do B, Yoshiura K, Yuasa K, et al (1993) Multimodality imaging of cervicofacial actinomycosis. Oral Surg Oral Med Oral Pathol 76:772–782
Schade G, Ussmuller J, Leuwer R (1998) Value of duplex ultrasound in diagnosis of parotid tumors. Laryngorhinootologie 77:337–341
Schurawitzki H, Gritzmann N, Fezoulidis J, Karnel F, Kramer J (1987) Value and indications for high-resolution real time sonography in nontumor salivary gland diseases. Rofo Fortschr Geb Roentgenstr Neuen Bildgeb Verfahr 146:527–531
Shimizu M, Ussmuller J, Donath K, et al (1998) Sonographic analysis of recurrent parotitis in children: a comparative study with sialographic findings. Oral Surg Oral Med Oral Pathol Oral Radiol Endod 86:606–615
Shimizu M, Ussmuller J, Hartwein J, Donath K (1999) A comparative study of sonographic findings of tumorous lesions in the parotid gland. Oral Surg Oral Med Oral Pathol Oral Radiol Endod 88:723–737
Shugar JMA, Som PM, Ryan JR, Jacobson AL, Bernard PJ, Dickman SH (1988) Multicentric parotid cysts and cervical adenopathy in AIDS patients. A newly recognized entity: CT and MR manifestations. Laryngoscope 98:772–775
Sigal R (1996) Oral cavity, oropharynx and salivary glands. Neuroimaging Clin N Am 6:379–399
Sigal R, Monnet O, De Baere T, et al (1992) Adenoid cystic carcinoma of the head and neck: evaluation with MR imaging and clinical pathologic correlation in 27 patients. Radiology 184:95–101
Silvers AR, Som PM (1998) Salivary glands. Radiol Clin North Am 36:941–966

Som PM, Biller HF (1989) High-grade malignancies of the parotid gland: identification with MR imaging. Radiology 173:823–826

Som PM, Shugar JMA, Sacher M (1988) Benign and malignant parotid pleomorphic adenomas: CT and MR studies. J Comput Assist Tomogr 12:65–69

Steiner E (1994) Ultrasound imaging of the salivary glands. Radiologe 34:254–263

Steiner E, Graninger W, Hitzelhammer J, et al (1994a) Color-coded duplex sonography of the parotid gland in Sjögren's syndrome. Rofo Fortschr Geb Roentgenstr Neuen Bildgeb Verfahr 160:294–298

Steiner E, Turetschek K, Wunderbaldinger P, et al (1994b) Imaging in parotid tumors: US versus MRI. Rofo Fortschr Geb Roentgenstr Neuen Bildgeb Verfahr 160:397–405

Takashima S, Takeuchi H, Morimoto S, et al (1991) MR imaging in Sjögren syndrome: correlation with sialography and pathology. J Comput Assist Tomogr 15:393–400

Takashima S, Morimoto S, Tomiyama N, Takeuchi N, Ikezoe J, Kozuka T (1992a) Sjögren syndrome: comparison of sialography and ultrasonography. J Clin Ultrasound 20:99–109

Takashima S, Nagareda T, Noguchi Y, et al (1992b) CT and MR appearances of parotid pseudo-tumors in Sjögren syndrome. J Comput Assist Tomogr 16:376–383

Teresi LM, Kolin E, Lufkin RB, Hanafee WN (1987a) MR imaging of the intraparotid facial nerve: normal anatomy and pathology. AJR Am J Roentgenol 148:995–1000

Teresi LM, Lufkin RB, Wortham DG, Abemayor E, Hanafee WN (1987b) Parotid masses: MR imaging. Radiology 163:405–409

Thackray AC, Lucas RB (1974) Tumors of the major salivary glands. In: Atlas of tumor pathology. Washington, DC, Armed Forces Institute of Pathology, pp 1–15

Thibault F, Halimi P, Bely N (1993) Internal architecture of the parotid gland at MR imaging: facial nerve or ductal system? Radiology 188:701–704

Thoron JF, Raffaelli CP, Carlotti B, et al (1996) Etude en échographie du plan veineux parotidien. J Radiol 77: 67–669

Trappe M, Marsot-Dupuch K, Le Roux C (1991) Study of the salivary glands in 1990. Ann Radiol 34:114–117

Traxler M, Gritzmann N (1986) Sonographic detection of salivary calculi of the sublingual gland. Rontgenblatter 39:328–329

Tunkel DE, Loury MC, Fox CH, Goins MA, Johns ME (1989) Bilateral parotid enlargement in HIV seropositive patients. Laryngoscope 9:590–595

Ussmuller J, Donath K, Shimizu M, Bergmann I (1997) Differential diagnosis of tumorous space-occupying lesions of the parotid gland: angiolymphoid hyperplasia with eosinophilia and Kimura disease. Laryngorhinootologie 76: 110–115

Varghese JC, Thornton F, Lucey BC, Walsh M, Farrell MA, Lee MJ (1999) A prospective comparative study of MR sialography and conventional sialography of salivary duct disease. AJR Am J Roentgenol 173:1497–1503

Vogl TJ, Dresel SHJ, Spath M (1990) Parotid gland: plain and gadolinium-enhanced MR imaging. Radiology 177:667–674

Vona S, Colombo E, Damiani G, Bianco R, Cornalba GP (1994) Salivary gland lesions in HIV-positive patients. Eur Radiol 4:434–438

Wagner W, Bottcher HD, Schadel A, Mollmann M (1987) Sensitivity and specificity of sonography in relation to the diagnosis of parotid tumors. Ultraschall Med 8:175–177

Whyte AM, Byrne JV (1987) A comparison of computed tomography and ultrasound in the assessment of parotid masses. Clin Radiol 38:339–343

Wooley AL, Wimberly LT, Royal SA (1998) Retained wooden foreign body in a child's parotid gland: a case report. Ear Nose Throat J 77:140–143

Yasumoto M, Nakagawa T, Shibuya H, Suzuki S, Satoh T (1993) Ultrasonography of the sublingual space. J Ultrasound Med 12:723–729

Yoshimura Y, Inoue Y, Odagawa T (1989) Sonographic examination of sialolithiasis. J Oral Maxillofac Surg 49:907–912

Yoshiura K, Yuasa K, Tabata O, et al (1997) Reliability of ultrasonography and sialography in the diagnosis of Sjögren's syndrome. Oral Surg Oral Med Oral Pathol Oral Radiol Endod 83:400–407

4 Lymph Nodes

Jean Noël Bruneton, Denis Matter, Nathalie Lassau, Olivier Dassonville

CONTENTS

J.N. Bruneton, MD
Service de Radiologie, Hôpital de l'Archet, 151, route de St.-Antoine Ginestière, B.P. 3079, F-06202 Nice Cedex 3, France
D. Matter, MD
Centre d'Imagerie Médicale, 85 route du Polygone, F-67100 Strasbourg, France
N. Lassau, MD
Département d'Imagerie Médicale, Institut Gustave-Roussy, F-94805 Villejuif Cedex, France
O. Dassonville, MD
Département d'ORL, Centre Antoine-Lacassagne, 33 avenue de Valombrose, F-06189 Nice Cedex 2, France

Proportionally speaking, the head and neck region of the human body contains the greatest number of lymph nodes (approximately 400–700).

Palpation remains the initial method of choice for examination of the neck, and can readily identify enlarged lymph nodes. However, even when palpation is performed by an experienced examiner, small nodes often escape detection. Furthermore, when enlarged lymph nodes are present, clinical examination is insufficient to determine the exact extent of nodal involvement, the presence of extracapsular spread, or vascular relationships.

Since the 1980s, sonography has demonstrated its utility for cervical node examination, in particular for the staging of ENT cancers and lymphoma (Bruneton et al. 1984; Bruneton et al. 1987). The limitations of imaging studies in general, and of sonography in particular, are related to the fact that an estimated 25%–40% of patients have micrometastases despite "normal" imaging studies (Dillon 1998; Van den Brekel et al. 1996).

4.1 Anatomy

The lymph nodes of the neck lie between the deep cervical fascia and the prevertebral fascia. The Rouvière classification in ten main groups, divided into three major chains (the pericervical collar, the deep cervical nodes, and the accessory chains), has been replaced by a system of levels aimed at standardization of neck dissection terminology (ROBBINS et al. 1991).

- Level 1: submental and submandibular nodes
- Level 2: high jugular nodes
- Level 3: midjugular nodes
- Level 4: low jugular nodes
- Level 5: spinal accessory and transverse cervical nodes
- Level 6: anterior cervical nodes

It should be noted that the retropharyngeal nodes and the parotid group of lymph nodes are not covered by this classification.

4.1.1 Level 1 Nodes

Level 1 corresponds to the submental and submandibular triangles. The submandibular nodes lie along the inferior aspect of the mandible, lateral to the anterior belly of the digastric muscle, and remain strictly extraglandular. The submental lymph nodes lie between the anterior bellies of the digastric muscles, beneath the mylohyoid muscle. Level 1 is the drainage region for the lymphatics of the lower lip, the anterior chin, the gingiva, the anterior portion of the floor of the mouth, the tip of the tongue, and the internal facial structures.

4.1.2 Level 2 Nodes

Level 2 corresponds to the high jugular region, which extends from the base of the skull to the hyoid bone. This is the level most frequently involved by cervical node metastases. The jugulodigastric node (principal node of Kuttner), the largest node of level 2, lies just inferior to the posterior belly of the digastric muscle. Large tumors of the oropharynx, posterior oral cavity, supraglottic larynx, or parotid gland metastasize initially to this level. Carcinomas of the hypopharynx, glottis, and anterior oral cavity also frequently metastasize to level 2 nodes.

4.1.3 Level 3 Nodes

Level 3 corresponds to the midjugular region, between the hyoid bone and the cricoid cartilage. This region is the first relay for hypopharyngeal, glottic, and subglottic carcinomas.

4.1.4 Level 4 Nodes

Level 4 corresponds to the low jugular region and extends from the cricoid cartilage to the clavicle. The infra-omohyoid nodes lie inferior to the tendon of the omohyoid muscle. Level 4 nodes drain the infraglottic region, the thyroid gland, and the cervical esophagus. The low jugular region is rarely the only level involved by head and neck tumors. Carcinomas of the anterior tongue and noncervical tumors (noncervical esophagus, lung, breast, stomach) also occasionally metastasize to level 4.

4.1.5 Level 5 Nodes

Level 5 corresponds to the posterior cervical triangle, behind the sternocleidomastoid muscle, and includes both the spinal accessory and transverse cervical chains. Solitary nodal metastases are infrequent at this level, except in case of nasopharyngeal cancer or a posterior skin cancer; in contrast, level 5 nodes are commonly involved during lymphoma.

4.1.6 Level 6 Nodes

Level 6, corresponding to the juxtavisceral area, includes superficial and deep sets of lymph nodes. The superficial nodes lie beneath the platysma. The prelaryngeal lymph nodes lie anterior to the cricothyroid membrane. The pretracheal lymph nodes drain lymph from the lower half of the thyroid. The paratracheal chain lies in the visceral space; the most numerous nodes are the intertracheoesophageal and recurrent nodes, which lie in the groove between the trachea and the esophagus. Level 6 nodes drain the supra- and infraglottic regions, piriform sinuses, thyroid gland, trachea, and esophagus.

4.1.7 Parotid Nodes

This nodal group, which is not covered by the classification by level, comprises nodes situated around and within the parotid gland. These lymph nodes drain the external auditory meatus, the integuments of the frontal, temporal, and midlateral regions of the face, the parotid gland, and the posterior oral cavity.

4.1.8 Retropharyngeal Nodes

The retropharyngeal group encompasses nodes situated in the retropharyngeal space, anterior to the long muscles of the head and neck. Always located above the hyoid bone, medial to the internal carotid artery, they can be visualized only by CT and MRI. The retropharyngeal nodes drain the cavum and the oropharynx (Richter and Feyerabend 1991; Sigal and Lamer 1999; Van den Brekel and Castelijns 1999).

4.2 Ultrasound Examination Technique

4.2.1 Gray-Scale Imaging

Sonographic examination is performed with 7.5–13 MHz electronic linear array or mechanical sector transducers. Very superficial nodes are often better assessed with higher frequency transducers (up to 20 MHz).

The superficial cervical lymph nodes are examined after localization of the common carotid artery (CCA) and the internal jugular vein (IJV). Axial scans obtained along the transverse axis of these vessels, starting from the lower neck, permit satisfactory evaluation of the vascular relationships of any nodal mass. Sonography depicts the nodes of levels 2, 3, and 4 that are situated anterior to the IJV and the CCA and the spinal chain nodes in the posterior triangle (level 5) located behind these two vascular landmarks. Sagittal scans are of lesser diagnostic value and serve essentially documentation purposes. The recurrent nodes situated inferior to and behind the thyroid gland can occasionally be visualized in patients who are able to hyperextend their neck, and by scanning during swallowing.

Whether during preoperative workup or, as is increasingly the case, prior to first-line chemotherapy, the exact location and size of any sonographically visible abnormal nodes must be reported as accurately as possible. Indication of findings on a diagram showing the various levels constitutes a helpful reference document allowing comparison with data obtained later on, during post-therapy follow-up, in a more helpful way than is possible with a written report.

Gray-scale imaging is sometimes considered insufficient, owing to its examiner-dependent nature. Beissert et al. (2000) proposed use of extended field-of-view sonographic sequences for cervical evaluation. Axial scanning sequences obtained at 1-cm intervals from the submandibular region down to the lower part of the neck are computer-processed to produce a large field-of-view image (like the contact scanning technique of the 1980s). However, technical difficulties exist for examination of the mandibular angle region. Furthermore, relatively thin slices are required to avoid excessive gaps in deep regions (risk of overlooking pathological centimeter-sized nodes). Individual neck anatomy must also be taken into account; exploration of thick necks is generally satisfactory whereas thin necks involve difficulties for transducer manipulation. The artifacts observed with this technique are the same as those encountered in conventional sonography (intralaryngeal air, blood vessel pulsation). The potential value of the technique is to allow comparison of serial studies using reproducible data. Compared with CT, this technique had a sensitivity of 92% for exploration of the entire neck for Beissert et al. (2000).

4.2.2 Doppler and Color Doppler (CD) Sonography

Wu et al. (1998) point out that analysis of vascular patterns and vascular density requires settings that provide the highest possible sensitivity without noise. These authors advocate use of a high-pass filter on 50 Hz, a pulse repetition frequency (PRF) on 800 Hz, moderate-to-long persistence, and a slow-sweep technique. Use of such settings allows measurement of velocities as low as 5 cm/s.

Tschammler and Hahn (1999) emphasized the importance of proper adjustment of the flow-mode, power, and threshold settings to avoid overlooking small vascular structures. These authors feel that detection of intranodal flow signals is more reliable in the presence of perinodal color artifacts, but without excessive noise.

Real-time examination allows determination of the plane in which the most intranodal vessels are visible. Longitudinal and axial scans are required to completely analyze all nodes visualized by conventional sonography.

Wu et al. (1998) utilized a dedicated software program to compute the "vascularity index", corresponding to the ratio between the number of colored pixels and the number of total pixels within a given lymph node section. Determination of the vascularity index requires averaging of the values for three transectional planes per node, a procedure that takes around 10 min per node.

CD and PD facilitate the localization of vascular structures. Along with analysis of nodal morphology, these techniques allow Doppler measurements of the peak systolic flow velocity (PSV), the resistive index (RI), and the pulsatility index (PI).

Owing to rapid technological advances, and depending on the unit used, preference may be given to CD or PD. However, PD has a number of advantages over CD: homogeneous noise appearance, less direction and velocity dependence, less temporal variance, higher sensitivity, and improved vessel contrast (Bude and Rubin 1996).

Analysis of vascular structures and Doppler measurements are helpful because malignant tumors secrete angiogenetic factors that stimulate neoangiogenesis, and the wall of a new blood vessel differs from that of a normal vessel in that it lacks a muscular layer. Tumor vessels tend to form shunts that Doppler sonography can demonstrate by measurement of the RI and PI. Interestingly, the first use of Doppler for examination of lymph nodes dates back to 1973 (Mountford and Atkinson 1973).

4.2.3 Ultrasound Contrast Agents

Intravenous D-galactose administration allows identification of vascular structures not visible by unenhanced CD examination. Moritz et al. (2000) recommend a concentration of 300 mg/ml. Use of 4 g allows injection of two or three smaller boli, each of which produces a scanning window of around 5 min. After a "blooming" effect that lasts several seconds, identification of increased numbers of smaller vessels is facilitated and vascular architecture is better delineated. This technique is without risk for the patient.

4.2.4 Ultrasound-guided Aspiration Cytology

This technique has gained popularity because cytological criteria are much more reliable than data provided by physical examination, sonography, CT, or MRI (Fig. 4.1). Compared with palpation-guided aspiration biopsy, US-guided fine-needle aspiration (FNA) has a 24.3% higher accuracy and reduces by 84% the number of inadequate samples (Robinson and Cozens 1999). US-guided FNA is also more sensitive than conventional sonography. In the study by Baatenburg de Jong et al. (1991), US-guided fine-needle aspiration biopsy (US-FNAB) had a sensitivity of 98% and a specificity of 95% versus 88% and 82%, respectively, for US. These figures were confirmed by Van den Brekel et al. (1991), who reported an accuracy of 89% for US-FNAB versus 70% for sonography for nodes ranging from 3 to 12 mm in diameter (these authors biopsied most nodes at least twice to obtain sufficient material).

CT and MRI provide information only on lymph node size – an unreliable criterion for malignancy because not all enlarged nodes are metastases. US-guided FNA thus appears to be an indispensable supplement for etiological diagnosis (Atula et al. 1997).

Except in the case of lymphomas, cytological FNA is generally sufficient for diagnosis, and in general does not involve any complications. In their series of 60 biopsies performed under US-guidance with a 15-G, 16-G, or 18-G cutting needle, Bearcroft et al. (1995) reported only one subclinical hematoma. Use of a US-guided biopsy gun fitted with a 1.2-mm biopsy needle improves the efficacy of aspiration cytology. Elvin et al. (1997) reported a nondiagnostic sampling rate with such medium-sized needle biopsies (MNB) of only 3% versus 25% for FNA, without any complications. MNB thus appears particularly indicated for the staging and follow-up of lymphomas (only two false-negative findings in 26 patients with malignant lymphoma reported by Elvin et al. 1997).

4.3 Gray-Scale Patterns

Since 1984, when we stated that only pathological nodes were visible sonographically (Bruneton et al. 1984), the development of very high frequency transducers capable of visualizing fine structural details has led to description of correlations between sonographic features and histological findings (Bruneton et al. 1994; Rubaltelli et al. 1990; Sakai et al. 1988; Vassallo et al. 1992). In a personal study using state-of-the-art equipment, one or more normal cervical lymph nodes were detected in two thirds of the sugjects, generally as oval structures with an echogenic hilum (Bruneton et al. 1994). Today, technological improvements

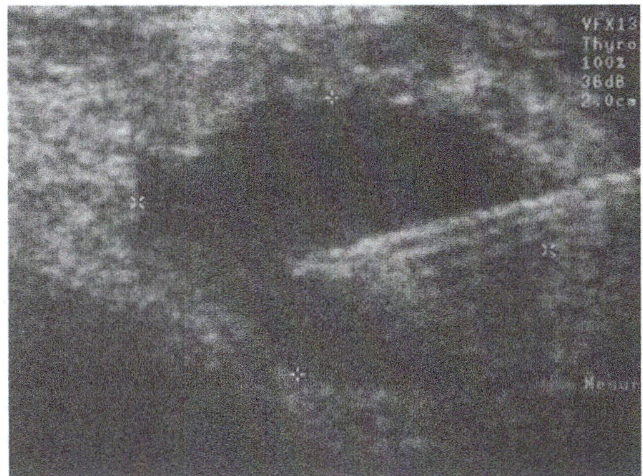

a

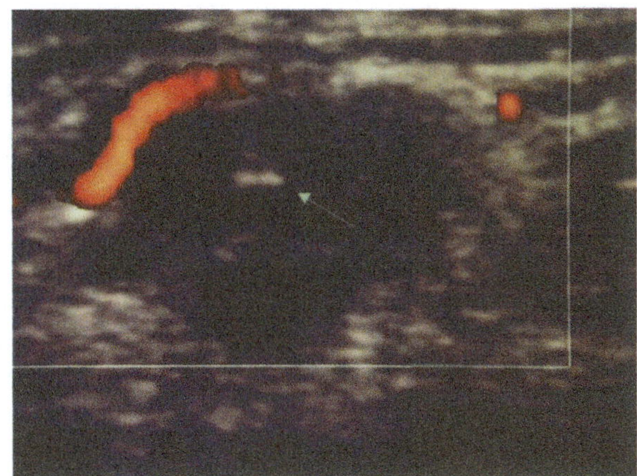

b

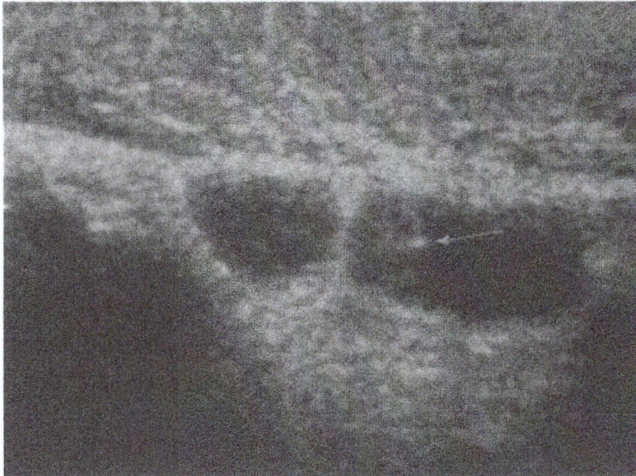

c

Fig. 4.1a–c. US-guided FNA of nodal metastases. **a** FNA of a nodal metastasis (1.5/1 cm between the *crosses*); the needle is clearly visible on the scan passing through the axis of the node. **b** Power Doppler visualization of the perinodal vascular pattern. The tip of the needle is visible within the node (*arrow*). **c** Presence of two small metastatic nodes; the tip of the needle is visible within one of the nodes (*arrow*)

are such that, aside from rare exceptions, cervical US consistently visualizes the normal lymph nodes.

A number of parameters must be evaluated for differentiation of benign and malignant nodes by gray-scale imaging: maximum transverse diameter, longitudinal/maximum transverse diameter ratio, nodal hilum, nodal cortex, nodal margins (in search of extracapsular spread), and nodal echotexture.

4.3.1 Maximum Transverse Diameter

This was the first discriminative criterion described in the literature (Bruneton et al. 1984): A maximum transverse diameter of 0.8 cm was considered the upper normal limit for reactive nodes. For Rainer et al. (1993), any node exceeding 2 cm in transverse diameter is obligatorily metastatic. However, used alone, this parameter appears both insufficient and inaccurate, because up to 42% of nodal metastases have a maximum transverse diameter smaller than 1 cm (Eichhorn et al. 1987). The maximum transverse diameter is thus unreliable for differentiation of reactive and metastatic lymph nodes (Moritz et al. 2000; Takeuchi et al. 1999).

No anatomic correlation has been published in the literature concerning lymphomatous nodes. However, a transverse diameter of 10 mm associated with multiple enlarged nodes can be considered diagnostic in a recognized context of lymphoma (Bruneton et al. 1987).

4.3.2 Longitudinal/Maximum Transverse Diameter Ratio

This is the essential morphological parameter, permitting relatively accurate differentiation of reactive and malignant nodes. Thanks to real-time multiplanar analysis, sonography is more accurate than MRI or CT for calculation of the L/T ratio (longitudinal (maximal) diameter of the node/largest transverse diameter perpendicular to the longitudinal diameter). Reactively enlarged and normal lymph nodes tend to be oval whereas malignant nodes appear rounded. Using a cut-off value of 2, the L/T ratio has a sensitivity of 81%–95% and a specificity of 67%–96% (Sakai et al. 1988; Steinkamp et al. 1994b; Vassallo et al. 1992). Chang et al. (1994) calculated a mean L/T value for malignant nodes of 1.4 versus 1.9 for benign nodes (p=0.001).

More recently, using the short-to-long axis (S/L) ratio, Ying et al. (1999) defined optimum cut-off values for the various cervical regions: submental nodes 0.5, submandibular nodes 0.7, parotid region nodes 0.5, upper cervical nodes 0.4, middle cervical nodes 0.3, posterior triangle nodes 0.4.

4.3.3 Echogenic Hilum

The hyperechoic central line characteristic of lymph nodes is also referred to as the hilum in studies comparing sonographic and histopathological data (Rubaltelli et al. 1990). This linear hyperechoic structure corresponds to the numerous interfaces formed by lymphatic sinuses that converge in the internal portion of the medulla, where they are supported by loose connective tissue. When the hilum has a normal thickness, fat plays no role in its echogenic character; in contrast, normal nodes containing overabundant fat have a much thicker hilum. Hilar thickening may also be secondary to an increase in the number of lymphatic sinuses and vessels following chronic inflammation (Vassallo et al. 1992).

An echogenic, thickened hilum is thus not always indicative of a reactive etiology: Certain inflammatory or neoplastic processes can also cause progressive enlargement of the hilum, which may acquire a peripheral position before ultimately disappearing. Metastatic nodes rarely present an echogenic central or peripheral hilum, and the majority of malignant nodes (76%–92%) have no hilum (Rubaltelli et al. 1990; Vassallo et al. 1992). However, in their study of 46 cervical lymph nodes with a linear echogenic hilum, Evans et al. (1993) diagnosed a malignancy in 58.7% and tuberculosis in 15.2%; the other 12 cases were benign. During treatment by radiotherapy or chemotherapy, massive fatty infiltration occasionally renders the nodes completely hyperechoic, thereby preventing sonographic demonstration of the hilum.

In a limited number of cases, a completely normal lymph node presents as a solid, very weakly echoic structure but without a hilum (Bruneton et al. 1995).

4.3.4 Nodal Cortex Thickness

The thickness of the nodal cortex (studied in particular by Vassallo et al. 1992) can be assessed sonographically only if a hilum is present to serve as a reference structure. A narrow cortex (thickness less than half the transverse diameter of the hilum) is encountered essentially in benign nodes; only 9% of malignant nodes with a hyperechoic central hilum have a narrow cortex. Concentric cortical widening is seen essentially in malignancies (70% of cases), but also occurs in benign conditions (enlarged peripheral lymphatic follicles). Eccentric cortical widening may be due to focal malignant cortical invasion or, more rarely, to a granuloma or focal cortical follicular hyperplasia (Vassallo et al. 1992).

4.3.5 Nodal Margins

Nodal margins are a poor criterion for discrimination. In the study by Moritz et al. (2000), 46% of nodal metastases had well-defined margins while 14% of reactively-enlarged (nontumoral) nodes were poorly delineated. Surface irregularities and blurred margins nearly always correspond to extracapsular rupture of nodal metastases, regardless of lesion size.

4.3.6 Nodal Echotexture

The internal echotexture of normal and reactively-enlarged lymph nodes is constant, consisting of a hypoechoic cortex and a hyperechoic hilum. A number of sonographic features have been related to various pathologies:

- Hypoechogenicity compared with the adjacent fat and connective tissue. This is the most frequent sonographic finding and does not permit differentiation of benign and malignant nodes. Markedly hypoechoic nodes may even appear pseudocystic, as in lymphoma, due to the homogeneous arrangement of the cell layers. Echogenicity tends to increase in response to chemotherapy owing to fibrotic changes.
- The homogeneous or heterogeneous echotexture of a node is also a weak parameter for differentiation; 11% of reactively enlarged (benign)

nodes were heterogeneous while 38% of metastatic nodes were homogeneous, according to Moritz et al. (2000).
- Isoechoic or even discretely hyperechoic echotexture in often large metastatic nodes; the coexistence of normal and tumoral zones creates numerous interfaces. Hyperechogenicity is also encountered in keratinized metastases (Nakayama et al. 1997).
- "Patchy" hypoechogenicity due to coagulation necrosis, associated with cystic degeneration in tuberculous nodes
- Pseudocystic appearance, due to complete necrosis of an often solitary cystic metastasis of occult papillary carcinoma of the thyroid (especially in children). The differential diagnosis for this classic, but rare, appearance, is a branchial cyst (Ahuja et al. 1998). In other cases, liquefaction necrosis of a metastatic node produces an anechoic appearance, but such nodes nearly always have surface irregularities that distinguish them from a noncomplicated cyst.
- Large cortical calcifications, in granulomatous disease, and nodal metastases after radiotherapy or chemotherapy
- Microcalcifications in nodal metastases of papillary or medullary thyroid carcinoma

4.3.7 Diagnostic Value of Imaging Parameters

Certain sonographic parameters are more helpful than others for differentiation of benign and malignant nodes. Multivariate analysis of the various sonographic criteria by Chikui et al. (2000) revealed that absent hilar echoes and increases in short axis length were the best predictors of metastatic cervical nodes.

Takeuchi et al. (1999) reported an accuracy rate of 98.6% for US differentiation of metastatic and benign nodes. Nodal metastases were hypoechoic in 69% of cases and isoechoic to the surrounding tissues in 31%; punctate bright echogenic spots were noted in 78%, there was no linear echogenic hilum, and 19% of the metastatic nodes exhibited a cystic pattern. In contrast, 92% of the benign nodes were hypoechoic, while 8% were isoechoic; none showed echoic spots or a cystic pattern, but 58% had a linear echogenic hilum.

Vassallo et al. (1993) used the L/T ratio (Solbiati ratio), cortical thickness, and analysis of the hilum to differentiate benign and malignant nodes. In their study, 82% of the nodes with a Solbiati ratio under 2, 81% of the nodes without an echoic hilum, and 70% of the nodes with eccentric cortical widening were malignant. In contrast, 72% of the nodes with a Solbiati ratio over 2, 86% with a wide hilum, and 91% with a narrow cortex were benign.

4.4 Pulsed Doppler and Color Doppler Sonography

Doppler studies, and color Doppler (CD) in particular, are hindered by the fact that they involve subjective analysis that sometimes gives discordant results. This problem is increasing, as technological improvements today increase the rate of demonstration of small vascular structures (Na et al. 1997). In addition, intranodal angioarchitecture has not yet been codified, and the number of vascular patterns described for benign and malignant nodes ranges from 4 (Wu et al. 1990) to 8 (Tschammler and Hahn 1999).

4.4.1 Pulsed Doppler

Doppler analysis of tumor vascularity is not always satisfactory. Determination of the PI and the RI is sometimes not possible, and results for benign and malignant nodes overlap considerably (Moritz et al. 2000). Furthermore, controversy exists as to the significance of Doppler values. The study of 43 untreated patients (including 13 with metastatic lymph nodes) by Choi et al. (1995) stands out, because these authors reported elevated PI and RI values for metastatic nodes compared with reactive nodes.

Chang et al. (1994) found that 81% of malignant lymph nodes had an RI less than 0.6, but the specificity of CD was only 81% because 19% of benign nodes also had an RI less than 0.6. The mean PSV was 16 cm/s in the malignant nodes versus 5.6 cm/s in the benign nodes. CD is also limited by the fact that vessels are visible in only 38% of benign nodes.

Taking into account the progressive improvements made in Doppler analysis, published results vary:
- Steinkamp et al. (1994a) used threshold values of 1.6 for the PI and 0.8 for the RI to differentiate benign and malignant etiologies with an accuracy of 91%. Differentiation of metastases and lymphomas was not possible, but these authors found that tuberculous nodes had lower RI and PI values than metastases.

- Na et al. (1997) reported cut-off values of 1.5 for the PI and 0.8 for the RI and achieved a specificity of 100% for malignancy, but the sensitivity of these thresholds was only 47% and 55%, respectively.
- According to Schroeder et al. (1998), neither measurement of flow velocity nor calculation of RI or PI values permitted reliable differentiation of malignant and benign lymph nodes.
- Issing et al. (1999) found that lymph node metastases produced higher Doppler signals than reactive nodes; use of an RI threshold value of 0.6 for metastases increased the specificity of color flow imaging to 92% (p=0.001).

Analysis of Doppler studies in the literature reveals the heterogeneity of results. Along with the subjective nature of Doppler studies and the technological improvements that permit depiction of increasingly smaller vascular structures, it must be remembered that not all small vessels in metastatic nodes appear abnormal hemodynamically.

4.4.2 Color Doppler and Power Doppler

Regardless of the technique used, the aim of Doppler studies is visualization of nodal vascularity for morphological analysis or hemodynamic study. The diagnostic value of CD remains controversial, and Chikui et al. (2000) attribute more importance to gray-scale data than to CD findings. Moritz et al. (2000) emphasized the fact that vessels cannot always be identified in enlarged lymph nodes. This may justify use of contrast media in certain situations.

Tshammler and Hahn (1999) classified nodal angioarchitecture using eight criteria:

- Type 1: hilar vessels visible at one of the poles or at the deepest point
- Type 2: longitudinal vessels coursing parallel to the long axis of the lymph node; these vessels arise from the hilar vessels
- Type 3: peripheral branches that course centripetally towards the nodal cortex; these branches originate from a longitudinal vessel
- Type 4: intranodal color spots representing short venous or arterial segments
- Type 5: aberrant central vessels that form an angle of over 30° with the longitudinal axis of the lymph node and never originate from a longitudinal vessel
- Type 6: displacement of intranodal vessels
- Type 7: focal absence of flow signals compared with the remainder of the node
- Type 8: subcapsular vessels that do not originate from hilar or longitudinal vessels

For Tshammler et al. (1998), types 1–4 suggest a benign (reactive) etiology whereas types 5–8 are indicative of a malignant process. According to them, only 9.6% of reactive nodes exhibit a malignant vascular pattern (types 5–8) whereas 77.6% of malignant nodes present at least one vascular criterion of malignancy.

Wu et al. (1998) classified nodal vascularity in four patterns:

- Hilar type, with or without secondary branches (corresponding to types 1 and 3 of Tshammler and Hahn 1999)
- Spotted type, arterial or venous vessel signals (corresponding to type 4 of Tshammler and Hahn 1999)
- Peripheral type, perinodal pattern of multiple vascular signals (corresponding to type 8 of Tshammler and Hahn 1999)
- Mixed type (association of more than one type of vascular distribution)

Using this classification, Wu et al. (1998) found that 83% of benign nodes were avascular or had a hilar-type vascular pattern, whereas 78% of malignant cervical nodes were of the nonhilar type (mixed in 47%, spotted in 20%, and peripheral in 11%). The difference between these two groups is statistically significant (p<0.01). Wu et al. (1998) consider avascular nodes and nodes with a hilar-type pattern benign; nodes with the three other patterns are considered malignant. Although this classification has a sensitivity of 83% and a specificity of 78% for malignant lymphadenopathy, lymphomatous nodes also commonly exhibit a hilar-type vascular pattern (Wu et al. 1998).

Steinkamp et al. (1999) described three types of perfusion: central, peripheral, and hilar. They classed the intensity of perfusion using a semi-quantitative scale of 0 (no perfusion) to 3 (high perfusion). In their study, reactively enlarged nodes showed intense hilar perfusion (82.1%), whereas nodal metastases exhibited mainly peripheral flow (84.7%) of grade 1–3 intensity. Lymphomatous nodes were highly perfused, displaying both central and peripheral color signals (90.9%).

Along with morphological analysis, Wu et al. (1998) advocate semi-quantitative assessment of vascular distribution using a vascularity index. Benign nodes had a mean maximum vascularity index of

0.048 versus 0.169 for malignant nodes, a statistically significantly difference ($p<0.01$). Combination of a vascularity index +0.09 and a malignant (nonhilar) vascular pattern had a positive predictive value for malignant cervical lymphadenopathy of 91%; although sensitivity was an unacceptably low 58%, specificity was as high as 97%. The poor sensitivity is attributable to the fact that metastatic tumor cells require a certain amount of time to cause measurable vascular changes. In addition, the sensitivity of CD does not always allow detection of early vascular modifications (Wu et al. 1998).

Delorme et al. (1997) attributed a prognostic value to CD findings, as highly vascular lymph nodes were correlated with an unfavorable prognosis.

4.4.3 Contrast Agents

Moritz et al. (2000) advocate intravenous contrast agent administration during Doppler studies to increase the number of identifiable vessels, a parameter poorly analyzed by conventional B-scan ultrasound.

CD studies using D-galactose injection constantly report improved analysis of nodal vascularity. In particular, intranodal vascular structures not visible prior to injection are seen in 23%–50% of cases after contrast enhancement (Maurer et al. 1999; Moritz et al. 2000; Schroeder et al. 1998, 1999). As CD detects only a small portion of the vascularity of certain nodes, this can lead to confusion with a tumor defect, even if the node is of normal size. Application of a signal-enhancing agent in such cases may provide complementary information that confirms or rules out a hypothesis of partial tumor invasion.

According to Moritz et al. (2000), reactively enlarged (inflammatory) nodes typically show hilar vessels coursing from the periphery to their center, with branches visible in the center of larger lymph nodes. Metastatic nodes had predominantly peripheral vessels with multiple branches that traversed the capsule and ran toward the center of the node; hilar vessels were absent. Giovagnorio et al. (1997) reported better results with PD, which improved the sensitivity of vascular exploration.

Intravenous administration of contrast medium during CD improves differentiation of benignity and malignancy. For Moritz et al. (2000), conventional B-scan ultrasound had a diagnostic accuracy of only 79%; addition of CD improved the accuracy rate to 84%, while application of a contrast enhancer resulted in an overall diagnostic accuracy of 99%. Contrast-enhanced CD corrected the diagnosis for 14% of lymph nodes, leading to a change in therapeutic management for 10% of the patients. These authors recommend application of a contrast enhancer predominantly for nodes <10 mm, as these are the nodes for which conventional vascular exploration is not always satisfactory. Future technological improvements will undoubtedly modify this approach.

4.5 Etiological Diagnosis

4.5.1 Normal and Reactive Nodes

Except in those rare instances where no small echogenic hilum is present, the normal lymph node is easily identified sonographically within the more echoic surrounding connective tissue and fat. Occasionally, these oval structures with a transverse diameter of only 2 or 3 mm are nearly anechoic, but a small echogenic hilum can be visualized. Owing to technological advances, CD now often visualizes the hilar vascular distribution or at least one vessel coursing towards or away from the hilum (Fig. 4.2).

Reactively enlarged nodes are usually the sequelae of a recent or long-standing, acute or chronic inflammatory process and are sonographically indistinguishable from normal nodes. According to Schroeder et al. (1998), reactive nodes are nearly always oval; only 4% in their series were rounded (Figs. 4.3 and 4.4).

Schroeder et al. (1998) and William et al. (1996) have described several sonomorphological features for benign reactive lymph nodes:

- A homogeneous echotexture corresponding histologically to very moderate inflammatory changes (34.6%–37.7%)
- Presence of a linear echogenic hilum representing less than one third of the maximum nodal diameter, indicating increased fibrosis (43.4%–52.1%)
- Presence of a distinct echoic hilum extending to more than one third of the maximum nodal diameter, reflecting fatty replacement of the hilar tissue (10.9%–18.9%). William et al. (1996) described nearly complete lipomatous atrophy in 2.4% of nodes, imaged as central echogenicity with a small peripheral echogenic border corresponding to the remaining parenchyma.

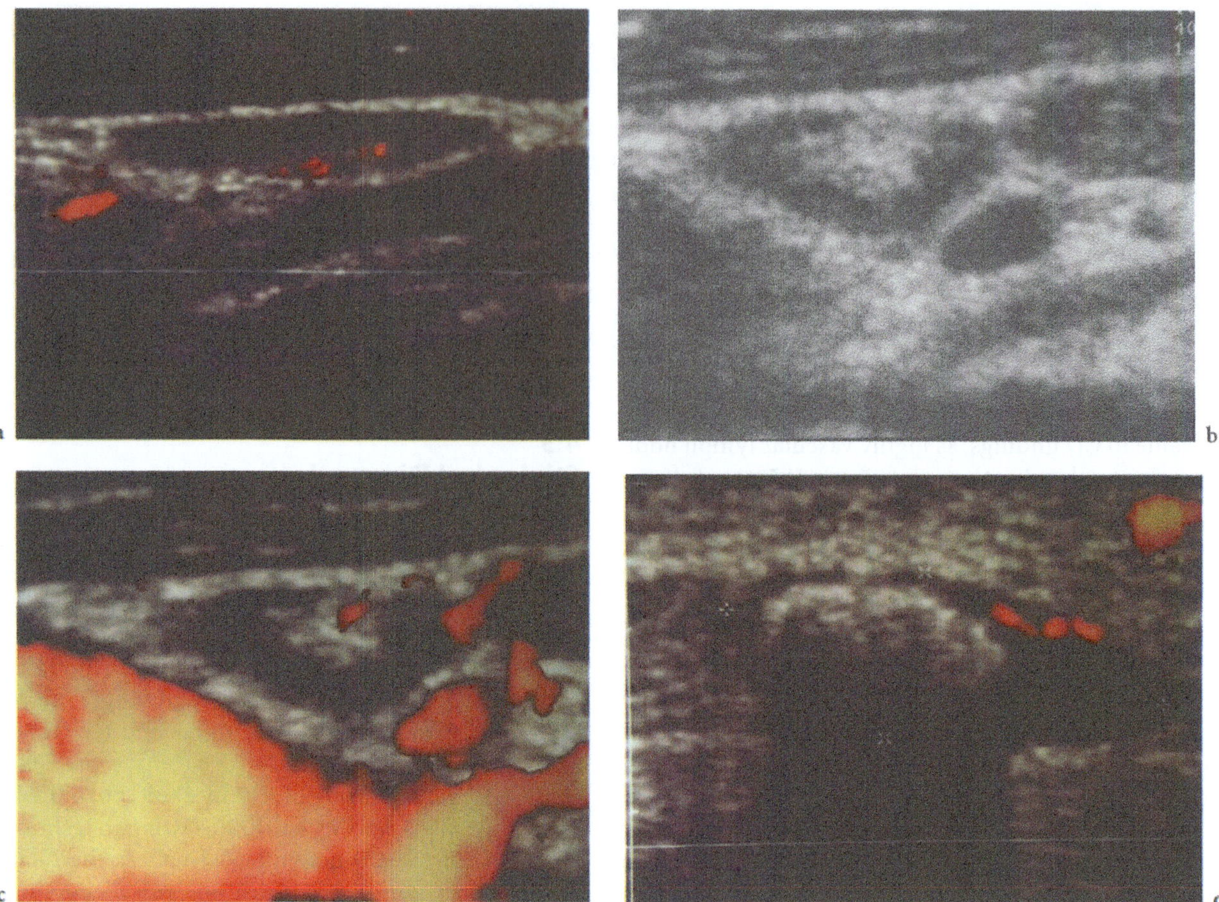

Fig. 4.2a–d. Normal lymph node **a** Oval shape, with a hilar-type vascular pattern. **b** Association of an echogenic hilum and a solid, but less echogenic cortex. **c** Same patient as in (**b**), PD reveals the presence of vascular structures within the echogenic hilum. **d** Rare normal variant with a hyperechoic hilum causing strong posterior attenuation, PD study reveals penetration of the vascular structure into the hilum

Nodal vessels are not always visible, and D-galactose-enhanced color duplex sonography permits visualization of vessels with a benign sonomorphology (SCHROEDER et al. 1999). Reactive nodes are often highly vascular and typically show intense hilar perfusion (82.1% for STEINKEMP et al. 1999).

4.5.2 Metastatic Nodes

Cervical nodal metastases are not always sonographically distinguishable from normal lymph nodes; in patients with head and neck cancer, 25%–40% of "normal-sized" nodes on imaging studies actually contain micrometastases (DILLON 1998).

Schematically, any suspicious small node at grayscale examination (rounded node, absence of an echoic hilum) should prompt US-guided FNA (Fig. 4.5). If a node appears normal on sonograms but color Doppler reveals a defect, complementary analysis is required (US-guided FNA or contrast-enhanced analysis of nodal vascularity).

Inversely, clearly malignant nodes require topographic study rather than an etiological workup; particular attention should be paid to determination of vascular relationships, particularly with the CCA and the IJV.

Sonography is a highly sensitive technique for examination of nodal metastases. DANNINGER et al. (1999) reported a sensitivity of 96% and a specificity of 69%. Causes of false-positive findings include a concomitant inflammatory process or a history of diagnostic (biopsy of the primary tumor) or therapeutic procedures (dental extractions) (MENDE et al. 1996). Diagnostic criteria suggesting malignancy

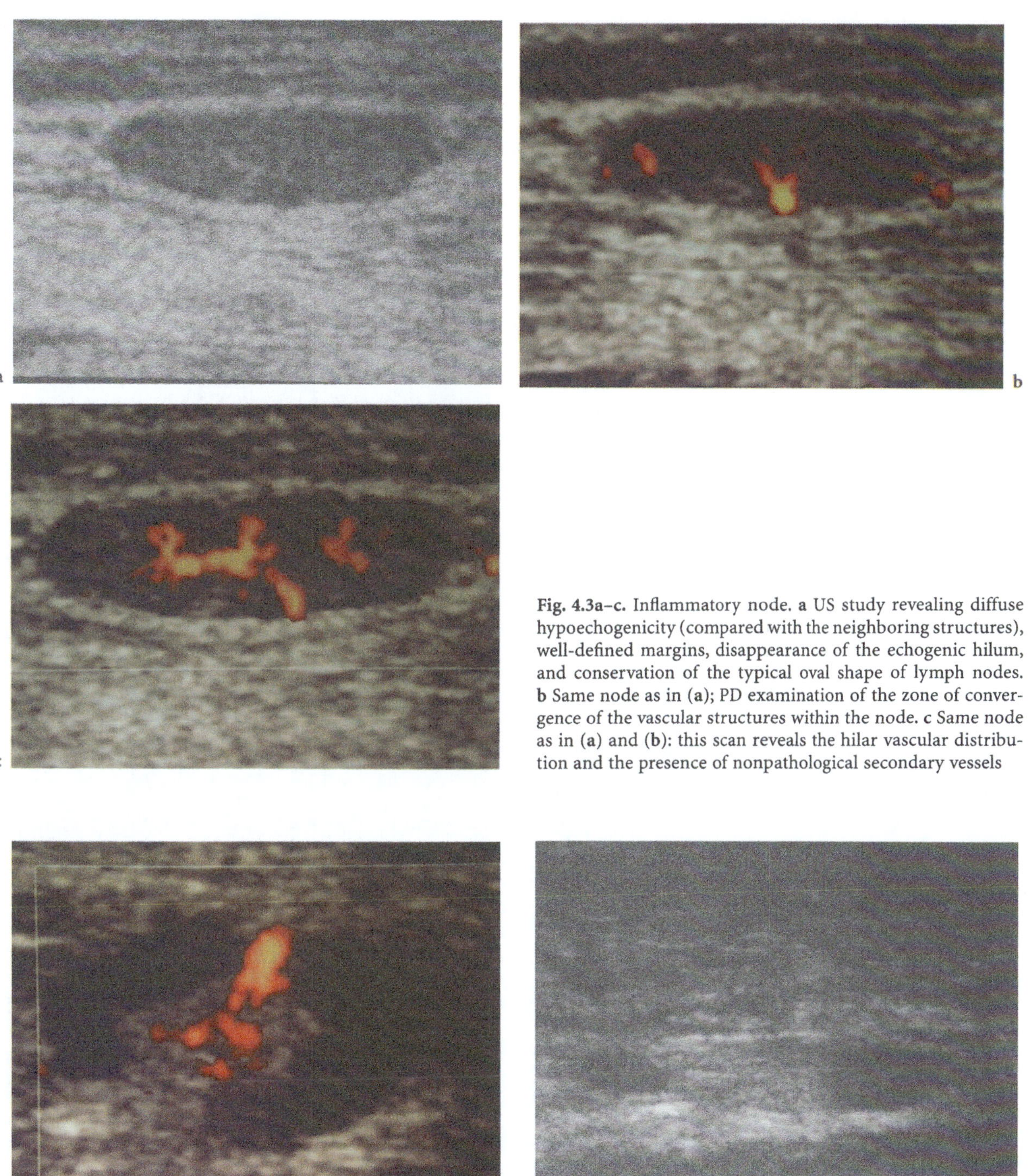

Fig. 4.3a–c. Inflammatory node. **a** US study revealing diffuse hypoechogenicity (compared with the neighboring structures), well-defined margins, disappearance of the echogenic hilum, and conservation of the typical oval shape of lymph nodes. **b** Same node as in (**a**); PD examination of the zone of convergence of the vascular structures within the node. **c** Same node as in (**a**) and (**b**): this scan reveals the hilar vascular distribution and the presence of nonpathological secondary vessels

Fig. 4.4a,b. Inflammatory nodes. **a** Harmoniously enlarged submandibular node; color Doppler reveals hypervascularity at the level of the echogenic hilum. **b** The inhomogeneous appearance of the subcutaneous space was due to radiotherapy; the two small nodal masses visualized were considered benign after FNA

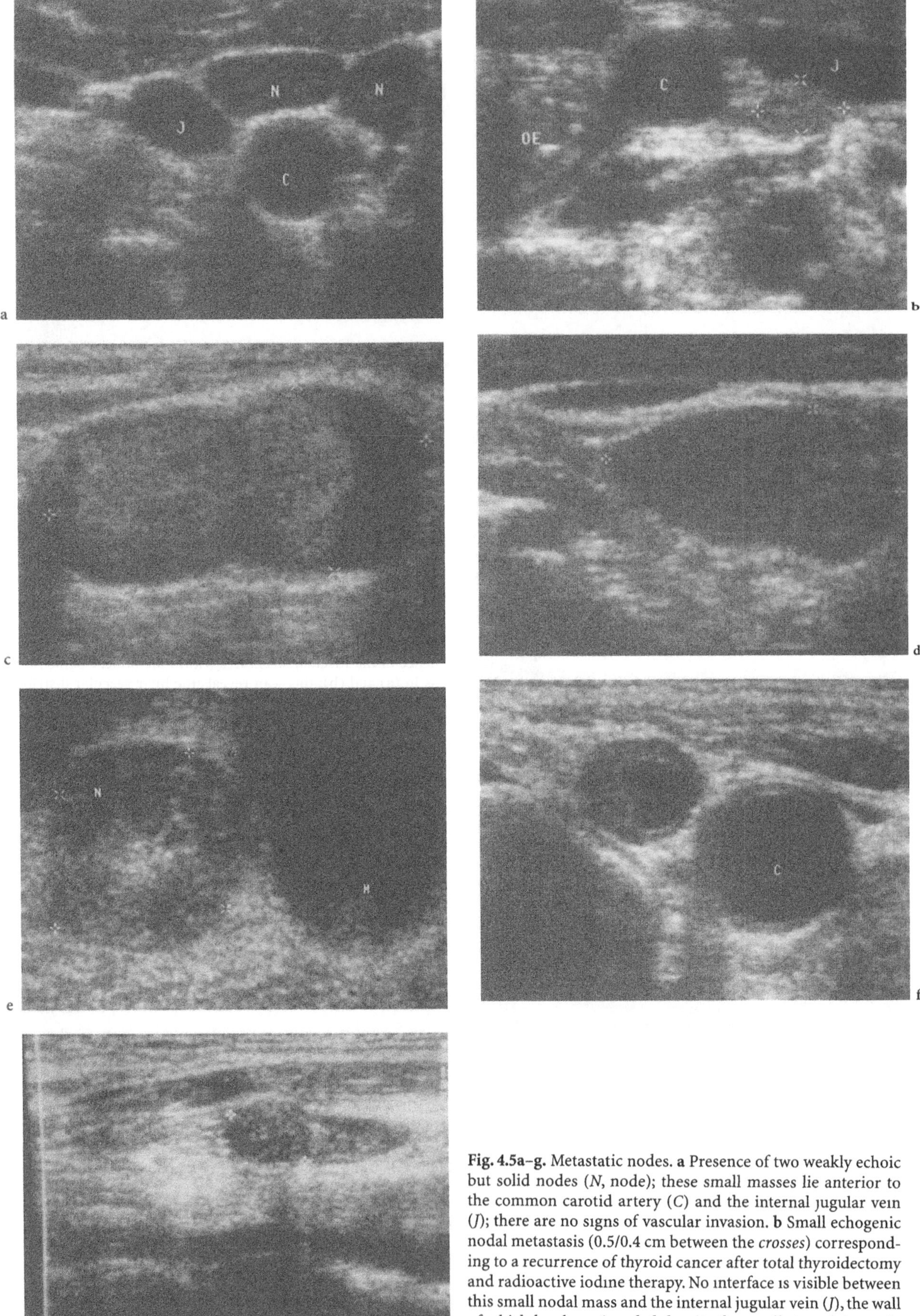

Fig. 4.5a–g. Metastatic nodes. **a** Presence of two weakly echoic but solid nodes (*N*, node); these small masses lie anterior to the common carotid artery (*C*) and the internal jugular vein (*J*); there are no signs of vascular invasion. **b** Small echogenic nodal metastasis (0.5/0.4 cm between the *crosses*) corresponding to a recurrence of thyroid cancer after total thyroidectomy and radioactive iodine therapy. No interface is visible between this small nodal mass and the internal jugular vein (*J*), the wall of which has been invaded despite the small size of the node (*OE*, esophagus; *C*, common carotid artery). **c** Cluster of two

for small nodal masses include tiny inhomogeneous internal echoes reflecting fibrosis and necrosis (Naito 1990) and a fluid-like zone indicative of necrosis. Necrosis has an elevated diagnostic value for metastasis, regardless of nodal shape, and is considered a prognostic factor, as necrosis reflects poor oxygenation, which suggests resistance to chemotherapy and radiotherapy (Janot et al. 1993).

As mentioned previously, malignant nodes only occasionally have a hilar-type vascular pattern; in contrast, a predominantly peripheral perfusion pattern (grades I–III) is suggestive of metastasis (Steinkamp et al. 1999) (Fig. 4.6).

Extracapsular spread should be suspected for all nodes with irregular contours. Sonographic examination of large nodes requires use of a Valsalva maneuver to dilate the IJVs, thereby improving assessment of any venous compression (Fig. 4.7). IJV thrombosis due to adenopathies is suggestive of metastasis regardless of node size, because in a personal series such thrombosis corresponded to metastases in 75 cases and to lymphoma in only three (Bruneton et al. 1990). Nodal compression of the IJV, which is evaluated better during breath-holding than during a Valsalva maneuver, occurs with both metastasis and lymphoma, and this finding has no diagnostic value. Inflammatory processes rarely cause IJV thrombosis.

Invasion of the carotid artery typically corresponds to end-stage disease (Fig. 4.8). Gritzmann et al. (1990) imaged such invasion as focal hypoechogenic transformation of the arterial wall. Palpation and swallowing during real-time scanning can assist evaluation of vascular involvement, in particular arterial invasion.

4.5.3 Lymphomatous Nodes

Although lymphomatous nodes vary in size, sonography typically demonstrates a well-delineated mass with weak echogenicity or even fluid-like images (Ishii et al. 1992). Less common US features include spotty, linear, or dendritic hypoechoic areas (Sakai et al. 1991). Even large lymphomatous nodes rarely produce vascular invasion, and venous involvement is especially uncommon (Bruneton et al. 1990).

In the absence of a recognized primary cancer, in particular a head and neck tumor, US examination of the neck must be completed by exploration of the supraclavicular regions. Detection of similar nodal lesions is suggestive of a thoracoabdominal cancer or lymphoma. In most cases, however, when cervical and supraclavicular nodal involvement is detected, the primary tumor has already been diagnosed. This should suggest the possibility of lymphoma, and prompt complementary US examination of the axillary and inguinal regions, as well as the deep abdominal nodes. At the cervical level, lymphomas have a propensity for involvement of levels 1 (submental and submandibular region) and 5 (spinal region) (Ahuja et al. 1996b).

CD findings for lymphomatous nodes vary in the literature. Such nodes were highly perfused, with color signals in the center and periphery, for Steinkamp et al. (1999), whereas Wu et al. (1998) reported that lymph nodes may have a pseudo-inflammatory appearance, with a predominantly hilar vascular distribution pattern (Fig. 4.9).

4.5.4 Treated Nodes

Pretherapy workup and staging require accurate determination of both the size and location of involved nodes. Demonstration of vascular relationships is essential when surgery is envisaged. This parameter is of lesser importance when induction chemotherapy, combined or not with radiotherapy, is planned. The initial workup must provide objective morphological data allowing subsequent evaluation of response to therapy. Schafer et al. (1996) used sonographic volumetry for surveillance of cervical lymph nodes during radiotherapy. They reported a 50% reduction in node size after 3 weeks, corresponding to a mean tumor volume reduction of 1.3% per day. Size reduction under radiotherapy was less rapid for large lymph nodes.

nodal metastases creating a falsely reassuring image of a normal oval node (2.7/1.7 cm between the *crosses*); these lesions were actually nodal metastases of a papillary thyroid cancer. **d** Nodal metastasis (1.6/0.8 cm between the *crosses*): This nodal mass appears more or less oval, and its sonographic pattern does not allow definitive diagnosis in a patient with a head and neck cancer; FNA remains indispensable. **e** Axial scan revealing a rounded nodal mass (*N*) (1.2/1.1 cm between the *crosses* in the submandibular space lateral to the mandible (*M*); this sonographic image must not be mistaken for a normal node despite the presence of an intranodal echoic hilum. **f** Centimeter-sized node with a zone of central necrosis; this appearance is pathognomonic for a metastasis (*C*, common carotid artery). **g** Atypical small nodal mass with a morphologically normal extremity and a rounded extremity (6 cm between the *two crosses*) that is suspicious in a patient with head and neck cancer; surgical resection of the node confirmed that only the rounded portion was metastatic; the other extremity was composed of normal nodal tissue

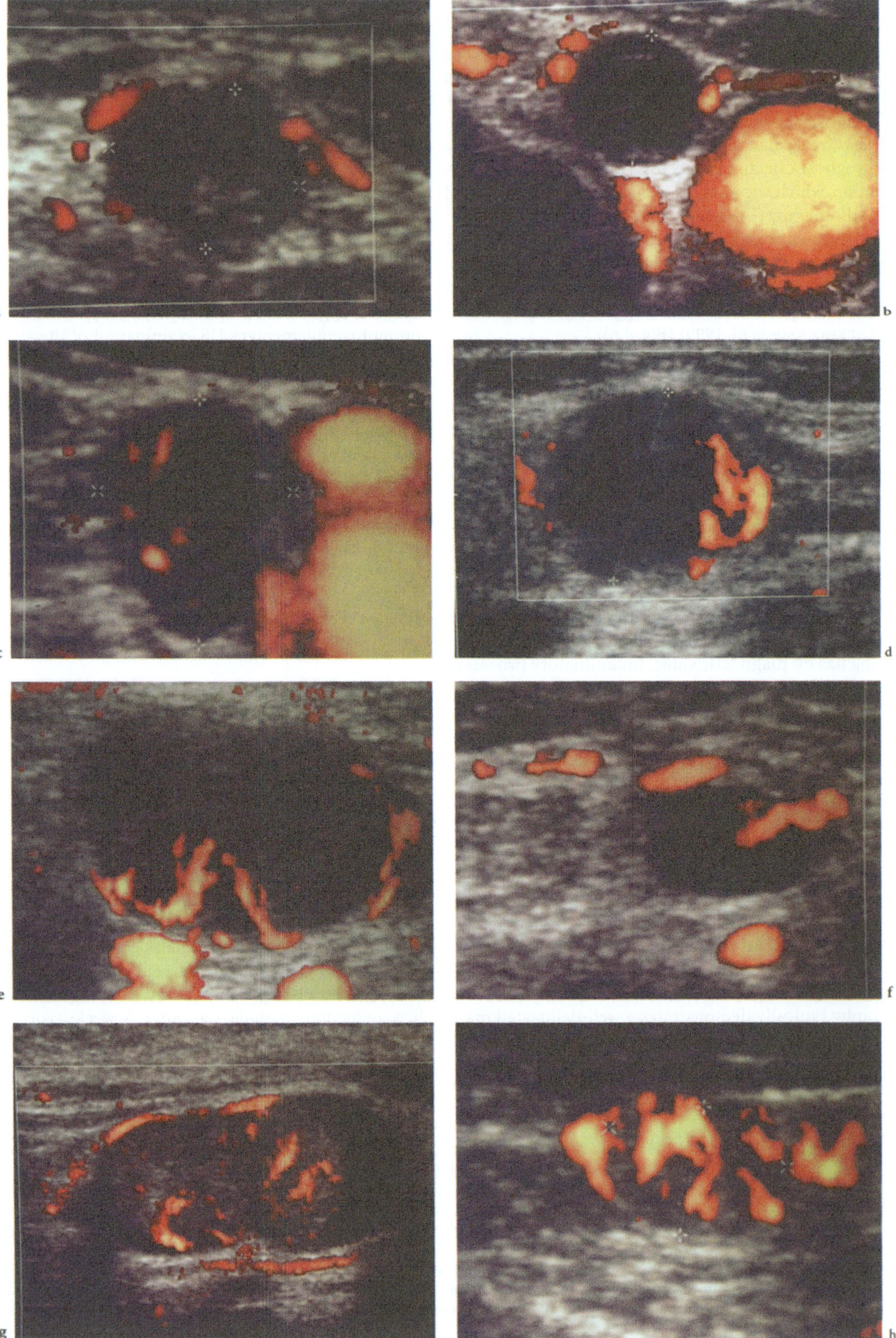

a
b
c
d
e
f
g
h

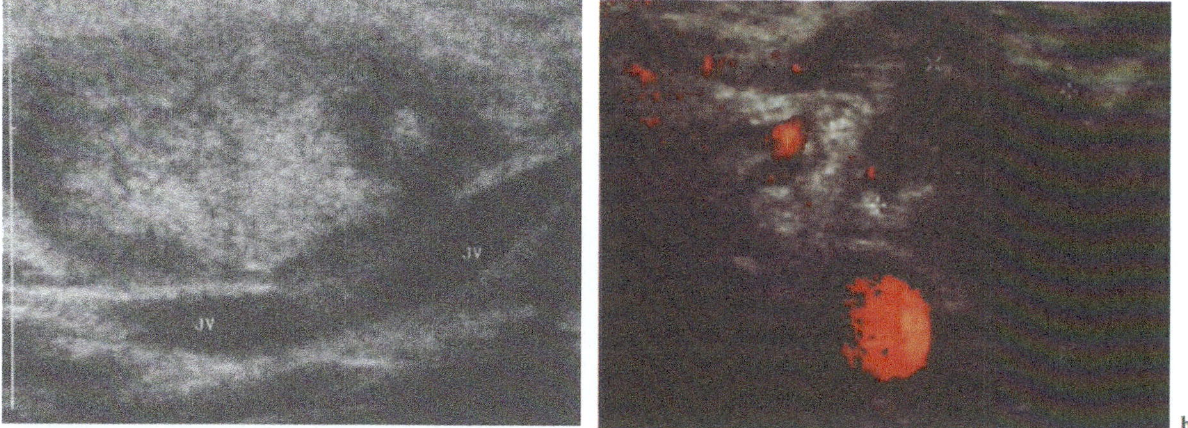

Fig. 4.7a,b. Relationship between nodal metastases and the internal jugular vein. **a** Large nodal metastasis (3.5 cm in greatest dimension) with a mixed vascular pattern and an essentially hyperechoic center; this tumoral lesion invaded and traversed the wall of the internal jugular vein (*JV*) over a distance of 1.2 cm. **b** Nodal mass (1.9/1.4 cm between the *crosses*) associated with complete occlusion of the internal jugular vein (axial scan with power Doppler)

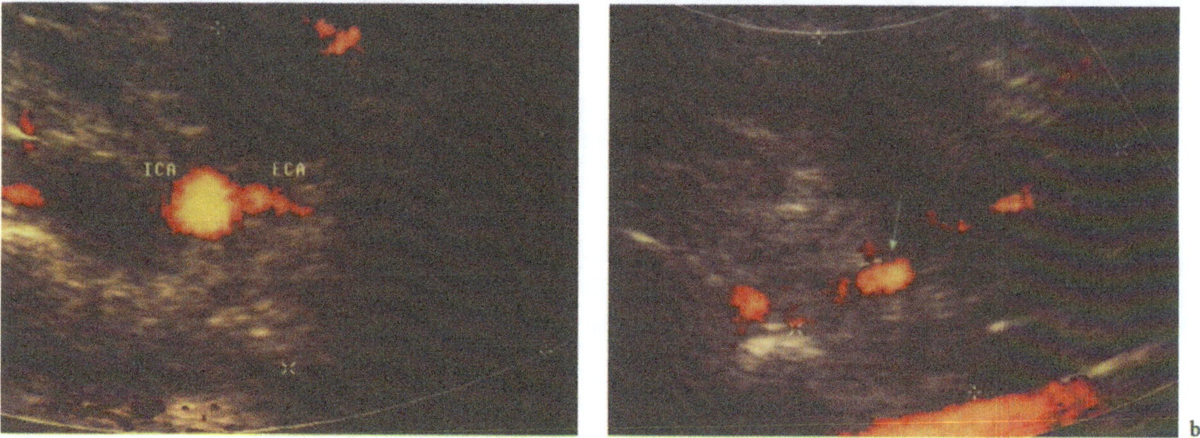

Fig. 4.8a,b. Massive right laterocervical invasion with arterial involvement (ENT cancer recurrence). **a** Invasion of the origin of the external carotid artery (*ECA*) by the tumor (5.4/4.1 cm between the *crosses*) (*ICA*, internal carotid artery). **b** Axial scan at a higher level revealing invasion of the right internal carotid artery (*arrow*) by the tumoral recurrence (4.6/4.5 cm between the *crosses*)

Fig. 4.6a–h. Vascular patterns of nodal metastases. **a** Small nodal metastasis (0.6/0.5 cm between the *crosses*) without any detectable tumor vascularity. **b** Nearly completely necrotic nodal metastasis (0.7 cm between the *two crosses*) without any vascularity detectable at PD (same patient as in Fig. 4.6f). **c** Anarchic intranodal vascularity associated with a rounded shape (0.8/0.7 cm between the *crosses*). **d** Intense focal peripheral vascularity in a small metastatic node (1.2 cm between the *two crosses*), contrasting with the avascular appearance of the quasi-totality of the node. **e** Nodal metastasis of a head and neck cancer: PD revealed peripheral vessels traversing the nodal capsule, a sign of capsular rupture that is often not detected by US. **f** Small (0.5 cm) nodal metastasis with an abnormal vascular pattern: the vessels traversing the capsule indicate capsular rupture despite the small size of the lesion. **g** Two clustered cervical nodal metastases of a papillary cancer: presence of both peripheral and internal tumoral vascularity is highly suggestive of metastases (same patient as in Fig. 4.5c). **h** Small hypervascular metastasis (0.8/0.6 cm between the *crosses*): this small mass was the only abnormality observed during follow-up of a thyroid cancer treated by thyroidectomy and radioactive iodine (nodal recurrence)

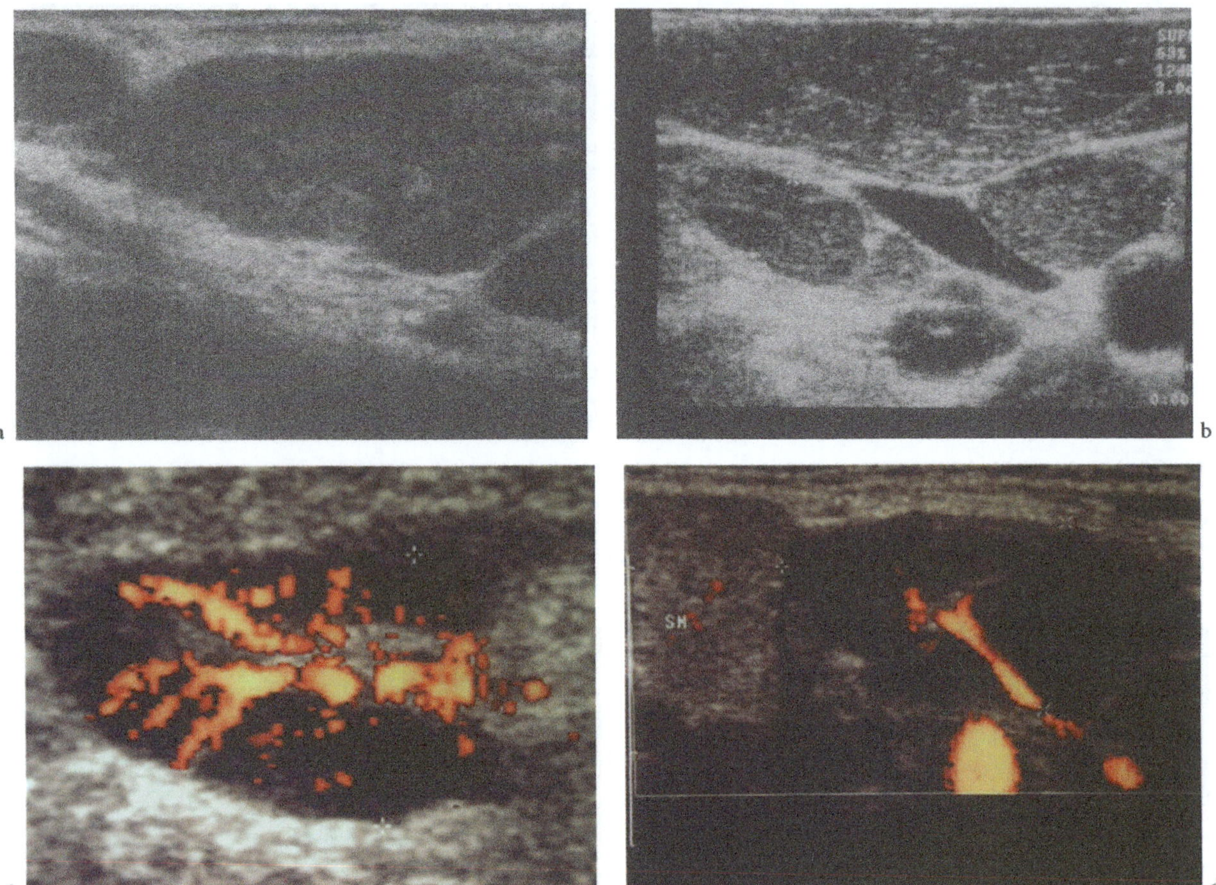

Fig. 4.9a–d. Lymphomatous nodes. **a** Multiple, roughly oval nodal masses with loss of the echogenic hilum, without any vascular impact. **b** Multiple cervical nodes surrounding the internal jugular vein, without any signs of invasion. **c** The diffuse (hilar and longitudinal) hypervascularity could have been mistaken for a common inflammatory node; the presence of other deep and superficial nodal masses corrected the diagnosis. **d** Submandibular (*SM*) lymphomatous node (2.3/1 cm between the *crosses*); PD revealed the essentially hilar vascular pattern, which has no discriminatory value

Modifications in node volume in response to therapy may be accompanied by morphological changes; for example, the appearance of focal or diffuse hyperechoic zones reflects progressive fibrosis. These changes are especially visible during the treatment of lymphoma. The appearance of small echoic zones (indicative of fibrosis) and calcifications can also be observed in metastatic nodes treated by radiotherapy (Fig. 4.10).

Ahuja et al. (1996a) observed the following features in nodes treated by radiotherapy: absence of a hilum in 97.9%, well-delineated margins in 85.3%, transverse diameter greater than 8 mm in 7.7%. These features do not rule out residual tumor, however, and if the clinical context requires an objective response, US-guided FNA is required (Fig. 4.11).

Search for recurrent disease in treated nodes may be helpfully performed with Doppler. Use of a PI cut-

Fig. 4.10a–g. Metastatic node treated by radiotherapy and/or chemotherapy. **a** Small, ill-defined nodal mass (1/0.5 cm between the *crosses*) containing numerous small echogenic structures reflecting calcified involution after radiotherapy (the node initially measured 2/1.5 cm). **b** Roughly rounded node containing numerous small echogenic structures reflecting post-therapy involution. PD revealed that this node (which was highly vascular prior to treatment) was now almost avascular; this finding, associated with the small echogenic structures, suggested post-radiotherapy fibrosis. **c** Cervical nodal metastasis of papillary cancer; the progressive appearance of internal hyperechogenicity during radiotherapy was associated with a reduction in size (here 2/1.3 cm). **d** Power Doppler analysis of a cervical nodal metastasis under chemotherapy; the node, which here measures 0.8 cm, presents punctate echogenic images and a marked decrease in vascularity; US-guided FNA revealed only fibrotic tissue. **e** Nodal calcification after cervical irradiation (1.1 cm between the *two crosses*); the lesion manifests as a convex echogenic mass associated with a posterior acoustic shadow. **f** Small residual nodal mass (0.6/0.6 cm between the *two crosses*) containing

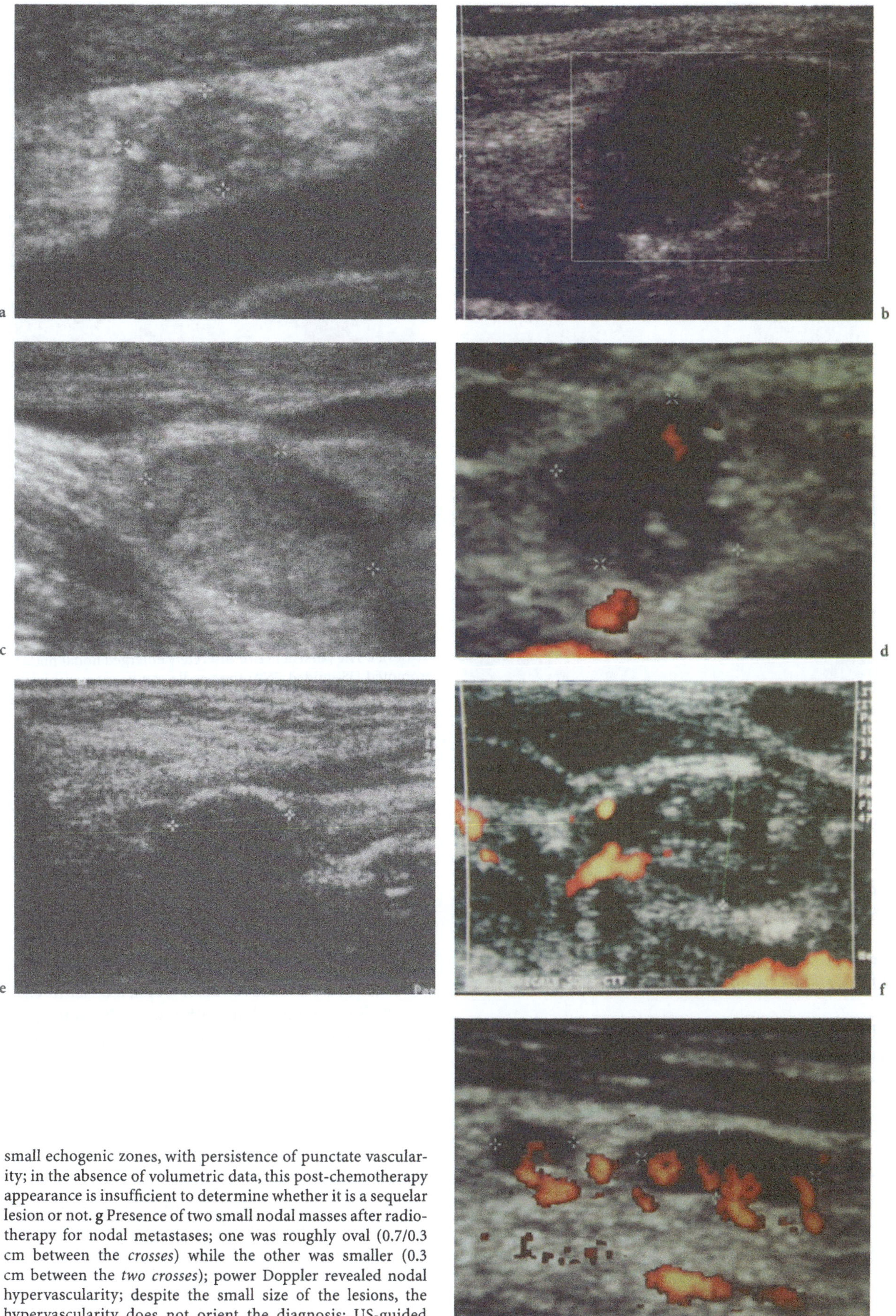

small echogenic zones, with persistence of punctate vascularity; in the absence of volumetric data, this post-chemotherapy appearance is insufficient to determine whether it is a sequelar lesion or not. **g** Presence of two small nodal masses after radiotherapy for nodal metastases; one was roughly oval (0.7/0.3 cm between the *crosses*) while the other was smaller (0.3 cm between the *two crosses*); power Doppler revealed nodal hypervascularity; despite the small size of the lesions, the hypervascularity does not orient the diagnosis; US-guided FNA is indispensable

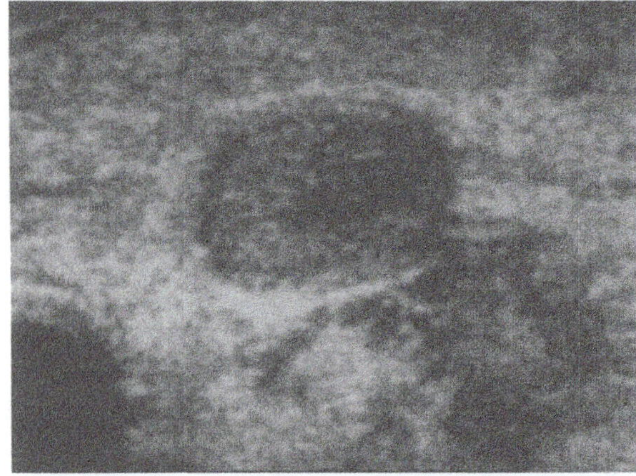

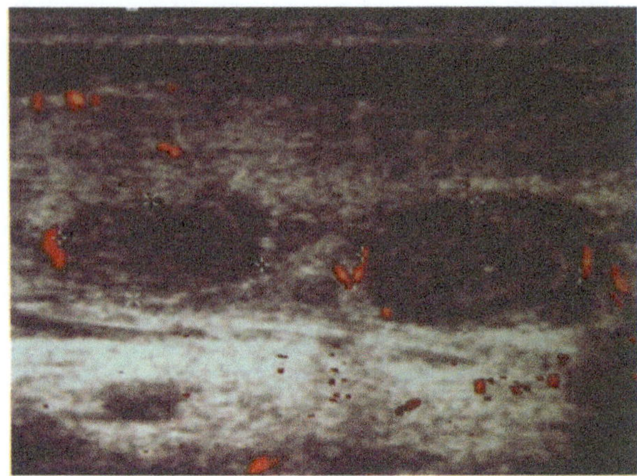

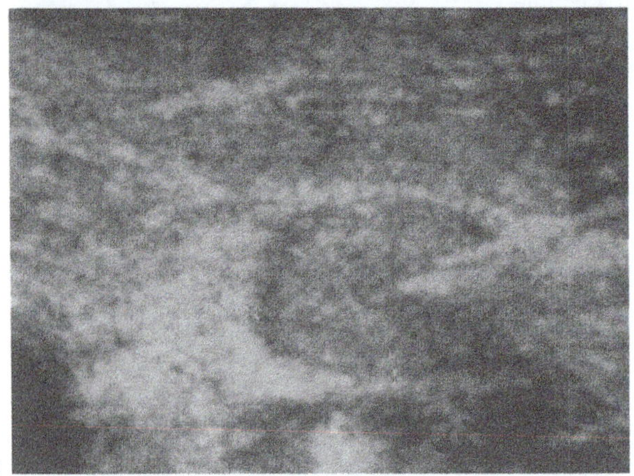

Fig. 4.11a–c. Nodal metastases under combined radiotherapy and chemotherapy. **a** This well-defined hypoechoic nodal mass containing more echogenic zones had diminished considerably in size following therapy. **b** Same patient as in (**a**): power Doppler revealed the absence of any suspicious hypervascularity in two nodes (1/0.5 and 1.1/0.7 cm between the *crosses*). **c** The persistence of discretely enlarged nodal masses prompted US-guided FNA; the needle can be seen within the lesion (1/0.6 cm between the *crosses*); analysis of the aspirate revealed the persistence of metastatic tissue

off value of 1.6 and an RI cut-off value of 0.8 had an accuracy of 96% for differentiation of benign and malignant lesions for Steinkamp et al. (1994c).

4.5.5 Specific Inflammatory Processes

4.5.5.1 Tuberculous Cervical Lymphadenitis

Tuberculous nodes have three typical sonographic appearances:

- Multiple, sharply marginated and hypoechoic rounded and oval nodal masses with posterior enhancement (an appearance indistinguishable from that of nodal metastases)
- Caseating necrosis, with ill-defined margins
- Cold abscesses, with an inhomogenenous echotexture and inhomogeneous acoustic shadowing (Winkelbauer et al. 1992). Occasionally, an anechoic mass with blurred borders may suggest a metastasis of melanoma.

All of these appearances may initially suggest a malignant etiology; additional diagnostic difficulties may exist when the presence of hyperechoic intranodal material creates a pseudo-hilum (Evans et al. 1993).

Despite the nonspecific morphological features of these lesions, their location may orient the diagnosis, because the posterior triangle is often affected (70% of cases for Ying et al. 1998).

Variable results have been reported with CD. Tuberculous lymphadenopathy was characterized by low vascularity in the study of Wu et al. (1998); seven of their 17 cases were avascular, seven had a hilar-type vascular pattern, one presented spots, and the vascularity index was consistently low. According to Na et al. (1997), CD analysis permits identification of at least one criterion of vascular pathology (Fig. 4.12).

Overall, except for extensive nodal involvement in a recognized context of tuberculosis, disease associated with small oval nodes creates diagnostic difficulties that render biopsy obligatory (Winkelbauer et al. 1992).

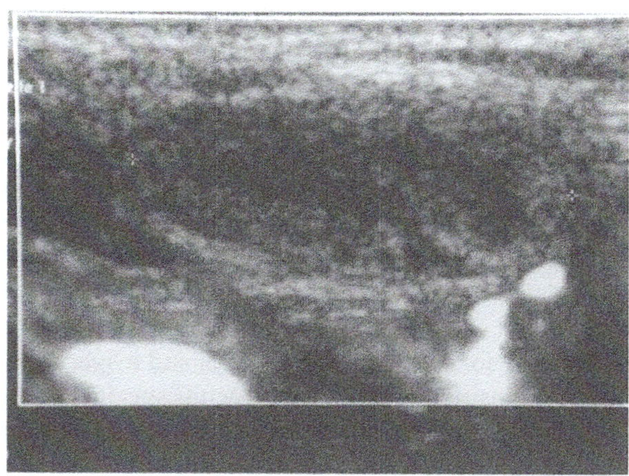

Fig. 4.12. Tuberculous cervical lymphadenitis: nonspecific weakly echogenic mass (caseation probable); power Doppler failed to reveal any intranodal vascularity

4.5.5.2 Histiocytic Necrotizing Lymphadenitis (Kikuchi Disease)

Described most commonly in Japan, this self-limited, benign lymphadenopathy resolves spontaneously over several weeks or months. The major differential diagnosis is lymphoma, and histological examination is required for conclusive diagnosis.

The hypoechoic lesions are surrounded by a thin hyperechoic rim. Multiple node clusters smaller than 2.5 cm in diameter are visualized (Fulcher 1993). The posterior triangle is usually the only cervical site (77% for Turner et al. 1983); the supraclavicular, intracarotid, and extracervical node chains are infrequent sites of involvement. Deep-seated abdominal nodes often go undetected (Miller and Perez-Jaffe 1999). PD never reveals a malignant type of nodal vascularity (i.e., spotted, peripheral, or mixed), and the enlarged cervical nodes exhibit a predominantly hilar-type pattern of hypervascularity (Wu et al. 1998).

4.5.5.3 Sarcoidosis

Radiological suspicion of mediastino-pulmonary sarcoidosis should prompt supraclavicular and cervical sonographic examination in search of the easily biopsied nodal masses present in slightly over 10% of patients with sarcoidosis (Lohela et al. 1996). The multiple hypoechoic lesions range from 1 to 3 cm in diameter and do not cause vascular compression (Fig. 4.13).

4.6 Other Imaging Modalities

4.6.1 Computed Tomography

The normal lymph node is homogeneous, and isodense to muscle. Cervical node examination requires administration of an iodinated contrast medium for opacification of the arteries and veins. A small, generally peripheral, echodense structure corresponding to the hilum is seen occasionally, but thin slices are required to rule out necrosis of a tumoral node. Any increase in the density of the peripheral fat should suggest inflammation or extracapsular spread.

In the literature, CT is reportedly less effective than US for the detection of metastatic cervical nodes, but results must be analyzed as a function of the equipment utilized. Cole et al. (1993) reported that US had a sensitivity of 81.3% and a specificity of 84.6% versus 78% and 93.8%, respectively, for CT. Furukawa et al. (1991) underscored the fact that sonography demonstrates more superficial lymph nodes than CT. Leicher-Duber et al. (1990) confirmed the slight superiority of sonography for preoperative lymph node staging, with a sensitivity of 90% versus 84% for CT and only 74% for palpation. The recent study on the N0 neck by Van den Brekel and Casteljins (1999) underscored the considerable variations in literature series, where sensitivity ranges from 14% to 83% while specificity varies from 78% to 100%. These data must be reexamined owing to the introduction of multislice CT units permitting rapid acquisition of millimeter slices that can be used to provide an objective document.

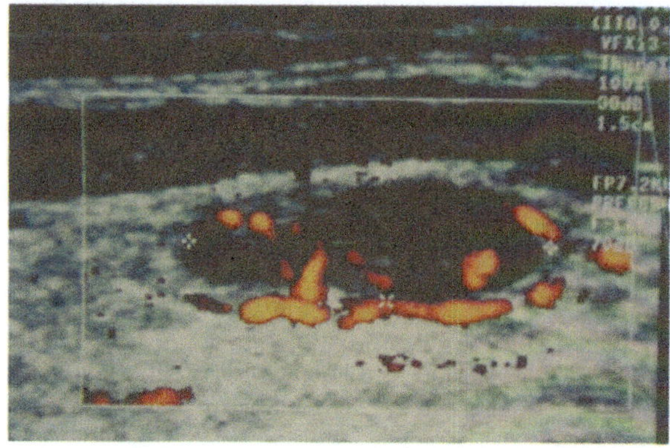

Fig. 4.13. Sarcoidosis: power Doppler did not differentiate between an inflammatory lesion and a tumoral lesion

There are no diagnostic CT criteria, and the maximum transverse diameter is the only useful information obtained. Following their work with ultrasonography, Van den Brekel et al. (1998) suggested 7 mm as the upper limit of normal for level-2 nodes and 6 mm for the other levels as a means of reducing the number of false-negative findings.

Morphologically, the presence of central nodal necrosis, even when only 3 mm in the long axis, is highly suggestive of metastasis. This parameter had a sensitivity of 74% and above all a specificity of 100% for Van den Brekel et al. (1990b).

Overall, head and neck cancers can be reliably staged by CT or MRI, as these modalities can visualize the superficial and deep cervical nodes. Ultrasonography is currently more accurate for superficial nodes, as it permits diagnostic analysis and can be used to guide FNA.

4.6.2 Magnetic Resonance Imaging

Like CT, standard MRI sequences provide merely volumetric data. Although MRI offers better contrast resolution than CT and permits multiplanar scanning, its efficacy for the evaluation of metastatic cervical nodes remains controversial (Sigal and Lamer 1999; Youssem and Hurst 1994), especially because units available in the 1990s were hampered by numerous artifacts (swallowing, respiration, and blood circulation).

On T_1-weighted sequences, the normal lymph node is typically isointense or discretely hyperintense to muscle and hypointense to fat. On T_2-weighted images, the normal node is hyperintense to muscle and discretely more intense than fat, but it is not uncommon for it to be isointense and indistinguishable from the surrounding fat. Necrosis is highly specific for metastasis and can be readily visualized on T_1-weighted sequences after intravenous administration of gadolinium. However, such highly specific necrosis is rare in small nodal metastases (Van den Brekel et al. 1990a).

Complementary methods can be used to improve MRI results: gadolinium-enhanced 3-D MR angiography (Georgi et al. 1999) allows visualization of enlarged inflammatory nodes and arterially supplied metastases, although demonstration of metastases with arteriovenous shunts and necrotic nodes with little blood supply is poor. Use of a specific iron-based contrast medium associated with a T_2-weighted sequence provides a signal specificity currently unavailable with unenhanced MRI (Sigal and Lamer 1999).

4.6.3 Scintigraphy

Positron emission tomography with 18 FDG (FDG-PET) appears to have a greater diagnostic accuracy than more conventional imaging modalities such as US and CT. Stokkel et al. (2000) reported the marked superiority of this method for preoperative staging: sensitivity was 96% versus 85% for CT and 64% for US-guided FNA. Fischbein et al. (1998) reported a sensitivity for nodal disease of 93% and a specificity of 77%; sensitivity reached 100% while specificity was 64% for detection of residual and recurrent disease at the primary site, which is particularly important.

Despite encouraging results with FDG-PET, other scintigraphic techniques have proven disappointing. [^{11}C] Methionine-positron emission tomography, in particular, has not proven helpful for follow-up of patients undergoing external-beam radiotherapy (Nuutinen et al. 1999). Similarly, injection of technetium 99m-labeled colloid around the primary tumor followed by analysis of the sentinel node by planar scintigraphy with a hand-held gamma camera has also generally proven disappointing (Koch et al. 1998).

4.7 Differential Diagnosis

The difficulties for differential diagnosis of enlarged cervical lymph nodes are related to the number of lesions (Bruneton et al. 1995). With the exception of neurofibromatosis (in which the multiple nodules are associated with cutaneous symptoms), multinodular disease nearly always corresponds to lymphadenopathy, regardless of whether there is any recognized clinical context.

The possibility that a solitary nonthyroid, nonsalivary, and nonvascular cervical mass is an enlarged lymph node should be entertained only in patients with recognized cancer or lymphoma. Sonographically, an anechoic nodule in the mid-jugulocarotid region, along the anterior belly of the sternocleidomastoid muscle, suggests a branchial or lymphoepithelial cyst. Thyroglossal duct cysts, in contrast, generally lie along the midline, in an infrahyoid or prehyoid position. Vascular swelling (aneurysm, phlebectasia) is readily identified by sonography. Solid solitary nodules may have a rare etiology such as neurofibroma; solitary sarcomatous lesions tend to be larger than nodal lesions. Chemodectomas have a suggestive topography, and CD demonstrates their characteristic hypervascularity.

4.8 Head and Neck Cancers

The presence of lymphadenopathy in patients with head and neck cancers is a well-recognized prognostic factor (CEREZO et al. 1992). Numerous studies have demonstrated the limitations of physical examination for detection of cervical nodal metastases in these patients, because false-negative findings are reported in approximately one third of all cases. Patients with head and neck cancer thus require more accurate nodal explorations; even when physical examination detects a nodal mass in the lateral neck of such a patient, it cannot determine whether there is any vascular involvement, in particular IJV thrombosis. As indicated previously, CT and MRI can both depict and characterize cervical nodes and, in 38%–67% of cases, correct the false-negative errors of palpation (SOM 1992; STERN et al. 1990; VAN DEN BREKEL and CASTELJINS 1999).

4.8.1 Pretherapy Workup and Staging

The accuracy of sonography alone never exceeds 70%, because any increase in sensitivity is associated with a decrease in specificity. VAN DEN BREKEL and CASTELJINS (1999) confirmed the accuracy of US-guided FNA for the N0 neck (accuracy 89%, sensitivity 76%, specificity 100%), and this technique should play an important role in therapeutic management. As early as the mid 1980s, HAJEK et al. (1986) reported that sonography modified the surgical strategy in 56% of cases by constantly demonstrating lesions that were more extensive than had been evaluated clinically; in the majority of cases more radical surgery proved necessary, and 14% of patients were considered inoperable. Whenever surgery is planned as the initial therapy, demonstration of any bilateral nodal and/or venous involvement is essential. Radical neck dissection has been increasingly replaced, at least as the first-line procedure, by induction chemotherapy or a chemoradiotherapy combination.

The benefits of sonography for the workup of superficial lymph nodes in patients with head and neck cancer is due essentially to the topographic accuracy of the technique (BRUNETON and NORMAND 1987):

- Detection of subclinical ipsilateral nodes
- Accurate analysis of the size of palpable nodes. A map indicating the number and size of nodes can be prepared as a reference document for the surveillance of patients managed nonsurgically. Precise volumetric analysis is thus extremely important for evaluation of response to therapy.
- Search for extracapsular spread. This is a significant prognostic factor, because patients with extracapsular spread had a 3-year survival rate of only 28.9% versus 73.4% in the absence of such spread (PRIM et al. 1999). However, extracapsular rupture is difficult to demonstrate for nodes with a transverse diameter smaller than 1 cm. CD demonstration of peripheral vessels traversing the nodal wall can aid diagnosis because this feature usually reflects capsular rupture.
- Analysis of vascular relationships. As indicated previously, US has an elevated sensitivity for detection of venous thrombosis and arterial wall invasion.
- Exploration of the contralateral cervical node-bearing regions. Metastatic spread to the contralateral neck is not uncommon and modifies the therapeutic protocol, as it corresponds to stage N2c disease. Contralateral pathological nodes are usually small, and the difference in sensitivity between US and physical examination is at a maximum in these cases (ATULA et al. 1996).

Opinions differ concerning the role of sonography for the clinically N0 neck. As indicated previously, the possible presence of micrometastases obligatorily limits the sensitivity of imaging techniques to a maximum of 75% (VAN DEN BREKEL 1996).

TAKES et al. (1998) found that CT had an accuracy comparable to that of US. However, because CT remains obligatory for the staging of the primary tumor, they consider additional investigation by US-FNA unnecessary.

4.8.2 Post-therapy Follow-up

Sonography is the ideal imaging modality for monitoring superficial metastatic nodes in patients with head and neck cancer who have not undergone surgery. In addition, because cutaneous thickening of the neck is not infrequent after radiotherapy, the quality of physical examination is reduced in such cases. Even when hindered by edema or fibrosis, US provides complementary data of better quality for monitoring purposes (Fig. 4.14).

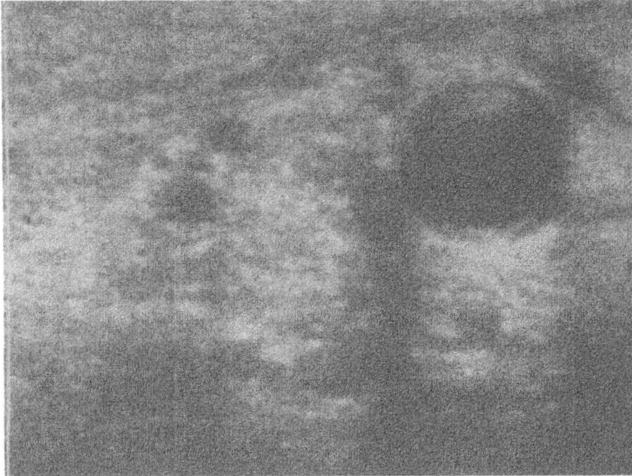
a

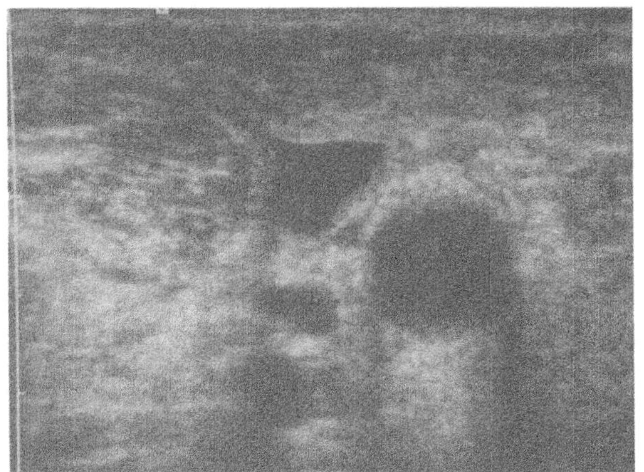
b

Fig. 4.14a,b. Radiochemotherapy protocols modify the sonographic appearance of the cervical region. **a** Radical neck dissection (removal of the nodes, the internal jugular vein, and the sternocleidomastoid muscle). **b** Functional neck dissection

Following induction chemotherapy or a combination of radiotherapy and surgery, therapeutic efficacy can be helpfully assessed by serial US studies (Schafer et al. 1996). More effective than clinical examination, sonography can provide data of prognostic value. In a personal series (Bruneton et al. 1984), only two of 33 patients in whom US revealed lesion stability or progression under treatment were still alive at 1 year. In contrast, only nine of 67 patients in whom US demonstrated an improvement in nodal status died in less than 12 months.

Postoperatively, reactive nodal enlargement may occur in the lateral cervical neck, independently of any nodal lesion. Sonography can be repeated in such cases at 2-week intervals for monitoring purposes. Progressive diminution in node size permits a malignant process to be ruled out (Szmeja et al. 1999).

In the long term, diagnosis of tumor or nodal recurrence is critical, because only early detection permits effective therapeutic management. In a series of 136 patients who had developed nodal recurrences, Szmeja et al. (1999) found that sonographic and surgical findings were highly correlated (95%), whereas physical examination had a very low sensitivity (14%) (Fig. 4.15).

Steinkamp et al. (1994a) proposed the use of CD to aid detection of recurrence in the lateral neck of treated patients.

Finally, for N0 neck patients who have undergone treatment only for their primary tumor, Van den Brekel et al. (1999) proposed systematic cervical US associated with physical examination: All suspicious nonpalpable nodes depicted sonographically undergo US-guided FNA, which allows early diagnosis of nodal involvement. The risk of overlooking occult metastases is reduced to only 18%, which is much better than with palpation alone.

4.9 Lymphoma

Superficial lymphadenopathy is the most frequent manifestation of lymphoma, during both initial staging and recurrence (Schein et al. 1975). Although usually larger in diameter than metastatic nodes, lymphomatous nodes have a soft consistency that reduces the accuracy of physical examination. Precise information on superficial node involvement can be obtained by US examination of the supraclavicular, axillary, and inguinal regions, in addition to the cervical region. In Hodgkin's disease (HD), US can demonstrate lymphomatous nodes overlooked by physical examination; above all, it increases the number of involved nodes visualized, which is a prognostic factor in HD. In non-Hodgkin's lymphoma (NHL), where the prognosis depends more on the histological disease type, optimized detection and evaluation of superficial node involvement improves analysis of response to therapy by increasing the number of evaluable targets (Young et al. 1978).

In HD, relapses tend to occur during the first 2 or 3 years. Whether associated or not with a deep site of involvement, superficial node recurrence is seen in 89%–95% of relapses (Bayle-Weisgerber et al. 1984). In NHL, 69% of relapses affect the lymph nodes (Schein et al. 1975; Weeks 1991). Regardless

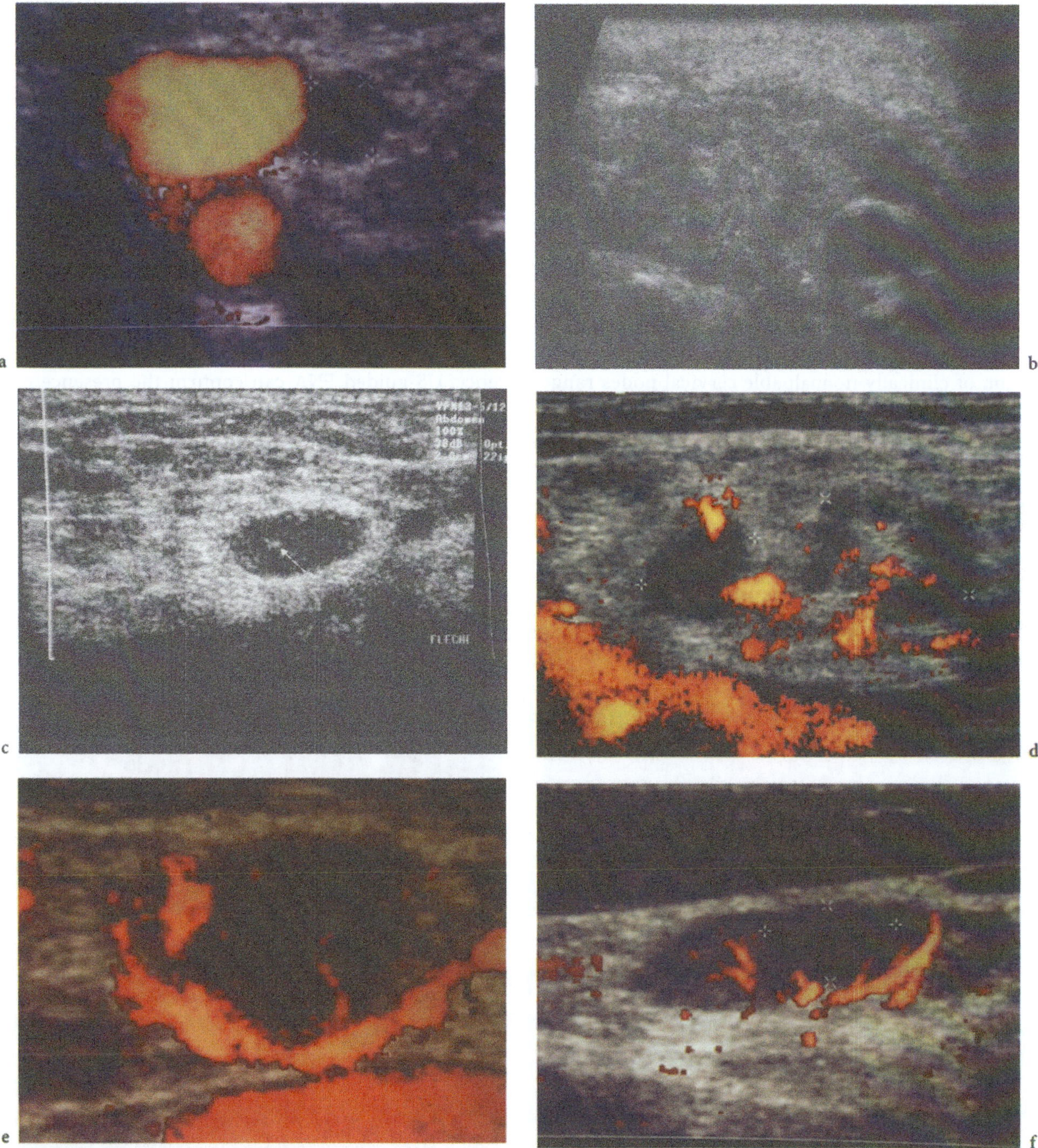

Fig. 4.15a–f. Post-therapy metastatic nodal recurrence. **a** Small nodal mass (0.5/0.5 cm between the *crosses*) in contact with the internal jugular vein; US-guided FNA confirmed the diagnosis of recurrence. **b** Large, diffuse nodal recurrence 6 months after neck dissection; owing to post-therapy modifications (surgery, radiotherapy), the margins of the recurrence are difficult to determine sonographically. **c** Demonstration of an oval nodal mass without an echogenic hilum and no specific features; FNA revealed an inflammatory node (the tip of the needle is indicated by an *arrow*). **d** Nodal recurrence in the form of two masses; the larger one (1.3 cm between the *two crosses*) has a reassuring echopattern (echogenic hilum and hilar vascularity) but the smaller one (0.9 cm between the *two crosses*) appears pathological (rounded shape and especially the presence of peripheral vessels penetrating the capsule). This image, characteristic of nodal metastasis, allowed affirmation of nodal recurrence despite the small size of the lesions. **e** Nodal recurrence (12 mm in greatest dimension): pathological vascular pattern with, in particular, the presence of capsular rupture (vessel arising from a peripheral vascular structure that perforates the capsule to supply the center of the node). **f** Oval nodal mass in a patient treated for a head and neck malignancy; power Doppler revealed the presence of an abnormal intranodal defect (0.7/0.4 cm between the *crosses*); US-guided FNA of the defect revealed the presence of metastatic tissue, thus confirming nodal recurrence

of the type of lymphoma, the superficial lymph nodes are the most common site of recurrent disease, the exact frequency of which is difficult to determine owing to progressive improvements in response rates to chemotherapy (Fig. 4.16).

In order to reduce the risk of false-positive findings, we advocate combined use of the transverse node diameter (minimum 1 cm) and the presence of multiple nodal lesions as the basis for diagnosis of nodal involvement in patients with lymphoma. Sonography has proven more sensitive than physical examination at both the cervical level and the other superficial node-bearing regions (Bruneton et al. 1987; Gerrits et al. 1994); the improvement in detection of clinically nonpalpable cervical nodes ranges from 10.8% to 13%. Using a biopsy gun fitted with a needle 1.2 mm in diameter for US-guided FNA, Elvin et al. (1997) successfully typed 92.3% of lymphomas without need for surgery.

Even minimally enlarged lymphomatous nodes often exhibit hypervascularity that helps identify their pathological character. In other cases, the hilar-type vascular pattern seen at power Doppler is less pronounced and not significantly different from that of reactive nodes (Wu et al. 1998). Whether by gray-scale imaging or CD, the purpose of sonography is to determine as accurately as possible the number of involved nodes, which is a significant prognostic factor for patients treated by radiotherapy alone (Goldwein et al. 1991).

Not all nodes affected by lymphoma require FNA, but histological proof is indispensable regardless of the histological type whenever US suggests recurrence. US-guided FNA can confirm the presence of disease recurrence and occasionally reveals transformation of the lymphoma from a less aggressive to a more aggressive type (this adverse course occurs in 20%–40% of all cases of NHL).

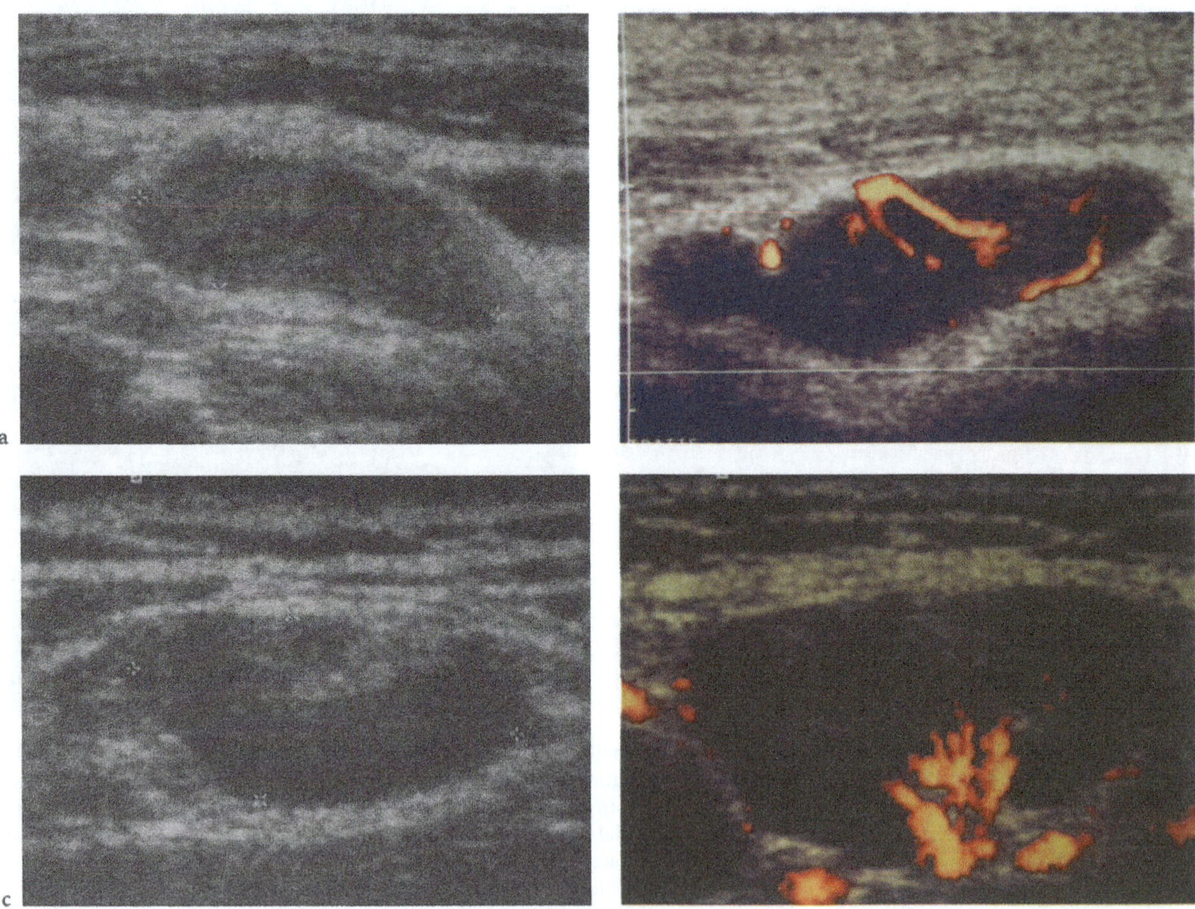

Fig. 4.16a–d. Sonographic follow-up of a treated nodal lymphoma. **a** Oval nodal mass (1.6/0.6 cm between the *crosses*) without an echogenic hilum and no specific features; FNA demonstrated the presence of lymphomatous tissue. b Color Doppler study of a treated nodal lymphoma; atypical vascularity related to disease recurrence. **c** Nodal recurrence of NHL (1.5/0.7 cm between the *crosses*); misleading appearance of an echogenic, peripheral pseudo-hilum. **d** Nodal recurrence of NHL; power Doppler demonstrated massive hypervascularity of the hilar region; this finding was judged insufficient to affirm a diagnosis of nodal recurrence; US-guided FNA demonstrated the presence of lymphomatous tissue

References

Ahuja A, Ying M, Leung JF, Metreweli C (1996a) The sonographic appearance and significance of cervical metastatic nodes following radiotherapy for nasopharyngeal carcinoma. Clin Radiol 10:698–701

Ahuja A, Ying M, Yang WT, Evans R, King W, Metreweli C (1996b) The use of sonography in differentiating cervical lymphomatous lymph nodes from cervical metastatic lymph nodes. Clin Radiol 51:186–190

Ahuja A, Ng CF, King W, Metreweli C (1998) Solitary cystic nodal metastasis from occult papillary carcinoma of the thyroid mimicking a branchial cyst: a potential pitfall. Clin Radiol 53:61–63

Atula TS, Grenman R, Varpula MJ, Kurki TJ, Klemi PJ (1996) Palpation, ultrasound, and ultrasound-guided fine-needle aspiration cytology in the assessment of cervical lymph node status in head and neck cancer patients. Head Neck 18:545–551

Atula TS, Varpula MJ, Kurki TJ, Klemi PJ, Grenman R (1997) Assessment of cervical lymph node status in head and neck cancer patients: palpation, computed tomography and low field magnetic resonance imaging compared with ultrasound-guided fine-needle aspiration cytology. Eur J Radiol 25:152–161

Baatenburg de Jong RJ, Rongen RJ, Verwoerd CD, Van Overhagen H, Lameris JS, Knegt P (1991) Ultrasound-guided fine-needle aspiration biopsy of neck nodes. Arch Otolaryngol Head Neck Surg 117:402–404

Bayle-Weisgerber C, Lemercier N, Teillet F, et al (1984) Hodgkin's disease in children: results of therapy in a mixed group of 178 clinical and pathologically staged patients over 13 years. Cancer 54:215–222

Bearcroft PWP, Berman LH, Grant J (1995) The use of ultrasound-guided cutting-needle biospy in the neck. Clin Radiol 50:690–695

Beissert M, Jenett M, Wetzler T, Hinterseher I, Kessler C, Hahn D (2000) Enlarged lymph nodes of the neck: evaluation with parallel extended field-of-view sonographic sequences. J Ultrasound Med 19:195–200

Bruneton JN, Normand F (1987). Cervical lymph nodes. In: Bruneton JN (ed) Ultrasonography of the neck. Springer, Berlin Heidelberg New York, pp 81–91

Bruneton JN, Roux P, Caramella E, Demard F, Vallicioni J, Chauvel P (1984) Ear, nose and throat cancer: ultrasound diagnosis of metastasis to cervical lymph nodes. Radiology 152:771–773

Bruneton JN, Normand F, Balu-Maestro C, et al (1987) Lymphomatous superficial lymph nodes: US detection. Radiology 165:233–235

Bruneton JN, Balu-Maestro C, Merran D, et al (1990) Rapports veineux des adénopathies cervicales. Revue d'une série de 300 cas. J Radiol 71:57–60

Bruneton JN, Balu-Maestro C, Marcy PY, Melia P, Mourou MY (1994) Very high frequency (13 MHz) ultrasonographic examination of the normal neck: detection of normal lymph nodes and thyroid nodules. J Ultrasound Med 13:87–90

Bruneton JN, Rubaltelli L, Solbiati L (1995) Lymph nodes. In: Solbiati L, Rizzatto G (eds) Ultrasound of superficial structures. High frequencies, Doppler and interventional procedures. Churchill Livingstone, Edinburgh, pp 279–301

Bude RO, Rubin JM (1996) Power Doppler sonography. Radiology 200:21–23

Cerezo L, Millan I, Torre A, Aragon G, Otero J (1992) Prognostic factors for survival and tumor control in cervical lymph node metastases from head and neck cancer. Cancer 69:1224–1234

Chang DB, Yuan A, Yu CJ, Luh KT, Kuo SH, Yang PC (1994) Differentiation of benign and malignant cervical lymph nodes with color doppler sonography. AJR Am J Roentgenol 162:965–968

Chikui T, Yonetsu K, Nakamura T (2000) Multivariate feature analysis of sonographic findings of metastatic cervical lymph nodes: contribution of blood flow features revealed by power Doppler sonography for predicting metastasis. Am J Neuroradiol 21:561–567

Choi MY, Lee JW, Jang KJ (1995) Distinction between benign and malignant causes of cervical, axillary, and inguinal lymphadenopathy: value of Doppler spectral waveform analysis. AJR Am J Roentgenol 165:981–984

Cole I, Chu J, Kos S, Motbey J (1993) Metastatic carcinoma in the neck; a clinical computerized tomography scan and ultrasound study. Aust NZ J Surg 63:468–474

Danninger R, Posawetz W, Humer U, Stammberger H, Jakse R (1999) Ultrasound investigation of cervical lymph node metastases: conception and results of a histopathological exploration. Laryngorhinootologie 78:144–149

Delorme S, Dietz A, Rudat V, Zuna I, Bahner ML, Van Kaick G (1997) Prognostic significance of color Doppler findings in head and neck tumors. Ultrasound Med Biol 23:1311–1317

Dillon WP (1998) Cervical nodal metastases: another look at size criteria. Am J Neuroradiol 19:796–797

Eichhorn T, Schroeder HG, Glanz H, Schwerk WB (1987) Histologically controlled comparison of palpation and sonography in the diagnosis of cervical lymph node metastases. Larynx Rhinol Otol 66:266–274

Elvin A, Sundstrom C, Larsson SG, Lindgren PG (1997) Ultrasound-guided 1.2-mm cutting-needle biopsies of head and neck tumours. Acta Radiol 38:376–380

Evans RM, Ahuja A, Metreweli C (1993) The linear echogenic hilus in cervical lymphadenopathy. A sign of benignity or malignancy? Clin Radiol 47:262–264

Fischbein NJ, Assar OS, Caputo GR, et al (1998) Clinical utility of positron emission tomography with 18F-fluorodeoxyglucose in detecting residual/recurrent squamous cell carcinoma of the head and neck. Am J Neuroradiol 19:1189–1196

Fulcher AS (1993) Cervical lymphadenopathy due to Kikuchi disease: US and CT appearance. J Comput Assist Tomogr 17:131–133

Furukawa M, Kaneko M, Mochimatsu I, Sawaki S, Igari H, Tsukuda M (1991) Comparative studies of diagnosis with US or CT of tree cervical lymph node metastases in head and neck cancer. Nippon Jibiinkoka Gakkai Kaiho 94:577–586

Georgi M, Gha J, Teubner J, Bolte R (1999) Lymph node imaging with ultra-rapid 3D MR angiography. Rofo Fortschr Geb Rontgenstr Neuen Bildgeb Verfahr 170:218–221

Gerrits CJ, Van Overhagen H, Van Lom K, Adrihansen HJ, Lowenberg B (1994) Ultrasound examination of pathological cervical lymph nodes in patients with non-Hodgkin's lymphoma and Hodgkin's lymphoma. Br J Haematol 88:826–828

Giovagnorio F, Caiazzo R, Avitto A (1997) Evaluation of vasculature patterns of cervical lymph nodes with power Doppler sonography. J Clin Ultrasound 25:71–76

Goldwein JW, Coia LR, Hanks GE (1991) Prognostic factors in patients with early stage non-Hodgkin's lymphomas of the head and neck treated with definitive irradiation. Int J Radiat Oncol Biol Phys 20:45–51

Gritzmann N, Grasi MC, Helmer M, Steiner E (1990) Invasion of the carotid artery and jugular vein by lymph node metastases: detection with sonography. AJR 154:411–414

Hajek PC, Salomonowitz E, Turk R, Tscholakoff D, Kumpan W, Czembirek H (1986) Lymph nodes of the neck: evaluation with US. Radiology 158:739–742

Ishii J, Fujii E, Suzuki H, Shinozuka K, Kawase N, Amagasa T (1992) Ultrasonic diagnosis of oral and neck malignant lymphoma. Bull Tokyo Med Dent Univ 39:63–69

Issing PR, Kettling T, Kempf HG, Heermann R, Lenarz T (1999) Ultrasound evaluation of characteristics of cervical lymph nodes with reference to color Doppler ultrasound. A contribution to differentiating reactive from metastatic lymph node involvement in the neck. Laryngorhinootologie 78:566–572

Janot F, Cvitkovic E, Piekarski JD, et al (1993) Correlation between nodal density in contrast scans and response to cisplatin-based chemotherapy in head and neck squamous cell cancer: a prospective validation. Head Neck 15:222–229

Koch WM, Choti MA, Civelek C, et al (1998) Gamma probe-directed biopsy of the sentinel node in oral squamous cell carcinoma. Arch Otolaryngol Head Neck Surg 124:455–459

Leicher-Duber A, Bleier R, Duber C, Thelen M (1990) Cervical lymph node metastases: a histologically controlled comparison of palpation, sonography and computed tomography. Rofo Fortschr Geb Rontgenstr Neuen Bildgeb Verfahr 153:575–579

Lohela P, Tikkakoski T, Strengell L, Mikkola S, Koskinen S, Suramo I (1996) Ultrasound-guided fine-needle aspiration cytology of non-palpable supraclavicular lymph nodes in sarcoidosis. Acta Radiol 37:896–899

Maurer J, Schroeder RJ, William K, et al (1999) Diagnostic value of signal-enhanced color Doppler sonography in reactively enlarged lymph nodes. Radiology 39:74–80

Mende U, Zoller J, Dietz A, Wannenmacher M, Born IA, Maier H (1996) Ultrasound diagnosis in primary staging of head-neck tumors. Radiology 36:207–216

Miller WT jr, Perez-Jaffe LA (1999) Cross-sectional imaging of Kikuchi disease. J Comput Assist Tomogr 23:548–551

Moritz JD, Ludwig I, Oestmann JW (2000) Contrast-enhanced color Doppler ultrasound for evaluation of enlarged cervical lymph nodes in head and neck tumors. AJR Am J Roentgenol 174:1279–1284

Mountford RA, Atkinson P (1973) Doppler ultrasound examination of pathologically enlarged lymph nodes. Br J Radiol 52:464–467

Na DG, Lim HK, Byun HS, Kim HD, Ko YH, Beak JH (1997) Differential diagnosis of cervical lymphadenopathy: usefulness of color Doppler sonography. AJR Am J Roentgenol 168:1311–1316

Naito K (1990) Analysis of cervical metastatic lymphadenopathy by ultrasonography. Nippon Igaku Hoshasen Gakkai Zasshi 50:918–927

Nakayama E, Ariji E, Shinohara M, Yoshiura K, Miwa K, Kanda S (1997) Computed tomography appearance of marked keratinisation of metastatic cervical lymph nodes: a case report. Oral Surg Oral Med Oral Pathol Oral Radiol Endod 84:321–326

Nuutinen J, Jyrkkio S, Lehikoinen P, Lindholm P, Minn H (1999) Evaluation of early response to radiotherapy in head and neck cancer measured with [^{11}C] methionine-positron emission tomography. Radiother Oncol 52:225–232

Prim MP, De Diego JI, Hardisson D, Madero R, Nistal M, Gavilan J (1999) Extracapsular spread and desmoplastic pattern in neck lymph nodes: two prognostic factors of laryngeal cancer. Aun Otol Rhinol Laryngol 108:672–676

Rainer T, Ofner G, Marckhgott E (1993) Ultrasound diagnosis of regional lymph node metastasis of the neck in patients with head-neck neoplasms: sonomorphologic criteria and diagnostic accuracy. Laryngorhinootologie 72:73–77

Richter E, Feyerabend T (1991) Normal lymph node topography, CT atlas. Springer, Berlin Heidelberg New York

Robbins KT, Medina JE, Wolfe GT, et al (1991) Standardizing neck dissection terminology. Official report of the Academy's Committee for Head and Neck Surgery and Oncology. Arch Otolaryngol Head Neck Surg 117:601–605

Robinson IA, Cozens NJ (1999) Does a joint ultrasound-guided cytology clinic optimize the cytological evaluation of head and neck masses? Clin Radiol 54:312–316

Rubaltelli L, Proto E, Salmaso R, Bortoletto P, Candiani F, Cagol P (1990) Sonography of abnormal lymph nodes in vitro: correlation of sonographic and histologic findings AJR Am J Roentgenol 155:1241–1244

Sakai F, Kiyono K, Sone S, et al (1988) Ultrasonic evaluation of cervical metastatic lymphadenopathy. J Ultrasound Med 7:305–310

Sakai F, Sone S, Kiyono K, et al (1991) Computed tomography of neck lymph nodes involved with malignant lymphoma: comparison with ultrasound. Radiat Med 9:203–208.

Schafer CB, Bartzsch OM, Feldmann HJ, Molls M, Allgauer M (1996) Ultrasound volumetry of cervical lymph nodes during radiotherapy as a method of therapy monitoring. Ultraschall Med 17:289–294

Schein PS, Chabner BA, Canellos GP et al (1975) Non-Hodgkin's lymphoma: patterns of relapse from complete remission after combination chemotherapy. Cancer 35:354–357

Schroeder RJ, Maurer J, Hidajat N, et al (1998) Signal-enhanced color-coded duplex sonography of reactively and metastatically enlarged lymph nodes. Rofo Fortschr Geb Rontgenstr Neuen Bildged Verfahr 168:57–63

Schroeder RJ, Maurer J, Gath HJ, William K, Hidajat N (1999) Vascularization of reactively enlarged lymph nodes analyzed by color duplex sonography. J Oral Maxillofac Surg 57:1090–1095

Sigal R, Lamer S (1999) Radio-anatomie des chaînes ganglionnaires de la sphère ORL. J Radiol 80:1816–1819

Som PM (1992) Detection of metastasis in cervical lymph nodes: CT and MR criteria and differential diagnosis. AJR Am J Roentgenol 158:961–969

Steinkamp HJ, Maurer J, Cornehl M, Knobber D, Hettwer H, Felix R (1994a) Recurrent cervical lymphadenopathy: differential diagnosis with color-duplex sonography. Eur Arch Otorhinolaryngol 251:404–409

Steinkamp HJ, Teske C, Knobber E, Schedel H, Felix R (1994b) Sonographie in der Tumornachsorge von Kopf-Hals-Tumorpatienten. Wertigkeit Sonomorphologischen Kriterien und des sonographischen M/Q-Quotienten. Ultraschall Med 15:81–88

Steinkamp HJ, Rausch M, Maurer J, et al (1994c) Color-coded duplex sonography in the differential diagnosis of cervical lymph node enlargements. Rofo Fortschr Geb Rontgenstr Neuen Bildgeb Verfahr 161:226–232

Steinkamp HJ, Teichgraber UK, Mueffelmann M, Hosten N, Kenzel P, Felix R (1999) Differential diagnosis of lymph node lesions. A semiquantitative approach with power Doppler sonography. Invest Radiol 34:509–515

Stern WBP, Silver CE, Zeifer BA, Persky MS, Heller KS (1990) Computed tomography of the clinically negative neck. Head Neck 12:109–113

Stokkel MP, Ten Broek FW, Hordijk Gj, Koole R, Van Rijk PP (2000) Preoperative evaluation of patients with primary head and neck cancer using dual-head 18 fluorodeoxyglucose positron emission tomography. Ann Surg 23:229–234

Szmeja Z, Wierzbicka M, Kordylewska M (1999) The value of ultrasound examination in preoperative neck assessment and in early diagnosis of nodal recurrences in the follow-up of patients operated for laryngeal cancer. Eur Arch Otorhinolaryngol 256:415–417

Takes RP, Righi P, Meeuwis CA, et al (1998) The value of ultrasound with ultrasound-guided fine-needle aspiration biopsy compared to computed tomography in the detection of regional metastasis in the clinically negative neck. Int J Rad Oncol Biol Phys 40:1027–1032

Takeuchi Y, Suzuki H, Omura K, et al (1999) Differential diagnosis of cervical lymph nodes in head and neck cancer by ultrasonography. Auris Nasus Larynx 26:331–336

Tschammler A, Hahn D (1999) Multivariate analysis of the adjustment of the colour duplex unit for the differential diagnosis of lymph node alterations. Eur Radiol 9:1445–1490

Tschammler A, Ott G, Schang T, Seelbach-Goebel B, Schwager K, Hahn D (1998) Lymphadenopathy: differentiation of benign from malignant disease-color Doppler US assessment of intranodal angioarchitecture. Radiology 208:117–123

Turner RR, Martin J, Dorfman RF (1983) Necrotizing lymphadenitis. A study of 30 cases. Am J Surg Pathol 7:115–123

Van den Brekel MWM (1996) US-guided fine-needle aspiration cytology of neck nodes in patients with N0 disease. Radiology 201:580–581

Van den Brekel MWM, Castelijns JA (1999) Radiologic evaluation of neck metastases: the otolaryngologist's perspective. Semin Ultrasound CT MR 20:162–174

Van den Brekel MWM, Castelijns JA, Stel HV, et al (1990a) Detection and characterization of metastatic cervical adenopathy by MR imaging: comparison of different MR techniques. J Comput Assist Tomogr 14:581–589

Van den Brekel MWM, Stel HV, Castelijns J, et al (1990b) Cervical lymph node metastasis: assessment of radiologic criteria. Radiology 177:379–384

Van den Brekel MWM, Stel HV, Castelijns JA, Croll GJ, Snow GB (1991) Lymph node staging in patients with clinically negative neck examinations by ultrasound and ultrasound-guided aspiration cytology. Am J Surg 162:362–366

Van den Brekel MWM, Van der Waal I, Meyer CJLM, Freeman JL, Castelijns JA, Snow GB (1996) The incidence of micrometastases in neck dissection specimens obtained from elective neck dissections. Laryngoscope 106:987–991

Van den Brekel MWM, Castelijns JA, Snow GB (1998) The size of lymph nodes in the neck on sonograms as a radiologic criterion for metastasis: how reliable is it? Am J Neuroradiol 19:695–700

Van den Brekel MW, Reitsma LC, Quak JJ, et al (1999) Sonographically guided aspiration cytology of neck nodes for selection of treatment and follow-up in patients with N0 head and neck cancer. Am J Neuroradiol 20:1727–1731

Vassallo P, Weinecke K, Roar N, Peters PE (1992) Differentiation of benign from malignant superficial lymphadenopathy: the role of high-resolution US. Radiology 183:215–220

Vassallo P, Edel G, Roos N, Naguib A, Peters PE (1993) In vitro high-resolution ultrasonography of benign and malignant lymph nodes. A sonographic-pathologic correlation. Invest Radiol 28:698–705

Weeks JC, Yeap BY, Canellos GP, Shipp MA (1991) Value of follow-up procedures in patients with large-cell lymphoma who achieve a complete remission. J Clin Oncol 9:1196–1203

William C, Maurer J, Steinkamp HJ, Vogl TJ, Felix R (1996) Differential diagnosis of cervical lymph node enlargements: ultrasound and histomorphology of reactive lymph nodes. Bildgebung 63:113–199

Winkelbauer F, Denk DM, Ammann M, Karnel F (1992) Sonographische Diagnostik der Halslymphknotentuberkulose. Ultraschall Med 13:28–31

Wu CH, Hsu MM, Chang YL, Hsieh FJ (1998) Vascular pathology of malignant cervical lymphadenopathy. Qualitative and quantitative assessment with power Doppler ultrasound. Cancer 83:1189–1196

Ying M, Ahuja A, Evans R, King W, Metreweli C (1998) Cervical lymphadenopathy: sonographical differentiation between tuberculous nodes and nodal metastatases from non-head and neck carcinomas. J Clin Ultrasound 26:383–389

Ying M, Ahuja A, Brook F, Brown B, Metreweli C (1999) Nodal shape (S/L) and its combination with size for assessment of cervical lympadenopathy: which cut-off should be used? Ultrasound Med Biol 25:1169–1175

Young RC, Canellos GP, Chabner BA, Hubbard SM, De Vita VT jr (1978) Patterns of relapse in advanced Hodgkin's disease treated with combination chemotherapy. Cancer 42:1001–1007

Youssem DM, Hurst RW (1994) MR of cervical lymph nodes: comparison of fast spin-echo and conventional spin-echo T2 W scans. Clin Radiol 49:670–675

5 Larynx and Hypopharynx

Patrick Chevallier, Pierre-Yves Marcy, Christopher Arens, Charles Raffaelli, Bernard Padovani, Jean Noël Bruneton

CONTENTS

P. Chevallier, MD
Service de Radiodiagnostic, Hôpital de l'Archet, 151 Chemin de St. Antoine de Ginestière, F-06200 Nice Cedex, France
P.Y. Marcy, MD
Service de Radiodiagnostic, Centre Antoine-Lacassagne, 33 avenue de Valombrose, F-06189 Nice Cedex 2, France
C. Arens, MD
HNO-Universitätsklinik, Justus-Liebig-Universität Giessen, Faulgenstraße 10, D-35394 Giessen, Germany
C. Raffaelli, MD
Service de Radiodiagnostic, Hôpital Pasteur, 30, avenue Voie Romaine, BP 69, F-06002 Nice Cedex 1, France
B. Padovani, MD
Professor of Radiology, Service de Radiodiagnostic, Hôpital Pasteur, 30, avenue Voie Romaine, BP 69, F-06002 Nice Cedex 1, France
J.N. Bruneton, MD
Professor of Radiology, Centre Antoine-Lacassagne, 33 avenue de Valombrose, F-06189 Nice Cedex 2, France

5.1 Introduction

Magnetic resonance imaging (MRI) and computed tomography (CT) are the imaging techniques of choice for examination of the larynx and hypopharynx. Since the pioneering research on vocal cord vibration using Doppler ultrasound conducted by Mensch in 1964, several other investigators have mentioned the potential utility of percutaneous or endoscopic sonography for analysis of the normal anatomy and pathologies of these organs. Few authors have described the use of high-frequency ultrasound (US) for examination of laryngeal anatomy and pathologies, however. The infrequency of such studies is probably due to unfamiliarity with the normal sonographic features of the larynx and hypopharynx and the various technical maneuvers that can be used to circumvent the factors that hamper sonographic examination of this region.

5.2 Percutaneous Sonography

5.2.1 Examination Technique (Fig. 5.1)

The patient is examined in the supine position, with the head slightly retroflexed, using a high-frequency transducer of at least 7.5 MHz.

Examination is initiated by instructing the patient to breathe quietly and regularly. Midline axial scanning is performed from the hyoid bone down to the inferior border of the cricoid cartilage. Owing to their midline location and the homogeneous nature of their calcification in the adult, these hyperechoic structures with strong posterior shadowing are readily identified. Recurrent midline axial scans are then obtained upward and downward through the spaces between the hyoid bone and the thyroid cartilage

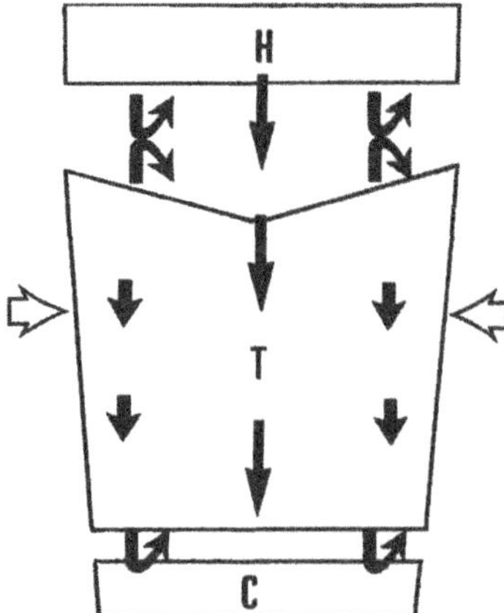

Fig. 5.1. Diagram of the hyoid bone (*H*) and the thyroid (*T*) and cricoid (*C*) cartilages. Sonographic protocol for examination of the larynx and hypopharynx during quiet breathing: 1, midline transverse axial scans from the hyoid bone down to the cricoid cartilage (*long arrows*); 2, recurrent axial scans through the thyrohyoid and cricothyroid membranes (*curved arrows*); 3, axial scans sweeping through each thyroid ala (*short arrows*); 4, transverse scans (*open arrows*)

(thyrohyoid membrane) and between the thyroid cartilage and the cricoid cartilage (cricothyroid membrane). Axial scans are also obtained at the level of each thyroid cartilage ala. This initial phase of US workup is completed by longitudinal scans along the anteroposterior axis of each ala of the thyroid cartilage, and by transverse scans. When necessary, workup is completed by examination of the cervical node-bearing areas, as described by Bruneton et al. (1987). These various steps are performed in B-mode, combined, when appropriate, with Doppler US to confirm the absence of physiological vascularity in certain anatomic zones (see Chap. 2).

The second part of the examination, performed in B-mode and/or Doppler mode, consists in dynamic evaluation of anatomic structures in all three planes of space during phonation of the sound "e" and during swallowing, completed when necessary by breath-holding/inspiration sequences or Valsalva maneuvers. Selection of the maneuvers and the scan plane(s) depends on the anatomic structure to be studied and the clinical context prompting US examination (see Sects. 5.2.3–5.2.6).

5.2.2 Normal Features

5.2.2.1 Larynx

5.2.2.1.1 Laryngeal Cartilages

The laryngeal cartilages are of two histological types: hyaline cartilages (thyroid cartilage, arytenoid cartilages except for the vocal processes, cricoid cartilage) and elastic cartilages (epiglottis, vocal processes of the arytenoid cartilages, and accessory cartilages) (Rebel et al. 1980). The elastic cartilages rarely undergo calcification, whereas the hyaline cartilages calcify or ossify starting at nodes of ossification in a fairly stereotyped order, as described by Waldaptel and Baclesse (Dulac 1974). Calcification initially progresses posteriorly, from the bottom upwards, then from back to front. Calcification of the thyroid and cricoid cartilages occurs earlier and is more complete in men than in women, probably due in part to hormonal factors. Cartilaginous ossification is not always symmetrical, and calcified and ossified hyaline tissues may be juxtaposed.

5.2.2.1.1.1 Thyroid Cartilage

The paired, shield-shaped thyroid cartilage (from the Greek *thyreos*, shield) that protects the other components of the larynx begins at the base of the tongue, at the level of vertebrae C-4 and C-5. The largest cartilage of the larynx, the thyroid cartilage is composed of two vertical quadrilateral plates, 3–4 cm in height. The anterior borders of these plates, which may be asymmetrical, meet in the midline to form a ventrally oriented acute angle that is larger in women than in men. The posterior aspects of the thyroid cartilage extend upward as the superior cornua, to which the lateral thyrohyoid ligaments are attached, and downward as the shorter inferior cornua, which join with the cricoid cartilage.

On midline axial sonograms, the two lateral alae typically form an asymmetrical, upside-down V. On near-midline transverse and longitudinal sonograms, the thyroid ala images, respectively, as a rectilinear band and an inwardly curved concave stripe.

The sonographic appearance of the thyroid cartilage varies with the degree of calcification (Fig. 5.2).

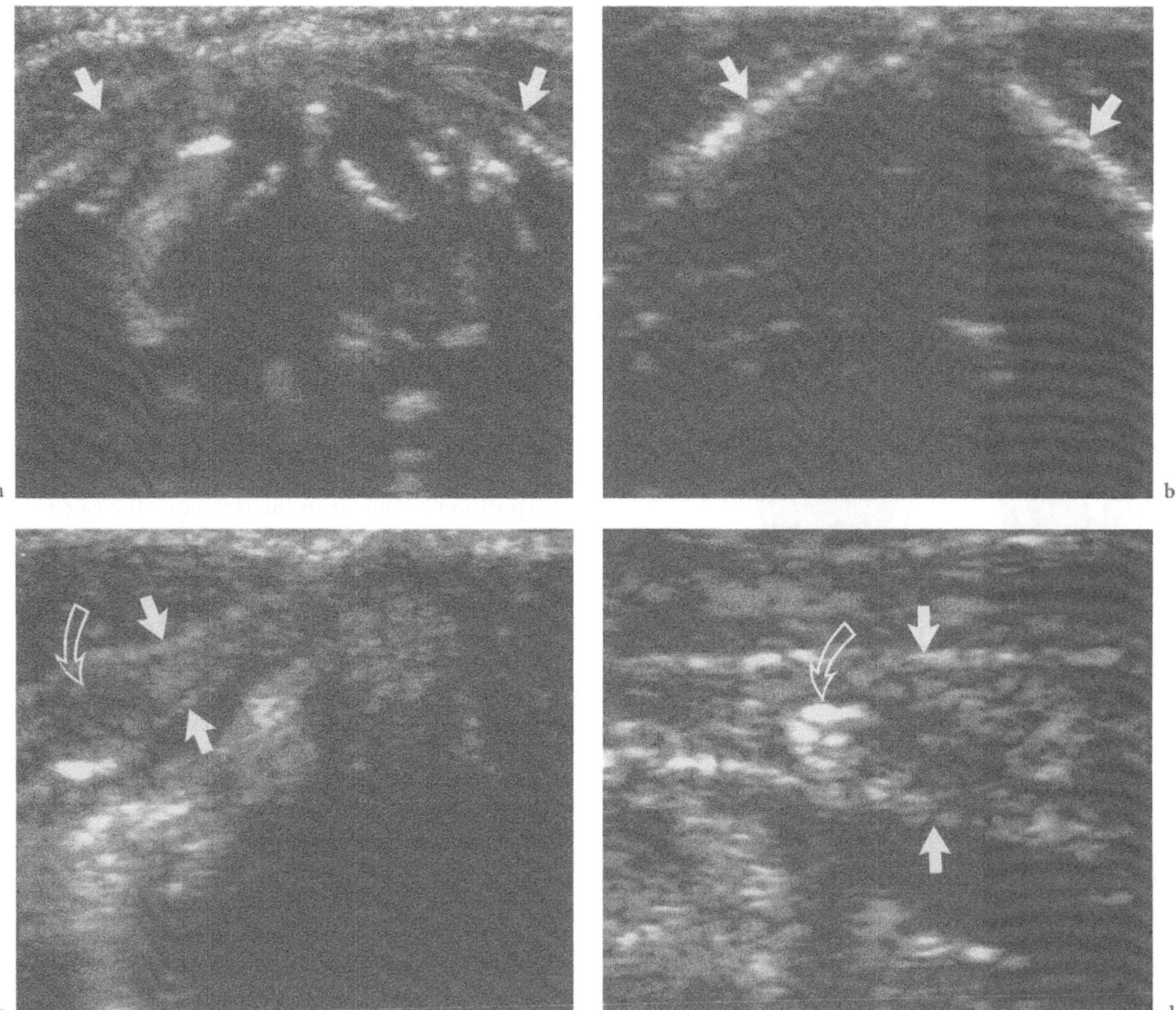

Fig. 5.2a–d. Axial sonograms: thyroid cartilage (*arrows*) at different stages of calcification. **a** Partial calcification with good visualization of the retrothyroid structures, **b** nearly complete calcification, **c** absence of calcification with a noncalcified node of ossification (*open arrow*), and **d** calcified node of ossification (*open arrow*)

Six sonographic stages have been described (CHEVALLIER et al. 1997), based on the research of WALDAPTEL and BACLESSE (DULAC 1974) (Fig. 5.3).

While still hyalinized, the thyroid cartilage comprises an inmost part (the medulla) that is isoechoic to the infrahyoid muscles and is delimited by two 1- to 2-mm-thick, hyperechoic parallel borders corresponding to the internal and external perichondria (such borders are absent on articular surfaces which have no perichondrial covering). Although the internal perichondrium is usually continuous, it is interrupted in around 10% of cases. Tumor spread across the thyroid cartilage thus cannot be affirmed solely on the basis of interruption of the border corresponding to the internal perichondrium on sonograms. The internal perichondrium remains fixed during dynamic maneuvers; this permits differentiation from the hyperechoic paraglottic or paralaryngeal fat that is mobile during such maneuvers. The internal and external perichondria of the midportion of the thyroid ala are occasionally transfixed by the superior laryngeal artery (CHEVALLIER et al. 1997; TROTOUX et al. 1986).

The nodes of ossification are usually calcified, and these hyperechoic nodular structures create posterior shadowing (Fig. 5.2d). When calcification has not yet begun, these nodes sometimes image as a pseudotumoral nodule (Fig. 5.2c). Once extensive calcifi-

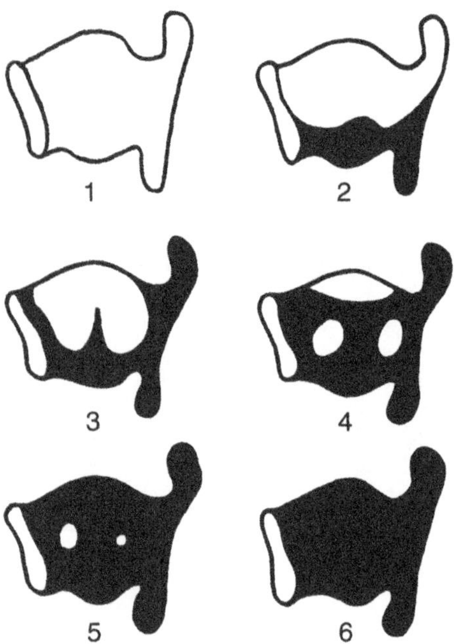

Fig. 5.3. The six sonographic stages of thyroid cartilage calcification

cation has occurred, hyperechoic lines appear in an asymmetrical manner within the medulla of the two cartilaginous plates; advanced stages of calcification (stages 5 and 6) render the thyroid cartilage globally hyperechoic (Fig. 5.2b).

Stage 1 calcification is never seen in the adult, because at least partial calcification of an inferior cornu has already occurred. Calcification is less than or equal to stage 3 in 90% of women and 40% of men; this permits satisfactory examination of all or part of the retrothyroid anatomic structures (except for certain intrinsic laryngeal muscles and the aryepiglottic folds) in 92.1%–98% of individuals (Chevallier et al. 1997). Endolaryngeal examination is more difficult once calcification is complete or nearly so (Chevallier et al. 1997; Derchi et al. 1992; Gritzmann et al. 1989; Valente et al. 1996); in such cases, optimum use must be made of the remaining windows of hyaline cartilage and specific scan planes (suprathyroid axial scans recurrent downward, infrathyroid axial scans recurrent upward, and retrothyroid longitudinal scans recurrent forward).

5.2.2.1.1.2
Arytenoid Cartilages

The small, roughly pyramidal arytenoid cartilages are paired symmetrical structures that average 15 mm in height. They are the point of convergence of the intrinsic laryngeal muscles and play a key role in laryngeal dynamics. Their broad base has two apophyses: a sharp, anteromedial process (the vocal process) and a rounded, posterolateral process (the muscular process). Their inferior aspect has an elliptical, concave articular surface that is related to the arytenoid surface of the cricoid cartilage.

On transverse axial sonograms through the midportion of the thyroid cartilage (Fig. 5.4) and on recurrent axial scans on either side of the thyroid cartilage, the arytenoid cartilages are hyperechoic to the vocalis muscles and are symmetrical in shape, size, and position on either side of the midline.

According to Gritzmann et al. (1989), the arytenoid cartilages are rarely if ever visible owing to the interposition of the air in the larynx or the calcified thyroid cartilage. However, Chevallier et al. (1997) reported visualization of the arytenoid cartilages in 94% of women and 64% of men. For the latter authors, the air in the larynx is not an obstacle to imaging because the arytenoid cartilages are located more laterally, and breath-holding or a Valsalva maneuver can markedly reduce the volume of laryngeal air.

5.2.2.1.1.3
Cricoid Cartilage

Lying immediately below the thyroid cartilage, the cricoid cartilage is an essential component of the laryngeal framework. The only circular cartilage of the upper airway, it provides a solid base for the other cartilaginous components of the larynx to which it is attached. The cricoid cartilage consists of an arch, or ring, ranging in height from 4 to 9 mm, and a broad posterior portion (lamina of cricoid cartilage) measuring 22–32 mm in height.

Described essentially in children (Garel et al. 1990, 1991, 1992), the cricoid cartilage images sonographically as a hypoechoic ring, the posterior portion of which is masked by the air in the larynx (Fig. 5.5).

The cricoid cartilage is a hyaline cartilage, like the thyroid cartilage. In adults, the sonographic features and the course of calcification of the two structures are similar, although there are several differences: The internal perichondrium of the cricoid cartilage is never interrupted, the nodes of calcification are not visible, and calcification is symmetrical.

In individuals whose thyroid cartilage is only minimally calcified, the lamina of cricoid cartilage may be visualized at the glottic-supraglottic level during breath-holding, because this maneuver considerably reduces the air in larynx at this level.

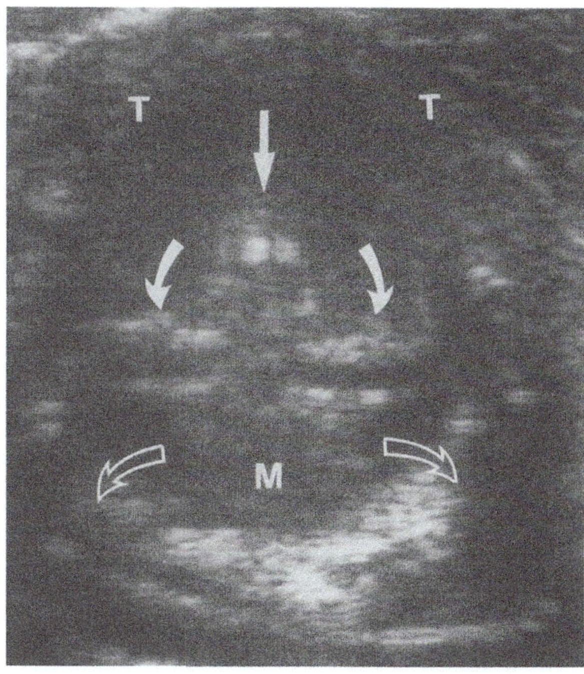

a

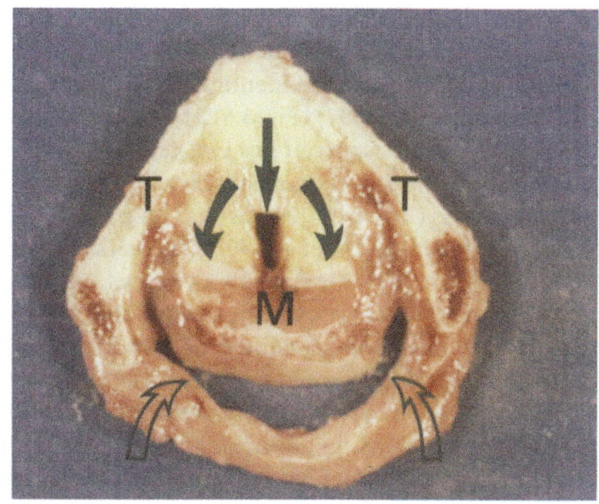

b

Fig. 5.4a,b. Axial views: (**a**) sonogram and (**b**) anatomic preparation through the mid portion of the thyroid cartilage (*T*). Visualization of the upper part of the arytenoid cartilages (*curved arrows*), the interarytenoid muscle (*M*), the vestibule of the larynx (*arrow*), and the hypopharynx (*open arrows*)

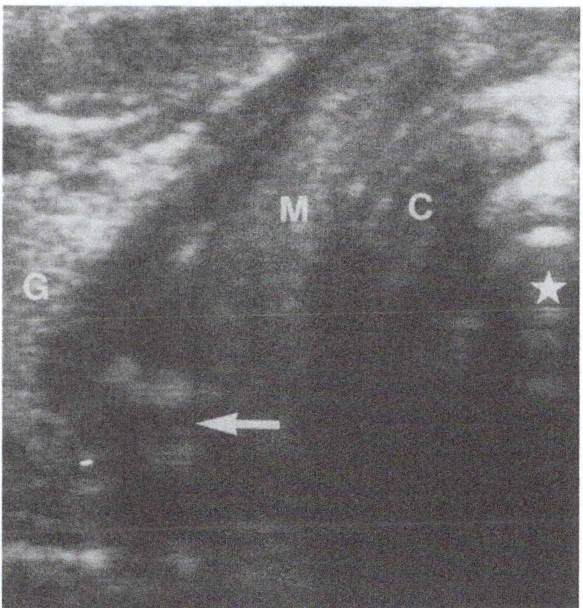

a

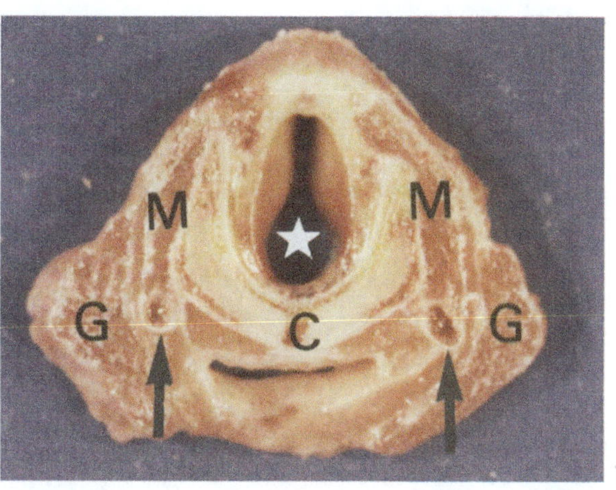

b

Fig. 5.5a,b. Axial views: (**a**) sonogram and (**b**) anatomic preparation through the lamina of the cricoid cartilage. *C* Cricoid lamina; *M* cricothyroid muscle; *arrows* inferior cornua of the thyroid cartilage; *G* thyroid gland; *star* subglottic airway

5.2.2.1.1.4
Epiglottic Cartilage

This thin, unpaired leaf-shaped plate of fibrocartilage ranges in height from 3 to 7 cm. At its apex, the ligamentous fibers forming the "stem" are attached to the angle of the thyroid cartilage, and in its lower third to the ligament of Broyles by the intermediary of the thyroepiglottic ligament. The free, lingual upper extremity of the epiglottic cartilage represents one quarter to one third of its entire height; its attached, inferior portion forms the posterior limit of the thyrohyoepiglottic space.

Sonographically, the free extremity of the epiglottic cartilage is rarely visible, owing to the shadow created by the hyoid bone (which is always ossified in the adult) and the presence of air in the region of the laryngeal margin. In contrast, the remainder of the epiglottic cartilage can be identified in 98% of cases (Chevallier et al. 1997) (Fig. 5.6). Hypoechoic to the thyrohyoepiglottic space, it lies in a central location, posterior to this space, on axial scans and is usually homogeneous (Böhme 1990; Chevallier et al. 1997; Clavier 1989; Derchi et al. 1992; Gritzmann et al. 1989; Valente et al. 1996). In 10% of cases, and particularly in individuals over the age of 70 years, the echotexture is inhomogeneous, probably due to fatty changes and/or calcium deposits (Chevallier et al. 1997). A hyperechoic border marks the posterior limit of the epiglottis in all cases for Clavier (1989) and in 75% of cases for Chevallier et al. (1997); this border, corresponding to the interface between the vestibular air and the epiglottic tissue, may be modified by dynamic maneuvers.

Depending on the segment, the thickness of the epiglottis varies on sonograms from 1.5 to 2.5 mm in women and from 1.8 to 3.4 mm in men (Chevallier et al. 1997). Probably due to its very slight thickness in children, pediatric radiologists have described the epiglottic cartilage as a hyperechoic stripe (Garel et al. 1990, 1991, 1992); actually, this stripe probably corresponds to the interface between the vestibular air and the epiglottic tissue rather than to the epiglottic cartilage itself.

Sonography often reveals a swelling on the lateral borders of the mid-segment of the epiglottic cartilage; sono-histological correlations indicate that this swelling corresponds to the insertion of the intrinsic muscles of the larynx (thyroepiglottic and aryepiglottic muscles) and the pharyngo-epiglottic ligament on the lateral surface of the epiglottis (Chevallier et al. 1997).

The epiglottis is usually evaluated by static imaging, although several publications have described evaluation of its movement during phonation using B-mode and M-mode techniques (Böhme 1988, 1990).

a

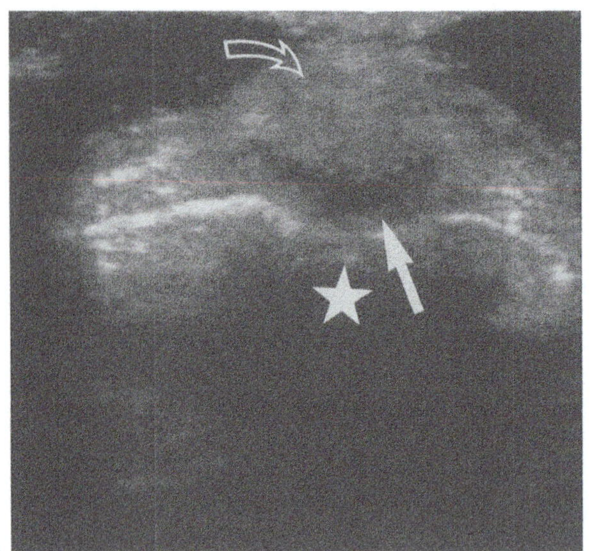

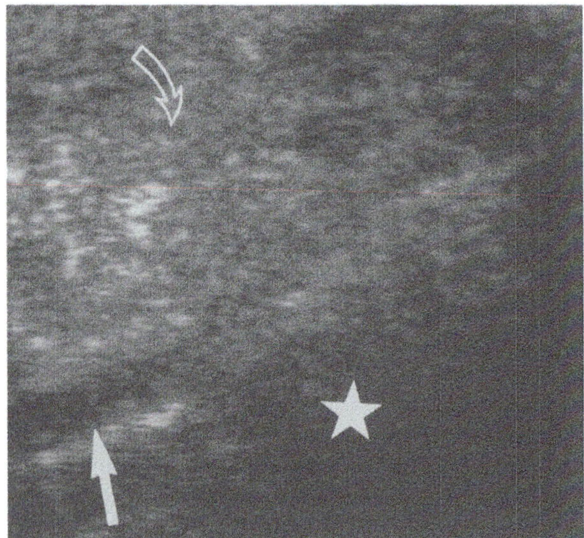

c

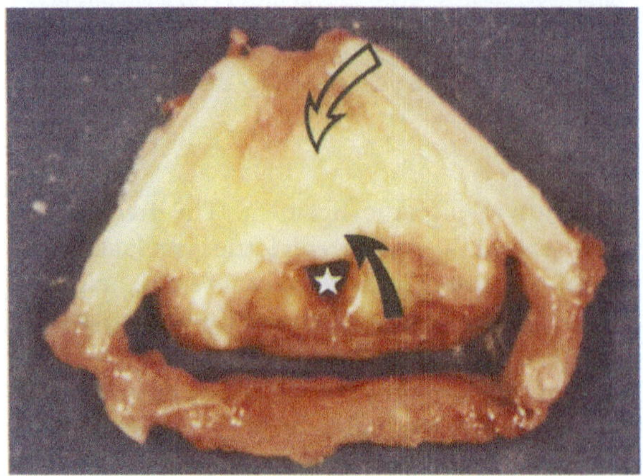

Fig. 5.6a–c. Axial (**a**) and midline transverse scans (**b**) and axial anatomic preparation (**c**) through the attached part of the epiglottic cartilage (*arrows*), which varies in thickness and usually has lateral bulges. This attached portion forms the posterior limit of the thyrohyoepiglottic space (*open arrows*), seen posteriorly as a hyperechoic border corresponding to its interface with the laryngeal lumen (*stars*)

5.2.2.1.2
Fat-containing Spaces

On transverse scans, the thyrohyoepiglottic space appears more or less triangular, with its base oriented superiorly. It is bounded superiorly by the hyoepiglottic membrane, anteriorly by the hyoid bone, the thyrohyoid membrane, and the superior part of the thyroid cartilage, and anteriorly by the anterior aspect of the attached portion of the epiglottic cartilage. This space is divided into right and left pre-epiglottic spaces by the midline, the vertical pre-epiglottic membrane. Open laterally, the thyrohyoepiglottic space continues laterally and posteriorly as the paralaryngeal space, located between the muscular and mucosal structures medially and the thyrohyoid membrane and the thyroid ala laterally. In the glottic (endolaryngeal) region, the thyrohyoepiglottic space is continuous with the fatty connective tissue of the paraglottic space.

5.2.2.1.2.1
Thyrohyoepiglottic Space

Although consistently accessible to US examination, the inferior portion of the thyrohyoepiglottic space may be masked if the thyroid cartilage is highly calcified, i.e., stage 5 (Chevallier 1995; Clavier 1989).

The thyrohyoepiglottic space is hyperechoic to the adjacent structures and is generally homogeneous (Böhme 1990; Chevallier et al. 1997; Clavier 1989; Derchi et al. 1992; Gritzmann et al. 1989) (Fig. 5.6). Discrete inhomogeneity is seen occasionally, particularly in men over the age of 70 years or during Valsalva maneuvers due to the reduction of its anteroposterior diameter (Chevallier 1995). Inhomogeneity may be related to a modification in the distribution of collagen fibers, which is one of the factors that determines the echogenicity of fat (Spencer et al. 1995). The septum separating the two pre-epiglottic spaces is not visible, probably owing to the similarity or insufficient difference in the acoustic impedance of these structures.

No vascularity is demonstrable by Doppler US (Chevallier 1995), despite the existence of several tiny vessels arising from a branch of the superior laryngeal artery and an inconstant, pre-epiglottic venous arcade.

5.2.2.1.2.2
Paralaryngeal and/or Paraglottic Fat

This fat, which is mobile during respiration, images as a hyperechoic border along the internal perichondrium of the ala of the thyroid cartilage. Doppler examination demonstrates vascularity in over one half of cases (Chevalier et al. 1997) (Fig. 5.7).

5.2.2.1.3
Ligaments, Membranes, and Folds

The *thyroepiglottic ligament* constitutes the inferior prolongation of the epiglottic cartilage (Clavier 1989). In approximately 10% of cases, this hypoechoic structure contains uniformly scattered hyperechoic spots (Chevallier 1995) that may correspond to air bubbles or, more probably, to the numerous glandular structures that dissociate the elastic and collagen fibers of this ligament (Guerrier et al. 1979). The thyroid insertion of the thyroepiglottic ligament corresponds to the *anterior commissure*, which images as a hyperechoic spot (Fig. 5.8) (Chevallier et al. 1997).

The *aryepiglottic folds* correspond to the elevation of the fibroelastic mucous membrane of the larynx by the aryepiglottic ligaments; these folds extend from the apex of the arytenoid cartilage on each side to the lateral surface of the epiglottis. Sonographically, the aryepiglottic folds are isoechoic to the fat in the thyrohyoepiglottic space; they are only partially visible owing to the constant interposition of air between their medial aspect and the posterior surface of the epiglottis.

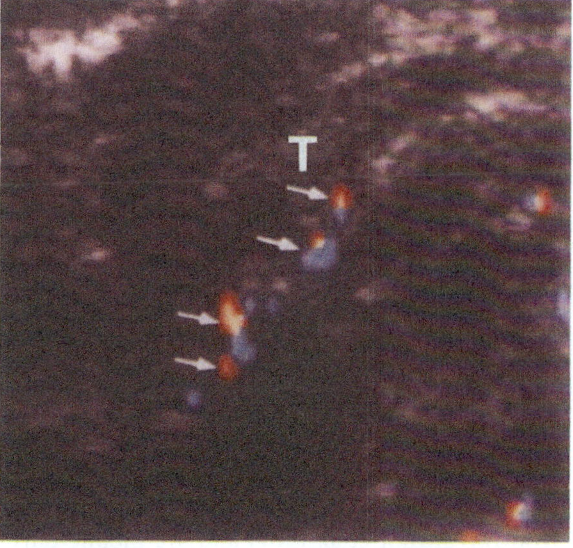

Fig. 5.7. Doppler examination: axial scan showing the vascularity of the paralaryngeal fat (*arrows*); *T* thyroid cartilage

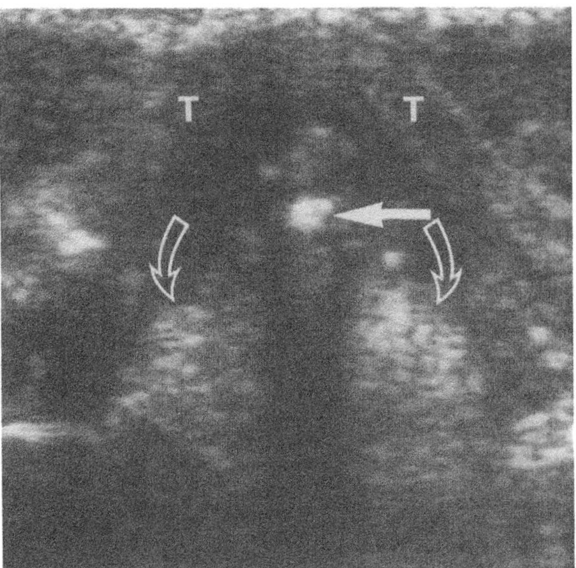

Fig. 5.8. Axial scan through the level of the anterior commissure *(arrow)* and the vestibular folds *(open arrows)*; *T* thyroid cartilage

The *thyrohyoid membrane* is consistently distinguishable sonographically as a hypoechoic border that should be rectilinear, without any gaps (CHEVALLIER et al. 1997).

5.2.2.1.4
Vestibular Folds

The vestibular folds (false vocal cords) are completely or partially visible in 96.1% of women and 71.8% of men (CHEVALLIER et al. 1997).

These variably shaped folds of mucous membrane are attached ventrally to the angle of the thyroid cartilage; they open out laterally and posteriorly, and terminate dorsally on the anterolateral surface of the arytenoid cartilages.

In both adults and children, the vestibular folds manifest sonographically as paired, symmetrical triangles with an anterior base that are hyperechoic to the vocalis muscles (CARP and BUNDI 1992; CHEVALLIER et al. 1997; GAREL et al. 1990; RAGHAVENDRA et al. 1987; UEDA et al. 1989) (Fig. 5.8). Their echogenicity has been related to their glandular and fat contents. The vestibular folds are a helpful landmark for localization of the subjacent vocal cords (RAGHAVENDRA et al. 1987) and are mobile during respiration (CHEVALLIER et al. 1997). Doppler US may reveal vascular signals within the folds.

5.2.2.1.5
Ventricles of the Larynx

The laryngeal ventricles are small (2-cm-long) pouches of mucous membrane that extend laterally between the vestibular folds and the vocal folds. From their anterosuperior portion arises a vertical fibrous pouch, the laryngeal saccule, that extends upward between the vestibular fold and the thyroid cartilage.

The laryngeal ventricles are visible sonographically in 38.5% of men and 92.1% of women (CHEVALLIER et al. 1997) as strongly hyperechoic spots or lines anterior to the midline; they are symmetrical on either side of the midline in 84% of cases (Fig. 5.9). A circular pattern of hyperechoic spots is observed in 7%–8% of cases, particularly in women over the age of 60 years (CHEVALLIER 1995); this US pattern may correspond to bilateral saccular dilatation, a normal variant (BROYLES 1959). The hyperechogenicity may be due partly to the air in this region; this would explain the modification of the appearance of the ventricles during dynamic maneuvers. As for the thyroepiglottic ligament, this hyperechogencity might also be due in part to the mucus-secreting glands in the chorion of the saccular mucosa (these 60–70 glands express a mucoid secretion that lubricates the vocal cords) (MYSSIOREK and PERSKY 1989).

5.2.2.1.6
Vocal Cords

Thin folds of mucous membrane forming the glottic level, the vocal cords (vocal folds) correspond to the internal layers of the inferior thyroarytenoid muscles and the inferior thyroarytenoid ligaments or vocal ligaments. The rima glottidis is an elongated opening that can be divided into two segments: an anterior portion between the vocal folds (the vocal glottis) and an intercartilaginous posterior portion lying between the medial surfaces of the arytenoids (the respiratory glottis). The sites of union of the two vocal cords are referred to as the anterior and posterior commissures.

5.2.2.1.6.1
Static Examination

On axial sonograms, the vocalis muscles appear triangular, with their summit facing anteriorly; hypoechoic to the vestibular folds, these muscles are symmetrical and usually homogeneous (CARP and BUNDI 1992; CHEVALLIER et al. 1997; DERCHI et al. 1992; GRITZMANN 1989; OOI 1991; SCHINDLER et al. 1990)

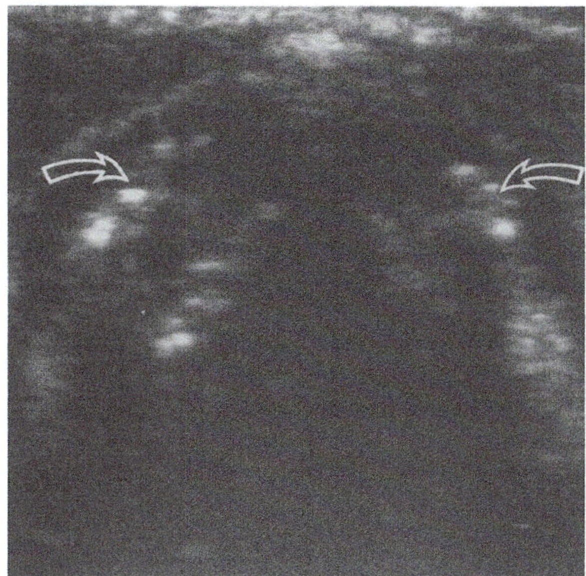
a

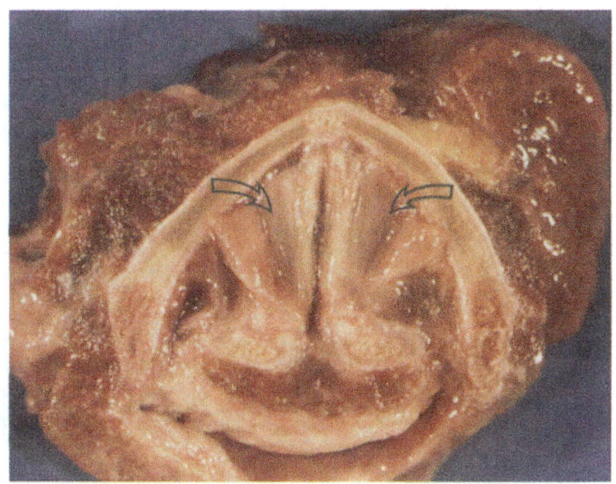
b

Fig. 5.9a,b. Axial scans: (a) sonogram and (b) anatomic preparation through the laryngeal ventricles (*open arrows*)

(Fig. 5.10). In highly favorable study conditions, the vocal cords may appear fringed (Chevallier et al. 1997; Miles 1989). In less than 10% of cases, a hyperechoic anteroposterior line may mimic a duplicate vocal cord (Chevallier et al. 1997). This line may correspond to the junction between the vocalis muscle and the other intrinsic laryngeal muscle fibers lying alongside the ligamentous portion of the vocal cord, as described by Salvi in 1901 (Terracol and Griener 1971).

On axial scans oblique superiorly and anteriorly, the vocal ligament images as an oblique hyperechoic line, oriented anteromedially, lying alongside the vocalis muscle (within the vocal fold) and forming its medial limit. The vocal ligament is not visible in children (Garel et al. 1990, 1992); it is discontinuous in more than 50% of adults and is more frequently identified than the vocalis muscle in men (Chevallier et al. 1997). This variability in sonographic presentation may be due to age-related histological changes in structure (Fresnel-Elbaz 1995). The anterior sesamoid cartilages are visible in 10% of individuals as punctate enhancement of the anterior portion of the vocal ligament.

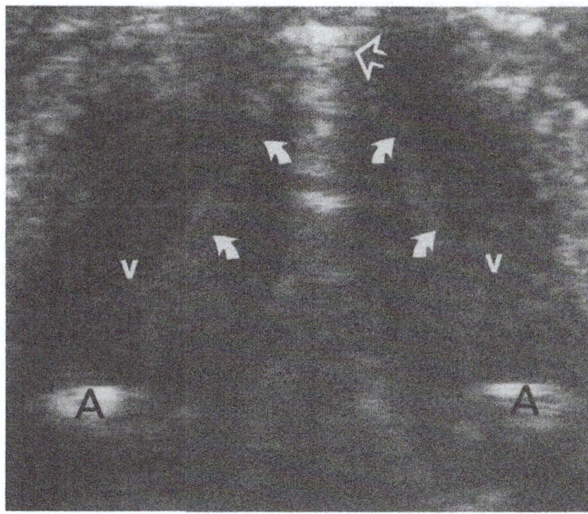

Fig. 5.10. Axial scan through the vocal cords (*v*). Visualization of the vocal ligaments (*arrows*), the anterior commissure (*open arrow*), and the arytenoid cartilages (*A*)

As for visualization of the other retrothyroid anatomic structures, demonstration of the vocal cords depends on the degree of calcification of the thyroid cartilage; it is thus both gender and age dependent. The vocal cords are visualized in 94.1% of women and 43.6% of men (Chevallier et al. 1997).

5.2.2.1.6.2
Dynamic Examination

B-mode Imaging. During "quiet" breathing or a "deep inspiration/breath-holding" sequence, the vocal cords are subject to movements of abduction (inspiration) and adduction (expiration, breath-holding). These sonographically demonstrable movements should be symmetrical (Chevallier et al. 1997; Ooi et al. 1995; Raghavendra et al. 1987; Schindler et al. 1990); movements are slow enough to allow interpretation during real-time examination (Fig. 5.11). When the vocal ligament is visible, its vibration can be identified during phonation (Fig. 5.12).

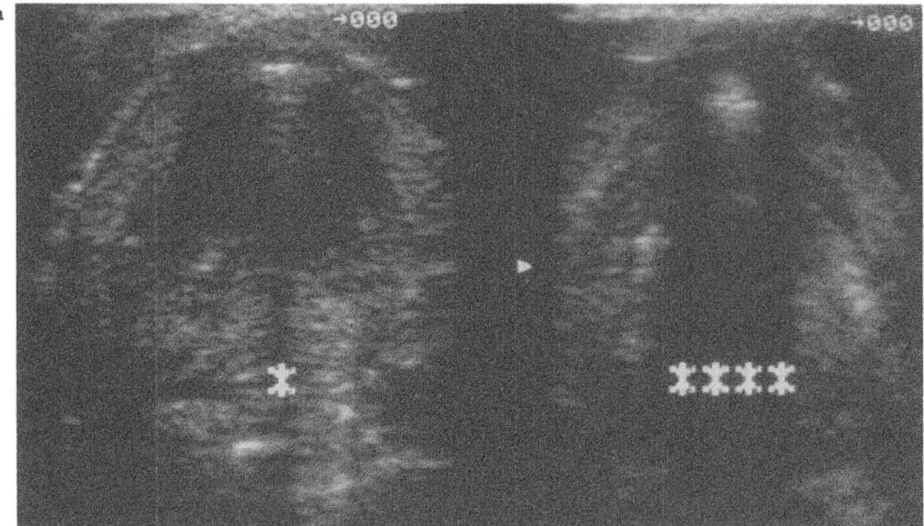

Fig. 5.11a,b. Axial scans at the glottic level during breath-holding (**a**) and inspiration (**b**), with abduction of the vocal cords and opening of the rima glottidis during inspiration (*asterisks*)

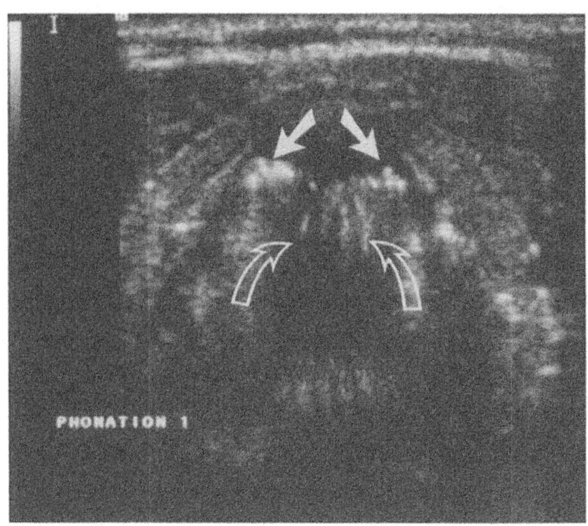

Fig. 5.12. Axial scan through the vocal ligaments (*open arrows*) that vibrate during phonation of the sound "e" and through the air-filled laryngeal ventricles (*arrows*)

Continuous Doppler US. Analysis of vocal cord vibration by continuous Doppler was occasionally described in the 1960s (Hertz et al. 1970; Mensch 1964; Minifie et al. 1968). The vibratory cycle and the frequency and amplitude of vibrations were analyzed in the same manner as during electrolaryngography (hence the term ultrasonolaryngography).

Pulsed Doppler. Pulsed Doppler examination of the vocal cords (Fig. 5.13) is performed in a transverse axial plane. A study window measuring at least 5 mm^2 is positioned on a vocal cord localized by B-mode imaging, or merely by estimation (mid-height of the thyroid cartilage, several millimeters to one side of the midline), during phonation. The signal is recorded during phonation of the sound "e" using a high pulse repetition frequency (PRF) and band pass filter; the contralateral vocal cord is examined in the same manner, as identically as possible (phonation, position of the study window, angulation of the transducer with respect to the skin) (Chevallier 1995).

The recorded signal is composed of a succession of positive and negative peaks compared with the baseline (Chevallier 1995; Schindler et al. 1990). These peaks reflect the horizontal movements of the vocal cords (abduction/adduction), stretching of the vocal cords, and undulation of the mucosa that also participates in vibration of the vocal cords.

The frequency of these peaks cannot be analyzed in 40% of women because they occur too rapidly; the frequency varies from 8 to 29 peaks/s in men. This frequency does not correspond to the fundamental modal frequency; it is merely a relative frequency allowing comparison of the two vocal cords (in the middle register, the vocal cord vibration cycle [number of open/close cycles per second] is in the range of 220–240 in women and 110–130 in men).

The greater the intensity of phonation and the lower the degree of thyroid cartilage calcification, the higher the amplitude of the peaks. This is analogous to results obtained on sonograms or electrolaryngograms, where the spectral amplitude corresponds to the intensity of the voice expressed in decibels. Here again, the numerical value of this vocal parameter cannot be determined by pulsed Doppler US. In contrast, the spectral amplitude of the two vocal cords can be compared.

a 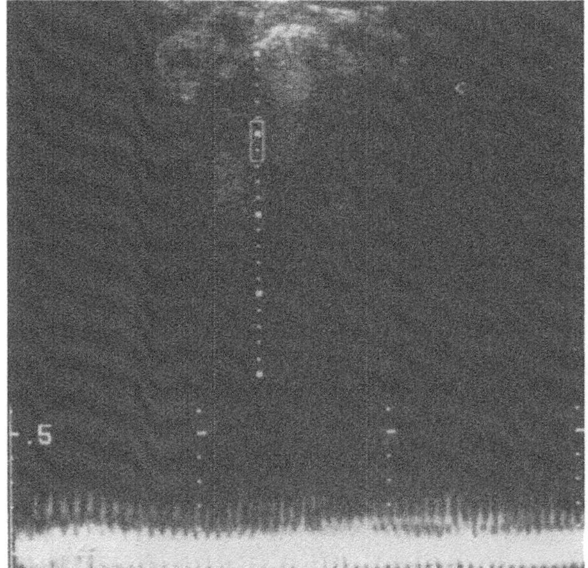

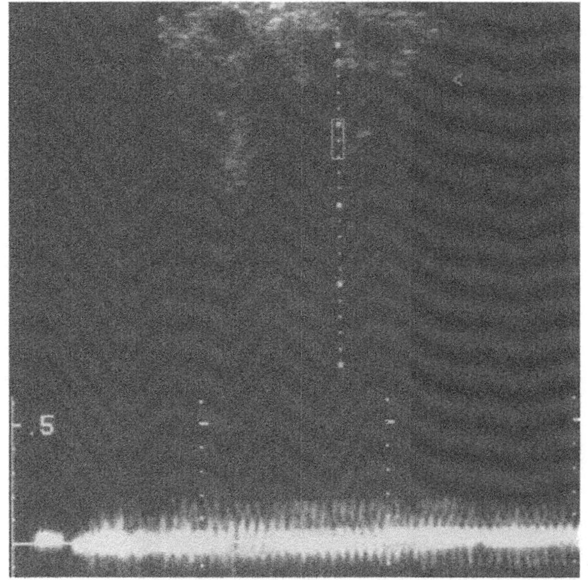 b

Fig. 5.13a,b. Pulsed Doppler recording of vibration of the right (**a**) and the left (**b**) vocal cords during phonation of the sound "e". The spectrum obtained is composed of a succession of peaks, the frequency and amplitude of which are symmetrical and can be superimposed on a baseline spectrum

As on electrolaryngograms, "stains" created by difficult-to-systematize anarchic vibrations superimposed on the basic waveform may create artifacts on the Doppler waveform (Peneygre and Lelièvre 1989).

The spectra of the vocal cords are asymmetrical in nearly 10% of healthy individuals (Chevallier 1995). Such false-positive findings are probably multifactorial and underscore the relative difficulty of Doppler examination of both vocal cords under strictly identical conditions. Pulsed Doppler appears independent of the degree of calcification of the thyroid cartilage.

Color Doppler and Power Doppler. Color Doppler and power Doppler studies provide colored images reflecting the phenomena that occur during phonation. These colored images probably reflect both laryngeal airflow due to the expiration of air from the lungs, as suggested by Ooi et al. (1995), who were the first to describe this technique, and the interrelated phenomena of airflow and vibration of the structures that compose the phonatory apparatus.

Examination is performed during phonation of the sound "e", using an acoustic window that includes the entire endolarynx. The PRF is set between 6 and 12.5 kHz, depending on the degree of calcification of the thyroid cartilage. Axial scans are obtained during sustained and regular phonations strictly perpendicular to the long vertical axis of the larynx, passing successively through the thyrocricoid membrane (recurrent upward towards the base of the arytenoid cartilages) and through the anterior commissure (first horizontal, then recurrent upward) (Chevallier 1995).

Scanning opposite the base of the arytenoid cartilages permits identification of two symmetrical round or oval colored spots (Fig. 5.14). These spots may correspond to the complex movements of the base of the arytenoid cartilages and the posterior portion of the vocal cords (Chevallier 1995). This scan plane appears the most effective because the colored spots are obtained rapidly, easily, and in a consistently reproducible manner.

The colored stripe with a long anteroposterior axis visible on horizontal scans through the anterior commissure may correspond to the glottic-supraglottic column of air. The anterior and posterior bulges visualized probably represent the air turbulence in the region of the anterior and posterior commissures. This colored stripe is surmounted by a symmetrical, anteriorly convex crescent that creates a "mushroom" appearance (Chevallier 1995; Ooi et al. 1995) (Fig. 5.15). This colored crescent, which may be the translation of the airflow in the saccules, is detected in only 62.5% of patients (Chevalier 1995).

In 62.5% of cases, recurrent scans upward through the anterior commissure reveal two symmetrical, parallel, colored stripes with a long anteroposterior axis, each of which presents an anterior bulge (Chevallier 1995) (Fig. 5.16). These stripes may be the direct translation of vocal cord vibration; the anterior bulge may represent the ventricular airflow. As

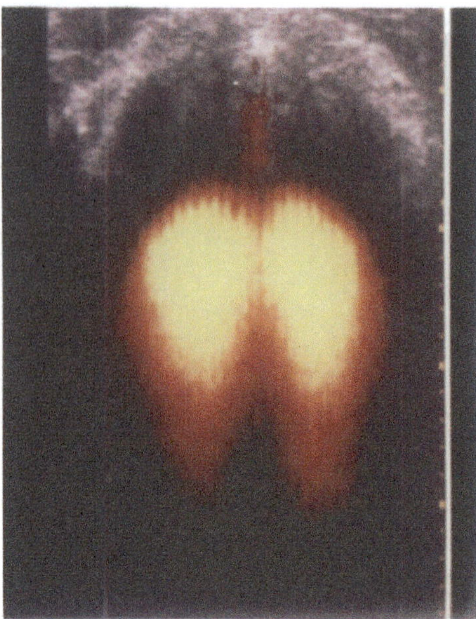

Fig. 5.14. Power Doppler axial scan at the level of the arytenoid cartilage during phonation of the sound "e". Two symmetrical colored spots are visualized

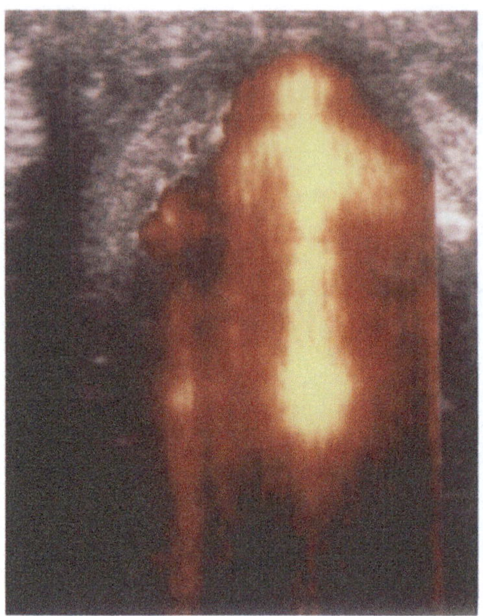

Fig. 5.15. Power Doppler study: axial scan through the rima glottidis and the ventricles during phonation of the sound "e". The colored crescent may be the tranbslation of the airflow induced by phonation

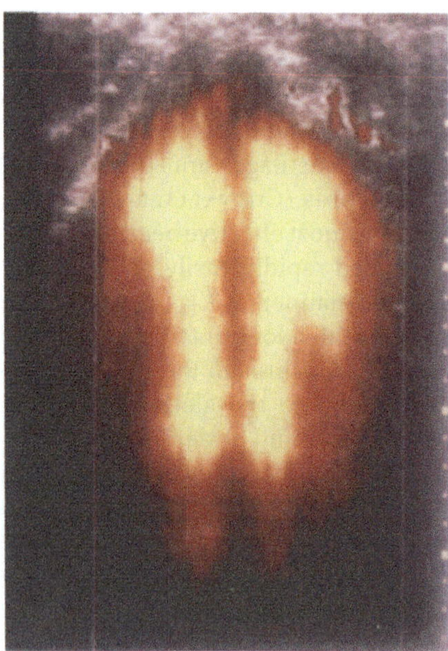

Fig. 5.16. Power Doppler axial scan through the vocal cords and the laryngeal ventricles during phonation of the sound "e". The colored stripes with anterior bulges may correspond to vibration of the vocal cords and the airflow in the ventricles

on horizontal scans, these colored stripes are seen in only 62.5% of patients (Chevallier 1995).

Color Doppler and power Doppler studies are independent of the degree of calcification of the thyroid cartilage. Compared with color Doppler, power Doppler appears merely to improve the definition of the colored images.

5.2.2.2 Valleculae

These depressions, one on each side of the median glossoepiglottic fold, represent the boundary between the larynx and the pharynx and can be identified in nearly 85% of cases (Chevallier et al. 1997). Recurrent axial US scans upward through the thyrohyoid membrane reveal a succession of hyperechoic spots forming a fine, discontinuous straight or posteriorly concave line (Chevallier et al. 1997; Clavier 1989). In 15% of cases, the valleculae are hypoechoic to the base of the tongue, but they are always symmetrical.

5.2.2.3 Piriform Sinuses

The unpaired, funnel-shaped hypopharynx is continuous above with the oral pharynx; below, it continues as the esophagus. Depressions in the lateral walls form the piriform sinuses, elongated spaces running along the posterior borders of the larynx and bounded medially by the aryepiglottic fold, which represents the summit of the laryngopharyngeal wall.

The sonographic features of the piriform sinuses are extremely varied owing to the juxtaposition of their component tissue layers and their contents of air and mucus (Figs. 5.4, 5.17). Hyperechoic air is visible in the anterior angle of the sinuses; the distribution of air always changes in a symmetrical manner during a Valsalva maneuver. In healthy individuals, it is not possible to accurately identify the various tissue layers composing the wall of the piriform sinuses.

Lateral axial scans generally suffice. Longitudinal scans can be obtained by placing the transducer opposite the posterior part of each thyroid ala (Fig. 5.17c); when the latter structures are only minimally calcified, such scans improve visualization of the effect of Valsalva maneuvers (Chevallier et al. 1997). Gritzmann et al. (1989) underscored the utility of examination during deglutition or while the patient swallows water. However, the modifications in sonographic anatomy caused by these maneuvers are too extensive and too rapid for real-time analysis (Chevallier et al. 1997). Videotape recording thus appears mandatory.

The piriform sinuses can be identified at least partially in 98% of women and 67% of men (Chevallier 1995).

5.2.3
Tumors

5.2.3.1
Malignant Tumors

Nearly 90% of all malignant tumors of the larynx and hypopharynx (Figs. 5.18–5.20) are squamous cell

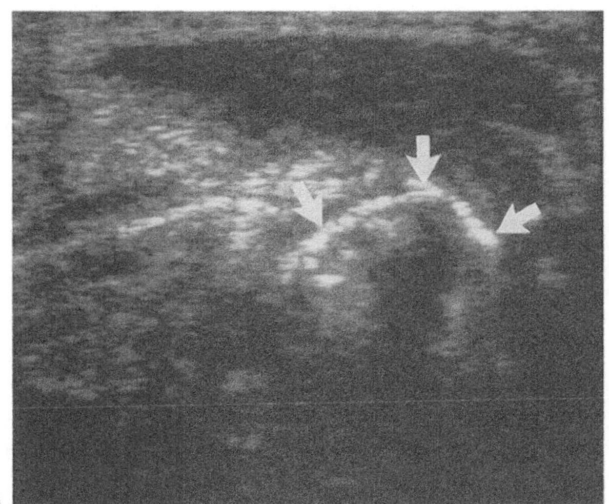

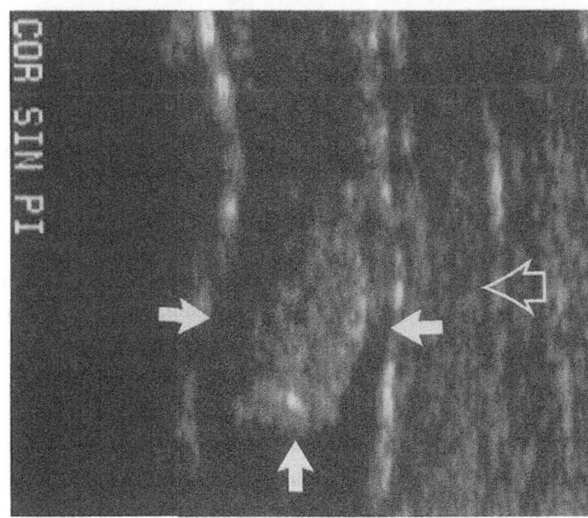

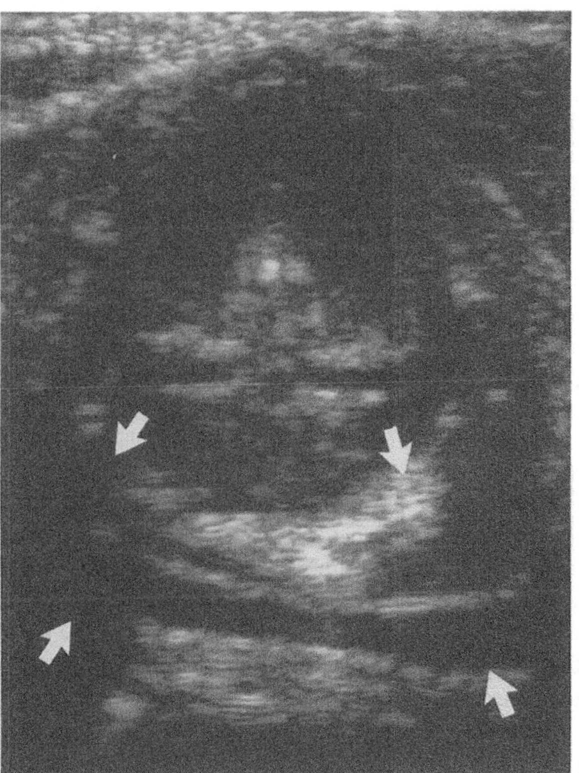

Fig. 5.17a–c. Axial scans (**a**, **b**) and transverse scan (**c**) through the piriform sinuses (*arrows*) during quiet breathing; *open arrow* thyroid ala

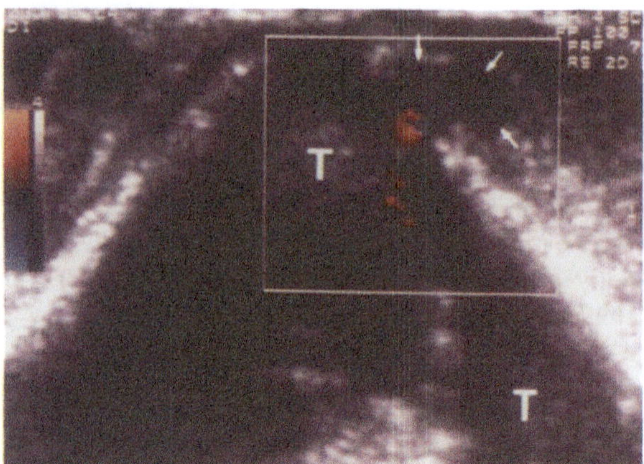

Fig. 5.18. Axial scan. Tumor mass (*T*) at the level of the left paralaryngeal fat and the thyrohyoepiglottic space extending through the left thyroid ala (*arrows*). Color Doppler demonstrates the vascularity of this transcartilage tumor spread

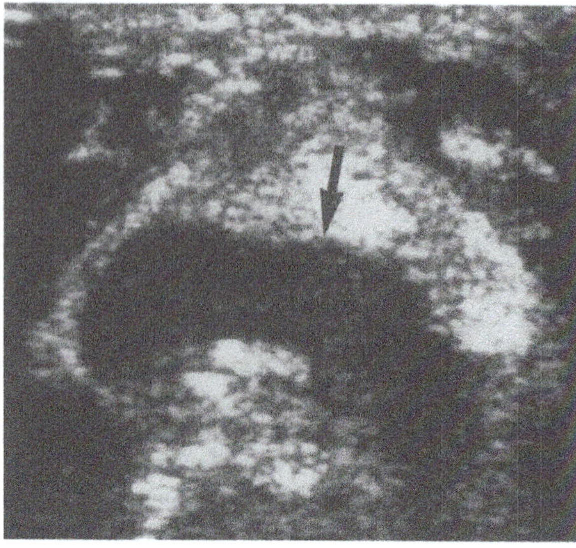

Fig. 5.19. Axial scan revealing tumor invasion of the attached portion of the epiglottis (*arrow*), which measures more than 10 mm at its thickest point

carcinomas related to alcohol and/or tobacco abuse. The entire aerodigestive tract can be involved, and 5%–10% of patients develop multiple synchronous or metachronous lesions (Henrot et al. 1999).

In a series of 40 patients with a laryngeal neoplasm, Zbären et al. (1996) compared the accuracy of tumor staging by clinical examination, endoscopy, MRI, and CT with histopathological examination of the surgical specimen. Tumors were correctly classified by an association of clinical examination and endoscopy in 57.5% of cases, by an association of clinical examination and CT in 80% of cases, and by an association of clinical examination and MRI in 87% of cases. CT and/or MRI are thus indispensable complements to clinical examination for accurate tumor classification using the TNM staging system (Hermanek and Sobin 1988) and for detection of any co-existent tumors that might modify management.

Despite the satisfactory results achieved with CT and MRI, these techniques are not always adequate, yet few investigators have evaluated the potential benefits of US for laryngeal tumors. In contrast, for hepatic tumors, for which CT and MRI are also highly effective, the complementarity of US is well-established.

Laryngeal tumors were first evaluated by US by in the late 1970s (Noyek et al. 1977). Few additional studies have been published since then (Chevallier 1995; Clavier 1989; Derchi et al. 1992; Erkan et al. 1993; Gritzmann et al. 1989; Gritzmann 1992; Loveday et al. 1994; Rothberg et al. 1986). As most of these reports concerned advanced laryngeal tumors (TNM stage T3 or T4), US successfully demonstrated the tumor mass in nearly all cases. The majority of tumors were hypoechoic to the adjacent tissues, but isoechoic and hyperechoic masses were also described. Hyperechoic intratumoral spots, corresponding to areas of necrosis, have also been observed. Malignant laryngeal tumors are most prevalent in men (95%–97.5% of cases) aged 45–70 years; as extensive calcification of the thyroid cartilage is frequent in this population, visualization of small tumors is difficult (Chevallier 1995).

High-frequency sonography is reportedly both highly sensitive and highly specific (close to 100% in both cases) for the detection of tumor spread to the thyrohyoepiglottic space, the subglottic region, the middle segment of the epiglottis (Fig. 5.19), and other nearby anatomic structures. The accuracy of US is lower for tumors involving the piriform sinuses (Fig. 5.20).

Sonographic search for cartilaginous tumor involvement is particularly interesting because, in the TNM classification, hypopharyngeal and laryngeal tumors are classed T4 whenever such spread has occurred. MRI appears more sensitive than CT in this setting (89%–94% versus 46%–67%) but less specific (74%–84% versus 87%–91%) because it overestimates the degree of cartilaginous involvement (Becker 2000; Declercq et al. 1998). In addition, despite the excellent negative predictive value of MRI, chemical shift artifacts can create phantom images of the cartilaginous cortex (Sakai et al. 1990). In the literature, the sensitivity of sonography varies from 73%–100%; specificity ranges from 82%–100%. Possible US findings include a gap in the border cor-

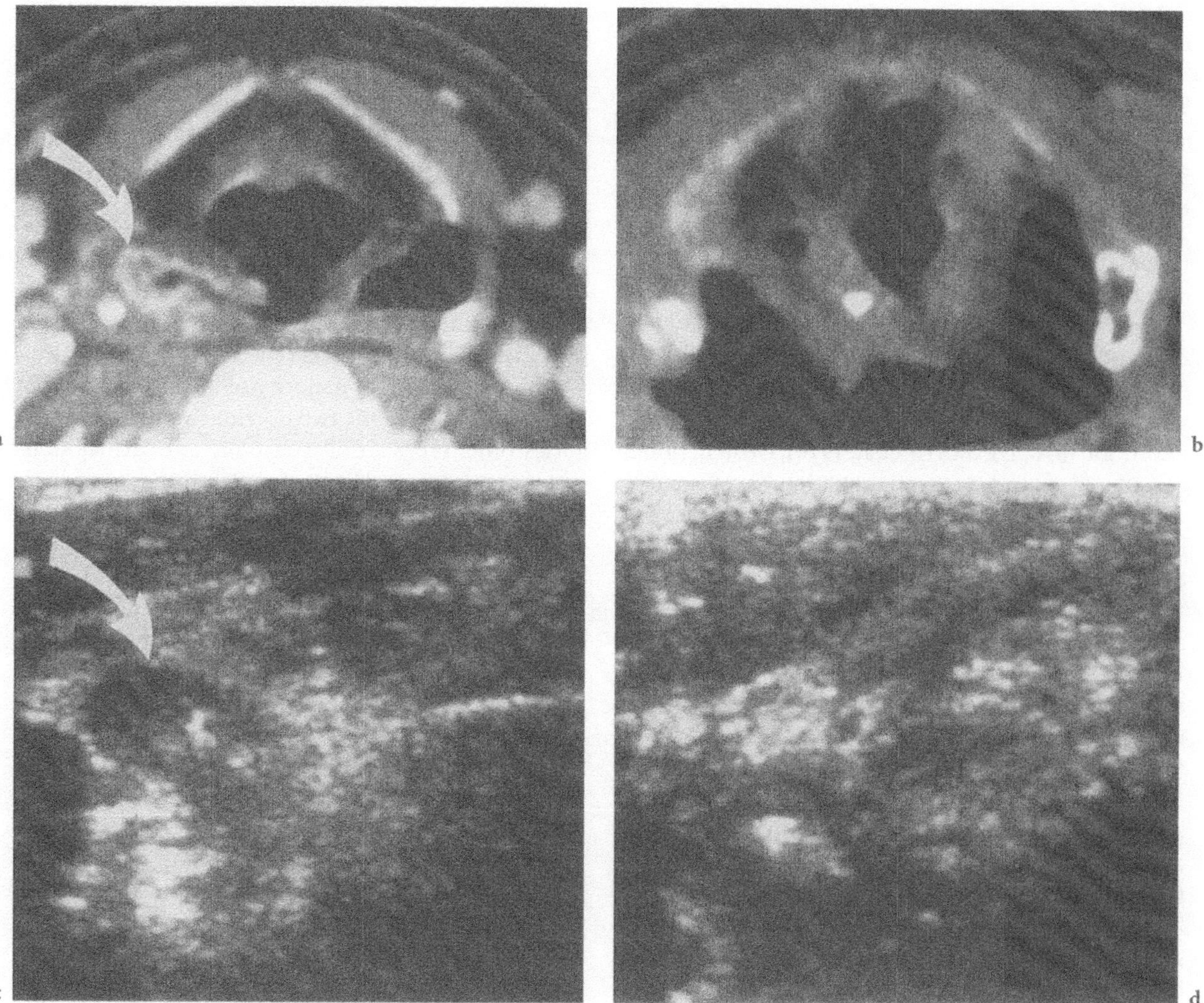

Fig. 5.20a–d. Axial CT (**a, b**) and US scans (**c, d**) of a right piriform sinus tumor (*arrows*) during breath-holding (**a, c**) and a Valsalva maneuver (**b, d**)

responding to the paralaryngeal fat or the border representing the internal perichondrium, intracartilaginous continuity of the tumor mass, or Doppler demonstration of intracartilaginous vascularity (Chevallier 1995) (Fig. 5.18).

Use of pulsed Doppler and power Doppler to study vocal cord vibration also appears interesting, because such studies have higher sensitivity than other imaging techniques; involvement of the vocalis muscle is difficult to evaluate by CT (Piekarski et al. 1999) and MRI can be degraded by kinetic artifacts.

Sonography can accurately evaluate the various lymph node groups, except for the deep juxtavisceral chains, which cannot be visualized (Bruneton et al. 1984; Bruneton et al. 1987). The size and morphological information provided by US, CT, or MRI may be insufficient. Specificity can be improved by US-guided aspiration biopsy (Henrot et al. 1999) and Doppler measurement of the resistive and pulsatility indexes (Na et al. 1997).

Sonography is unsuited to screening for metastases because squamous cell carcinomas of the head and neck metastasize predominantly to the lungs.

Overall, in a neoplastic setting, the natural obstacles to the use of laryngeal and hypolaryngeal sonography (air and calcification of the thyroid cartilage) can usually be overcome. Along with its high spatial and contrast resolution, high-frequency sonography permits dynamic examination and analysis of tissue vascularity. These advantages make it a potential complement to CT and MRI for the staging of laryngeal and hypopharyngeal tumors.

5.2.3.1
Laryngeal Cysts

Laryngeal cysts (Fig. 5.21) are benign lesions that were first recognized as a clinical entity at the end of the nineteenth century (CANUYT 1939). Most authors use the classification of DE SANTO (DE SANTO et al. 1970) that distinguishes retention cysts and saccular (appendicular) cysts, based on lesion size, location, and relations with the laryngeal mucosa.

Retention cysts (mucous cysts) predominate (76% of cases) (DE SANTO et al. 1970); they develop following the obstruction of glandular canaliculi that prevents the normal outflow of mucus (ALTMEYER and FECHNER 1978; DE SANTO et al. 1970). Obstruction is considered secondary to inflammation, as reflected by the high number of patients who report a history of laryngitis (ALTMEYER and FECHNER 1978). Retention cysts may occur at any point in the larynx except at the free border of the vocal cords, which do not contain any glands (OPHIR and LIFSCHITZ-MERCER 1989). For certain authors, the most frequent site is the lingual part of the epiglottis (ALTMETER and FECHNER 1978; KAWASAKI et al. 1983) whereas for others it is the vocal cord (DE SANTO et al. 1970; OPHIR and LIFSCHITZ-MERCER 1989). Retention cysts are usually smaller than 1 cm in diameter. Multiple lesions and association with a malignant laryngeal tumor are rare (SINGH et al. 1988).

Saccular cysts, which account for 24% of all laryngeal cysts (DE SANTO et al. 1970), are also referred to as congenital and embryonal laryngeal cysts (ALTMEYER and FECHNER 1978), owing to their prevalence in newborns and young children. They may have a congenital origin (fourth branchial arch anomaly) or an acquired cause (stenosis of the laryngeal saccule, or herniation of the saccule into the ventricle). These cysts occur at the supraglottic level, in the region of the laryngeal saccule. While laryngoceles and saccular cysts have the same origin, and can occur in similar locations (internal and mixed types), laryngoceles contain air, whereas cysts do not. Saccular cysts tend to measure at least 1 cm in diameter and are usually larger than retention cysts (DE SANTO et al. 1970).

Although the great majority of laryngeal cysts can be classed in one of the two previously described categories, other types are also encountered: cartilaginous cysts (ALTMEYER and FECHNER 1978; BURGESS and YIM 1985), oncocytic cystadenomas (LUNDGRER et al. 1982; OPHIR and LIFSCHITZ-MERCER 1989), cystic lymphangioma (LEROUX-ROBERT and DE BRUX 1976).

Laryngeal cysts may be asymptomatic or they may be accompanied by dysphonia, dysphagia, dyspnea, or a sensation of discomfort in the throat.

No prospective imaging study to date has evaluated the incidence of this pathology, which remains uncertain. In the studies of NEW and ERICH (1938) and HOLINGER and JOHNSON (1951), laryngeal cysts represented, respectively, 4.3% of 722 and 6.1% of 1197 benign laryngeal tumors. In contrast, CHEVALLIER et al. (1998) observed laryngeal cysts in 6.7% of healthy individuals. A discrete masculine predominance has been reported (ALTMEYER and FECHNER 1978; KAWASAKI et al. 1983).

a

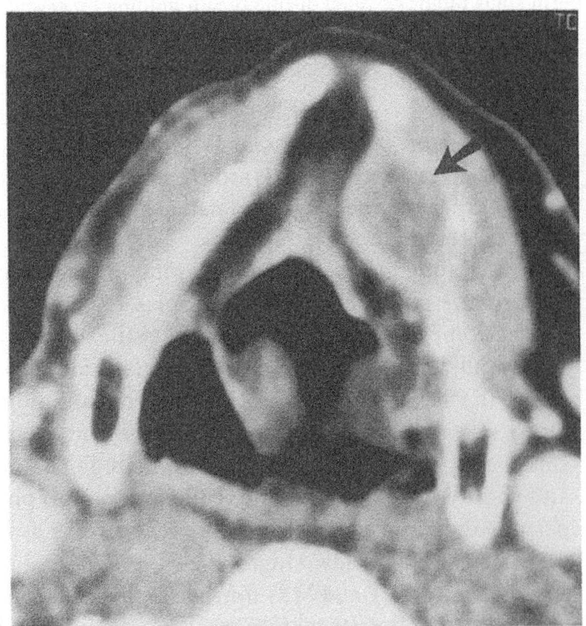

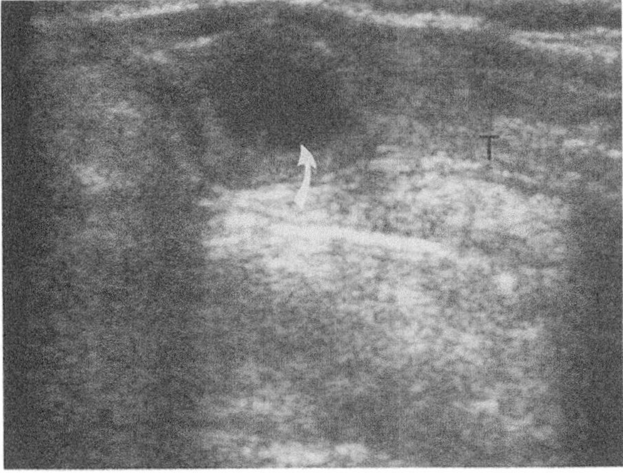

Fig. 5.21a,b. Cartilaginous cyst (*arrows*) arising in the left thyroid ala: **a** CT, **b** US, *T* thyroid cartilage

The sonographic features of laryngeal cysts are poorly known, owing to the few publications on the subject and the small study populations (CHEVALLIER et al. 1998; SHITA et al. 1999; YOUSSEFZADEH et al. 1993). Mucus-containing cysts appear anechoic or hypoechoic and are well-delimited by a hyperechoic border, resulting in posterior enhancement of the ultrasonic beam. Calcification of the hyaline cartilages (especially the thyroid cartilage) may be a limiting factor for visualization of certain cysts (it was the cause of the only failure in the study of YOUSSEFZADEH et al. 1993). However, when local conditions are favorable, cysts 2–3 mm in diameter may be visible sonographically (CHEVALLIER et al. 1998). Like hepatic and renal cysts, laryngeal cysts are usually readily diagnosed by US. A cyst located in a thyroid ala must not be mistaken for the transthyroid course of the superior laryngeal vascular pedicle (a rare possibility) or transcartilaginous tumor spread; in the first case, care must be taken to determine whether the structure is round or tubular, and whether a vascular signal is detectable on Doppler imaging; in the second case, US demonstration of the integrity of the internal perichondrium and the paralaryngeal fat and posterior reinforcement of the ultrasound beam are findings in favor of a cystic etiology. The differential diagnosis for saccular cysts is a laryngocele, but the latter usually contains air that is readily identified sonographically.

5.2.4 Laryngoceles

A laryngocele (Fig. 5.22) is an anomalous air-containing sack formed by ballooning of an expansion of the ventricular saccule of the larynx (CANALIS et al. 1977; STELL and MARAN 1975). Men between the ages of 50 and 60 years are affected primarily, but the true incidence is unknown because these lesions are often asymptomatic. STELL and MARAN (1975) estimated the annual incidence at 1 per 2,500,000 population in England.

Three varieties are distinguished (CANALIS et al. 1977; GIOVANNIELLO et al. 1970): (a) internal laryngoceles, located beneath the vestibular fold and the internal strap muscle, which remain strictly endolaryngeal; (b) external (exolaryngeal) laryngoceles, following herniation of the air-containing pouch through the thyrohyoid membrane, communicating by a thin channel with the undilated ventricle; and (c) mixed laryngoceles (association of an internal and an external laryngocele on the same side).

Mixed laryngoceles are more common (44%–50%) than the internal (21%–40%) or external (26%–34%) types (CANALIS et al. 1977; STELL and MARAN 1975). Unilateral laryngoceles predominate (80%) (STELL and MARAN 1975).

The ventricle is covered by a pseudostratified ciliated epithelium rich in mucus glands (KOTBY et al.

a

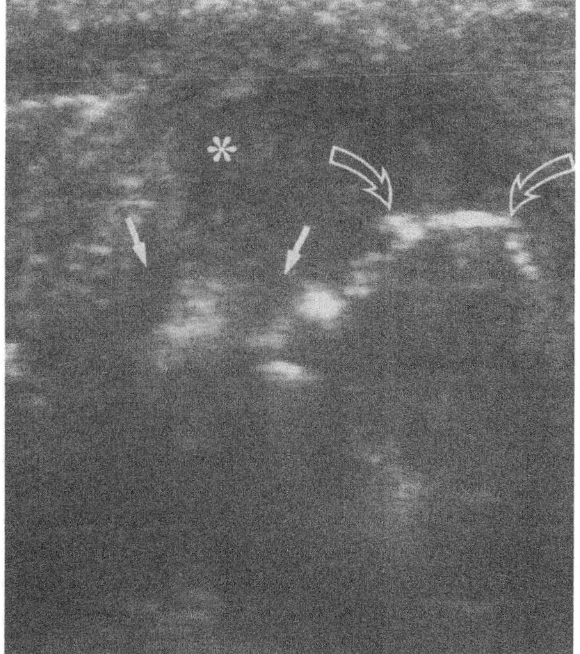

b

Fig. 5.22a,b. Laryngocele (*open arrows*) on CT (**a**) and US (**b**). Epiglottis (*arrows*) and the thyrohyoepiglottic space (*asterisk*)

1991); this explains why laryngoceles are filled with air and mucus. In contrast, saccular cysts contain only mucus because they do not communicate with the laryngeal lumen.

A congenital theory and an acquired theory have been proposed to explain the onset of these lesions. A congenital anomaly could explain those laryngoceles observed in newborns or infants, and a congenital defect (long sacculus, hypotonia of the thyroepiglottic and aryepiglottic muscles) could predispose to their development in adults (Detsouli et al. 1994). Acquired causes include repeated hyperpressure in the supraglottic airway, as occurs in certain occupations (glassblowers, wind-instrument players, etc.), or pathologies (chronic cough, obstruction of the laryngeal saccule by a tumor, an inflammatory process, or fibrosis) (Micheau et al. 1978).

Clinical findings depend to a great extent on the size of the lesion. Internal laryngoceles tend to be asymptomatic but may cause dysphonia, dysphagia, pain, or dyspnea; dyspnea generally occurs when the laryngocele suddenly or very rapidly increases in volume following a violent effort with the glottis closed or a coughing spell, or, less often, secondary to formation of a laryngopyocele (Detsouli et al. 1994; Stell and Maran 1975). The external variety manifests as an intermittent, reducible swelling in the lateral neck that reappears during straining, thereby confirming its communication with the laryngeal airway (Canuyt 1939). Mixed laryngoceles associate the clinical signs of external and internal types.

Several studies have described sonographic demonstration of the various types of laryngocele (Chevallier 1995; Heppt et al. 1990; Hubbard 1987; Morgan and Emberton 1994; Vierzen et al. 1994).

On axial sonograms, internal laryngoceles manifest as an air-filled mass in the place of the homolateral laryngeal saccule. External or mixed laryngoceles image sonographically as an inhomogeneous laterocervical mass containing variable proportions of air and fluid. The mass lies opposite the thyrohyoid membrane, which is not visible; in contrast, this membrane can always be identified in the normal state (Chevallier et al. 1997).

Complementary dynamic examination is required to search for the communication between the air-filled or air- and water-filled mass with the laryngeal channel. Application of pressure may reduce the volume of the laryngocele, producing gurgling and hissing sounds (Bryce's sign); in contrast, a Valsalva maneuver may increase the volume of the laryngocele. These signs may be absent with laryngeal tumors if the neoplastic tissue obstructs the communication (Chevallier 1995) or if the Valsalva maneuver is not performed energetically enough. In such cases, it is impossible sonographically to differentiate an external or mixed laryngocele from an air- and water-filled cervical mass of another origin.

5.2.5 Pharyngoceles

A pharyngocele (hypopharyngeal diverticulum) (Fig. 5.23) is a benign, anomalous pouch formed by hernial protrusion of the mucous membrane through a defect in the hypopharynx, particularly at the junction of the esophagus and the pharynx, where the muscular coat may be weak (Norris 1979).

Like laryngoceles, pharyngoceles are rare. Often asymptomatic, their true incidence is unknown, as they have been described only infrequently in the literature (Van de Ven and Schutte 1995). As for laryngoceles, augmentation of the air pressure in the cervical airway favors their development. Clinical symptoms may include dysphagia, dysphonia, cervical pain, weight loss, regurgitation, or a cervical mass (Norris 1979; Van de Ven and Schutte 1995).

The sonographic features of the hypopharynx are usually pleomorphic, owing to the juxtaposition of its component tissue layers and its variable contents of air and mucus (Chevallier et al. 1997). However, under normal conditions, the air in the anterior angle of the two piriform sinuses is always symmetrical (Chevallier et al. 1997). In patients with a pharyngocele, the piriform sinuses appear asymmetrical. A hyperechoic mass with the US features of air and ring-down artifacts is seen on the affected side, in place of the piriform sinus; the mass may even deform the ala of the thyroid cartilage (Chevallier et al. 2000). Transverse axial scans are the most helpful, although they may contain artifacts in patients with a highly calcified thyroid cartilage. In such cases, the pathological piriform sinus is best examined in a longitudinal plane, posterior to the homolateral ala of the thyroid cartilage (Gritzmann et al. 1989). Apart from these anatomic and static considerations, the communication between the abnormally located air and the piriform sinus can be identified by the modification in the distribution of this air during compression of the mass or during Valsalva maneuvers, as described for laryngoceles (Chevallier et al. 2000; Hubbard 1987; Vierzen et al. 1994).

The major differential diagnosis is a laryngocele, although in the latter, the distribution of air in the

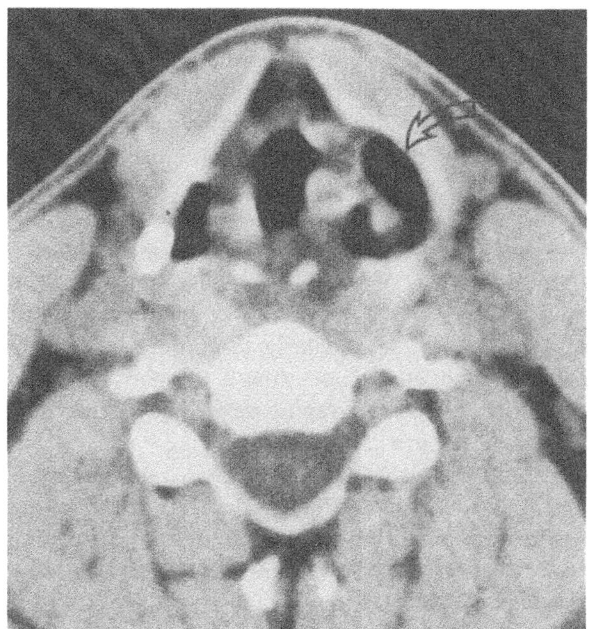

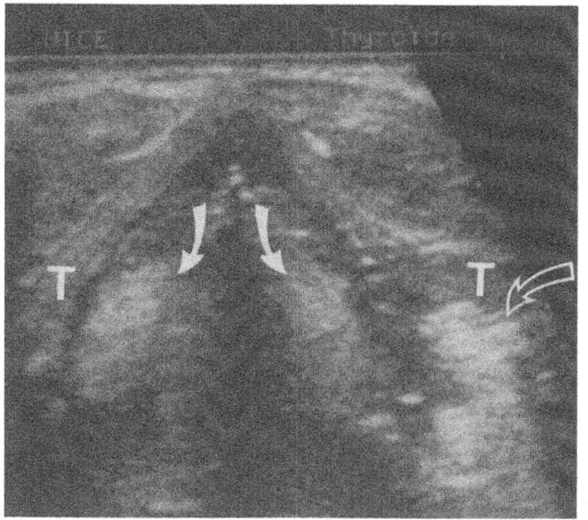

Fig. 5.23a,b. Left pharyngocele (*open arrows*) with deformation of the homolateral thyroid ala on CT (**a**) and US (**b**); *arrows* vestibular folds

piriform sinuses is symmetrical and the abnormal pouch of air lies in a more anterior position.

5.2.6 Vocal Cord Dysfunction

Vocal cord dysfunction has a number of etiologies, but traumatic (iatrogenic or not), tumoral, and idiopathic causes predominate (PARNELL and BRANDEBURG 1970). Lesions of neurogenic origin are peripheral in 90% of cases (AGHA 1983), occurring between the jugular foramen and the point of entry of the nerve structures into the larynx; intralaryngeal neurogenic lesions are rare (PARNELL and BRANDEBURG 1970). Central nervous system etiologies include tumors of the base of the skull, meningoradiculitis, and bulbar lesions (Wallenberg syndrome, acute polioencephalitis, syringobulbia, tumors).

Unilateral recurrent laryngeal nerve paralysis accounts for 90% of cases; left-sided involvement predominates because the course of the recurrent nerve is longer on that side. Clinical symptoms range from hoarseness to aphonia, sometimes occurring only when the patient is tired. However, an estimated 30%–50% of patients with unilateral recurrent laryngeal nerve paralysis are asymptomatic (COLLAZO-CLAVELL et al. 1995).

Laryngoscopy reveals an immobile vocal cord in a paramedian or median position, an intermediate position, or, occasionally, in complete abduction. The slight movements of the arytenoid cartilage seen on occasion are due to contraction of the interarytenoid muscle or mobilization of the cartilage following contact with its contralateral fellow (PENEYGRE and LELIÈVRE 1989). With time, the arytenoid cartilage tilts forward, the vocal cord atrophies, and the unaffected vocal cord may cross the midline.

At stroboscopy, the paralyzed vocal cord is located at a lower level; the ventricle on the homolateral side is wider and the vestibular fold is more salient.

On electromyography, vocal cord paralysis manifests as an increase in the contractions of the motor unit potentials of the vocalis muscle due to temporal and spatial summation.

CT findings in patients with vocal cord paralysis include: vocal cord in an abnormal position, dislocation of an arytenoid cartilage, dilated piriform sinus, rotation of the thyroid cartilage, clear visualization of only one ventricle (AGHA 1983). When vocal cord dysfunction is secondary to tumor spread, CT can demonstrate this invasion in proximity of a vocal cord, an arycricoid articulation, or the presumed course of a recurrent laryngeal nerve. However, CT cannot directly visualize the anomalous vibration of the vocal cord.

5.2.6.1 *B-mode Ultrasound*

Vocal cord dysfunction should be suspected initially whenever US reveals an asymmetry in vocal cord position during breath-holding or an asymmetry in the degree of calcification of the arytenoid cartilages (these cartilages are normally almost always symmetrical in position and degree of calcification) (CHEVALLIER 1995). A search must also be made for any reduction in the movement of the cartilage (abduction/adduction) during respiration or a mass syndrome in the region of the vocal cord (CHEVALLIER 1995). These US findings have considerable diagnostic value (CARP and BUNDI 1992; LOVEDAY et al. 1994; OOI 1991), although errors may occur due to poor visualization or nonvisualization of the glottis owing to extensive calcification of the thyroid cartilage (CHEVALLIER 1995). Furthermore, in contrast to the situation in children (GAREL et al. 1991, 1992), calcification of the thyroid cartilage in adults generally prevents direct identification of static or dynamic anomalies of the vocal cords or anomalies in the position of the dense echo produced by the air in the glottis. Visualization of a tumoral mass opposite the cervical course of one or both recurrent nerves is a feature suggesting vocal cord dysfunction of neurogenic and peripheral origin.

5.2.6.2
Pulsed Doppler

Few reports have been published on the use of pulsed Doppler US (Figs. 5.24, 5.25) to search for vocal cord dysfunction (CHEVALLIER 1995; SCHINDLER et al. 1990). Pulsed Doppler examination may reveal a reduced spectral amplitude on the pathological side compared with the unaffected side, and a less regular frequency with a different vibratory cycle (increase or decrease in the number of open/close cycles per second).

These parameters appear to vary with the duration of vocal cord involvement. In patients with long-standing paresis or paralysis, spatial recruitment of muscle fibers may increase rather than decrease the spectral amplitude; similarly, temporal recruitment may produce "stains", creating a Doppler spectrum similar to electromyographic recordings of the vocalis muscle (CHEVALLIER 1995).

Although pulsed Doppler is not dependent on the extent of thyroid cartilage calcification, it cannot be recommended for routine screening for bilateral and symmetrical involvement at this time because normal values for spectral frequency and amplitude have not yet been established.

5.2.6.3
Color Doppler and Power Doppler

Preliminary research appears to indicate excellent concordance between color Doppler (Figs. 5.25–5.27) and endoscopy (CHEVALLIER 1995; OOI et al. 1995). The colored spot that appears during phonation near the base of the arytenoid cartilages and the colored stripe located in the region of the vestibular fold

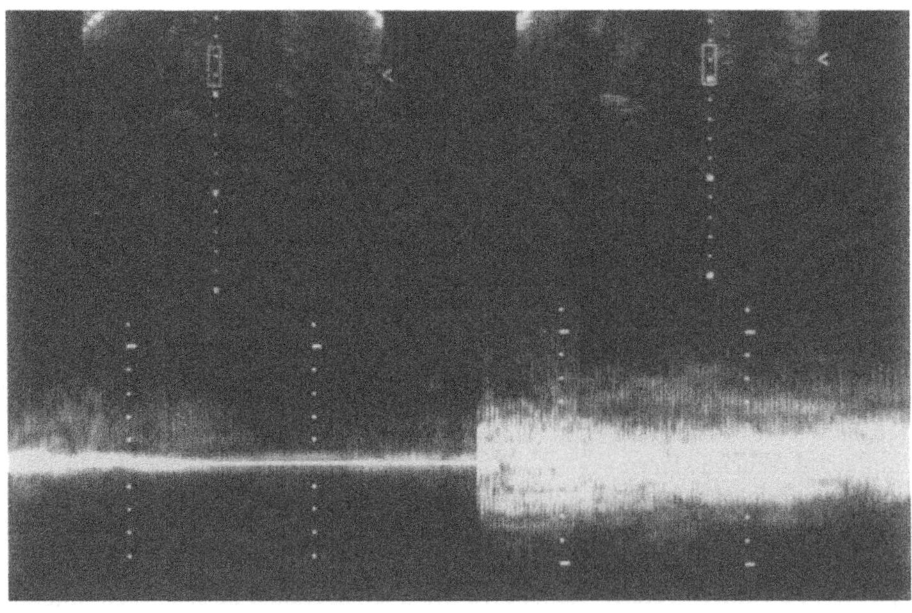

Fig. 5.24. Paresis of the right vocal cord related to tumor invasion. On pulsed Doppler, during phonation of the sound "e", the spectrum has a lower amplitude and is less regular on the affected side

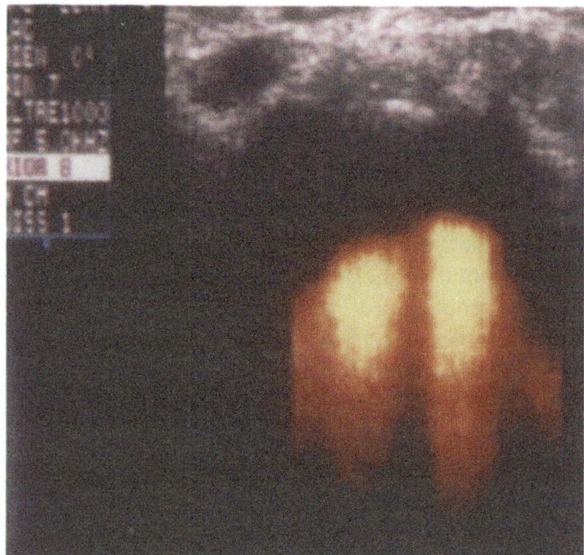

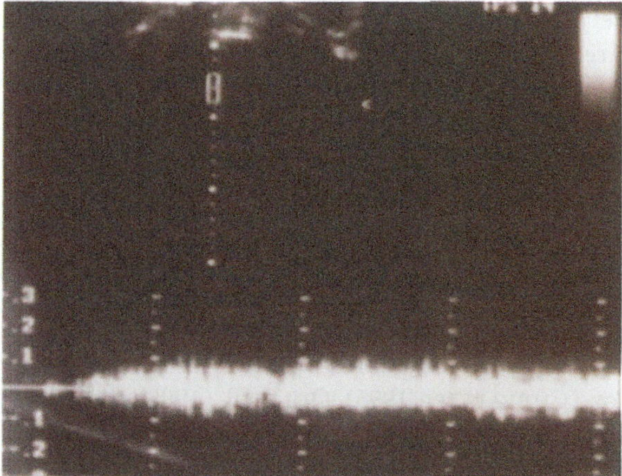

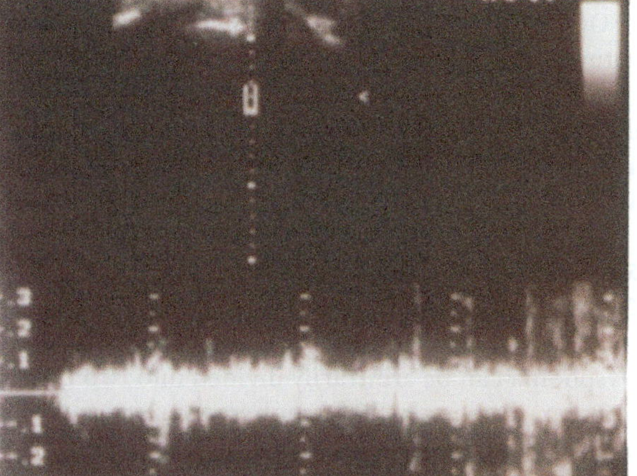

Fig. 5.25a–c. Long-standing paresis of the left vocal cord in a patient with Wallenberg syndrome. Asymmetry of the colored spots on power Doppler (**a**) and the spectra on pulsed Doppler (**b**, **c**) recorded during phonation of the sound "e". The spot on the affected side is larger; the stains on the spectral recording may be related to spatial and temporal muscle fiber recruitment

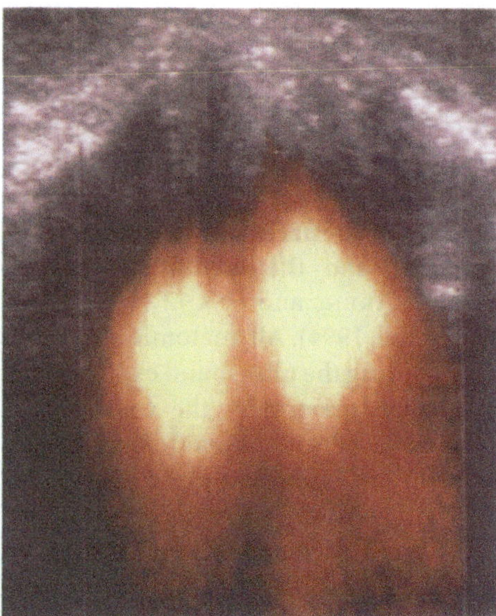

Fig. 5.26. Post-traumatic luxation of the right arytenoid cartilage demonstrated by a power Doppler axial scan. The surface area of the colored spot on the right is smaller and lies in a more posterior position than the contralateral spot

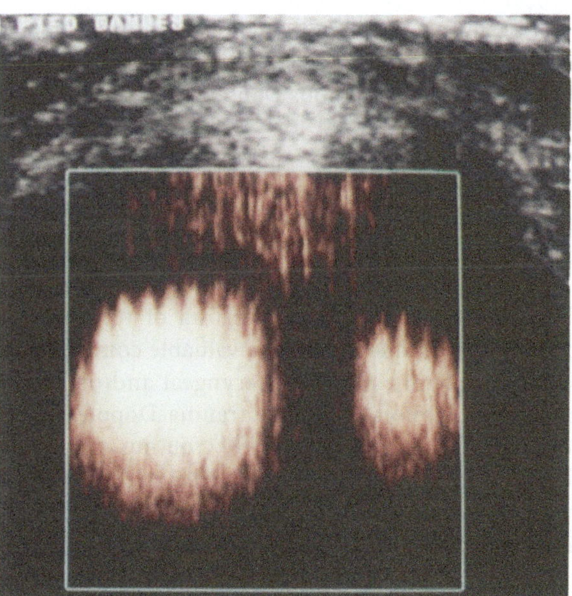

Fig. 5.27. Tumor invading the left side of the glottic region: power Doppler axial scan. The colored spot on the left is smaller than the contraleral spot

are usually smaller on the pathological side compared with the unaffected side. This appearance is not pathognomonic, however. In cases of long-standing involvement, the colored zones may actually be larger on the pathological side (as on pulsed Doppler study), owing to spatial and temporal recruitment of the muscle fibers (Chevallier 1995). In addition, when a mass syndrome exists at the level of the pathological vocal cord, the asymmetry in the surface area of the colored zone on the pathological side may be accompanied by an asymmetry in position (Chevallier 1995). Ooi et al. (1995) described the presence of an asymmetrical colored triangle in the region of the rima glottidis during the initial phase of phonation.

Owing to its qualitative rather than quantitative nature, color Doppler cannot distinguish paresis from paralysis. While power Doppler is indicated primarily to improve delimitation of the colored zones, it also has increased sensitivity for detection of slow airflows (Chevallier 1995).

5.2.6.4
Conclusion

Dysphonia can be arbitrarily divided into two types: complex dysphonia that requires accurate analysis of the various components of the voice (frequency, intensity, and tone), and less complex dysphonia secondary to recurrent laryngeal nerve involvement or a vocal cord mass syndrome.

For complex dysphonia, neither pulsed Doppler, color Doppler, nor power Doppler currently provides sufficient data. Continuous Doppler, the sonographic technique initially used for research on vocal cord vibration, may merit re-evaluation in this setting.

For less complex cases of dysphonia US appears more effective, in particular owing to the absence of dependency of Doppler results on the extent of thyroid cartilage calcification. Although several pitfalls exist concerning interpretation of results, this dynamic technique might be a valuable complement to other imaging studies of laryngeal and/or hypopharyngeal tumors or cervical trauma. Doppler studies might also prove useful for routine screening for asymptomatic recurrent laryngeal nerve involvement, as occurs in patients with benign thyroid disease, where the preoperative incidence has been estimated at 0.7% (Collazo-Clavell et al. 1995).

5.3
Endolaryngeal Sonography

5.3.1
Examination Technique

High-frequency endolaryngeal sonography, like endovascular sonography (Essop et al. 1993), requires use of a small-caliber catheter (from 8-French for a 20-MHz probe to 10-French for a 10-MHz probe). Larger probes may injure endolaryngeal structures during the examination.

Endolaryngeal ultrasound examination is performed during microlaryngoscopy. Following administration of the anesthesia, the endotracheal tube is placed just above the carina. The larynx is then visualized with a laryngoscope. The larynx is next flooded with 0.9% saline to obtain sufficient tissue connection and to prevent the retention of air bubbles in the anterior commissure. An increased cuff pressure is not felt to be necessary for a sufficient seal with the tracheal mucosa to prevent saline from flooding the bronchi. Afterwards, the high-frequency ultrasound catheter is hooked up to a 30° laryngoscopy endoscope and inserted into the larynx to monitor the position of the ultrasound tip during the examination. This endosonographic technique provides 360° cross-sections, from the trachea up to the epiglottis tip, that are recorded on videotape (Arens et al. 1998; Arens and Glanz 1999, Arens et al. 1999).

5.3.2
Normal Features

High-frequency endolaryngeal sonography reportedly permits identification of the laryngeal mucosa, the pre- and paraglottic spaces, the vocal ligament, the vocalis muscle, and the laryngeal cartilages (Arens et al. 1998; Arens and Glanz 1999; Arens et al. 1999; Zech et al. 1994). All anatomic structures can be visualized during the ultrasound examination. As on percutaneous sonography, the vocalis muscles appear hypoechoic; the vestibular folds, the internal perichondrium of the thyroid cartilage, and the laryngeal cartilages are hyperechoic.

The field of view of the very high frequency probes used is limited in depth and is restricted to exploration of the first 2.5 cm. Artifacts may also occur owing to the difference in acoustic impedance between the endolaryngeal saline and the laryngeal mucosa or the presence of air bubbles, especially near the anterior commissure.

No incidents have occurred in the more than 100 examinations performed so far, and in particular there have been no reports of inhalation of the saline instilled into the larynx.

5.3.3 Pathological Features

Endolaryngeal sonography can demonstrate all laryngeal neoplasms defined as T2, T3, or T4 in the TNM classification (Arens and Glanz 1999, Arens et al. 1999). Tumor spread to the thyroid cartilage is visualized, as on percutaneous sonograms, as a break in the hyperechoic border corresponding to the internal perichondrium. Nevertheless, errors in interpretation are possible opposite zones of transition between calcified cartilage and hyaline cartilage (Arens and Glanz 1999, Arens et al. 1999). For laryngeal neoplasms classed T1, endolaryngeal sonography can visualize only those tumors larger than 3 mm and/or those extending to the vocal ligament.

Lesions related to chronic laryngitis, epithelial dysplasia, or a microinvasive cancer are not accessible to sonography with 10- to 20-MHz miniprobes at the moment. Laryngeal cysts are readily identified as anechoic or hypoechoic lesions. Endolaryngeal US also permits measurement of the diameter and length of the larynx or trachea in case of stenosis (Figs. 5.28–5.32).

5.4 Conclusion

Endolaryngeal US examination is hampered essentially by difficulties of a technical nature, whereas percutaneous sonography is confronted primarily with anatomical obstacles. These difficulties can often be overcome, however.

Its noninvasiveness, widespread availability, and low cost are the main advantages of percutaneous ultrasound, which can be used either alone or as a complement to other imaging modalities that are insufficient even when used in association. Percutaneous US can provide decisive complementary data for optimum management of certain laryngeal or hypopharyngeal tumors; it also appears highly accurate for the workup of unilateral vocal cord dysfunction and can diagnose pharyngoceles, laryngoceles, and laryngeal cysts without the need for another imaging technique. While these affirmations must be taken with caution owing to the relatively few publications on the subject, they merit consideration owing to the high potential offered by sonographic contrast agents and the constant technical improvements made in ultrasound equipment.

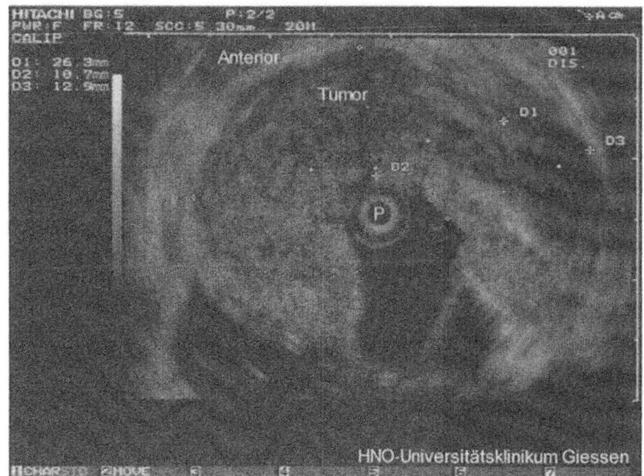

Fig. 5.28a,b. Endosonography (20 MHz) of epiglottic carcinoma. **a** Small tumor of the upper third of the epiglottis starting to invade the cartilage. *Tu* tumor; *P* probe; D1=0.6 cm; D2=1.4 cm. **b** Large epiglottic carcinoma infiltrating the pre-epiglottic space. *P* probe; D1=2.6 cm; D2=1.1 cm; D3=1.3 cm

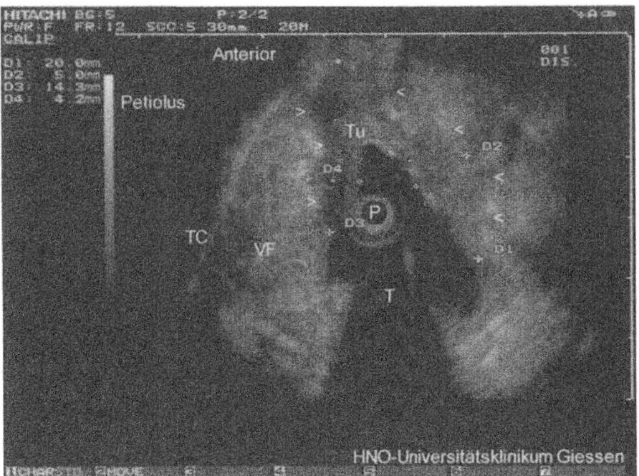

Fig. 5.29. Endosonography (20 MHz) of a petiolus carcinoma: The tumor involves both vestibular folds and the petiolus. *P* probe; *T* tube; *TC* thyroid cartilage; *Tu* tumor; *VF* vestibular fold; D1=2 cm; D2=0.5 cm; D3=1.4 cm; D4=0.4 cm

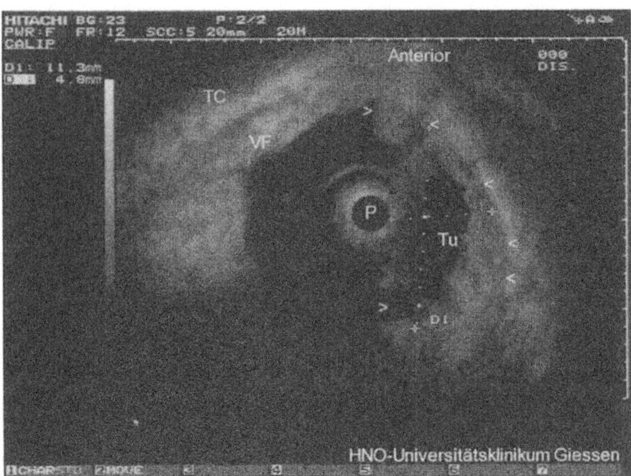

Fig. 5.30. Endosonography (20 MHz) of vestibular fold carcinoma: weakly echogenic tumor of the right vestibular fold without infiltration of the thyroid cartilage. *P* probe; *TC* thyroid cartilage; *Tu* tumor; *VF* left vestibular fold; D1=1.1 cm; D2=0.5 cm

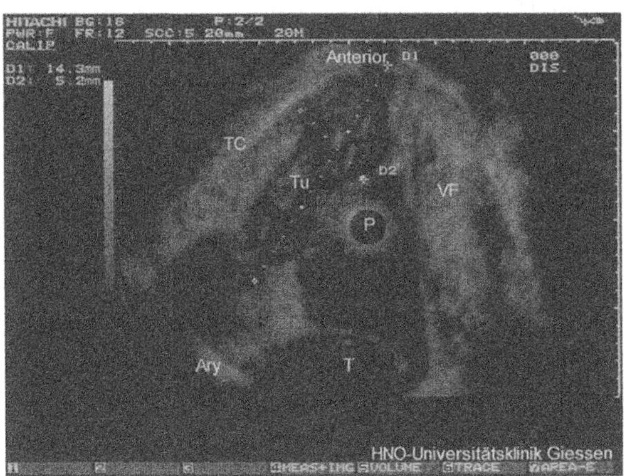

Fig. 5.31. Endosonography (20 MHz) of left vocal fold carcinoma with subglottic extension. *TC* thyroid cartilage; *Tu* tumor; *VF* right vocal fold; *Ary* aryteroid cartilage; *P* probe; *T* tube; D1=1.4 cm; D2=0.5 cm

High-frequency endoluminal sonography of the larynx and hypopharynx has become a useful diagnostic tool, supplementing microlaryngoscopy in the assessment of different laryngeal lesions, especially laryngeal cancer, even though its field of action is insufficient for examination of structures located more than 2.5 cm from the probe and too imprecise for examination of the mucosa. Here again, new technical developments should improve the accuracy of the method.

References

Agha FP (1983) Recurrent laryngeal nerve paralysis: a laryngographic and computed tomographic study. Radiology 148:149–155

Altmeyer VL, Fechner RE (1978) Multiple epiglottic cysts. Arch Otolaryngol 104:673–675

Arens C, Glanz H (1999) Endoscopic high-frequency ultrasound of the larynx. Eur Arch Otorhinolaryngol 256:316–322

Arens C, Eistert B, Glanz H, Waas W (1998) Endolaryngeal high-frequency ultrasound. Eur Arch Otorhinolaryngol 255:250–255

Arens C, Malzahn K, Dias O, Andrea M, Glanz H (1999) Endoscopic imaging techniques in the diagnosis of laryngeal cancer and its precursor lesions. Laryngorhinootologie 78:685–691

Becker M (2000) Neoplastic invasion of laryngeal cartilage: radiologic diagnosis and therapeutic implications. Eur J Radiol 33:216–229

Böhme G (1988) Echolaryngography. A contribution to the methods for sonographic assessment of the larynx. Laryng Rhinol Otol 67:551–558

Böhme G (1990) Ultraschalldiagnostik der Epiglottis. HNO 38:355–360

Broyles EN (1959) Anatomical observations concerning the laryngeal appendix. Ann Otol Rhinol Laryngol 68:461–470

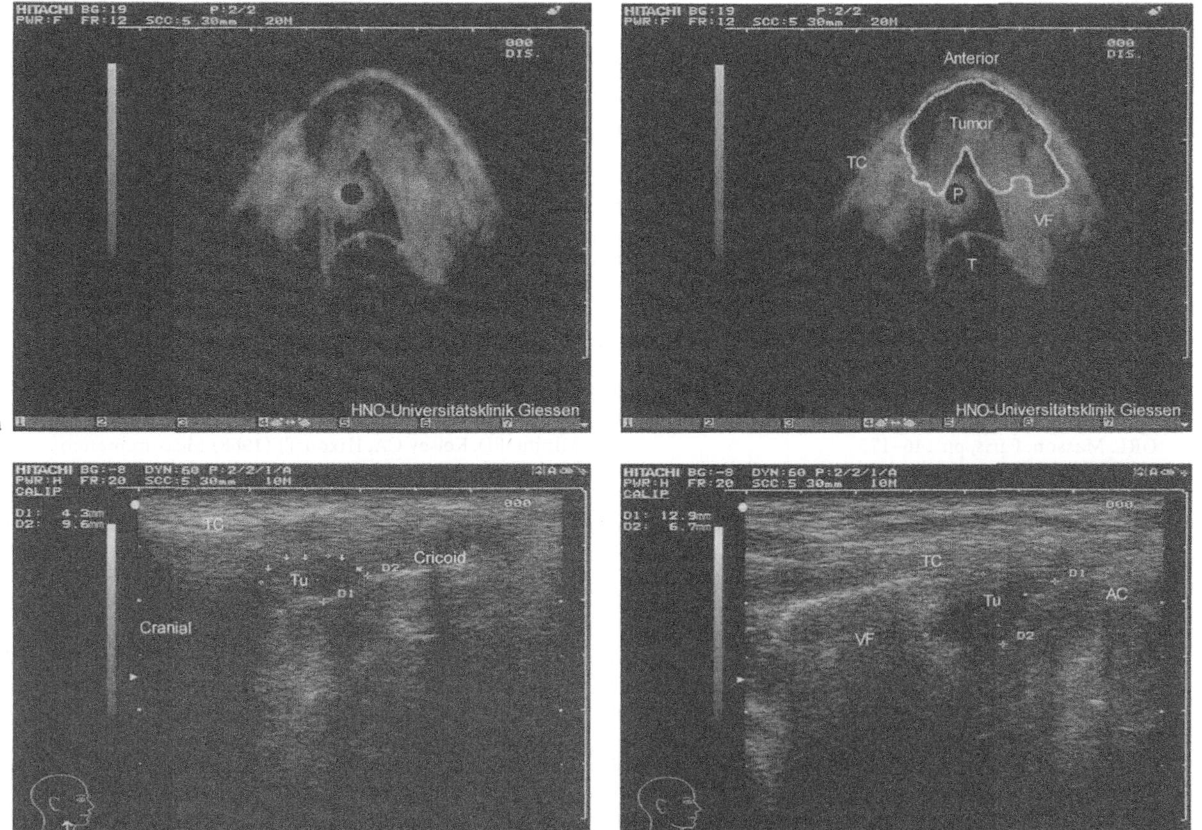

Fig. 5.32a–d. Patient presenting with cancer of the anterior commissure. **a** and **b** Endosonography (20 MHz): native picture (**a**) and picture with legend (**b**). *TC* thyroid cartilage; *VF* vocal fold; *P* probe; *T* tube. **c** External ultrasonography (20 MHz) showing the tumor (*T4*) between the cricoid and the thyroid cartilage (*TC*) at the cricothyroid ligament (D1=0.4 cm; D2=1 cm) **d** External ultrasonography (10 MHz) of the right vocal fold. *Tu* tumor; *TC* thyroid cartilage; *VF* vocal fold; *AC* anterior commissure; D1=1.3 cm; D2=0.6 cm

Bruneton JN, Roux P, Caramella E, Demard F, Vallicioni J, Chauvel P (1984) Ear, nose, throat cancer: ultrasound diagnosis of metastasis to cervical lymph nodes. Radiology 152:771–773

Bruneton JN, et al (1987) Medical ultrasound equipment, examination technique, and ultrasonography of the normal neck. In: Bruneton JN (ed) Ultrasonography of the neck. Springer, Berlin Heidelberg New York, pp 1–21

Burgess LP, Yim DW (1985) Laryngeal cysts of the thyroid cartilage. Arch Otolaryngol 111:826

Canalis RF, Maxwell DS, Hemenway WG (1977) Laryngocele: an updated review. J Otolaryngol 6:191–199

Canuyt G (1939) Les maladies du larynx. Masson, Paris, p 804

Carp H, Bundi A (1992) A preliminary study of the ultrasound examination of the vocal cords and larynx. Anesth Analg 75:639–640

Chevallier P (1995) Echographie du larynx et de l'hypopharynx chez l'adulte. Aspects normaux et applications potentielles en pathologie. Thèse de médecine,Nice, p 173

Chevallier P, Padovani B, Marcy PY, Chevallier A, Bruneton JN (1997) Echographie du larynx et de l'hypopharynx chez l'adulte. Aspects normaux. JEMU 18:53–67

Chevallier P, Marcy PY, Padovani B, Raffaelli C, Coussement A, Bruneton JN (1998) Aspect échographique des kystes laryngés. JEMU 19:385–388

Chevallier P, Motamedi JP, Marcy PY, Foa C, Padovani B, Bruneton JN (2000) Sonographic discovery of a pharyngocele. J Clin Ultrasound 28:101–103

Clavier A (1989) Echographie de la loge HTE: application en cancérologie. Thèse de médecine, Paris V, France, p 108

Collazo-Clavell ML, Gharib H, Maragos NE (1995) Relationship between vocal cord paralysis and benign thyroid disease. Head Neck 17:24–30

Declercq A, Van den Hauwe L, Van Marck E, Van de Heyning PH, Spanoghe M, De Schepper AM (1998) Patterns of framework invasion in patients with laryngeal cancer: correlation of in vitro magnetic resonance imaging and pathological findings. Acta Otolaryngol 118:892–895

Derchi LE, Dellepiane M, Giannoni M, Guglielmetti G, Ameli F (1992) Sonography in laryngeal tumors. Radiol Med (Torino) 83:224–229

De Santo LW, Devine KD, Weiland LH (1970) Cysts of the larynx: classification. Laryngoscope 80:145–176

Detsouli M, Chelly H, Essaadi M, Mokrim B, Touhami M, Benchekroun Y (1994) La laryngocèle comme étiologie de la détresse respiratoire. Ann Otolaryngol Chir Cervicofac 111:476–478

Dulac GL (1974) Pathologie pharyngo-laryngée. In: Dulac GL (ed) Traité de radiodiagnostic,vol XVII. Masson, Paris, pp 313–388

Erkan M, Tolu I, Aslan T, Güney E (1993) Ultrasonography in laryngeal cancers. J Laryngol Otol 107:65–68

Essop AR, Scott PJ, Tweddle AC, Rees MR, Williams GJ (1993) The surgical implications of endoluminal coronary ultrasound. Am Heart J 125:882–884

Fresnel-Elbaz E (1995) Exploration de la phonation In: Courtat P, Peytral C, Elbaz P (eds) Explorations fonctionnelles en ORL. Masson, Paris, pp 146–175

Garel C, Legrand I, Elmaleh M, Contencin P, Hassan M (1990) Laryngeal ultrasonography in infants and children: anatomical correlation with foetal preparations. Pediatr Radiol 21:164–167

Garel C, Hassan M, Legrand I, Elmaleh M, Narcy P (1991) Laryngeal ultrasonography in infants and children: pathological findings. Pediatr Radiol 21:164–167

Garel C, Contencin P, Polonovshi JM, Hassan M, Narcy P (1992) Laryngeal ultrasonography in infants and children: a new way of investigating. Normal and pathological findings. Int Ped Otorhinolaryngol 23:107–115

Giovanniello J, Grieco V, Bartone NF (1970) Laryngoceles. AJR Am J Roentgenol 108: 825–829

Gritzmann N (1992) Diagnostic imaging of laryngeal cancer, with special consideration of high-resolution sonography (in German). Wein Klin Wochenschr 104: 234–242

Gritzmann N, Traxler M, Grasl M, Pavelka R (1989) Advanced laryngeal cancer: sonographic assessment. Radiology 171:171–175

Guerrier Y, Andrea M, Paco J (1979) L'épiglotte et ses amarrages. Cah ORL 14:793–803

Henrot P, Stines J, Walter F, Pierucci, Troufléau P, Blum A, Roland J (1999) Optimisation des techniques d'imagerie dans l'exploration des tumeurs du pharynx, du larynx et de la cavité buccale. J Radiol 80:233–250

Heppt W, Born A, Maier H (1990) Use of B-mode sonography in the diagnosis of laryngocele. Laryngorhinootologie 69:378–380

Hermanek P, Sobin LH (1988) Classification TNM des tumeurs des voies aériennes supérieures. In: Hermanek P, Sobin LH (eds) Classification des tumeurs malignes. Springer, Paris, pp 20–29

Hertz CH, Lindström K, Sonesson B (1970) Ultrasonic recording of the vibrating vocal folds. Acta Otolaryngol (Stockh) 69:223–230

Holinger PH, Johnston KC (1951) Benign tumors of the larynx. Ann Otol 60:496–509

Hubbard C (1987) Laryngocele. A study of five cases with reference to radiological features. Clin Radiol 38: 639–643

Kawasaki H, Kuratomi K, Mitsumasu T (1983) Cysts of the larynx: a 10-year review of 94 patients. Auris Nasus Larynx 10 [Suppl]:47–52

Kotby MN, Kirchner JA, Kahane JC, Basiouny SE, Elsamaa M (1991) Histo-anatomical structure of the human laryngeal ventricule. Acta Otolaryngol (Stockh) 111: 396–402

Leroux-Robert J, De Brux J (1976) Histopathologie ORL et cervicofaciale. Leroux-Robert J, De Brux J (eds) Masson, Paris, pp 90–91

Loveday EJ, Bleach NR, Van Hasselt CA, Metreweli C (1994) Ultrasound imaging in laryngeal cancer: a preliminary study. Clin Radiol 49:676–682

Lundgrer J, Olofsson J, Hellquist H (1982) Oncocytic lesions of the larynx. Acta Otolaryngol (Stockh) 94:335–344

Mensch B (1964) Analyse par exploration ultrasonique du mouvement des cordes vocales isolées. Compt Rend Biol 12:2295

Micheau C, Luboinski B, Sancho H, Cachin Y (1978) Modes of invasion of cancer of the larynx. A statistical, histological, and radioclinical analysis of 120 cases. Cancer 38: 346–360

Miles KA (1989) Ultrasound demonstration of vocal cord movements. Br J Radiol 62:871–872

Minifie FD, Kelsey CA, Hixon TJ (1968) Measurement of vocal fold motion using ultrasonic Doppler velocity monitor. J Acoust Soc Am 43:1165–1169

Morgan NJ, Emberton P (1994) CT scanning and laryngoceles. J Laryngol Otol 108:266–268

Myssiorek D, Persky M (1989) Laser endoscopic treatment of laryngoceles and laryngeal cysts. Otolaryngol Head Neck Surg 100:538–541

Na DG, Lim HK, Dyun HS, Kim HD, Ko YH, Baek JH (1997) Differential diagnosis of cervical lymphadenopathy: usefulness of color Doppler sonography. AJR Am J Roentgenol 168:1311–1316

New GB, Erich JB (1938) Benign tumors of the larynx. Arch Otolaryngol 28:840–846

Norris CW (1979) Pharyngoceles of the hypopharynx. Laryngoscope 89:1788–1807

Noyek AM, Holgate RC, Wortzman G, et al (1977) Sophisticated radiology in otolaryngology: II. Diagnostic imaging: non-roentgenographic (non-X-ray) modalities. J Otolaryngol 6:95–117

Ooi LLPJ (1991) B-mode real-time ultrasound assessment of vocal cord function in recurrent nerve palsy. Ann Acad Med Singapore 21:214–216

Ooi LLPJ, Chan HS, Soo KC (1995) Color Doppler imaging for vocal cord palsy. Head Neck 17:20–23

Ophir D, Lifschitz-Mercer B (1989) Oncocytic cystic lesions of the upper respiratory tract. Ear Nose Throat 68: 237–244

Parnell FW, Brandeburg JH (1970) Vocal cord paralysis. A review of 100 cases. Laryngoscope 80:1036–1044

Peneygre R, Lelièvre G (1989) Paralysies laryngées. Encycl Med Chir (Paris). Oto-rhino-laryngologie; 20675 A10:8p

Piekarski JD, Héran F, Williams M (1999) Imagerie du larynx tumoral. J Radiol 80:209–221

Raghavendra BN, Horii SC, Reede DL, Rumancik NM, Persky M, Bergeron T (1987) Sonographic anatomy of the larynx with particular reference to the vocal cords. J Ultrasound Med 6:225–230

Rebel A, Basle M, Racadot J (1980) Cartilage, os, ossification. In: Coujart R (ed) Précis d'histologie humaine. Masson, Paris, pp 205–210

Rothberg R, Noyek AM, Freeman JL, Steinhardt MI, Stoll S, Goldfinger M (1986) Thyroid cartilage imaging with diagnostic ultrasound. Arch Otolaryngol Head Neck Surg 112:503–515

Sakai F, Gamsu G, Dillon WP, Lynch DA, Gilbert TJ (1990) MR imaging of the larynx at 1.5 tesla. J Comput Assist Tomogr 14:60–71

Schindler O, Gonella MC, Pisani R (1990) Doppler ultrasound examination of the vibration speed of vocal folds. Folia Phoniatr 42:265–272

Shita L, Rypens F, Hassid S, Vermeylen D, Struyven J (1999) Sonographic demonstration of a congenital laryngeal cyst. J Ultrasound Med 18:665–667

Singh YN, Misra K, Agarwal S, Rai D (1988) Multiple laryngeal cysts: association with malignancy (report of two cases with review of literature). Indian J Cancer 25:157–164

Spencer GM, Rubens DJ, Roach DJ (1995) Hypoechoic fat: a sonographic pitfall. AJR Am J Roentgenol 164:1277–1280

Stell PM, Maran AGD (1975) Laryngocele. J Laryngol Otol 89:915–924

Terracol J, Griener GF (1971) Le larynx. Bases anatomiques et fonctionnelles. Doin, Paris

Trotoux J, Germain MA, Bruneau X (1986) La vascularisation du larynx. Révision des données anatomiques classiques à partir d'une étude anatomique de 100 sujets. Ann Oto Laryng 103:389–397

Ueda D, Yano k, Okuno A (1989) Ultrasonic imaging of the tongue, mouth and vocal cords in normal children: establishment of basic scanning positions. J Clin Ultrasound 21:431–439

Valente T, Farina R, Minelli S, Pinto A, Rossi G, Tecame S, Caranci F (1996) The echographic anatomy of the larynx and the perilaryngeal structures. Radiol Med (Torino) 91:231–237

Van de Ven PM, Schutte HK (1995) The pharyngocele: infrequently encountered and easily misdiagnosed. J Laryngol Otol 109:247–249

Vierzen PBJ, Joosten FBM, Marnie JJ (1994) Sonographic, MR and CT findings in a large laryngocele: a case report. Eur J Radiol 18:45–47

Youssefzadeh S, Steiner E, Turetschek K, Gritzmann N, Kursten R, Franz P (1993)Sonographie von Larynxzysten. Rofo Fortschr Geb Rontgenstr Neun Bildgeb Verfahr 159:38–42

Zbären P, Becker M, Laeng H (1996) Pretherapeutic staging of laryngeal cancer: clinical findings, computed tomography and magnetic resonance imaging versus histopathology. Cancer 77:1263–1273

Zech M, Scherer M, Maier H, Heppt W (1994) Endosonographie des Larynx. Eur Arch Otorhinolaryngol 136 [Suppl}

6 Doppler Ultrasound of the Carotid and Vertebral Arteries

Charles Raffaelli, Christine Tran, Nicolas Amoretti

CONTENTS

C. Raffaelli, MD
Service de Radiodiagnostic, Hôpital Pasteur, 30, avenue Voie Romaine, BP 69, 06002 Nice Cedex 1, France
C. Tran, MD
Service de Radiodiagnostic, Hôpital Pasteur, 30, avenue Voie Romaine, BP 69, 06002 Nice Cedex 1, France
N. Amoretti, MD
Service de Radiodiagnostic, Hôpital Pasteur, 30, avenue Voie Romaine, BP 69, 06002 Nice Cedex 1, France

6.1 Introduction

Ischemic cerebrovascular accidents (ICVA), commonly referred to as stroke, remain a major public health problem, despite their decline in frequency in industrialized countries (Klag et al. 1989). One third of stroke patients die, and permanent disabilities are common. Patients with a history of transient ischemic attacks (TIA) have a 20-fold higher risk of stroke than the general population; the spontaneous risk of stroke following a TIA is 4%–10% of patients per year (Leonberg and Elliott 1981). Eighty percent of ICVAs are due to atherosclerosis, and the majority of atherosclerotic lesions involve the extracranial segments of the cerebral arteries. Thromboembolism of cardiac origin accounts for only 20% of ICVAs.

Treatment of atherosclerotic lesions is based on endarterectomy; this procedure is of recognized efficacy for symptomatic patients with high-grade stenosis (more than 70% reduction in diameter), in whom it reduces the incidence of stroke. In contrast, surgery has not yet been proven effective in individuals with moderate stenosis (30%–70% diameter reduction), and it is ineffective in patients with low-grade stenosis (less than 30% reduction in diameter) (ESCT 1991; NASCET 1991). Stenoses of the subclavian artery and innominate artery are usually treated by percutaneous transluminal angioplasty.

Most atherosclerotic lesions of the carotid, vertebral, and subclavian arteries are accessible to color Doppler sonography. This atraumatic imaging technique is the first-line modality for examination of symptomatic patients and to screen for atherosclerotic lesions of the cerebral arteries in high-risk individuals.

6.2 Carotid Arteries

6.2.1 Normal Anatomy

The right common carotid artery (CCA) arises from the brachiocephalic artery, dorsal to the right sternoclavicular joint (Fig. 6.1). The left CCA arises directly from the superior portion of the aortic arch, posterior to the brachiocephalic artery. Each artery ascends to the base of the neck, covered by the homolateral sternocleidomastoid muscle and accompanied by the internal jugular vein (IJV) and the vagus nerve.

In its cervical portion, the common carotid artery (CCA) lies in front of the anterior border of the sternocleidomastoid muscle. The CCA divides into the internal and external carotid arteries; the bifurcation usually lies between the level of vertebrae C-4 and C-6 but is often lower in the elderly. In 90% of individuals, the internal carotid artery (ICA) is posterior to the external carotid artery (ECA), in 10% the ICA lies medial to the ECA, and on rare occasion the ICA courses anteromedial to the ECA (Prendes et al. 1980).

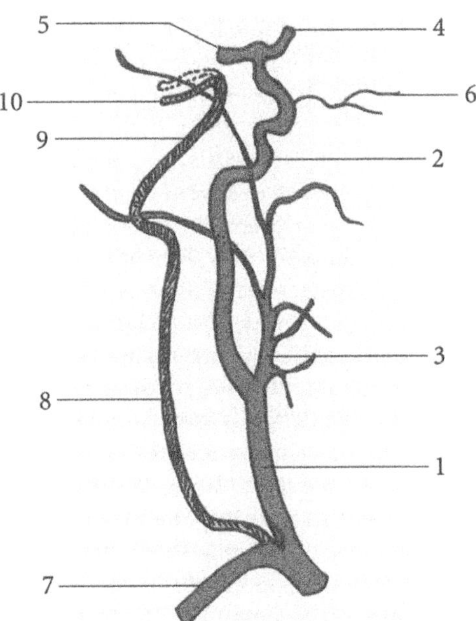

Fig. 6.1. Arteries of the neck and head (right lateral view). *1* right common carotid artery, *2* right internal carotid artery; *3* right external carotid artery; *4* right anterior cerebral artery; *5* right sylvian artery; *6* right ophthalmic artery; *7* right subclavian artery; *8* right vertebral artery; *9* basilar trunk; *10* right posterior cerebral artery

The area of the carotid bifurcation is usually dilated, and its caliber is larger than that of the CCA at this point. Termed the carotid bulb, this expansion typically includes the origin of the ICA, and especially its posterior portion. The ICA then ascends superiorly and medially to enter the base of the skull; the ICA does not give off any branches from its cervical portion.

In contrast, the ECA immediately gives off multiple branches of variable origin. The first branch, the superior thyroid artery, arises soon after the bifurcation.

The internal and external carotid systems have several collateral pathways that can maintain blood supply in case of ICA thrombosis. The chief communication is through the ophthalmic artery, which arises from the ICA and is anastomosed to the external carotid network via its internal nasal branch.

6.2.2 Clinical Considerations

Stroke is the consequence of interruption of the blood supply to a portion of the brain; the clinical consequences are directly related to the cerebral region affected and the efficacy of compensatory mechanisms.

Cerebrovascular insufficiency can be classed in four stages as a function of severity:

- Stage I disease: asymptomatic lesions, regardless of their extent
- Stage II disease: presence of neurological signs such as TIAs or a deficit reversible in less than 3 weeks. Stage IIa corresponds to complete resolution of symptoms; mild neurological deficits persist in stage IIb.
- Stage III and stage IV disease: progressive stroke (stage III) or established stroke (stage IV), regardless of possible ulterior resolution

The clinical symptoms of ischemia affecting the areas supplied by the carotid are variable, including monocular visual disturbances, speech disorders, impaired consciousness, facial paresthesia, hemiparesis, and hemiplegia.

Atherosclerotic stenoses predominate and are promoted by a variety of factors: arterial hypertension, diabetes mellitus, smoking, hypercholesterolemia, genetic factors. The majority of atherosclerotic lesions occur at bifurcations or in curved vascular segments. The most frequent mechanism of stroke is embolism from an atherosclerotic carotid lesion (Carr et al. 1996).

Stenoses greater than 75% in cross-sectional area significantly reduce arterial blood flow, and a correlation has been established between the severity of stenosis and the onset of stroke. In patients with moderate stenosis, cardiac arrhythmia or reduced arterial flow can potentiate the effects of stenosis and lead to stroke. Focal modifications in atheromatous plaque, such as intraplaque hemorrhage or local thrombosis, are other aggravating factors.

Stroke can also be caused by embolism from the heart or the aorta, as seen in patients with endocarditic arrhythmia or myocardial ischemia with mural thrombosis. Paradoxical embolism, which originates in a systemic vein, is secondary to a defect such as a patent foramen ovale. A pathology affecting the ascending aorta (aneurysm or dissection) is another possible cause.

During the late 1980s and 1990s, three major randomized trials were conducted to determine the efficacy of endarterectomy for carotid stenosis (ACAS 1995; ESCT 1991; NASCET 1991). Endarterectomy was found to have a prognostic benefit for stenosis, expressed in diameter, of at least 60% (ACAS 1995) to 70% (NASCET 1991), whether symptomatic or not.

Endarterectomy was shown to reduce the risk of ipsilateral stroke by 53%–84% compared with medical treatment. Findings also suggested that the prognostic benefit of surgical treatment increases with the degree of stenosis (NASCET 1991). In patients with a long life expectancy, surgery has also proven beneficial for stenosis of 50% (Barnett et al. 1998).

These trials also defined the technique for angiographic measurement of carotid stenosis.

6.2.3 Examination Technique and Normal Findings

6.2.3.1 General Examination Conditions

6.2.3.1.1 Ultrasound Equipment

Use of a high-frequency linear transducer is the rule; while sector transducers are easier to handle, linear probes provide images of better quality. A frequency of 7–8 MHz is a good compromise, combining sufficient spatial resolution with acceptable image quality. Probes that emit over a wide range of frequencies can also be very effective, provided the range is not too wide (in particular towards frequencies higher than 10 MHz) so as not to compromise the depth of exploration.

Lower frequencies (close to 5 MHz) permit satisfactory exploration in depth for patients with a thick neck. High frequencies are useful when examining very thin individuals and children (Cattin and Bonneville 1995). The high spatial resolution achieved with frequencies of 10 MHz or more allows detailed analysis of atheromatous plaque, but the limited depth of exploration prevents exhaustive examination.

A low-frequency sector transducer is sometimes helpful for examination of individuals with a thick neck when the carotid bifurcation is located high in the neck. The loss of resolution is compensated by the depth of exploration; when conditions are favorable, the course of the ICA can be followed up to its entry into the base of the skull.

Duplex sonography is the preferred mode of exploitation of color Doppler signals for the carotid vessels; triplex ultrasound scanning is rarely used because the frame rate is too slow.

6.2.3.1.2 Patient Positioning

No consensus has yet been reached concerning patient positioning, but the patient should be relaxed, with arms adducted, because contraction of the cervical muscles, particularly the sternocleidomastoid muscle, can hamper sonographic examination. The head must be hyperextended to access the region under the angle of the mandible; a pad can be placed under the neck to facilitate cervical extension. The patient can also be examined in a semi-reclining position. The examiner usually sits on the right side of the patient, whose head is positioned at the same level, or behind the patient's head. The patient is requested to refrain from speaking, to breathe calmly, and not to swallow. Pressure exerted by the transducer must be kept to a minimum to avoid eliciting a carotid sinus reflex that might evoke a vagal response. Examination of the contralateral carotid artery may be facilitated by having the patient turn his head; the head must be rotated no more than 15° to avoid excessive modifications of anatomic relationships. It is easier to examine each carotid artery separately; comparative study is of little value (Attlan et al. 1999; Cattin and Bonneville 1995; Zwiebel 1990).

6.2.3.2
Examination Procedure

6.2.3.2.1
Technical Parameters

Initial color Doppler settings should consist in a fairly high pulse repetition frequency (PRF) (approximately 40 cm/s), a high pass filter, and a high color priority, sensitivity, and persistence.

One of the difficulties is to obtain a satisfactory color image (ideal Doppler angle 0°) while conserving sufficient B-mode image quality (ideal insonation angle 90°). For axial imaging, the transducer must be angled in order to optimize the insonation angle. For sagittal scanning, electronic angulation (beam steering) should be used systematically. B-mode imaging permits rapid localization of the carotid arteries, the carotid bifurcation, and any atherosclerotic lesions.

Pulsed Doppler examination should always be performed on all three arteries (CCA, ICA, and ECA) plus any zone where color Doppler has revealed a flow anomaly.

The sample volume should be positioned in the center of vessels imaged in longitudinal section. Sample volume size can be adapted to vessel dimensions, although this is not obligatory (Hennerici and Neuerburg-Heusler 1998). Systematic angle correction is required for accurate velocity measurements (Zwiebel 1990). Ideally, measurements should be made using an insonation angle of 40°–70° to reduce the margin of error (Fig. 6.2). The spectrum obtained allows determination of the peak systolic velocity (PSV) and the resistive index (RI) calculated for an even number of cycles. In patients with highly pulsatile carotid arteries, it may be useful to increase the level of the high pass filter. Adjustment of the gain and the pulsed Doppler frequency can improve the spectral quality. Certain US units permit continuous real-time display of spectral hemodynamic parameters, provided a good-quality signal is recorded. Spectral quality depends closely on the Doppler angle and the quality of B-mode imaging of the vessel being examined. On some ultrasound units, the emission power can be increased to obtain a better signal; this possibility should obviously never be used for examination of the ophthalmic arteries. Pulsed Doppler examination can also be performed using highly recurrent axial scans to reduce the Doppler angle. This technique provides spectra of satisfactory quality when the ICA and the ECA lie very high, but the flow velocities recorded are necessarily only approximate (Paivansalo et al. 1996). Determination of the PSV in the CCA is of considerable importance for quantification of ICA stenosis. Measurement must be made at a distance from the bifurcation with appropriate angle correction; the sample volume must also be correctly centered (Zwiebel 2000a).

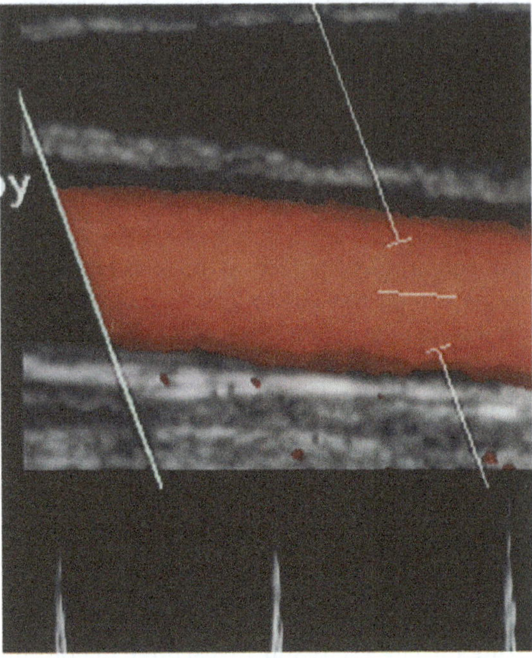

Fig. 6.2. Common carotid artery: Beam steering permits optimization of the insonation angle; the sample volume is positioned in the center of the vessel

6.2.3.2.2
Common Carotid Artery

Transverse B-mode scans obtained by placing the transducer opposite the anterior border of the sternocleidomastoid muscle allow analysis of the CCA. The carotid bifurcation, the ECA, and the ICA are then localized. Recurrent retroclavicular scans on the right side permit easy assessment of the brachiocephalic artery and the ostia of the right CCA and the right subclavian artery. The aortic arch and the emergence of the supra-aortic arterial trunks are occasionally visible.

6.2.3.2.3
Internal Carotid Artery and External Carotid Artery

On B-mode imaging, it is advisable to begin examination with sagittal scans in order to analyze the carotid bifurcation (Fig. 6.3). Axial localization of the direc-

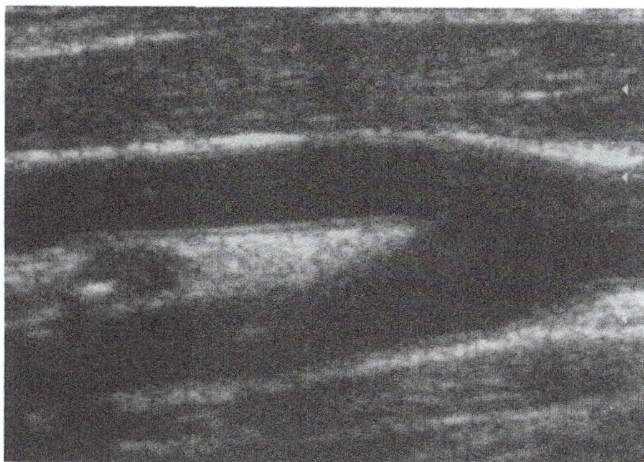

Fig. 6.3. Carotid bifurcation: oblique longitudinal scan obtained using a posterolateral approach

tion of the ICA and the ECA permits sagittal scans aligning the CCA, the ICA, and the ECA. A posterolateral approach, from behind the sternocleidomastoid muscle, is the most effective means of obtaining the best incidence; contralateral rotation of the head is often indispensable (Zierler et al. 1987). However, ideal scans cannot always be obtained when the configuration of the bifurcation is not favorable (Cattin and Bonneville 1995; Zwiebel 2000a). Systematic axial scanning permits evaluation of any atherosclerotic plaque.

Color Doppler sonography is initiated in the axial plane; the CCA, ICA, and the ECA are slowly scanned as far as possible using a recurrent submandibular approach. This allows determination of the direction and the morphology of the ICA, and in particular a search for loops or folds. Examination is continued using longitudinal scans; beam steering ensures an appropriate beam-vessel angle (40–70°) allowing optimum pulsed Doppler examination.

6.2.3.2.4 Ophthalmic Arteries

Examination of the carotid arteries is completed by analysis of the ophthalmic arteries. Several different incidences can be used to record signals at various levels in the ophthalmic artery (Dauzat 1991a). With the transducer placed on the closed eye, axial scans obtained using a posterointernal orientation permit signals in the terminal portion of the ophthalmic artery to be recorded. Other incidences are possible using a supraocular or transocular approach (Cattin and Bonneville 1995). On color Doppler, the PRF is reduced to 9 cm/s. The scan must visualize the optic nerve behind the eyeball. In the normal state, the ophthalmic artery can be localized close to the optic nerve (Fig. 6.4).

Pulsed Doppler of the ophthalmic artery must be performed at least 1 cm from the posterior pole of the eyeball in order to avoid recording the signals from a ciliary or retinal artery (flow in these structures is always anterograde).

6.2.3.3 Normal Findings

6.2.3.3.1 Normal Arterial Wall

High-frequency sonography of the carotid wall reveals three different structures (Nolsoe et al. 1990; Picano et al. 1988): a very thin, hyperechoic internal line formed by the interface between the intima and the circulating blood, a central zone of low echogenicity corresponding to the intima and the media (Pignoli et al. 1986), and an external hyperechoic zone corresponding to the adventitia (Fig. 6.5). Clear visualization of the intimal reflection on a longitudinal scan reflects proper positioning through the center of the vessel (Poli et al. 1988; Wolverson et al. 1983).

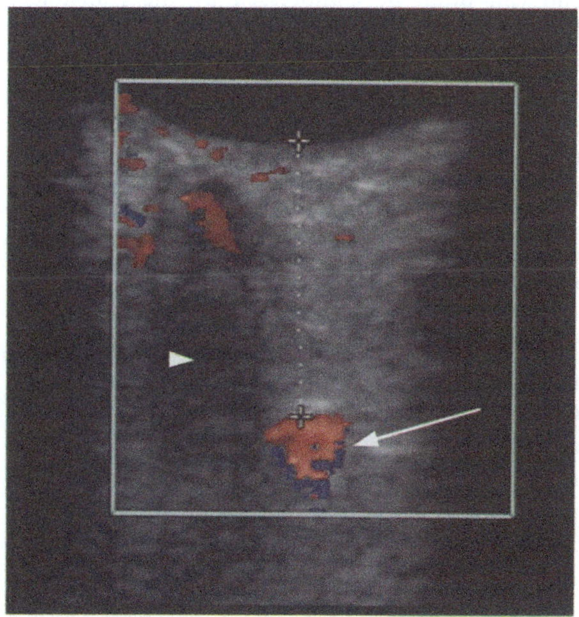

Fig. 6.4. Axial scan of the orbit showing the ophthalmic artery (*arrow*) located 1.4 cm from the posterior pole of the eyeball, near the optic nerve (*arrowhead*)

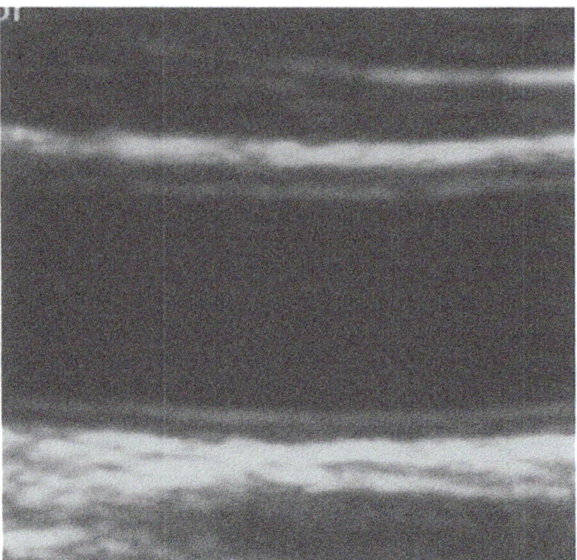

Fig. 6.5. Normal carotid wall

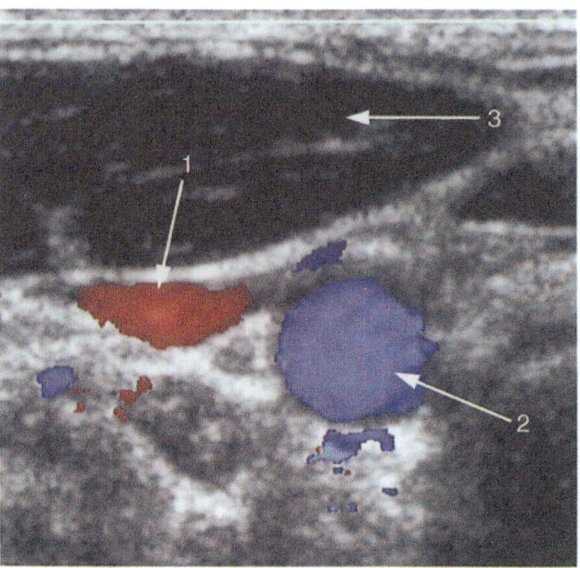

Fig. 6.6. Axial scan revealing the internal jugular vein (*1*), the common carotid artery (*2*), and the sternocleidomastoid muscle (*3*)

6.2.3.3.2 Common Carotid Artery

The diameter of the CCA is globally smaller than that of the carotid bulb. The waveform of the normal CCA is mixed, as this artery supplies both the viscera and the muscles. The diastolic component is constant, but of moderate intensity.

The internal jugular vein lies lateral to the CCA and can often be compressed by the transducer (Fig. 6.6). The waveform of the CCA is intermediate between those of the ICA and the ECA. In normal conditions, flow in the CCA is laminar (Fig. 6.7); the brightest colors, corresponding to the highest velocities, are homogeneously distributed at the center of the vessel (Zwiebel 2000a).

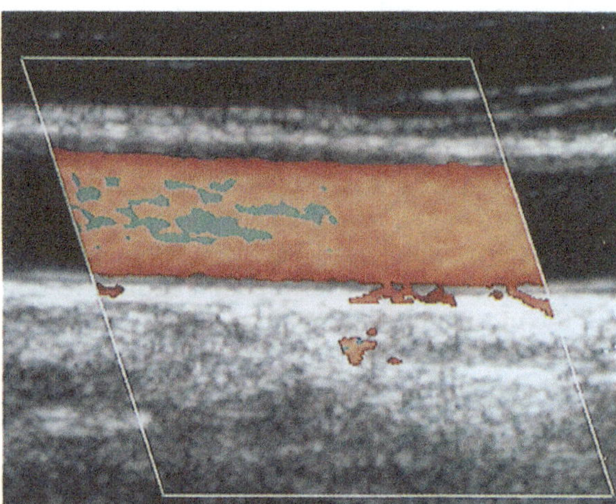

Fig. 6.7. Laminar flow in a normal common carotid artery: the brightest colors correspond to the highest velocities distributed within the center of the vessel

6.2.3.3.3 Carotid Bifurcation

The carotid bifurcation is extremely variable in topography but usually lies opposite vertebrae C3–4. On occasion, the carotid bifurcation is not visible at this level. A very high-lying bifurcation is accessible to examination by a low-frequency probe. An intrathoracic carotid bifurcation or agenesis of the ICA are exceedingly rare possibilities (Cattin and Bonneville 1995).

The carotid bulb manifests as a dilatation at the level of the bifurcation (Fig. 6.8); physiologic slowing of the blood flow at this point shows up as darker colors and a lower PSV. The flow reversal generally observed along the posterior wall of the carotid bulb (Fig. 6.9) (Zierler et al. 1987) is a normal finding. Flow reversal typically extends onto the posterior wall of the origin of the ICA; most marked in early systole, it may also persist into diastole. At the carotid bulb, flow reversal can be demonstrated during an average of 22% of the total cycle length (range 8%–80%) over a mean length of 14 mm in longitudinal section (6.1–22 mm). The zone of flow separation represents

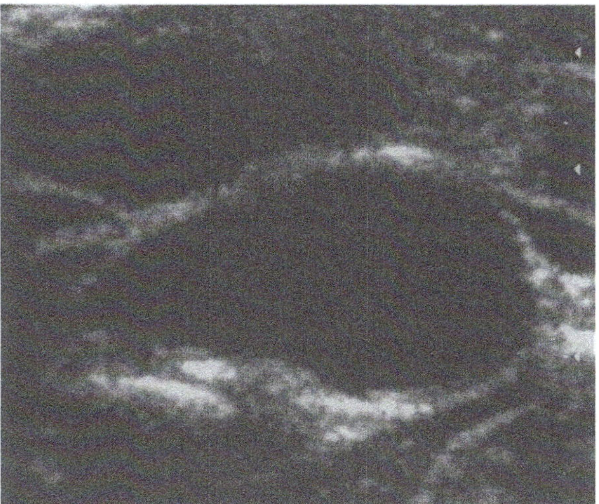

Fig. 6.8. Axial scan showing the carotid bulb and the origin of the right ICA

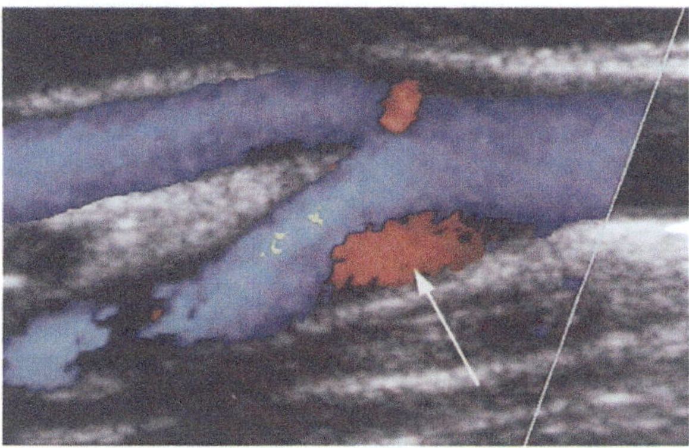

Fig. 6.9. Color Doppler: longitudinal scan of a normal carotid bifurcation. Physiologic posterobulbar reflux *(arrow)*

on average 33% (range 8%–64%) of the cross-sectional area of the carotid bulb (Middleton et al. 1988a). Unfamiliarity with the phenomenon of flow separation, which has been implicated in the formation of atheromatous plaque, can lead to diagnostic errors. Although its exact pathophysiology remains uncertain, absence of normal flow separation suggests the existence of atherosclerotic plaque in the carotid bulb.

6.2.3.3.4 Internal Carotid Artery

Spectral analysis of the ICA reveals a low resistance waveform with a sharp systolic peak that decreases slowly, and marked antegrade flow in diastole that results in a low resistive index, comparable to that of a visceral artery (Fig. 6.10). The normal waveform is characterized by a regular low-resistance stage

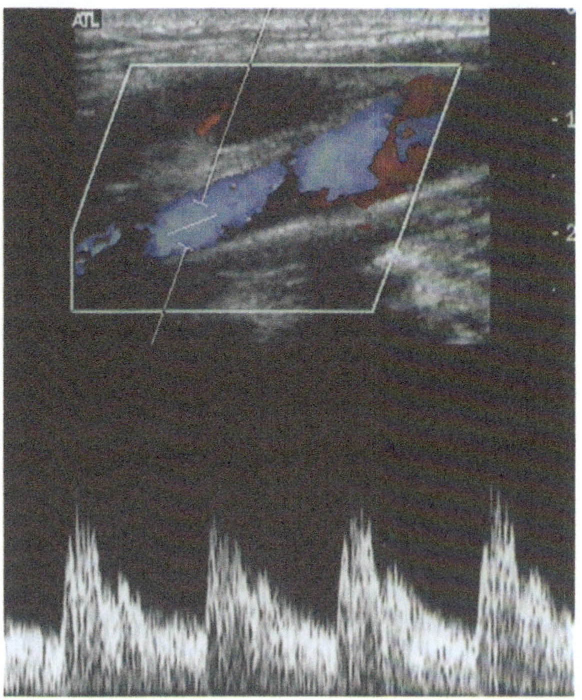

Fig. 6.10. Internal carotid artery: normal spectral pattern

and distribution of brightness towards the high and medium frequencies, which is materialized by the presence of a dark window under the systolic peak. The position of the sample volume (SV) has considerable influence on the spectrum obtained; a narrow sample volume gives a frequency spectrum in which the areas of brightness are themselves concentrated in a narrow band (Cattin and Bonneville 1995). The PSV of the ICA varies from 54 to 88 cm/s; it never exceeds 120 cm/s in normal individuals (Zwiebel 2000a).

6.2.3.3.5 External Carotid Artery

The spectral pattern of the ECA, which supplies the muscles, is characterized by a high resistance flow with a sharp systolic peak and very low flow in diastole that gives an RI close to 1 (Fig. 6.11). The PSV of the ECA never exceeds 115 cm/s in normal individuals (Zwiebel 2000a).

6.2.3.3.6 Ophthalmic Arteries

The spectrum of the ophthalmic artery is often similar to that of the ICA, although the diastolic component is not as marked.

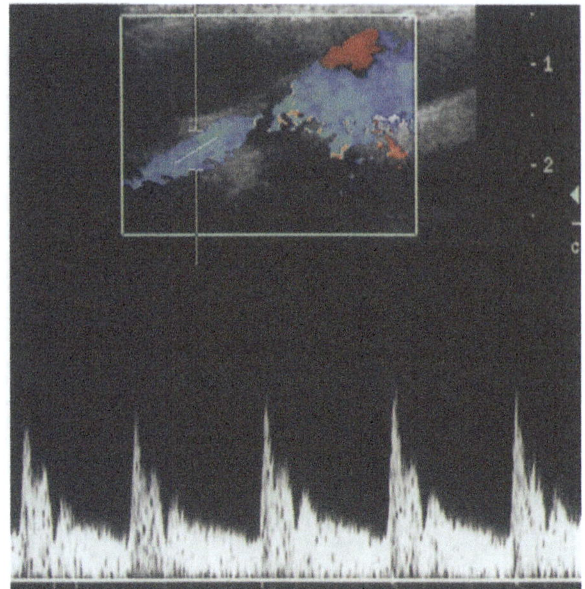

Fig. 6.11. External carotid artery: normal spectral pattern

6.2.3.4
Technical Difficulties

6.2.3.4.1
Calcified Plaque

When calcified plaque completely reflects the ultrasound beam, color signals may be absent opposite the affected vascular segment (Fig. 6.12). In such cases, a signal can sometimes be obtained by modifying the approach to the vessel or by increasing the color Doppler emission power. The vessel can also be evaluated by pulsed Doppler, which has better sensitivity than color Doppler. Because flow disturbances are usually maximal immediately distal to plaque, positioning the sample volume at this level permits satisfactory evaluation of any stenosis (Carroll 1991). It is also possible to search for indirect signs of ICA stenosis beyond the site of calcified plaque.

6.2.3.4.2
Differentiation of the ICA and the ECA

Although sometimes difficult, differentiation of the ICA and the ECA is mandatory because isolated ECA stenoses usually have no pathological consequences. When diagnostic difficulties are encountered, a number of features may facilitate vessel identification (Attlan et al. 1999; Hennerici and Neuerburg-Heusler 1998; Zwiebel 1990):

- Larger luminal diameter of the ICA (Fig. 6.13)
- Orientation of the ICA usually posterolateral to the ECA, and generally adjacent to the IJV
- Multiple and early branching vessels of the ECA, whereas the cervical ICA has none (Fig. 6.14); the trunk of the ECA is often shorter than 1 cm. The superior thyroid artery frequently lies posterior to the CCA and often allows localization of the ECA.
- High resistance flow pattern in the ECA, sometimes with transient diastolic flow reversal, contrasting with the marked diastolic flow of the ICA
- Modulation of the ECA waveform when the ipsilateral superficial temporal artery is tapped with a finger

a 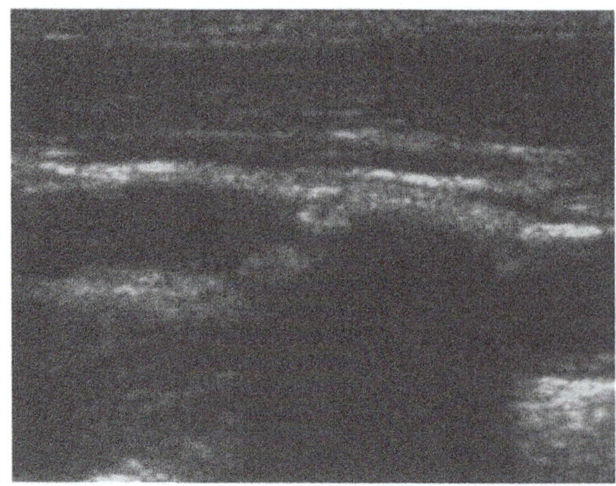

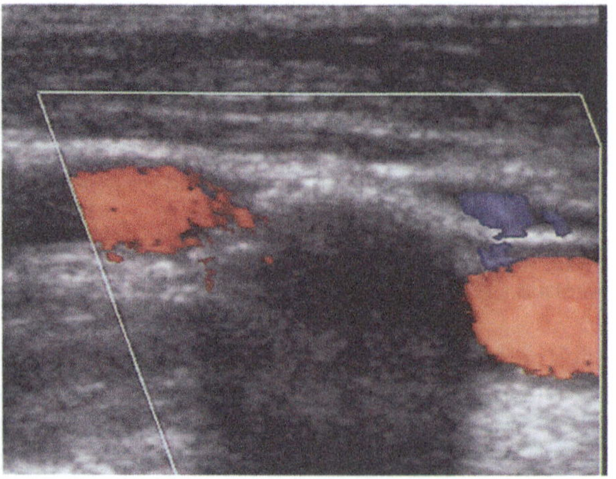 b

Fig. 6.12a,b. Calcified plaque with posterior acoustic shadowing (a) responsible for nonvisualization of flow at color Doppler (b)

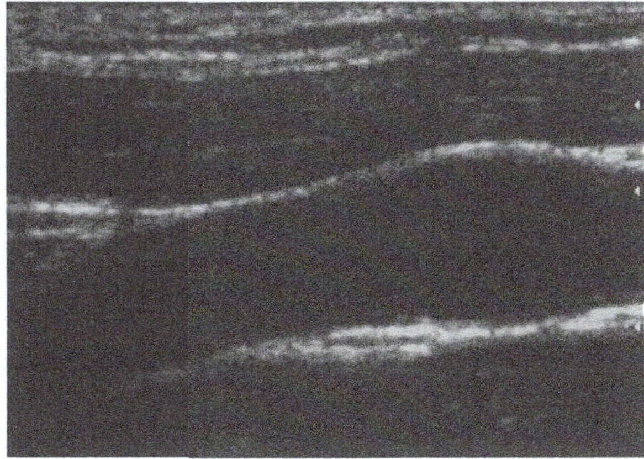

a

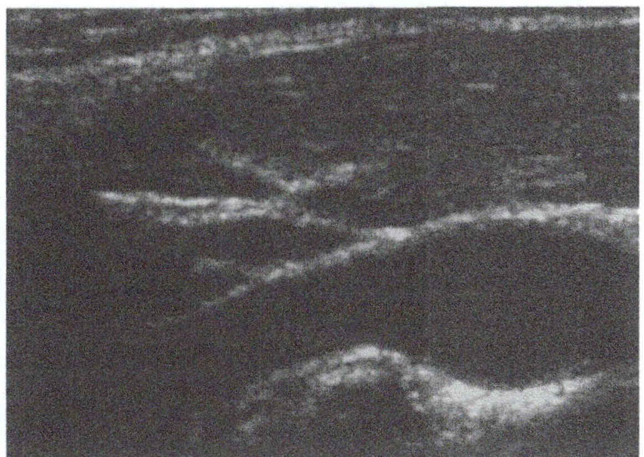

b

Fig. 6.13a,b. Longitudinal scan of the origin of the internal carotid artery (**a**) and the external carotid artery (**b**)

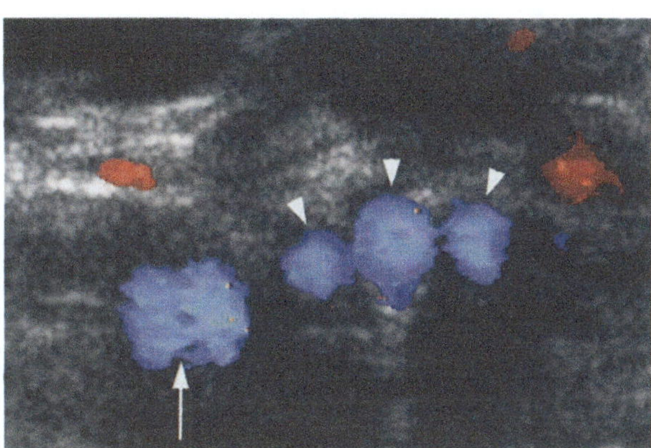

Fig. 6.14. Axial scan demonstrating the right internal carotid artery (*arrow*) and the branches of the external carotid artery (*arrowheads*)

6.2.3.4.3
Impact of Noncarotid Pathologies

Cardiopathies may have an impact on carotid and vertebrosubclavian waveforms. Such anomalies must not be mistaken for a carotid pathology.

Aortic valve cardiopathies cause modifications that are often evident. Aortic narrowing leads to an increase in the systolic elevation time, with a drop in the carotid PSV and the end-diastolic velocity (EDV). Aortic insufficiency manifests as a drop in the carotid EDV and a rise in the resistive index and the pulsatility index. The subclavian arteries often present a holodiastolic reflux (CATTIN and BONNEVILLE 1995).

An elevation in flow velocities may be observed in the territory supplied by the ECA in patients with hyperthyroidism or Paget's disease (ATTLAN et al. 1999).

6.2.3.5
Specific Technical Modalities

6.2.3.5.1
Power Doppler

Power Doppler is an original mode of exploitation of the Doppler signal in which the amplitude of the returned signal is recorded. The color imaging obtained is more sensitive than standard color Doppler and much less dependent on the insonation angle; these features result in improved anatomic detail and better delineation of the vascular walls (Fig. 6.15) (RUBIN et al. 1994). The images are monochromatic, usually red or orange, with the lighter colors corresponding to the highest velocities. Unlike color Doppler, power Doppler does not provide any hemodynamic information and cannot determine the direction of flow. Settings are difficult to adjust, and the technique requires specific training. A high gain must be used by adjusting the high pass filter and the scale of velocities. When the gain is too high, colored coding of the hyperechoic interfaces appears. Awareness of this potential artifact is necessary to avoid diagnostic errors. Power Doppler is also highly sensitive to movement, which can be a problem for carotid explorations.

During Doppler US of the cervical and cerebral vessels, power Doppler may prove useful for better delimitation of atheromatous plaque but remains merely a complement to color Doppler. Power Doppler can also better demonstrate tortuous arteries and vascular loops (CATTIN and BONNEVILLE 1995). The homogeneous colorization and the better anatomic details achieved with power Doppler can improve the credibility of Doppler examination by providing

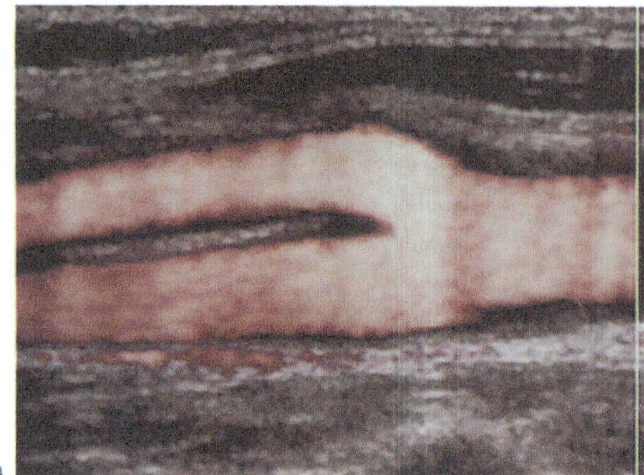
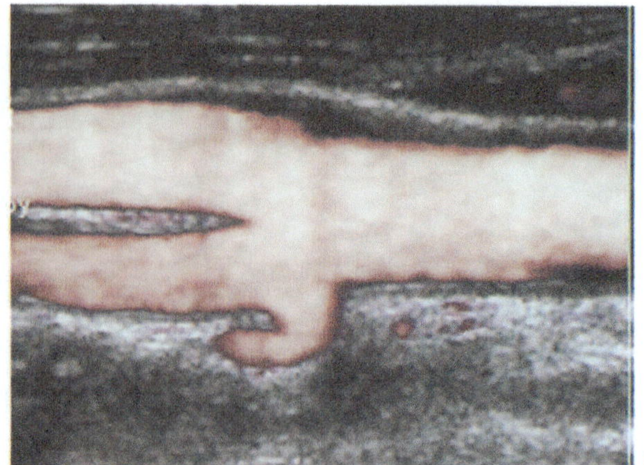

Fig. 6.15a,b. Power Doppler study of the carotid bifurcation provides improved delimitation of the vascular walls (a). The origin of the superior thyroid artery (b) permits identification of the ECA, which in this example lies posteromedially

the referring physician with angiographic-like documents. Power Doppler is also often performed during injection of contrast material.

6.2.3.5.2 Extended Field of View (FOV) US Systems

The Siemens Siescape Panoramic Imaging technology and the Acuson FreeStyle Extended Imaging display capability permit continuous free-hand acquisition of a structure that extends considerably beyond the field of the transducer. Power Doppler or color Doppler flow capability can be added. The scanned images obtained also help to improve the credibility of sonography because they resemble the documents obtained with other imaging techniques.

6.2.3.5.3 B-flow System

The B-flow system developed by General Electric is a new technique for exploitation of the returned signal that is completely different from the Doppler mode. It permits visualization of blood flow in B-mode with excellent sensitivity (Fig. 6.16).

6.2.3.5.4 Sono-CT

Sono-CT (ATL) is a system that allows oblique acquisitions for each transducer element by phase shift; this feature extends imaging possibilities beyond the usual rectangular (FOV) of linear transducers. Although the image obtained appears similar, reverberation artifacts are considerably reduced (Fig. 6.17). The higher lateral resolution considerably improves image quality at the lateral borders of the field. The system has recently been extended to sector transducers and associated with harmonic tissue imaging. Sono-CT limits artifacts affecting the carotid wall and can thus better define atheromatous plaque, and particularly plaque of low echogenicity.

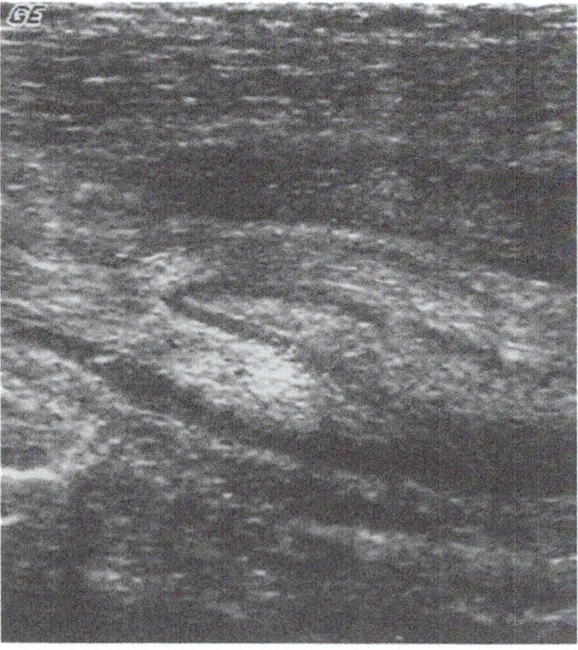

Fig. 6.16. B-flow system: carotid bifurcation

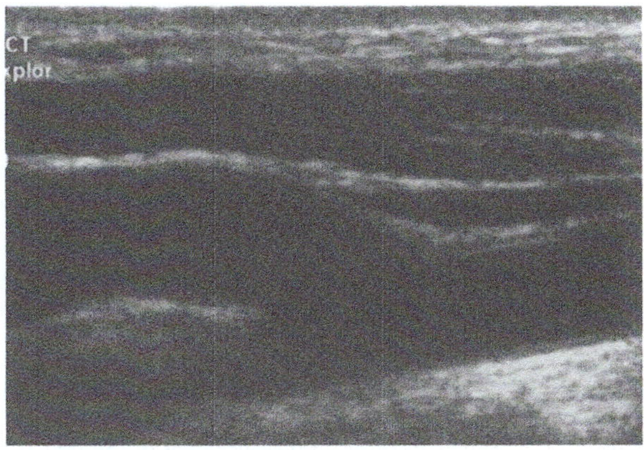

Fig. 6.17. Sono-CT: carotid bifurcation

6.2.3.5.5
Ultrasound Contrast Agents

Ultrasound contrast agents can be used to enhance the returning echo of flowing blood on both B-mode imaging and color Doppler (Albrecht et al. 1998; Schwartz et al. 1994). The indications and the agents themselves are in constant evolution.

The utility of contrast agents for Doppler US of the renal arteries and transcranial Doppler is evident, as these products enhance the signal from deep arteries or arteries protected by strongly attenuated structures. Although the cervical arteries are superficial and easily accessible to Doppler US, difficulties persist for analysis of calcified plaque with acoustic shadowing, evaluation of plaque surface characteristics, demonstration of very slow residual flow in cases of apparent thrombosis, and accurate quantification of stenosis. Contrast agents thus have a potential application in approximately 10% of examinations, but only small series of patients have been studied to date (Deklunder et al. 1998).

Because artifacts related to an increase in the endovascular signal (blooming) can be a problem, the enhancement period remains short, and flow velocity measurements are increased by approximately 5% (Fig. 6.18) (Abidlgaard et al. 1996).

Initial results reveal better efficacy for the study of carotid plaque and the description and quantification of stenoses (Furst et al. 1996; Sitzer et al. 1996a).

6.2.3.6
Synthesis and Documentation of Results

The examination report must include a minimum of hard-copy documents, and possibly a videotape recording. B-mode imaging should include a longitudinal image of the carotid bifurcation and images of any pathological areas. Spectral recordings should be provided for the CCA, ECA, ICA, and ophthalmic artery. Color Doppler images and spectral recordings are required for any pathological areas (stenoses, folds). By convention, sagittal scans are shown with the distal segment of the carotid on the left of the screen.

6.2.4
Atherosclerotic Carotid Plaque

6.2.4.1
Definition

Sonography is the only technique for in vivo structural analysis of atherosclerotic plaque available for routine use. The efficacy of MRI in this setting is currently under investigation (Saloner et al. 1996).

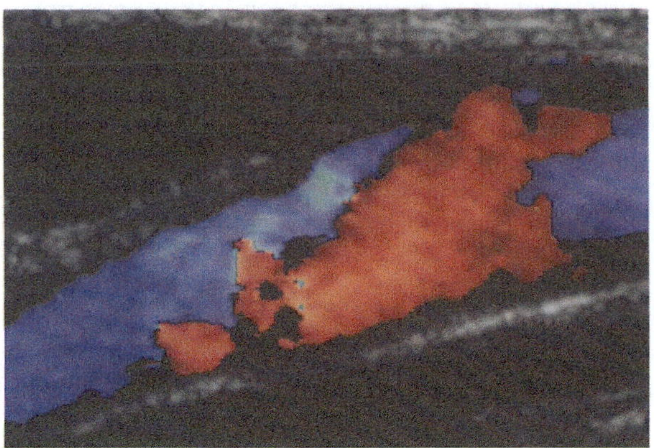

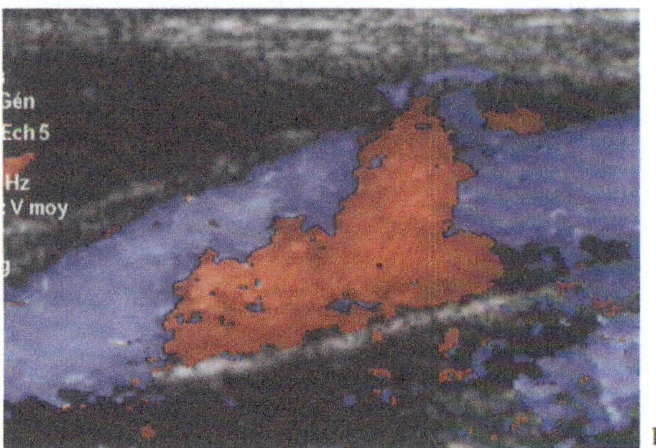

Fig. 6.18a,b. Carotid bulb and the internal carotid artery before (**a**) and after (**b**) injection of an ultrasound contrast agent. The signal is enhanced but perivascular artifacts are present

Atherosclerotic carotid plaque is a material of variable echogenicity that thickens the vessel wall, thereby reducing the diameter of the arterial lumen. Carotid plaque can be detected by measuring the distance between the adventitia and the intimal reflection that comprises the intima and the media (intimal-medial thickness, IMT) (Fig. 6.19). The IMT measures less than 1.2 mm in normal individuals without plaque (Zwiebel 2000b).

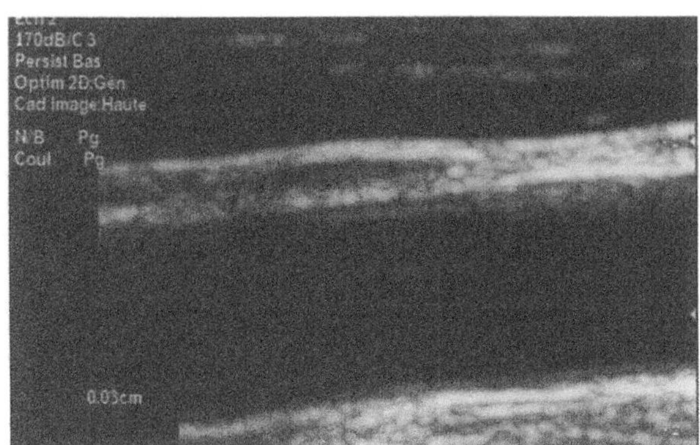

Fig. 6.19. Normal carotid wall: measurement of the IMT (0.3 mm)

6.2.4.2 *Pathological Anatomy*

The formation of atherosclerotic plaque involves three endothelium-mediated processes (Gibbons and Dzau 1994; Ross and Glomset 1976):
- Migration of smooth muscle cells into the subendothelial layers
- Intra- and extracellular lipid accumulation
- Development of a collagen-rich fibrous matrix

The surface characteristics of plaque are just as variable (Marcade 1996):
- Smooth (flat) plaque covered by a collagenous fibrous capsule
- Irregular plaque with a fixed appearance, often calcified
- Ulcerated plaque with a more or less deep defect that exposes the subjacent atheromatous material
- Septated plaque with cavities that remain endothelialized but may contain parietal thrombi.

The structure of carotid plaque may change suddenly or progressively as the result of various degenerative processes: intraplaque hemorrhage, necrosis, rupture of the fibrous capsule, intimal rupture leading to ulceration (Carr et al. 1996).

Intraplaque hemorrhage may occur following rupture of vasa vasorum or focal dissection; hemorrhage causes an increase in the volume of the plaque, and the subsequent ischemia makes the fibrous capsule and the endothelial layer fragile. This increases the risk of intimal rupture.

Rupture of the fibrous capsule or the intima can result in embolization due to shedding of plaque contents, or it may indirectly cause embolization following adherence of thrombus or platelets to the exposed plaque surface (Zwiebel 2000b).

The natural history of carotid plaque may include repeated cycles of injury and subsequent repair. The extent and the frequency of such cycles appear to be correlated with the size of the plaque and the frequency of neurological symptoms (Bassiouny et al. 1977).

Topographically, atherosclerotic ICA plaque usually occurs in the concavity of the carotid bulb, with the residual channel facing the external carotid artery. The spur of the carotid bifurcation is often spared (Marcade 1996).

6.2.4.3 *Detection and Analysis*

Carotid plaque is usually detected and analyzed by B-mode imaging (optimal insonation angle 90°). Longitudinal scans are particularly useful because they show a long vascular segment that may include the CCA, the carotid bifurcation, and the ICA. However, use of an insonation angle tangential to the plaque may lead to overestimation of the plaque (Fig. 6.20). Strictly axial scans, less subject to such errors, should thus be obtained systematically, although it may be difficult to obtain an insonation angle for the ICA close to 90° on axial scans when the carotid bifurcation is high-lying. Longitudinal scans can also underestimate the extent of plaque (Bluth 1996).

Settings (overall gain, gray scale) are critical, and must be adjusted during the examination so as not to overlook lesions with low echogenicity.

In addition to their value for demonstration of hemodynamic disturbances, color Doppler and especially power Doppler should be performed systematically to evaluate carotid plaque. The considerable technological progress made in these techniques today permits excellent delineation of plaque, thereby optimizing the search for anechoic lesions. Power Doppler improves analysis of plaque surface characteristics (Fig. 6.21) (De Bray et al. 1996; Griewing et al. 1996) and measurement of the residual channel (Steinke et al. 1996).

3-D data acquisition with power Doppler of the region of interest improves analysis of plaque sur-

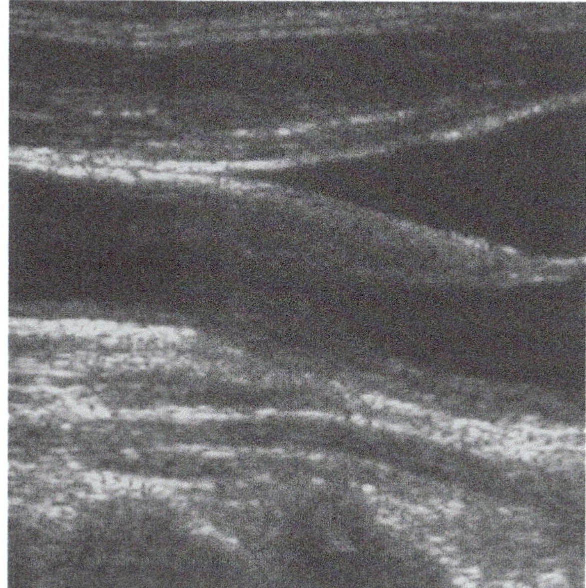

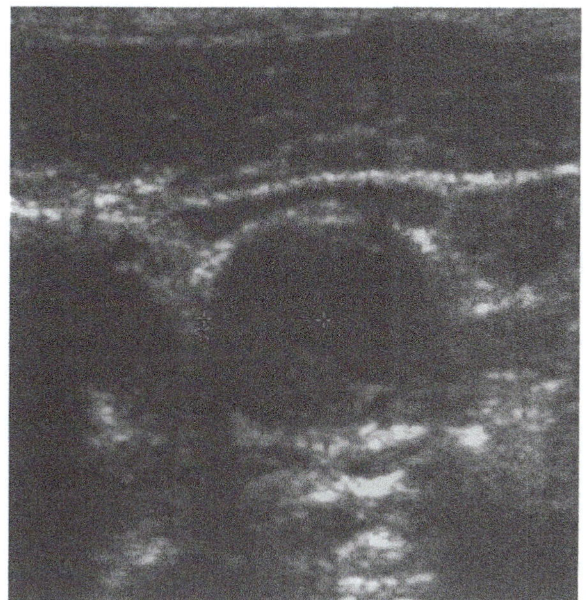

Fig. 6.20a,b. Evaluation of carotid plaque by B-mode imaging. The plaque is ill-defined and overestimated in the longitudinal plane (**a**); evaluation is optimal in the axial plane (**b**)

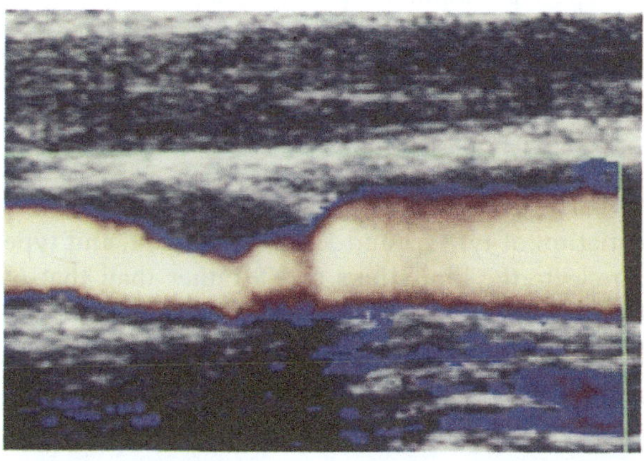

Fig. 6.21. Power Doppler permits better analysis of carotid plaque surface characteristics

face features. This technique opens the way for more accurate quantification of lesions, namely from a volumetric standpoint (Kessler and Griewing 1996).

Other techniques can also be used, such as ultrasonic densitometry that provides a structural projection of the plaque, allowing detection of hemorrhage (Nicolaides 1996; Persson et al. 1996). Analysis of the physical parameters of the returning signal permit an approach to certain plaque properties such as density, viscoelasticity, and anisotropy (Arbeille 1996).

Injection of an ultrasound contrast agent coupled with color Doppler improves study of the plaque surface and has a sensitivity of up to 83% for the detection of ulceration (Sitzer et al. 1996a).

Use of ultrasound contrast agents with the B-flow system has given promising results.

6.2.4.4 *Description*

Carotid plaque is characterized by three sonographically evaluable parameters: extent, contents, and surface. Extent refers to the topography of plaque, including indication of the artery or arteries affected, the length, and its possible circumferential character. Maximum plaque thickness is evaluated on transverse images. Plaque contents are evaluated in terms of overall echogenicity and homogeneity.

The first difficulty for evaluation of echogenicity is to select a reference; the description varies considerably, depending on whether the sternocleidomastoid muscle (SCM) or the circulating blood is used for comparison (Cesari et al. 1996; Zwiebel 2000b).

For comparison with the sternocleidomastoid muscle, three echo patterns can be defined:

- Low-echogenicity plaque, which is sometimes difficult to detect with B-mode imaging; color Doppler and power Doppler are more sensitive (Fig. 6.22). Echo-poor plaque can be mistaken for a parietal thrombus or myointimal hyperplasia (Cattin and Bonneville 1995).

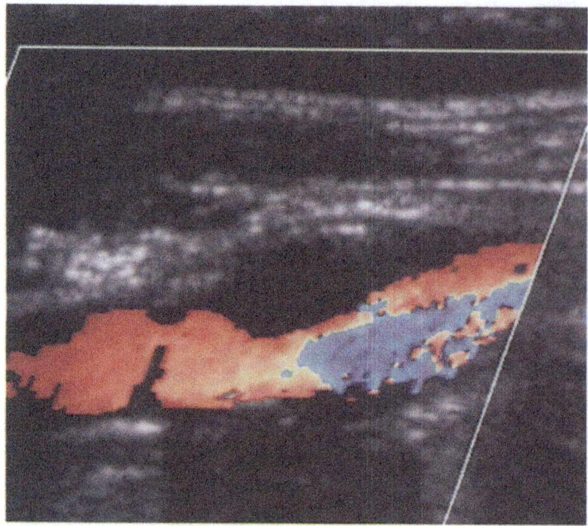

Fig. 6.22. Internal carotid artery: color Doppler reveals anechoic plaque (type 1) responsible for moderate stenosis not seen at B-mode imaging

- Strong echogenicity (calcified plaque) with distal acoustic shadowing. B-mode imaging is highly sensitive for the detection of calcifications at least 1 mm in diameter (Fig. 6.24). A twinkling artifact may be observed on color Doppler and must not be confused with an aliasing phenomenon.

Carotid plaque is often heterogeneous, and includes areas of varying echogenicity that must each be described. Sonographic heterogeneity appears to be correlated with plaque size (ZWIEBEL 2000b).

Plaque surface features, as imaged by B-mode imaging or color or power Doppler, are described in terms of irregularity and defects or cavities.

A constellation of findings is suggestive of ulceration (Fig. 6.25): cavity situated in the center of the plaque (this feature excludes pseudocavities in adjacent plaque), and cavity with irregular margins, intracavity flow on color Doppler (this rules out a hypoechoic zone or an anechoic mural thrombus).

6.2.4.5
Classification

The most commonly used semi-quantitative classification is that of GRAY-WEALE, modified by GEROULAKOS and NICOLAIDES (GEROULAKOS et al. 1993; GRAY-WEALE et al. 1988; WIDDER et al. 1990):

- Type 1: uniformly anechoic plaque detected by color coding of the endoluminal border or the echogenic border of the intimal reflection
- Type 2: predominantly hypoechoic or anechoic plaque (over 50% of the surface area)
- Type 3: predominantly echoic plaque (over 50% of the surface area)
- Type 4: homogeneously echoic plaque
- Type 5: calcified plaque; classification impossible owing to extensive acoustic shadowing

This classification has several drawbacks: Differentiation of types 2 and 3 can be difficult, and type 5 reflects the limitations of US rather than that of the classification itself. A simpler classification distinguishes homogeneous plaque (corresponding to

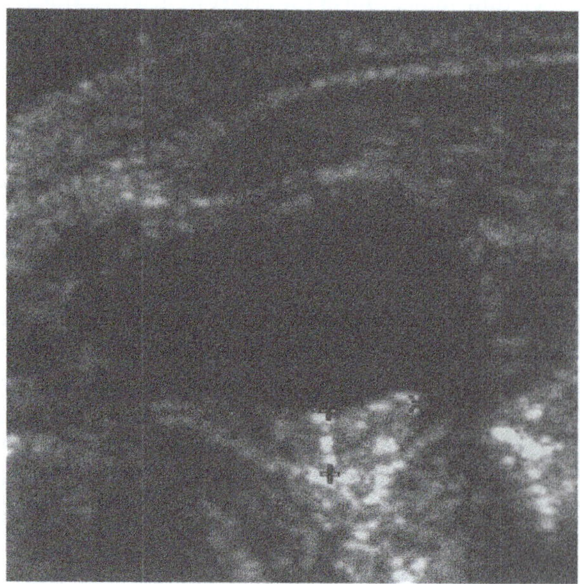

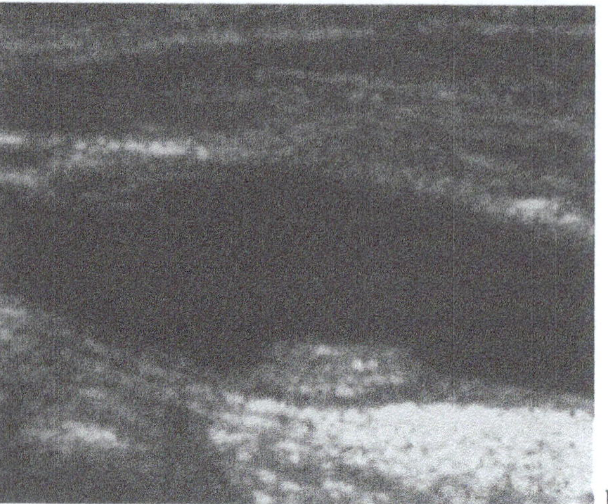

Fig. 6.23a,b. Small homogeneous echoic plaque with smooth contours (type 4)

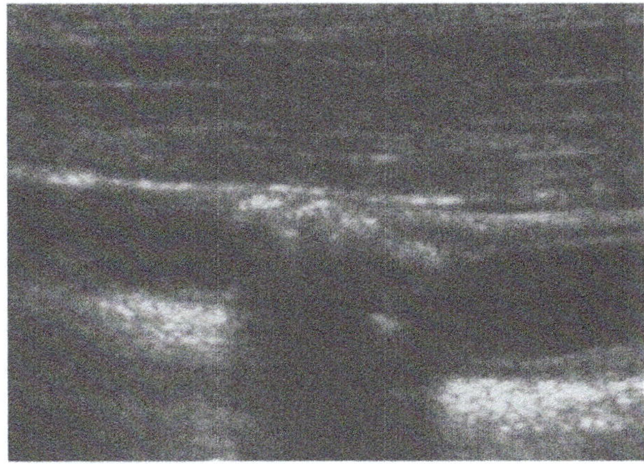
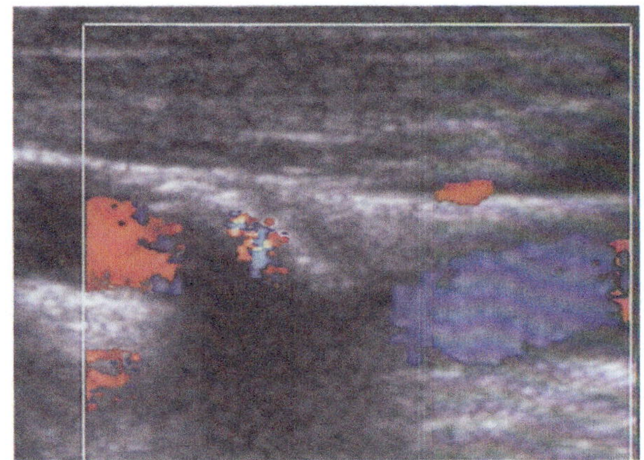

a b

Fig. 6.24a,b. Calcified plaque (type 5) with a twinkling artifact on color Doppler (**b**)

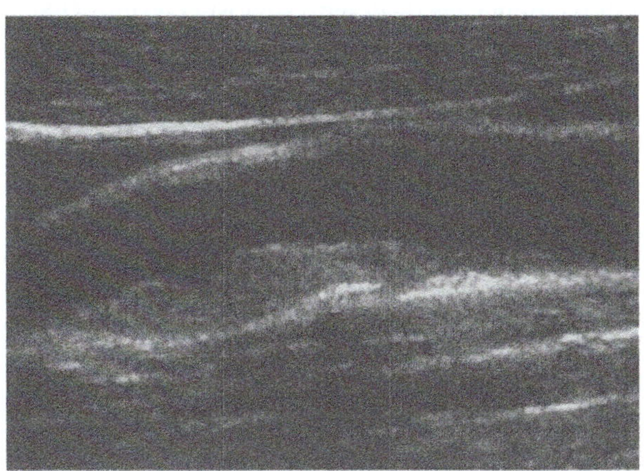
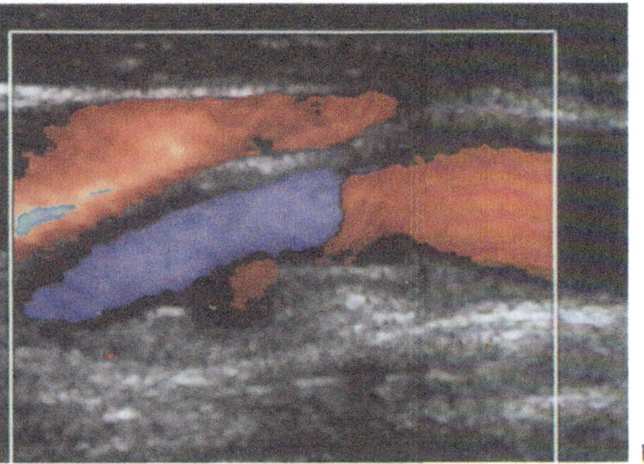

a b

Fig. 6.25a,b. Posterobulbar plaque with a central defect and loss of the intimal reflection on B-mode imaging (**a**). Color Doppler reveals turbulent flow in this depression (**b**). Appearance is suggestive of ulcerated plaque

types 1 and 4) and heterogeneous plaque (corresponding to types 2 and 3) (Bluth 1996).

6.2.4.6
Anatomic and Clinical Correlations

6.2.4.6.1
Sonoanatomic Correlations

Numerous investigators have attempted to correlate the sonographic features of plaque with plaque composition determined by examination of endarterectomy specimens. Various studies have compared plaque surface characteristics on sonograms with examination of surgical specimens or angiographic findings.

Following somewhat disappointing early results (Ratiff et al. 1985; Wolverson et al. 1983), the correlation between US data and histopathological findings is today considered satisfactory (Leys 1996). All studies taken together, mean sensitivity is 89.9% and mean specificity 67.8% (Reilly 1996).

Hypoechoic or anechoic plaque may be of purely lipid origin; this is especially true for smooth homogeneous plaque. Intraplaque hemorrhage or necrotic zones can also create hypoechoic or anechoic images (Bendick et al. 1988; Feeley et al. 1991).

Heterogeneous plaque (Fig. 6.26) corresponds in 65% of cases to the presence of a hemorrhagic component and in 35% to areas of necrosis or fat (Bluth et al. 1986). More than 90% of type 1 and type 2 lesions are partially hemorrhagic or ulcerated (Goes et al. 1990). A hyperechoic zone in plaque of lower echogenicity may correspond to post-hemorrhage fibrosis.

Homogeneous echoic plaque has a fibrous tissue origin; in the literature, it is detected with a sen-

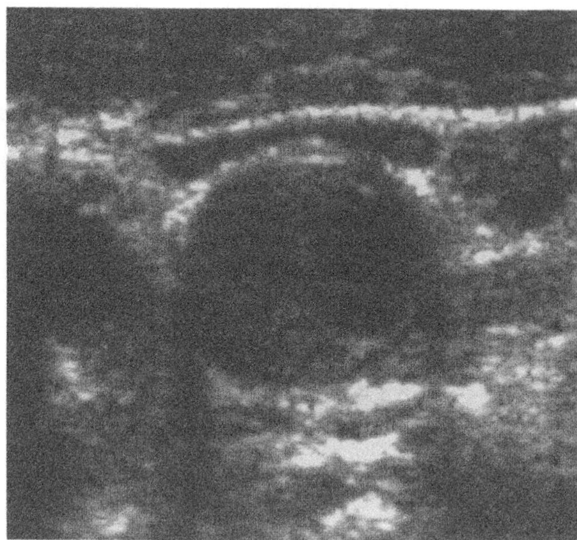

Fig. 6.26. Inhomogeneous plaque with an anterior hypoechoic component

sitivity of 71%–97% (Baud et al. 1988; Baud and Lemasle 1995; Bluth et al. 1986; Gray-Weale et al. 1988; Reilly et al. 1993; Sillesen 1995). Less than 30% of homogeneous plaque contains a hemorrhagic component. Presence of an organized thrombus can lead to diagnostic errors owing to the variability of echogenicity (anechoic or hyperechoic) (Baud et al. 1988; Bendick et al. 1988).

No correlation has been found between the degree of stenosis and plaque characteristics (Sterpetti et al. 1988), although Avril et al. (1991) reported a high frequency of type 1 or 2 plaque in tight stenoses.

Despite its relatively moderate efficacy for the detection of ulceration, Doppler US is sometimes more accurate than angiography, namely for plaque causing minimal lumen narrowing (Comerota et al. 1990; O'Donnell et al. 1985; O'Leary et al. 1987; Sitzer et al. 1996b). In the literature, sensitivity ranges from 33% to 67% and specificity from 31% to 84%. Diagnosis is complicated by the fact that ulcerated lesions undergo re-endothelialization within a short period (sometimes less than 3 weeks) (Lusby et al. 1982).

6.2.4.6.2 Anatomoclinical Correlations

The vascular risk of anechoic or hypoechoic plaque is currently well-established (Bock et al. 1993; Johnson et al. 1985; Langsfeld et al. 1989; Sterpetti et al. 1988). These observations corroborate the risk related to intraplaque hemorrhage, and in certain cases to lipid accumulation within plaque (Feeley et al. 1991). A correlation has also been established between ipsilateral TIA or ICVA and the presence of heterogeneous plaque (Cave et al. 1995; Iannuzzi et al. 1995).

Ulcerated or hemorrhagic carotid plaque is found in 50%–70% of patients with carotid ICVAs. Intraplaque hemorrhage is more extensive in symptomatic stenoses. The presence of ulcerations has been shown to be emboligenic (Bartinsky et al. 1981; Zukowski et al. 1984).

The risk of associated ICVA is 3–9 times lower with echoic homogeneous plaque than with hypoechoic plaque; in contrast, existence of a tight stenosis apparently multiples this risk only threefold (Bock et al. 1993; Sterpetti et al. 1988). Calcified plaque appears to have a risk similar to that of type 4 plaque. However, most recent studies on the benefit of endarterectomy have dealt with stenosing lesions (ESCT 1991; NASCET 1991). In the absence of prospective studies on sufficiently large populations, the echostructural features of atherosclerotic carotid plaque are insufficient to serve as the basis for surgical decisions, even though plaque echostructure appears just as important as the degree of stenosis. Evaluation of the risk linked to plaque requires new techniques such as transcranial Doppler to search for cerebral microemboli (high-intensity transient signals, HITS) (Sitzer 1995).

6.2.4.6.3 Reproducibility of Ultrasound

Inter- and intraobserver reproducibility are better in the more recent studies, owing to the consensus concerning the definition of semi-quantitative criteria for evaluation of carotid plaque (Li et al. 1996; Sutton-Tyrrell et al. 1992). Reproducibility is very good for the detection of weakly echoic stenoses and analysis of the surface of smooth or cavitated plaque, but it remains only moderate for overall analysis of echostructure (essentially difficulties in differentiation between types 2 and 3 plaque) (Baud et al. 1996).

6.2.4.7 Surveillance of Carotid Plaque

Surveillance of carotid plaque will undoubtedly become important as medical therapies are developed for atherosclerosis. In the early stage of the disease, isolated noncalcified plaques are often observed, predominantly on the posterior surface of the carotid bulb (Middleton et al. 1988b). Atherosclerotic plaque has undergone modifications in two thirds of patients after 24 months of follow-up and has regressed in two thirds of these cases (Arbeille et al. 1996). Hypoechoic or heterogeneous plaque appears more susceptible than homogeneous echoic plaque to transformation (Baud and Lemasle 1993; Sterpetti et al. 1988).

6.2.4.8 Synthesis and Documentation of Results

Analysis of atherosclerotic ICA plaque must be meticulous; findings must be documented objectively and cautiously, owing to the limitations of sonographic exploration. The examination report should indicate the carotid bulb diameter, the exact location of the plaque, its extension in height, and maximum plaque thickness on axial scans orthogonal to the vessel explored.

The echostructure should be described either using the Gray-Weale classification or, more simply, by indicating the type of plaque (heterogeneous, homogeneous, calcified). Plaque surface characteristics should be defined using the terms "irregular" or "cavitated" rather than "ulceration", as true ulceration may not actually be present.

6.2.5 Carotid Stenosis

6.2.5.1 Basic Diagnostic Features

While the diagnosis of ICA stenosis is often suggested by the appearance of the atherosclerotic plaque, spectral analysis remains the main diagnostic technique and is the basis for quantification.

Stenoses have well-defined Doppler features. On color Doppler, the stenotic zone is localized by the presence of elevated velocities that cause reverse coding of the highest velocities (Fig. 6.27) (aliasing phenomenon). Such so-called direct features exist starting with mild narrowing of at least 40%.

Indirect signs are observed when narrowing is more severe and include post-stenotic turbulence characterized by random reversal of the color coding. Post-stenotic flow reversal phenomena also occur along the vascular walls.

Careful spectral analysis with angle correction confirms acceleration of the flow velocity at the site of the stenosis (Fig. 6.28). Distal to the stenosis, spectral analysis reveals areas of turbulence, with partial reversal of the systolic flow, and dissipation of the velocities responsible for disappearance of the dark systolic window. Definition of qualitative parameters based on indirect signs also allows evaluation of stenosis (Table 6.1).

A certain number of diagnostic errors can be attributed to unfamiliarity with basic diagnostic features. The most serious error is confusion of the ECA and the ICA. A systematic search for the criteria described previously in case of stenosis is the only way to eliminate this source of error. Another possible error is confusion of occlusion and prethrombotic stenosis; this is often due to improper PRF and color-gain settings. In the postoperative setting, cervical hematomas that often contain air bubbles considerably hamper Doppler study, and can be responsible for false-positive errors.

a
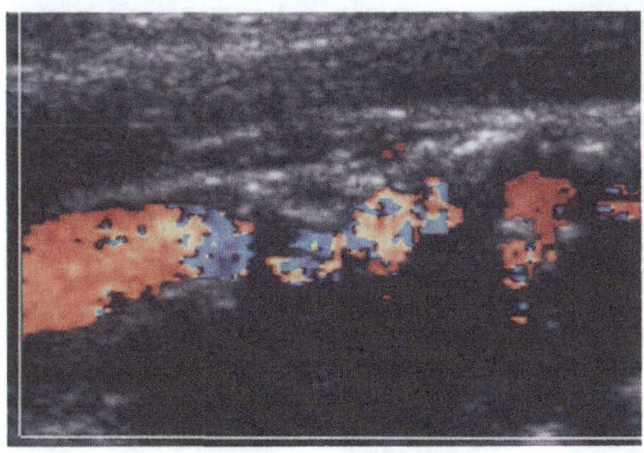

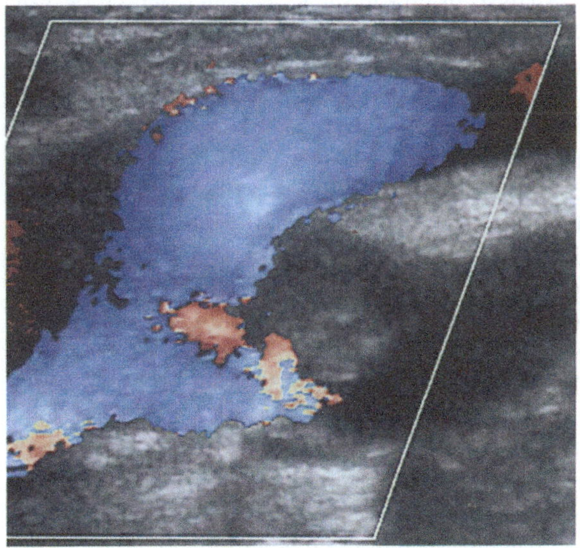
b

Fig. 6.27a,b. Color Doppler: carotid stenoses (aliasing phenomenon)

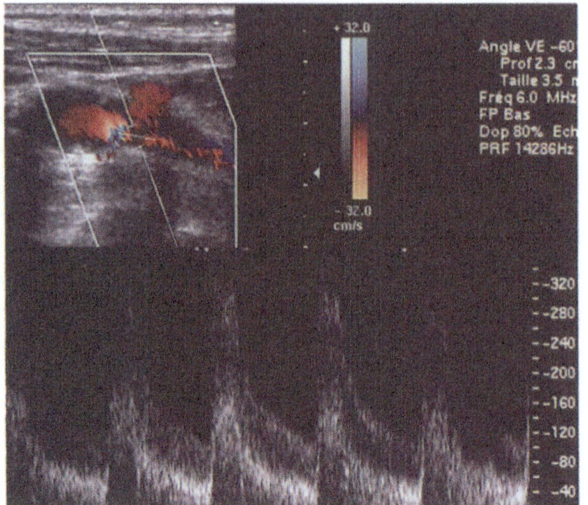

Fig. 6.28. Tight stenosis of the internal carotid artery; spectral analysis revealing acceleration of the flow velocity (PSV 3.2 m/s, EDV 1.2 m/s)

Table 6.1. Semi-quantitative evaluation of the degree of stenosis

Degree of stenosis (surface area)	Doppler signs
<50%	Disappearance of the physiologic posterobulbar reflux
	Post-stenotic reflux along the vessel walls
	Marginal post-stenotic turbulence
	Post-stenotic jet
	Post-stenotic spectral broadening
>75%	Post-stenotic turbulence
	Broadening (>50%) of the post-stenotic spectrum
>95%	Massive turbulence
	Perivascular vibratory artifact
	Complete disappearance of the dark systolic window
	Reduction of post-stenotic flow modulation
Prethrombotic	Extensive reduction in the post-stenotic flow on comparative study
	Reduced post-stenotic turbulence
Thrombosis	Absence of flow
	Sometimes minimal alternating flow that may simulate residual flow

6.2.5.2
Quantitative Parameters

Three zones must be examined whenever stenosis is suspected: the prestenotic region, the stenosis itself, and the post-stenotic area.

6.2.5.2.1
Prestenotic Region

This zone corresponds essentially to the CCA for stenoses of the ICA. Stenoses of the CCA or the innominate artery are rare and occur predominantly near the ostium (Brunholzl and von Reutern 1989).

Analysis of flow in the CCA is an essential part of Doppler US examination of the cervical vessels; the normal flow has a low resistivity (low pulsatility), like all other visceral arteries. Reference measurements concerning the CCA in case of ICA stenosis must be made at a distance from the carotid bifurcation owing to the variation in velocity as a function of the sampling site, namely proximal to the bifurcation (Lee et al. 2000). When the ICA presents a tight stenosis, the ICA waveform features high resistivity (high pulsatility) or even a decrease in the amplitude of the systolic peak. The flow in the CCA decreases compared with the flow in the contralateral CCA (Fig. 6.29).

In case of an ostial stenosis of the CCA the flow in the CCA is damped, with a reduction of the peak systolic amplitude (which is broadened), and can increase in the diastolic component. These anomalies are also observed in the ICA and the CCA (Breslau

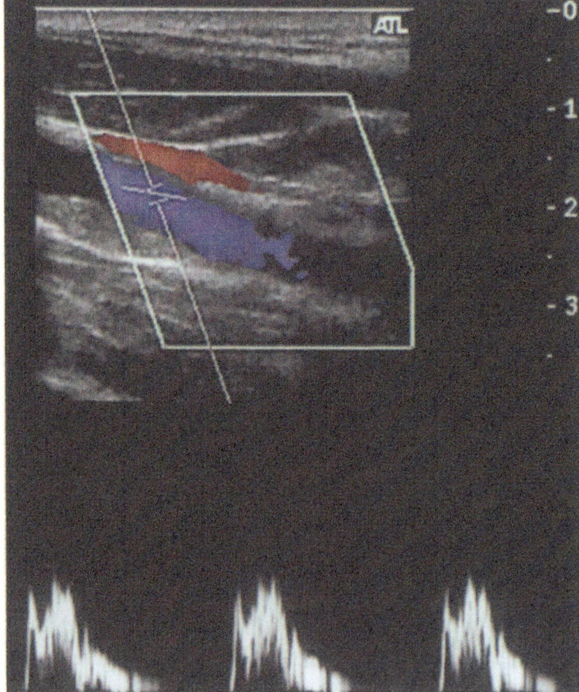

Fig. 6.29. Tight prethrombotic stenosis of the internal carotid artery. The CCA waveform reveals high-resistance flow with a drop in the PSV and disappearance of the diastolic component

et al. 1982). Comparison with the contralateral CCA is the only valid approach, because the flow in the CCA can vary greatly as a function of systemic circulatory parameters.

6.2.5.2.2 Stenotic Zone

B-mode imaging is the most accurate technique for detection and description of stenosing atherosclerotic lesions. The chief sign on color Doppler is acceleration of the flow velocity in the stenotic lumen, which manifests as an aliasing phenomenon; this sign is observed only when stenosis is greater than 40% (Fig. 6.30).

Three cardinal Doppler parameters must be acquired during spectral analysis (ZWIEBEL 2000c): the peak systolic velocity (PSV), the end-diastolic velocity (EDV), and the systolic velocity ratio (SVR). The SVR corresponds to the ratio between the systolic peak at the site of stenosis and the systolic peak measured in the CCA at a distance from the bifurcation.

The PSV must be measured along the entire stenotic zone, localized by the aliasing phenomenon on color Doppler, because the maximum value may be limited to a very short segment (Figs. 6.31, 6.32). Measurements made too hastily risk underestimating the SVR and thus the stenosis. Elevation of the PSV is well-correlated with the degree of stenosis (BLUTH et al. 1988; LANGLOIS et al. 1984). However, a drop in the

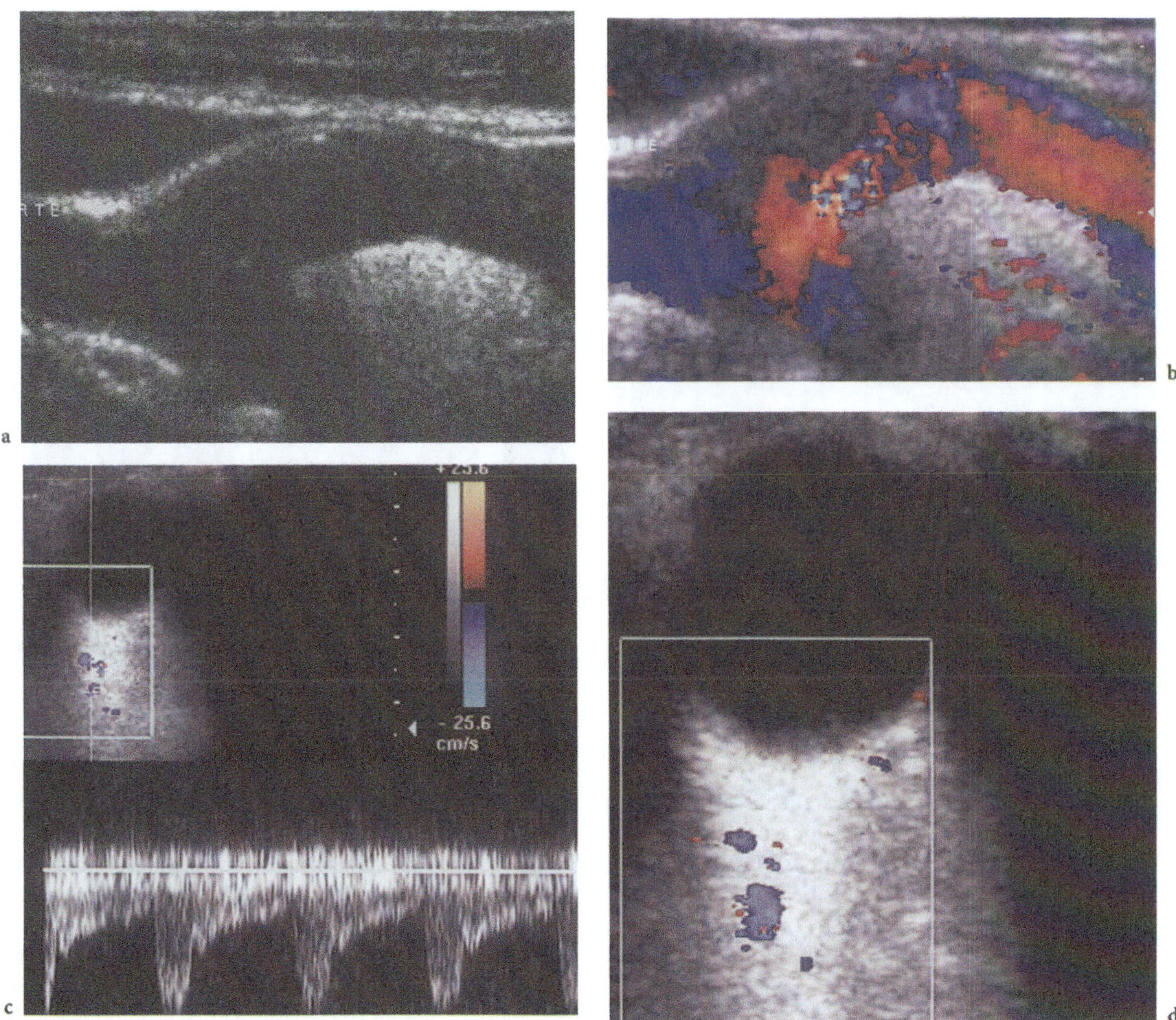

Fig. 6.30a–d. Tight stenosis of the ICA with type 1 plaque (**a**). Aliasing phenomenon on color Doppler (**b**). Flow reversal in the ophthalmic artery (**c** and **d**)

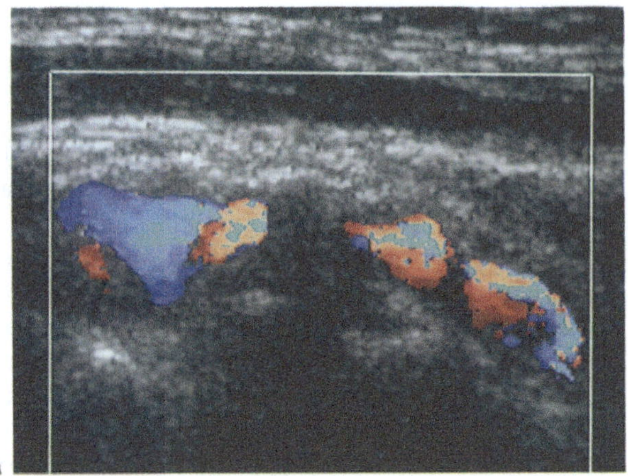

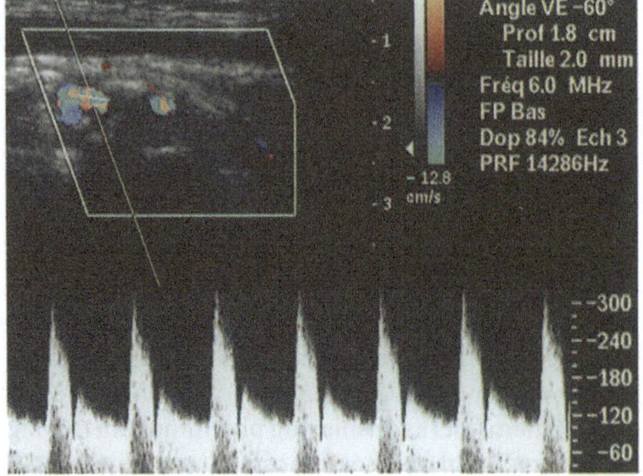

Fig. 6.31a,b. Long, tight stenosis of the ICA with calcified plaque. The aliasing phenomenon is visible despite the acoustic shadowing produced by the plaque (a). The spectral pattern near the plaque reveals acceleration of the flow velocity (more than 3 m/s) (b)

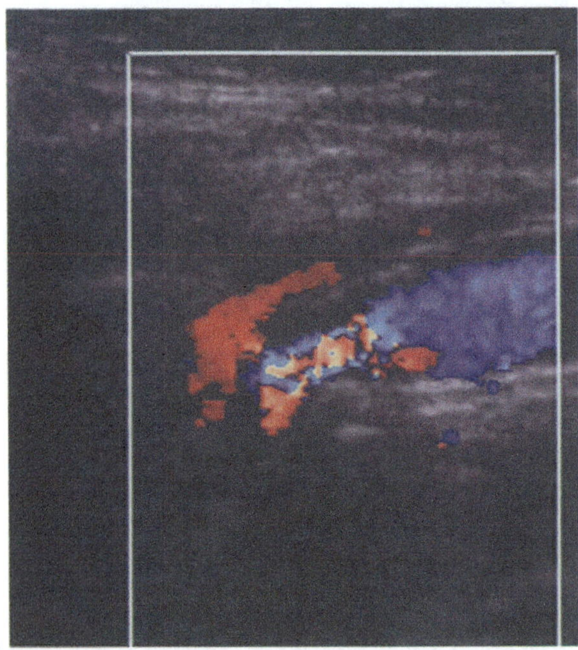

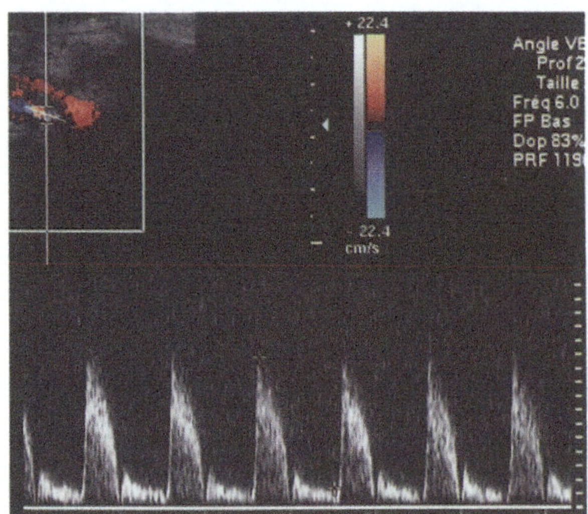

Fig. 6.32a,b. Stenosis of the ECA. Aliasing phenomenon on color Doppler (**a**). Spectral pattern revealing acceleration of the flow velocity (more than 2 m/s) (**b**)

PSV is observed in high-grade stenoses, and this can lead to an erroneous diagnosis of carotid occlusion.

For a given degree of carotid stenosis, the PSV can vary greatly among patients because this parameter depends on the length of the stenotic segment, its geometry, and individual hemodynamic factors (Moneta et al. 1995). Existence of an associated stenosis of the CCA, or the presence of collateral pathways related to contralateral carotid stenosis, can also produce lower PSV values that may result in underestimation of the stenosis (Abu Rahma et al. 1995; Beckett et al. 1990).

The EDV remains normal when arterial stenosis is less than 50%, owing to the absence of a pressure gradient across the stenosis during diastole. When stenosis exceeds 50%, a pressure gradient appears, and the EDV increases in proportion to the severity of the gradient, which rises rapidly once lumen narrowing exceeds 70% (Zwiebel 2000c). This parameter remains valid even for high-grade stenoses.

The SVR was developed to reduce errors due to variations in the PSV, and this parameter appears more effective for quantification of stenosis (Moneta et al. 1993). Calculation of the SVR can be very difficult for high-grade stenoses when the PSV is very high, as this may exceed the possibilities of the ultrasound unit. A unit equipped with a high PRF or continuous Doppler mode may prove helpful in such cases. The SVR is occasionally pathological in an otherwise normal individual.

Use of the DVR is hampered by an excessively high rate of false-positive errors (Lee et al. 1999).

6.2.5.2.3 Post-stenotic Zone

The post-stenotic zone is characterized by a drop in the intra-arterial pressure that produces relatively low flow velocities and nonlaminar flow. These flow disturbances are more or less proportional to the severity of luminal narrowing (Zwiebel 2000c). The resultant spectral broadening has been the subject of numerous attempts at quantifying the degree of stenosis, although results to date are inconclusive (Kalman et al. 1985).

Spectral broadening is proportional to the degree of stenosis, but does not allow quantification. Disappearance of the dark spectral systolic window (Fig. 6.33) suggests a stenosis greater than 50% in diameter but is not sufficiently specific (ESCT 1991). Complete signs of spectral broadening (elevated amplitude, low frequency signals, flow reversal, poor definition of the spectral border) suggest stenosis greater than 70%. In certain cases, and namely for stenosis on calcified plaque with acoustic shadowing that prevents analysis of the affected site, post-stenotic spectral broadening may be the sole diagnostic feature.

6.2.5.3 Doppler US Quantification of Carotid Stenosis

The essential step of quantifying carotid stenosis is hindered by two difficulties. First of all, several different methods exist for calculating the percentage of stenosis. Second, the validity and reproducibility of Doppler measurements remain controversial.

Stenosis can be expressed as a percentage reduction in diameter or cross-sectional area. Diameter reduction is most commonly used, particularly for defining therapeutic indications, because the same measurement is used in angiography. Moreover, owing to the variable geometry of stenosing plaque, no correlation exists between the percentage of diameter reduction caused by stenosis and the stenosed cross-sectional surface area.

On angiograms, the percentage of stenosis is defined by the ratio of the diameter of the circulating channel at the site of stenosis to the diameter of the ICA beyond the carotid bulb (NASCET 1991). The velocimetric criteria of stenosis in Doppler US are based essentially on angiographic data. Use of the carotid bulb diameter as a reference (ESCT 1991) can result in underestimation of the percentage of stenosis. In many studies, considerable uncertainly reigns about the techniques used to measure stenosis.

Multiple reports have described the efficacy of Doppler US for grading stenoses expressed in terms of diameter reduction as a function of velocimetric parameters and the SVR (Table 6.2). Unfortunately, the considerable differences among the equipment and techniques used for velocity measurement prevent valid comparison.

The sensitivity and specificity of Doppler US for the diagnosis of high-grade stenoses (more than 70% in diameter) remain controversial, ranging from 70% (Ackerman and Candia 1994; Ringelstein 1995) to more than 90% (Hoskins 1996; Howard et al. 1996; Steinke et al. 1990). The multiple sources of

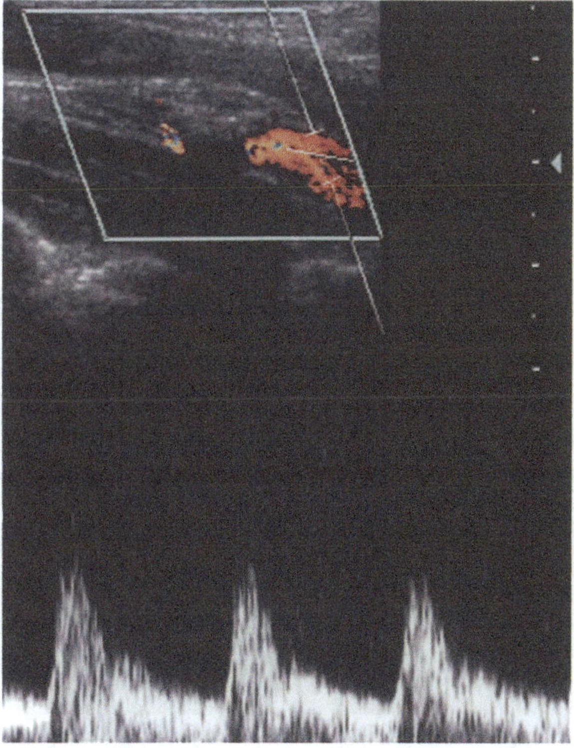

Fig. 6.33. Post-stenosis recording in the ICA; broadening of the systolic peak with disappearance of the dark systolic window

Table 6.2. Quantitative criteria for evaluation of the degree of stenosis

Reference	Stenosis (%)	PSV (cm/s)	EDV (cm/s)	SVR
Bluth et al. 1988	40–59	<130	<40	<1.8
	60–79	130–250	40–100	1.8–3.7
	80–99	>250	>100	>3.7
Robinson et al. 1988	<50	<150	<50	<2
	50–70	150–225	50–75	2–3
	>70	>225	>75	>3
Fraught et al. 1994	50–69	<130	<100	
	70–99	>130	>100	
Sidhu and Allan 1997	50–59	>130	<40	<3.2
	60–69	>130	40–110	3.2–4
	80–95	>230	110–140	>4
	95–99	>230	>140	>4

PSV peak systolic velocity; *EDV* end diastolic velocity; *SVR* systolic velocity ratio

error and variability in Doppler US measurements (namely velocity measurements) may explain this discordance.

Whenever possible, diameter ratios should be calculated directly using the duplex mode for color Doppler or power Doppler, even though results have not yet been completely validated (Fig. 6.34). In practice, such ideal evaluation is confronted with several difficulties: absence of direct access to the site of stenosis (calcifications, very high-lying topography), poor delineation of the arterial wall at the site of stenosis on B-mode imaging, defective fill-in of the residual channel on color Doppler. When the values obtained do not confirm velocimetric data, repeat measurements are advisable.

6.2.6 Carotid Occlusion

6.2.6.1 Etiologies

Most carotid occlusions are related to pre-existent atheroma. Other possible causes include carotid dissection or fibromuscular dysplasia. Occlusion of the ICA is by far the most frequent. The ECA and CCA may also be occluded, but involvement of the CCA is ten times less common than that of the ICA (Lee et al. 1996).

6.2.6.2 Positive Diagnosis

6.2.6.2.1 Occlusion of the ICA

Four cardinal signs are found on Doppler US (Mattos et al. 1992; Zwiebel 2000d): loss of axial

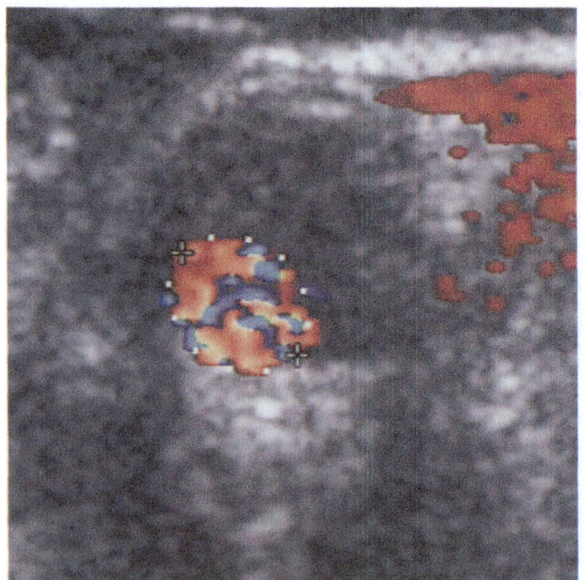

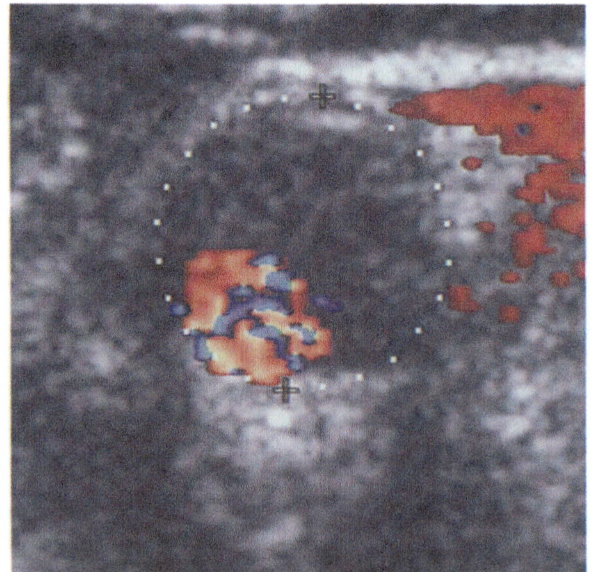

Fig. 6.34a,b. Spectral pattern of the CCA revealing high-resistance flow, with disappearance of the diastolic component (**a**). Thrombosis of the ICA with a recent echoic thrombus (**b**)

pulsatility in the ICA, luminal filling by the echoic thrombotic material, reduction of the vascular caliber in long-standing occlusions, and absence of flow demonstrable by color Doppler, even when settings are adjusted, in particular by lowering the PRF and the band pass filter (Fig. 6.35).

No correlation has been established between the age of a thrombus and the age of an occlusion (Maiuri et al. 1990). Owing to the absence of collaterals, thrombosis of the ICA often extends to the ostium.

The thrombotic material sometimes presents pulsations mimicking residual flow; the "back-and-forth" character and very low velocity are suggestive. In acute forms, an ICA stump that has conserved a reduced, alternating flow is demonstrated. The considerable reduction in the caliber of the ICA observed in old occlusions may lead to confusion with a thrombosis of the ECA, especially because the ECA is often voluminous, with a low resistance flow (Fig. 6.36) (Borstein et al. 1988; Bridgers 1989). The upstream impact on flow and reduction of the diastolic velocity in the CCA causes an elevation in the resistive index and a moderate reduction in the systolic peak. Owing to collateral mechanisms, the ECA may present a marked diastolic flow similar to the flow of the ICA, with which it must not be confused. The homolateral ophthalmic flow is reversed in 75% of cases.

Differentiation of a complete thrombosis from a prethrombotic stenosis can be difficult because a small residual channel may escape rapid analysis of imaging features (Gortler et al. 1994; Zwiebel and Crummy 1981). Any suspected occlusion should be assessed by lowering the PRF and the band pass filter to a minimum. Detection of a residual channel has a therapeutic interest because endarterectomy remains possible in such patients. Differential diagnosis is usually possible with modern US units (Kirsch et al. 1994; Steinke et al. 1990). More sensitive than color Doppler, power Doppler provides interesting data (Lee et al. 1996). Use of a low-frequency transducer permits evaluation of nearly the entire exocranial segment of the ICA. Although false-positive errors of occlusion occur in 15% of cases, use of ultrasound contrast agents appears to reduce this frequency (Abildgaard et al. 1996; Sitzer et al. 1993).

6.2.6.2.2
Occlusion of the CCA

Occlusion of the CCA is often characterized by clinical symptoms and is frequently associated with an ICVA (Fig. 6.37) (Chang et al. 1995). The ICA may remain patent owing to the existence of contralateral collaterals that revascularize the termination of the CCA and the ICA through the intermediary of the ECA supplied by the contralateral ECA. The ECA and certain of its branches show retrograde flow in such cases. This possibility should always be considered in case of CCA thrombosis because surgical revascularization is possible in such situations (Erickson et al. 1989; Zwiebel 2000d). The flow in the ICA is then often very diminished or even pseudovenous and must not be mistaken for venous flow with a reverse direction. Isolated occlusions or stenoses of the CCA should prompt a search for inflammatory or radiation-induced arteritis.

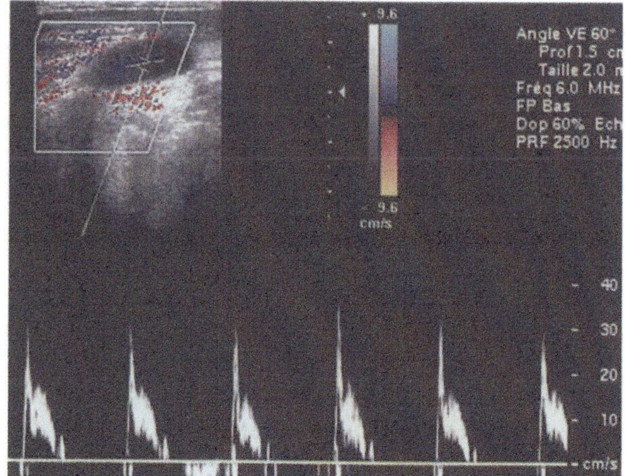

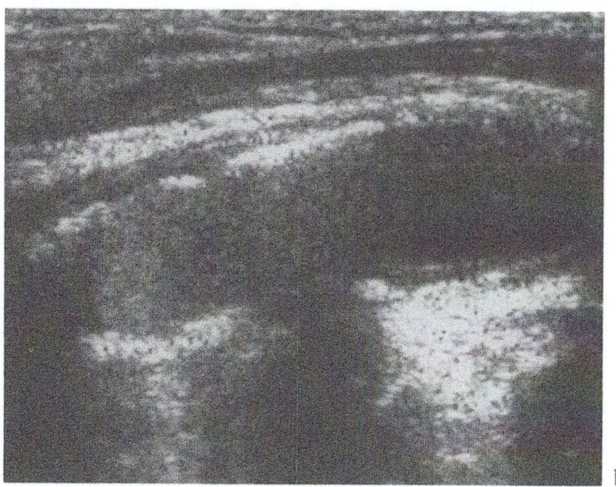

Fig. 6.35,a,b. ICA thrombosis. **a** CCA spectral pattern revealing high resistivity and disappearance of the diastolic component. **b** ICA thrombosis with a recent echoic thrombus

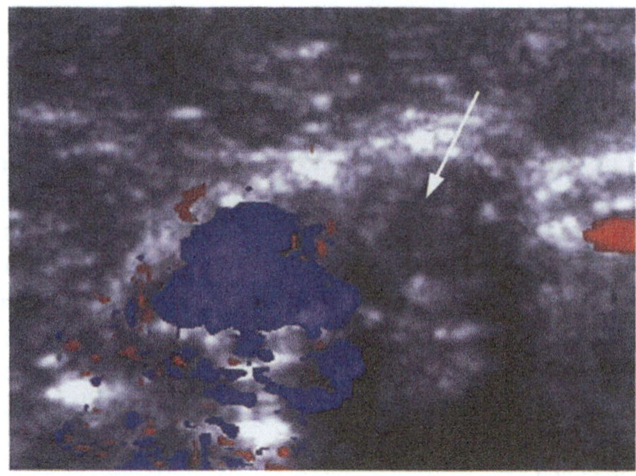

Fig. 6.36. Thrombosis of the ICA (*arrow*). The ECA remains patent (*arrowhead*)

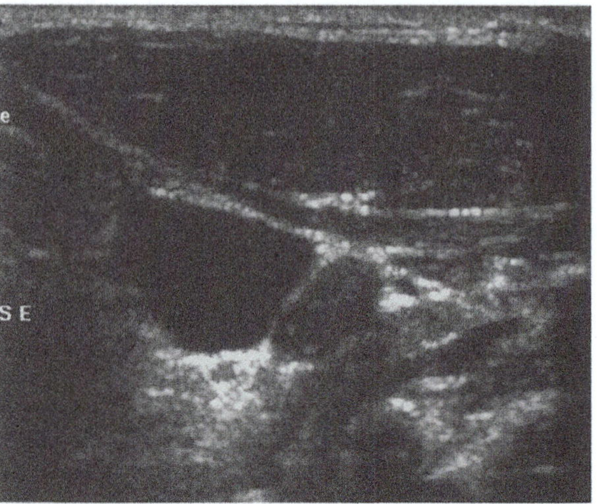

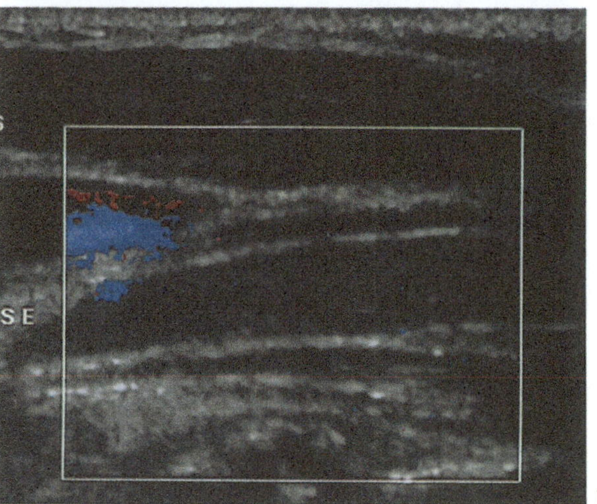

Fig. 6.37a,b. Long-standing thrombosis of a very small caliber CCA

6.2.7 Carotid Dissection

6.2.7.1 *Etiological Factors*

Longitudinal splitting of the arterial wall due to hemorrhage creates a circulating or thrombotic false channel (O'Dwyer et al. 1980; Van Damme et al. 1990). Cleavage usually affects the intima and part of the media. Fibromuscular dysplasia, certain connective tissue diseases (Marfan syndrome, Ehlers-Danlos syndrome), mucoid degeneration of the media, and arterial hypertension all promote dissection but are not the sole causes (Andersen 1980; Manelfe et al. 1974).

A traumatic origin is sometimes discovered. Severe trauma may result in extensive carotid dissection. More often, a careful history elicits mention of a nonroutine physical exercise involving the cervical spine, responsible for a pure internal carotid dissection or extension of an aortic dissection towards the CCA (Sellier et al. 1983).

"Spontaneous" dissections are a frequent cause of stroke in young individuals. The history sometimes reveals an episode of minor trauma (cervical manipulation, prolonged cervical hyperextension). The dissection usually occurs near the origin of the ICA; the intraparietal hematoma extends upwards to variable degrees, splitting the media. Progressive dissection may involve the subadventitia, in which case it may cause a false aneurysm or produce the equivalent of stenosis, or even lead to ICA thrombosis. Clinical signs are suggestive: cervicalgia irradiating to the hemiface preceding a contralateral neurological deficit, characteristic association with a Claude-Bernard-Horner syndrome reflecting involvement of the sympathetic plexuses (Mokri et al. 1979). IVCAs are often of embolic origin following migration of mural thrombi that have formed at the site of intimal rupture.

6.2.7.2 *Positive Diagnosis*

The examination of reference is angiography with selective catheterization of the CCA (Hauser et al. 1984; Provenzale 1995). Angiographic findings are highly variable: more or less extensive stenosis, occlusion, double contour appearance due to opacification of a false channel in which blood flow continues. Angiography remains the only technique capable of formally identifying residual flow and demonstrating false aneurysms. Signs of dysplasia should be sought on the other cervical and cerebral vessels (PETRO et al. 1987).

Doppler US findings often suggest stenosis or occlusion, in which case the etiology is determined from the clinical context (Fig. 6.38).

Attentive analysis on B-mode imaging may reveal a thin echogenic line oscillating within the carotid lumen that corresponds to an intimal flap. Color Doppler reveals the residual flow or may demonstrate distribution of the flow between the true and the false channels. All types of appearance are possible: stenosis with thrombosis of the false channel, double channel with an intimal flap, parietal hematoma, proximal pseudo-aneurysm (DE BRAY et al. 1994). Detection of pseudo-aneurysms is important, particularly in patients receiving anticoagulant treatment; these lesions may be very extensive and compress the lumen of the ICA. A weakly echoic parietal hematoma is sometimes visualized (CATTIN and BONNEVILLE 1995).

Spectral analysis reveals flow disturbances in the homolateral CCA, which presents a drop in its systolic peak and marked reduction of the diastolic component due to the upstream obstacle; the resistive index is elevated compared with the contralateral CCA. The homolateral ECA may present a less resistive flow, with a drop in the resistive index when the ECA participates in a collateral network implicating the ipsilateral ophthalmic artery, in which the flow may be reversed (ZWIEBEL 2000d).

Arteriography remains indispensable for high-lying dissections that may be overlooked by Doppler US. The contralateral cervical and cerebral vessels must be examined systematically in search of dysplastic lesions.

Dissections of the CCA are generally the result of aortic dissections that have extended to the CCA (Fig. 6.39). The accessibility of this artery facilitates diagnosis by Doppler US, because the intimal flap and flow separation are clearly visible on color Doppler. The false channel often presents a slow flow that is out of phase on color Doppler and weakly echoic on B-mode imaging. The systolic peak is often biphasic.

6.2.8 Loops and Folds

These anomalies may be associated with atherosclerosis or may occur in a context of dysplasia. Color Doppler and especially power Doppler can reveal the internal carotid loops (Fig. 6.40). A low-frequency transducer may prove helpful to search for high-lying loops.

Two presentations are usually described: coiling (often bilateral, of congenital origin) and kinking (usually of atherosclerotic origin) (CATTIN and BONNEVILLE 1995). Color Doppler and power Doppler can easily demonstrate these anomalies, which are a source of error with continuous Doppler.

On color Doppler, the abrupt change in the flow direction often creates an aliasing phenomenon; this is related to a reduction in the Doppler angle, and should not be considered indicative of stenosis. Signs equivalent to stenosis must be sought (acceleration validated with angle correction, turbulence, downstream slowing), namely in atheromatous folds.

No correlation has been established between these anomalies and the onset of stroke.

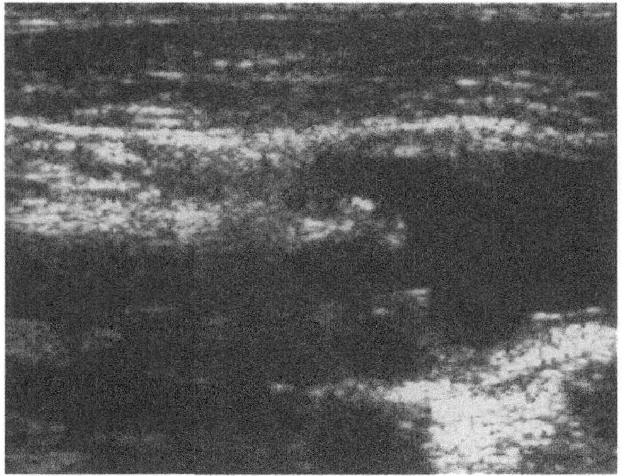
a

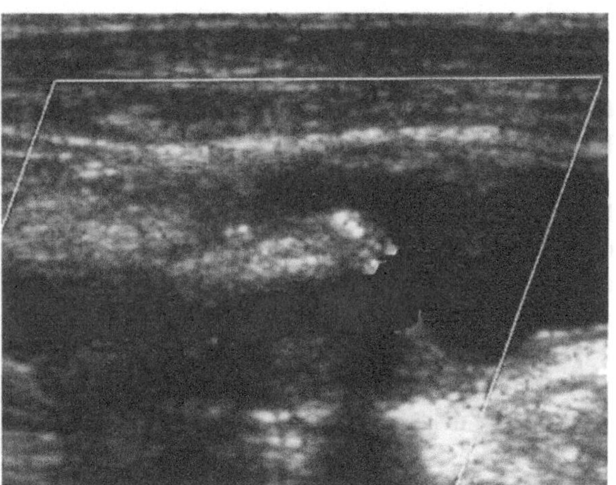
b

Fig. 6.38a,b. Dissection of the ICA from its origin, with thrombosis of the false channel

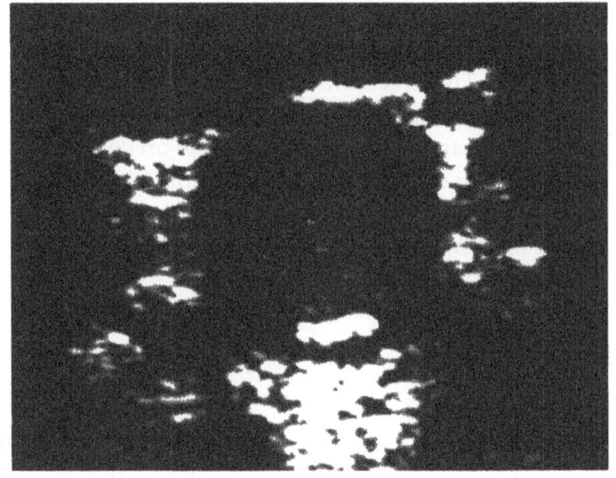
a

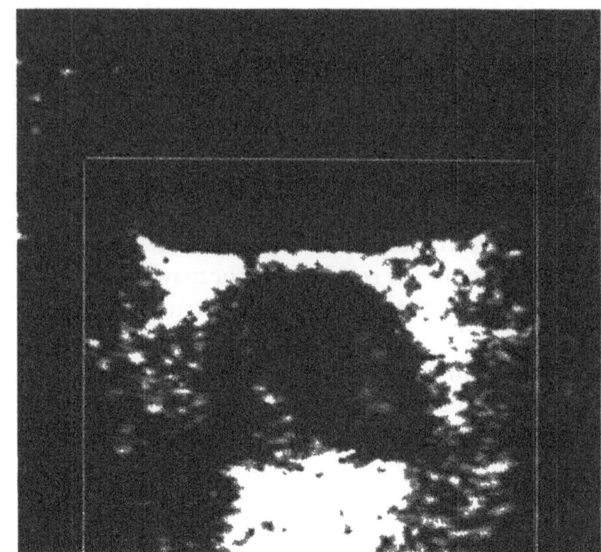
b

Fig. 6.39a,b. Dissection of the CCA following extension of an aortic dissection, with thrombosis of the false channel

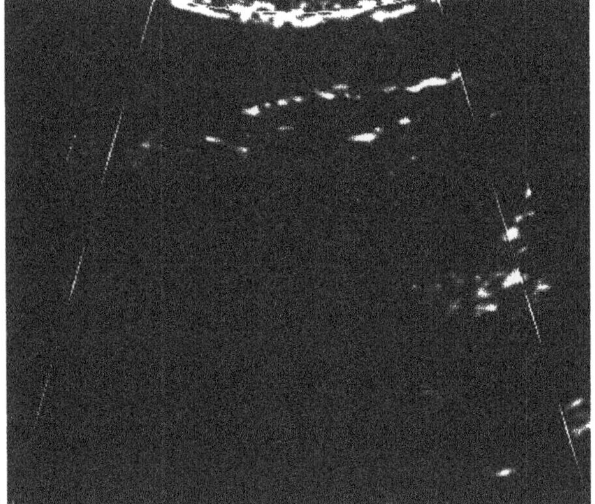
a

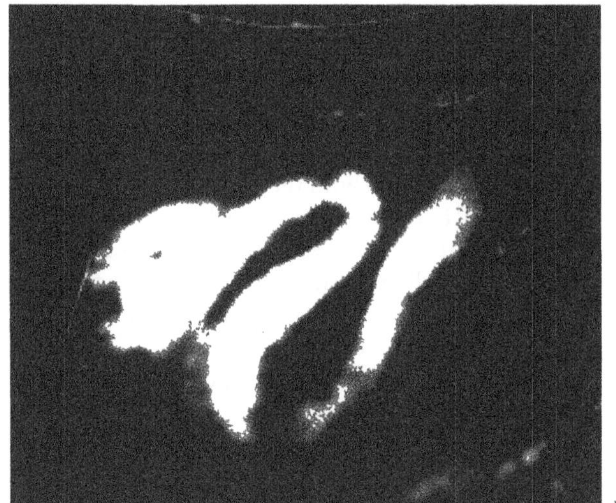
b

Fig. 6.40a,b. Loop of the ICA. Color Doppler study with a low-frequency transducer reveals the absence of stenosis (**a**). Power Doppler is not dependent on the insonation angle and thus permits better analysis (**b**)

6.2.9 Radiation-induced Arteritis

Diagnosis of radiation-induced arteritis is based on demonstration of arterial lesions in a territory irradiated at least 3 years previously (Cattin and Bonneville 1995). Irradiation for a head and neck cancer is the main cause; lesions are generally associated with infiltration of the soft tissues of the cervical region and cutaneous thickening. These fibrotic lesions essentially involve the media and the adventitia. Concomitant atheromatous lesions in these patients may be aggravated by irradiation (Dauzat 1991a).

Radiation-induced arteritis frequently affects the CCA, sometimes in a solitary manner. The most suggestive appearance is a succession of low-grade, concentric stenoses of the CCA that may be extensive, but often spare the carotid bifurcation.

Radiation-induced lesions image as homogeneous, hyperechoic thickening of the arterial wall (Fig. 6.41). Associated atheromatous lesions may be visible, owing to calcification or a heterogeneous pattern. The surface of these lesions (smooth or irregular) is accurately evaluated by color Doppler and power Doppler.

Radiation-induced arteritis can cause occlusion, and radiation-induced stenoses are a good indica-

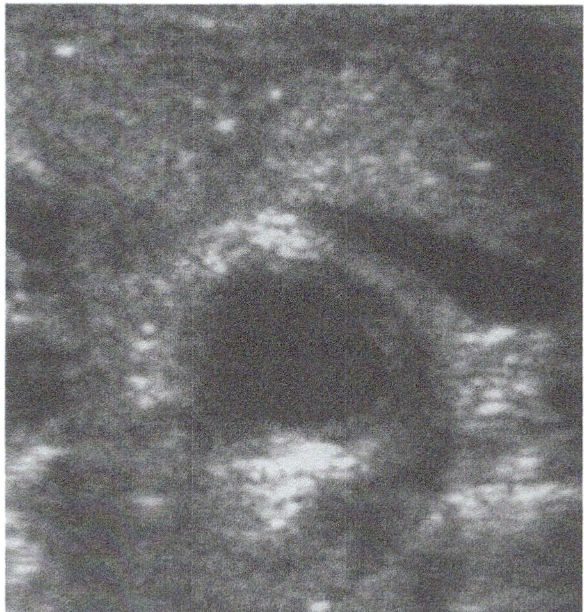

Fig. 6.41. Radiation-induced arteritis following irradiation for laryngeal cancer. Concentric thickening of the wall of the CCA

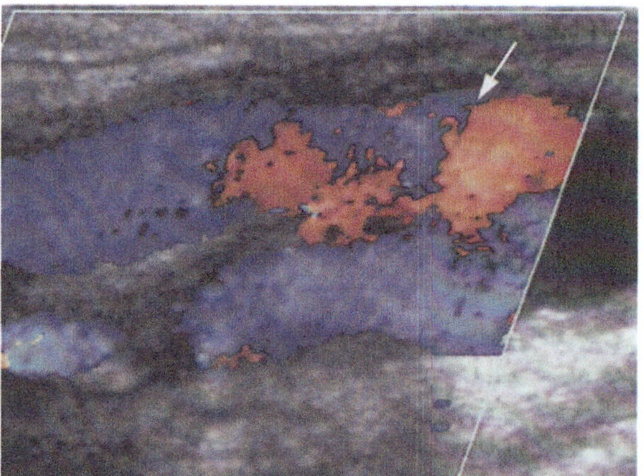

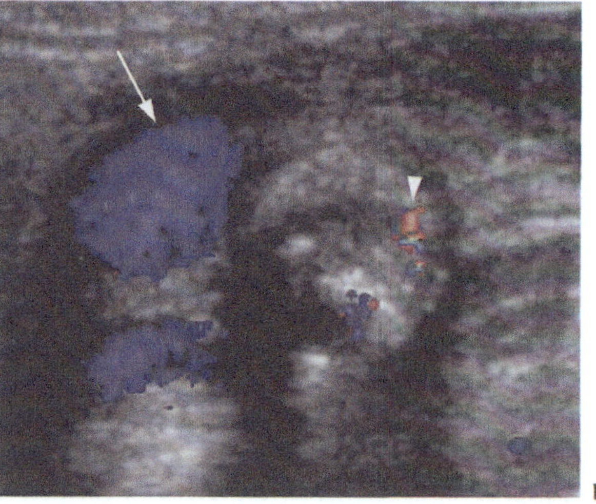

Fig. 6.42a,b. Verification of the patency of a carotid bypass (*arrow*). The anastomosis is clearly visible (**a**). The ICA is thrombosed, with partially calcified plaque and a twinkling artifact (**b**) (*arrowhead*)

tion for carotid angioplasty. Surgical treatment is extremely difficult (MELLIÈRE et al. 1990).

6.2.10 Post-operative Imaging Features

Color Doppler US may be very helpful for postoperative follow-up of patients managed by endarterectomy or a bypass procedure. Knowledge of the surgical technique used is essential (Fig. 6.42). During the early postoperative period, examination is rendered difficult by the surgical scar and tegmental infiltration, and a very posterior approach is mandatory.

After endarterectomy, 25% of patients have dilatation of the carotid bulb with significant marginal reflux, especially if a venous patch has been placed (DE BRAY et al. 1986). The hyperechoic internal border disappears up to the surgical margins; beyond this point the arterial wall has its usual appearance (Fig. 6.43) (DAUZAT 1991a). Echoic parietal thrombi may be present (MAROSI et al. 1986).

A search must be made for focal dissection with an intimal flap floating within the carotid lumen (CATTIN and BONNEVILLE 1995). Spectral recordings of the endarterectomy zone reveal flow turbulence that has no pathological signification in the early postoperative period and may persist for several months (ARBEILLE et al. 1989). Early postoperative stenoses have no particular features. Aside from detection of early postoperative complications, Doppler US is essential for follow-up owing to the possibility of carotid stenosis recurrence. Re-stenosis may be secondary to early intimal hyperplasia, which may be regressive and manifests as weakly echoic lesions (DE BRAY et al. 1989); recurrence of atheromatous lesions can result in late re-stenosis (ROHR-LE FLOCH et al. 1988).

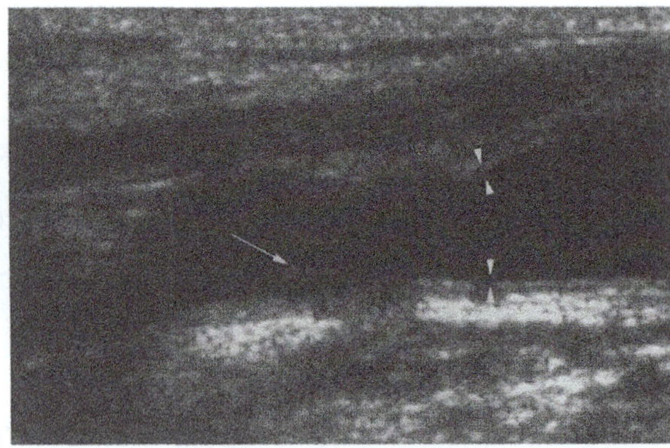
a

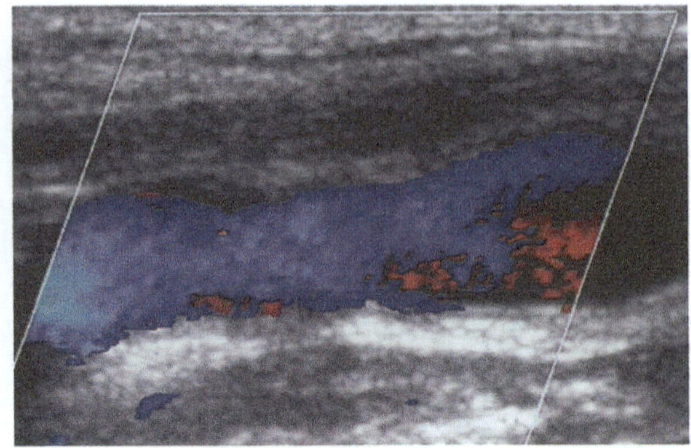
b

Fig. 6.43a,b. Post-endarterectomy appearance. The limits of the operated segment are clearly visible on B-mode imaging (*arrowheads*) (**a**). The intimal flap floating within the arterial lumen indicates focal dissection (*arrow*). Color Doppler reveals turbulent flow (**b**)

6.3 Vertebral Arteries

6.3.1 Normal Anatomy

Each vertebral artery (VA) arises from the homolateral subclavian artery. The vertebral ostium (V0) usually lies behind the clavicle, at the level of the posterior aspect of the subclavian artery (Fig. 6.1). The postostial course of the VA is often tortuous in older individuals. In this segment, termed V1, the vertebral artery is always accompanied by the vertebral vein, which is habitually anterior to the VA. The VA next penetrates the transverse foramen of vertebra C-6, then passes through the transverse processes of vertebral bodies C6–2. This rectilinear arterial portion is referred to as segment V2. During its passage through the transverse processes, the VA gives off small branches to the muscles and skeleton. These collaterals are anastomosed with the cervical arterial trunk arising from the branches of the thyrocervical trunk (TCT), which plays an important role in the event of VA occlusion. The VA then passes around the ipsilateral transverse process of vertebra C-1, forming a prominent loop directed posteriorly that corresponds to segment V3.Finally, the VA penetrates the occipital foramen in the posterior cranial fossa, where it joins with the contralateral VA, opposite the anterior surface of the cerebral trunk, to form the basilar trunk. This intracranial portion corresponds to segment V4. The VA is much smaller in diameter than the ICA and is asymmetric in size in 73% of normal individuals; the left VA is the dominant vessel in around 80% of such cases (Zwiebel 2000d). Hypoplasia of a VA is observed in 10% of subjects and is twice as frequent on the right side (Matula et al. 1977). Numerous possibilities for collateral flow exist for the VA; awareness of these compensatory mechanisms is essential to understanding the pathologies affecting these arteries (Hennerici and Neuerberg-Heusler 1998):

- Contralateral VA
- Circle of Willis: contralateral ICA (via the posterior communicating artery)
- Contralateral ECA (via the occipital artery)
- Homolateral subclavian artery (via the TCT).

6.3.2 Clinical Considerations

Vertebrobasilar insufficiency (VBI) is a complex entity of multifactorial origin without any specific clinical picture. Its pathogenesis is variable and is often unclear (Ausman et al. 1985). Owing to the great variability in symptoms, confusion is possible with other disorders producing similar neurological dysfunction (cardiac dysfunction, epilepsy, carotid stenosis, etc.).While atherosclerosis of the VA is the main cause of vertebrobasilar ischemia, other potential causes of VBI include hypotension, embolization, VA compression by osteophytes in segment V2, artery-to-artery steal syndromes, aneurysms of the VA or basilar trunk, direct involvement of the basilar trunk (occlusion, dissection), and occlusion of a portion of the distal arterial bed.

6.3.3 Examination Technique and Normal Findings

6.3.3.1 Subclavian Arteries

The subclavian arteries (SCAs) are visible and signals can be recorded over all or part of their course. The ostium of the right subclavian artery can be accessed using recurrent retroclavicular scans, but the ostium of the left SCA is rarely identifiable (Fig. 6.44).The SCA can be followed over its proximal and distal subclavian segments.

Owing to their primary destination towards the muscles, the subclavian arteries have high resistance waveforms with a protodiastolic reflux (Bendick and Jackson 1986; Touboul et al. 1986)

6.3.3.2 Vertebral Arteries

Localization of the vertebral arteries is more difficult, owing to their small size, their deep location, and their position within the transverse processes in segment V2. Examination requires longitudinal scans and a lower frequency transducer (5 MHz) than for carotid studies. Transducers with a high frequency or a wide frequency range including frequencies of more than 10 MHz often have insufficient sensitivity for color Doppler examination of individuals with a thick neck. Examination of the VA must be methodical to be effective; all three cervical levels must be examined, including spectral analysis.

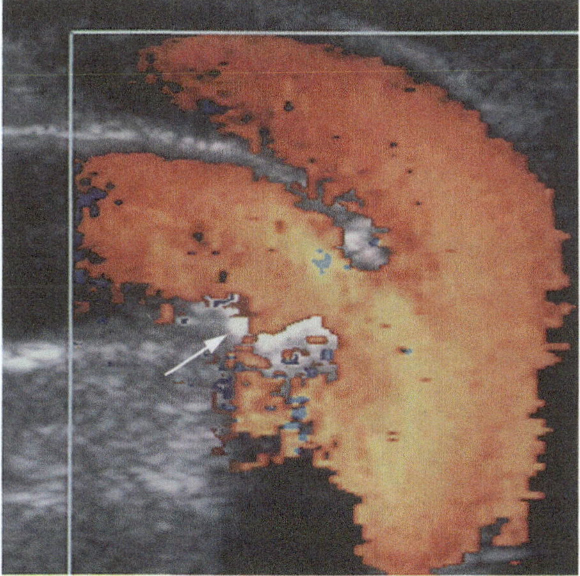

Fig. 6.44. Color Doppler: scan through the termination of the brachiocephalic arterial trunk revealing calcified plaque (*arrow*) at the ostium of the right subclavian artery. The ostium of the right CCA is also clearly visible

6.3.3.2.1 Segment V2

In practice, it appears more convenient to examine the V2 segment first. Identification of the transverse processes is an indispensable prerequisite. The CCA is first identified in the longitudinal plane in B-mode imaging. The transducer is then angled posteromedially and displaced slightly laterally until the transverse processes are seen (Bendick and Glover 1990). Color Doppler can then be performed with the PRF set lower than for carotid assessment.

Owing to the interposition of the bony structures, beam steering is not always contributory for evaluation of segment V2. If no signal is obtained, the PRF should be gradually lowered. On longitudinal scans, both vertebral vessels can often be imaged over several intertransverse process spaces (Fig. 6.45). The vertebral vein is usually visible anterior to the artery (Bartels et al. 1992). Color Doppler reveals the direction of flow in the VA, which is reversed compared with the adjacent vein; colorization is identical to that of the flow in the CCA. The diameter of the VA can then be measured. Cervical arthrosis with extensive osteophytosis can hinder or even prevent evaluation of segment V2 (Hennerici and Neuerberg-Heusler 1998).

The mean diameter of the vertebral artery in segment V2 is 4 mm. The pulsed Doppler waveforms of the VA are similar to those of the ICA (low resistance with an elevated diastolic component) (Fig. 6.46). The waveform pattern is symmetrical from one VA to another, but velocimetric data vary greatly owing to the frequent asymmetry of the VA. The peak systolic velocity (PSV) usually ranges from 20 to 40 cm/s; values less than 10 cm/s are considered pathological. Higher values are seen in patients with hypoplasia, stenosis, or occlusion of the contralateral VA (Bendick and Glover 1990).

6.3.3.2.2 Segments V0 and V1

Segment V1 and the ostium (V0) are examined using oblique axial or sagittal scans after localization of the vertebral artery as it enters C-2 (Fig. 6.47). The ostium is visible in 90% of cases on the right side and in 67% on the left side, lying on the posterosuperior

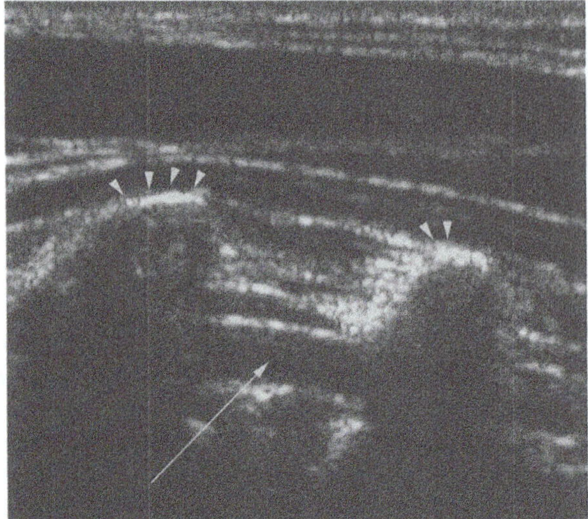

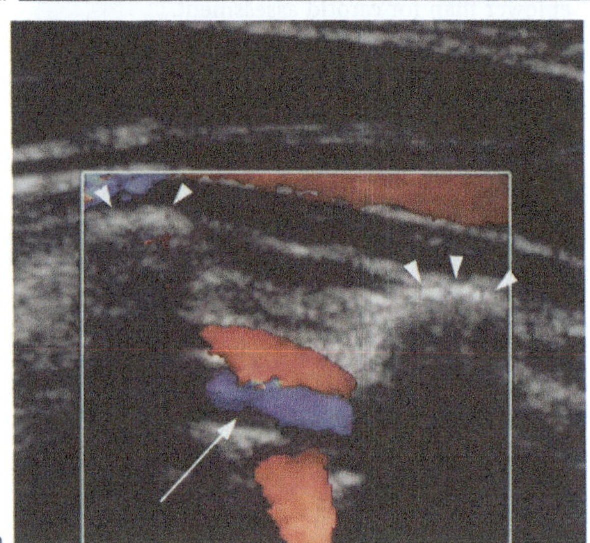

◁ **Fig. 6.45a,b.** Vertebral artery: segment V2. B-mode (**a**) and color Doppler (**b**). The vertebral artery (*arrow*) is always located posterior to the vertebral vein. The transverse processes are clearly visible (*arrowheads*)

Fig. 6.46. Spectral pattern of the vertebral artery in segment V2: low-resistance flow similar to that of an ICA

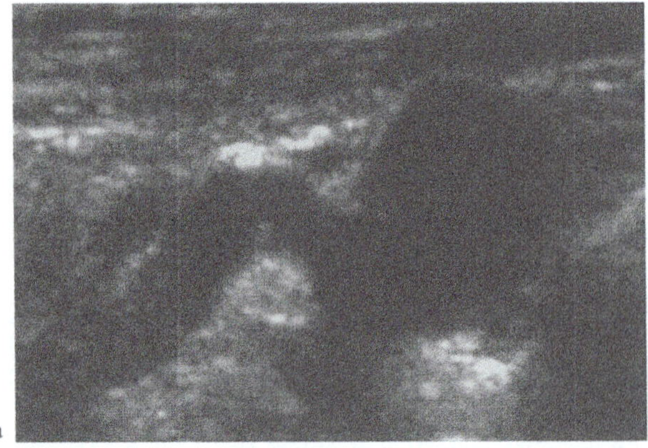

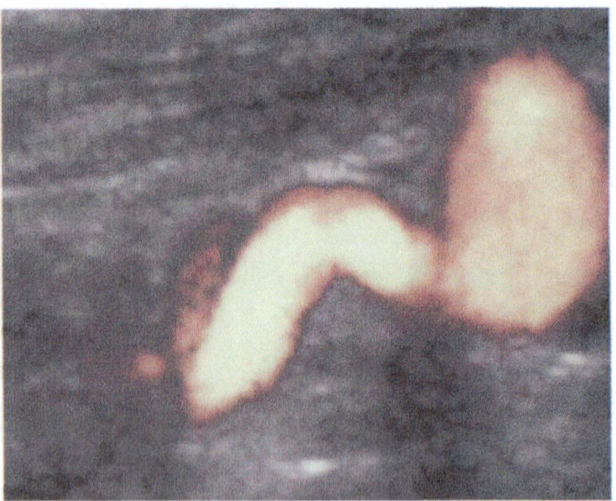

Fig. 6.47a,b. Right vertebral artery: longitudinal scan of the ost-ium (V0) and segment V1 in B-mode (**a**) and power Doppler (**b**)

surface of the homolateral subclavian artery (Trattnig et al. 1990). The posterior location of the ostium and the tortuous nature of the VA hamper examination. Segment V1 is tortuous in 39% of individuals (Matula et al. 1997). Power Doppler and a low-frequency transducer are helpful (Koga et al. 1999). On the left side, the vertebral artery may originate directly from the aortic arch. The right vertebral artery may arise from the origin of the right ICA. Confusion may arise between VA segment V1 and the subclavian branches to the neck, such as the TCT. Meticulous analysis of the arterial course and the pulsed Doppler waveform correct the diagnosis, because the TCT has a high resistance flow. The minor flow disturbances commonly observed in V0 and V1 have no particular significance (Zwiebel 2000d).

6.3.3.2.3
Segment V3

Segment V3 can also be visualized in 75% of cases as a loop behind the mastoid with an internal concavity (Fig. 6.48). The direction of flow varies very rapidly in this segment and can cause errors in velocity measurements. A low-frequency sector transducer with good color sensitivity is helpful. Confusion with the occipital artery is possible. Spectral analysis can correct the diagnosis because the occipital artery, a branch of the ECA, has a more resistive flow than the VA. In addition, only the occipital artery is compressible (Dauzat 1991b).

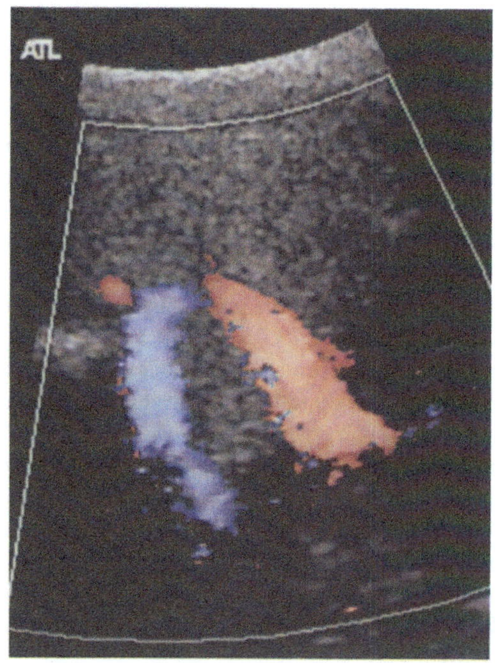

Fig. 6.48. Vertebral artery: segment V3 forms a posteriorly concave loop; examination performed with a low-frequency transducer (2–4 MHz)

6.3.3.3
Synthesis and Documentation of Results

Interpretation of Doppler studies of the VA requires caution; clinical findings and the examination conditions (and namely the exhaustive character of the study of the VA in its cervical course) must be indicated in the report.

Nonvisualization of a VA, which suggests an occlusion, should be interpreted in the light of technical conditions; failure to visualize the artery may actually be due to hypoplasia, agenesis of the VA, or even insufficiently sensitive ultrasound equipment. Direct visualization of the VA on B-mode imaging thus remains essential.

The following data should be reported (Zwiebel 2000d): spectrum of each SCA downstream of V0; visibility of each VA (nonvisualization of any cervical segment should be indicated); diameter of each VA in segment V2; spectrum of each VA in segment V2 with measurement of the PSV. Any anomalies observed should also be mentioned: nonvisible VA, diameter less than 2 mm, VA visible on B-mode imaging but no detectable flow on color Doppler, increased flow velocity, reduced flow velocity, abnormal flow direction.

6.3.4
Vertebral Artery Stenosis

Vertebral artery stenosis occurs primarily at the ostium and is usually due to atheromatous plaque. Aside from a few very favorable cases involving segments V0 and V1, analysis of the atherosclerotic lesion is not possible by B-mode imaging. Owing to the incomplete visibility of the artery at V0, search for indirect signs of stenosis is essential (Bluth et al. 1989). Doppler features are similar to those for carotid stenoses: accelerated flow velocity associated with turbulence. A PSV of more than 40 m/s is suggestive of stenosis greater than 50% (Bendick and Jackson 1986). The downstream flow is often diminished, with a drop in the PSV, a reduction in the resistive index, and broadening of the systolic peak.

Continuous Doppler is occasionally helpful when the vertebral ostium is inaccessible (Cattin and Bonneville 1995).

The second most common site of VA stenosis is segment V3. V3 stenoses, like lesions at high-lying sites (segment V4 or the basilar trunk), may be suggested by indirect signs concerning upstream flow (reduction in the PSV with elevation of the resistive index). The systolic peak is narrow and the diastolic component is reduced or absent (Bendick and Glover 1990).

Extrinsic compression of the VA may occur in segment V2 as the artery passes through the foramina of C1–6 owing to uncarthrosis. Signs of positional VBI exist in such cases. Doppler analysis reveals a brief acceleration, then sudden interruption of the VA in segment V3 when the head is rotated by several degrees (Attlan et al. 1999; Nakamura et al. 1998). Positional modifications in VA flow are observed in 17% of elderly patients with signs of VBI (Jargiello et al. 1998).

In contrast to carotid stenosis, accurate quantification of vertebral artery stenosis does not appear possible at this time.

6.3.5 Vertebral Artery Occlusion

Vertebral artery occlusion is often due to proximal atheromatous lesions; it may also occur secondary to a dissection (Ackerstaff et al. 1988). VA occlusion is frequently asymptomatic, owing to collateral mechanisms that involve the cervical branches of the ipsilateral thyrocervical trunk and the occipital artery, which often anastomose with the VA at the level of segment V3 (Cattin and Bonneville 1995).

B-mode imaging can directly reveal the echoic thrombosed arterial lumen (Fig. 6.49). Very often, the VA is not visible, and no signal is detected on color Doppler. A VA diameter of less than 2 mm and clear visibility of the vertebral vein are complementary diagnostic features. A recording of segment V3 is indispensable, using either continuous Doppler or a low-frequency transducer (Dauzat 1991b).

Distal VA occlusions are less common; they manifest essentially by indirect upstream signs, with high-resistance waveforms in segments V1 and V2, sometimes associated with transient reversal of the VA flow.

Differentiation of aplasia or severe hypoplasia from occlusion can be difficult. In cases of VA agenesis, no artery is seen on B-mode imaging of segments V1 and V2. Diagnosis of occlusion is based on color Doppler demonstration of the absence of flow, even with a minimum PRF and an elevated gain, whereas the VA is visible on B-mode imaging. When the ostium is visible, an initial residual stump with a retrograde flow may be observed. In case of hypoplasia, the flow in the VAs constantly has a reduced velocity and amplitude and elevated resistivity, the contralateral VA being of large diameter. Hypoplastic VAs usually do not rejoin the basilar trunk and terminate by a posteroinferior cerebellar artery (Attlan et al. 1999). A VA reperfused by collaterals owing to a subjacent occlusion presents a low-resistivity diminished flow.

Differentiation of VA occlusion from a very tight stenosis can also prove difficult (Visona et al. 1986).

6.3.6 Vertebral Artery Dissection

The vertebral artery is often subject to dissection owing to compression or stretching when the head is moved. All three levels of the cervical VA can be affected. The muscles, arthritic lesions (osteophytes), or even the atlas and axis may be implicated (Caplan et al. 1988). Combined cervical extension and rotation often modifies the vertebral flow, causing elevation of the pulsatility index that predominates during dextrorotation. This underscores the potential danger of cervical manipulation (Li et al. 1999).

In addition to severe trauma, minor trauma can also cause dissection (sports, professional activity

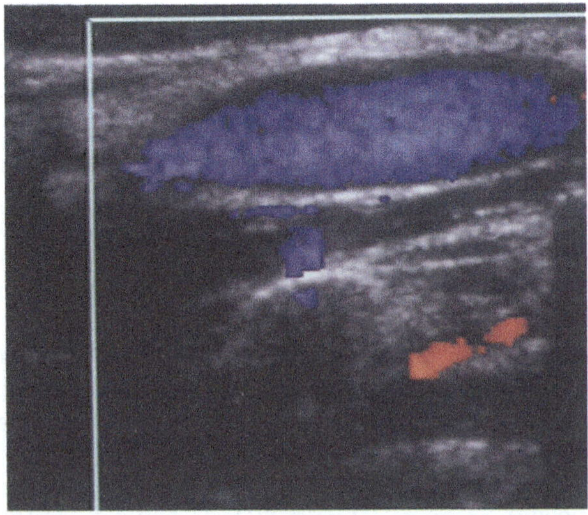

Fig. 6.49. Occlusion of a vertebral artery: absence of visible signal in segment V2; the vertebral artery is localized on B-mode and the vertebral vein presents a color signal

with prolonged or unusual cervical hyperextension, vertebral manipulation) (Chiras et al. 1985; Hart 1988; Frumkin and Baloh 1990). Like carotid dissections, certain lesions promote VA dissection: fibromuscular dysplasia, connective tissue disorders, mucoid degeneration of the media, arterial hypertension (Mokri et al. 1988).

The clinical picture is variable; cervicalgia is common, sometimes associated with occipital headaches followed by signs of ischemia in the affected vertebrobasilar territory. Female predominance has been noted. The severity of clinical symptoms and possible sequelae parallel intracranial extension of the dissection (De Bray et al. 1997). The termination of segments V2 and V3 are the sites of predilection (Fig. 6.50).

Angiography remains the gold standard of examination. Several presentations have been described (Greselle et al. 1987; Touboul et al. 1988): stenosis secondary to thrombosis of the false channel or compression by a false aneurysm related to a subadventitial dissection; occlusion; double circulating channel with intimal flap; false aneurysm possibly responsible for a parietal irregularity or stenosis.

Doppler US may permit diagnosis of dissections in segments V1 and V2 by revealing direct signs such as stenosis, ectasia, and, on rare occasion, an intimal flap with a double circulating channel (Bartels and Flügel 1996; Touboul et al. 1988). Anomalies exist on Doppler US in 94% of patients, but specific signs (segmental dilatation of the VA with visualization of the eccentric circulating channel) are seen in only 19% (De Bray et al. 1997).

The signs of VA stenosis or occlusion are often nonspecific, and only the clinical context suggests the diagnosis.

Doppler US is an excellent means of monitoring repermeabilization that permits adjustment of anticoagulant treatment.

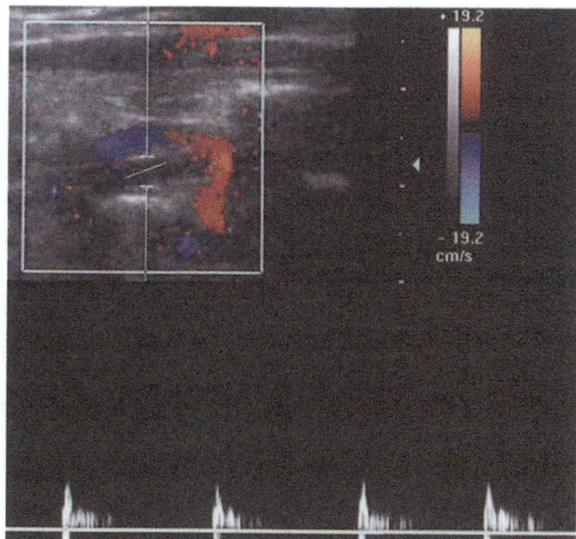

Fig. 6.50. Waveform of the vertebral artery in segment V2 presenting very slow flow velocities with disappearance of the diastolic component but without flow reversal. Appearance related to a high-lying dissection (segments V3 and V4)

6.3.7 Subclavian Steal

This particular form of VBI is caused by a high-grade atherosclerotic stenosis or occlusion of a subclavian artery proximal to the origin of the homolateral VA. Collateralization reverses the flow in the VA. Stenosis of the prevertebral segment of the SCA is left-sided in 85% of cases; only 15% of cases involve the right SCA or the innominate trunk.

Subclavian steal is usually asymptomatic; possible neurological deficits reflect involvement of the vertebrobasilar territory: bilateral visual disorders, headaches, auditory disorders, vertigo. They occur or are aggravated during an effort involving the upper limb on the side of the stenosis. Severe ischemic accidents in the vertebrobasilar territory occur especially when other arterial lesions are associated. The humeral arterial pressure is significantly reduced on the affected side, and there is often increased fatigability of the upper limb. Ischemic vertebrobasilar accidents are rare; collateral supply via the circle of Willis is always inadequate in such cases (Hennerici et al. 1988).

Doppler US is highly effective for diagnosis of subclavian steal; its sensitivity is markedly better than that of angiography, namely for early stages (Ackerstaff et al. 1984; Carroll and Holder 1990).

Signs vary with the extent of involvement; spectral analysis provides the most useful data; continuous Doppler is also of unquestionable interest in this pathology (Dauzat 1991b). The earliest symptom (stage I) is a notch in the systolic peak of the VA (Walker et al. 1982).

Transient steal (stage II) is characterized by reversal of the vertebral flow in systole; the diastolic flow remains orthograde, and on color Doppler has a to-and-fro pattern (alternation of the color of the AV flow).

Permanent steal (stage III) is related to complete vertebral flow reversal (Fig. 6.51); the vertebral artery and vein present the same coding on color Doppler (Attlan et al. 1999; De Bray et al. 1980).

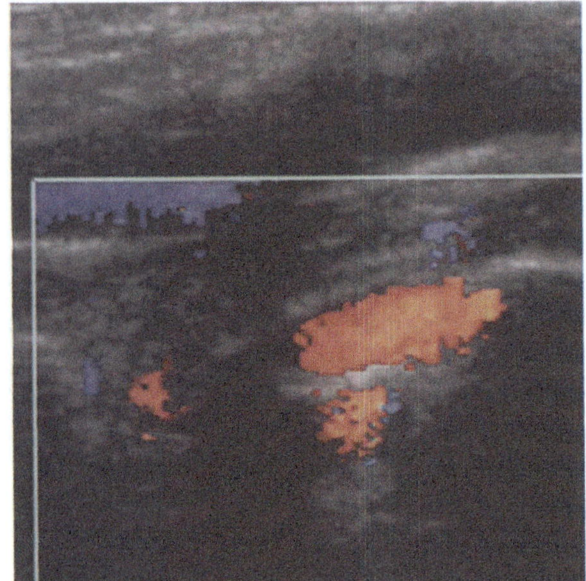

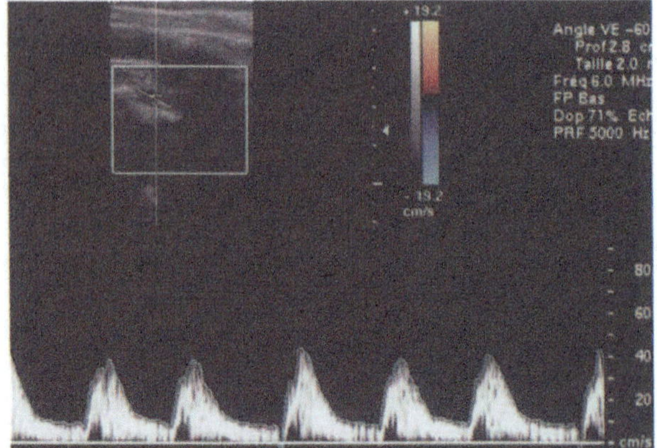

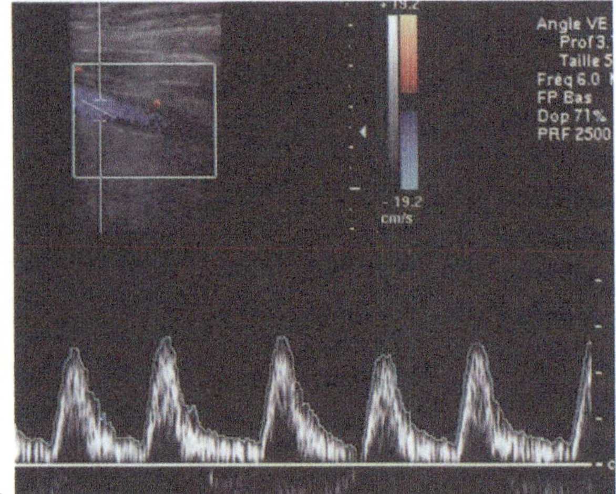

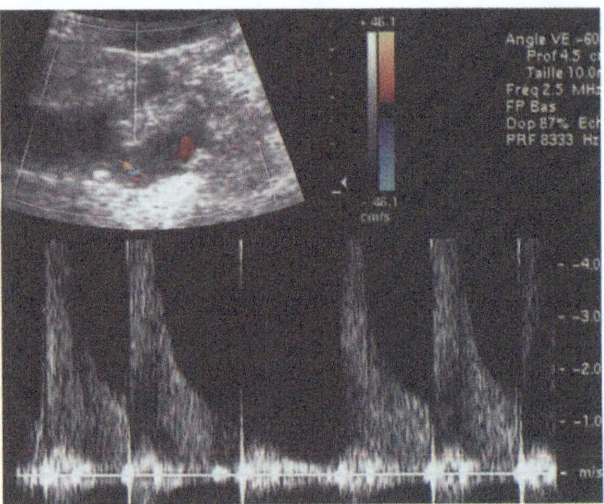

Fig. 6.51a–d. Vertebrosubclavian steal, stage III. Complete reversal of flow in the right vertebral artery (**a**) that has a slightly diminished spectral pattern (**b**). Appearance identical to the spectral pattern of the homolateral subclavian artery (**c**). Ostial stenosis of the right subclavian artery with acceleration of the flow velocity (more than 4 m/s) (**d**)

Provocation tests can be used. A blood pressure cuff is inflated on the side of the stenosis until blood flow is interrupted for 1 min at a value of more than two points compared with the humeral systolic pressure. Deflation of the cuff causes reactional hyperemia of the upper limb. Simultaneous recording of the homolateral VA reveals patent signs of steal, with flow reversal or merely an increase in the systolic notch. This test is of diagnostic interest only for stage I, when early steal must be distinguished from a stenosis of the vertebral ostium, both of which produce a systolic notch on spectral analysis (Cattin and Bonneville 1995). It is interesting as well for determination of whether the steal phenomena also affects the homolateral ICA (vertebrocarotid steal via the posterior communicating artery) or the contralateral ECA (via the occipital or ascending cervical arteries). These phenomena manifest as an increase in the diastolic velocities of the affected arteries when the cuff is deflated (Attlan et al. 1999).

Vertebral flow reversal is sometimes associated with a subjacent vertebral occlusion in patients with stenosis of the SCA, but without steal phenomena (Paivansalo et al. 1998).

Direct demonstration of a subclavian stenosis is easier on the right side, where the ostium is generally visible. Direct signs of stenosis include flow acceleration with broadening of the systolic peak and the presence of turbulence. Often, only indirect downstream signs are recorded: broadening of the systolic peak, disappearance of the protodiastolic reflux, global decrease.

6.3.8 Value and Limitations of Doppler US

Color Doppler US remains controversial for examination of the VA, owing to the small diameter of these arteries. All too often, examination is incomplete. Possibilities for error are numerous: confusion with other arteries, complexity of collateral networks, confusion of hypoplasia and occlusion, failure to demonstrate moderate or high-lying stenoses. Certain authors consider Doppler examination of the VA unnecessary or even inadvisable, as these vessels supply the cervical and cerebral territories, and they advocate angiography or MR angiography instead (ZWIEBEL 2000d). This attitude, often based on the results of studies prior to 1990 using continuous Doppler and pulsed Doppler, requires re-evaluation today. Technical progress in color Doppler imaging and systematic use of transcranial Doppler for segment V4 should permit vertebral Doppler studies to approach the diagnostic efficacy of carotid Doppler US (BARTELS and FLÜGEL 1993). Compared with digitized angiography, Doppler US has only moderate sensitivity for the detection of VA stenosis and occlusion (70%–90%). In contrast, its specificity is excellent (more than 95%) (WINTER et al. 1987). Results are even better in the most recent studies, in which color Doppler is used systematically and where sensitivity and specificity for the diagnosis of stenosis exceed 90% (BARTELS and FLÜGEL 1996; PFADENHAUER and MULLER 1995; SLIWKA et al. 1992). Greater than 90% sensitivity has also been reported for the diagnosis of dissection (BARTELS and FLÜGEL 1996). The association of power Doppler with color Doppler has a sensitivity of 90% and a specificity of 97% for the detection of VA anomalies (RIES et al. 1998). Doppler US is the most effective technique for the diagnosis of subclavian steal, with an accuracy of 100% (HENNERICI and NEUERBERG-HEUSLER 1998).

References

Abildgaard A, Egge TS, Klow NE, Jakobsen JA (1996) Use of sonicated albumin (Infoson) to enhance arterial spectral and color Doppler imaging. Cardiovasc Intervent Radiol 19:265–271

Abu Rahma AF, Richmond BK, Robinson PA (1995) Effect of contralateral severe stenosis of carotid occlusion on duplex criteria of ipsilateral stenoses: comparative study of various duplex parameters. J Vasc Surg 22:751–762

ACAS (Executive Committee for the Asymptomatic Carotid Atherosclerosis Study) (1995) Endarterectomy for asymptomatic carotid artery stenosis. JAMA 273:1421–1428

Ackerman RH, Candia MR (1994) Identifying clinically relevant carotid disease. Stroke 25:1–3

Ackerstaff RGA, Hoeneveld H, Slowikowski JM (1984) Ultrasonic duplex scanning in atherosclerotic disease of the innominate, subclavian and vertebral arteries. A comparative study with angiography. Ultrasound Med Biol 10:419–428

Ackerstaff RGA, Grosveld WJHM, Eikelboom BC, Ludwig JW (1988) Ultrasonic duplex scanning of the prevertebral segment of the vertebral artery in patients with cerebral atherosclerosis. Eur J Vasc Surg 2:387–393

Albrecht T, Urbank A, Mahler M (1998) Prolongation and optimization of Doppler enhancement with a microbubble US contrast agent by using continuous infusion. Preliminary experience. Radiology 207:339–347

Andersen CA (1980) Spontaneous dissection aneurysm of internal carotid artery associated with fibromuscular dysplasia. Am Surg 46:233–236

Arbeille P (1996) Sémiologie des paramètres physiques des ultrasons. JEMU 17:401

Arbeille P, Rabut H, Lapierre F, Bonithon MC (1989) Evolution du flux carotidien après endartériectomie. Artères Veines 8:165–168

Arbeille P, Bouin-Pineau MH, Philippot M, Aesch H (1996) Suivi des paramètres morphologiques des plaques d'athérome sur 24 mois. JEMU 17:337–341

Attlan E, Samson M, Melki P (1999) Troncs supra-aortiques cervicaux. In: Melki P, Hélénon O, Cornud F (eds) Echo-Doppler vasculaire et viscéral. Masson, Paris

Ausman JI, Shrontz CE, Pearce JE (1985) Vertebrobasilar insufficiency. A review. Arch Neurol 42:803–808

Avril G, Batt M, Guidoin R (1991) Plaques d'endartériectomie carotidienne: corrélations anatomo-cliniques. Ann Chir Vasc 5:50–54

Barnett HJM, Taylor DW, Eliosziw M (1998) Benefit of carotid endarterectomy in patients with symptomatic moderate or severe stenosis. N Engl J Med 26:1747–1752

Bartels E, Flügel KA (1993) Advantages of color Doppler imaging for the evaluation of vertebral arteries. J Neuroimaging 3:229–233

Bartels E, Flügel KA (1996) Evaluation of extracranial vertebral artery dissection with duplex color-flow imaging. Stroke 27:290–295

Bartinsky WS, Darbouze P, Nemen P (1981) Significance of ulcerated plaque in transient cerebral ischemia. Am J Surg 141:353–358

Bartels E, Fuchs HH, Flügel KA (1992) Duplex ultrasonography of vertebral arteries: examination, technique, normal values and clinical applications. Angiography 43:169–180

Bassiouny HS, Sakaguchi Y, Mikucki SA (1977) Juxtaluminal location of plaque necrosis and neoformation in symptomatic carotid stenosis. J Vasc Surg 26:585–594

Baud JM, Lemasle P, Gras C (1988) Evaluation du potentiel emboligène des plaques carotidiennes par l'écho-Doppler. A propos de 113 confrontation macroscopiques. J Mal Vasc 13:33–40

Baud JM, Lemasle P (1993) Devenir évolutif des plaques carotidiennes asymptomatiques peu sténosantes. Actualites Vasc Int 11:21–25

Baud JM, Lemasle P (1995) Quantification and assessment of the carotid lesions: stenosis degree and plaque volume. J Clin Ultrasound 23:113–124

Baud JM, De Bray JM, Delanoy P (1996) Reproductibilité ultrasonore dans la caractérisation des plaques carotidiennes. JEMU 17:377–380

Beckett WW, Davis PC, Hoffman JC (1990) Duplex Doppler sonography of the carotid artery: false-positive results in an artery contralateral to an artery with marked stenosis. AJR Am J Roentgenol 155:1091–1095

Bendick PJ, Jackson VP (1986) Evaluation of the vertebral arteries with duplex sonography. J Vasc Surg 3:523–530

Bendick PJ, Glover JL (1990) Hemodynamic evaluation of vertebral arteries by duplex ultrasound. Surg Clin North Am 70:235–244

Bendick PJ, Glover JL, Hankin R (1988) Morphologie de la plaque carotidienne: correlation de l'échographie et de l'histologie. Ann Chir Vasc 2:6–12

Bluth IE (1996) Evaluation and characterization of carotid plaque. JEMU 17:322–329

Bluth IE, Kay D, Merritt CRB (1986) Sonographic characterization of carotid plaque: detection of hemorrhage. AJNR Am J Neuroradiol 7:311–314

Bluth IE, Wetzner SM, Stavros AT (1988) Carotid duplex sonography: a multicenter recommendation for standardized imaging and Doppler criteria. Radiographics 8:487–506

Bluth IE, Merritt CRB, Sullivan MA, Bernhardt S (1989) Usefulness of ultrasound in evaluating vertebral arteries. J Ultrasound Med 8:229–235

Bock RW, Gray-Weale AC, Mock PA, Robinson DA (1993) The natural history of asymptomatic carotid artery disease. J Vasc Surg 17:160–171

Bornstein NM, Beloev ZG, Norris JW (1988) The limitations of diagnosis of carotid occlusion by Doppler ultrasound. Ann Surg 207:315–317

Breslau PJ, Fell F, Phillips DJ (1982) Evaluation of carotid bifurcation disease: the role of common carotid velocity waveform patterns. Arch Surg 117:58–60

Bridgers SL (1989) Clinical correlates of Doppler ultrasound errors in the detection of internal carotid occlusion. Stroke 20:612–615

Brunholzl CH, Von Reutern GM (1989) Hemodynamic effects of innominate artery occlusive disease: evaluation by Doppler ultrasound. Ultrasound Med Biol 15:201–204

Caplan LR, Baquis GD, Pessin MS, D'Alton J (1988) Dissection of intracranial vertebral artery. Neurology 38:868–877

Carr S, Farb A, Pearce WH (1996) Atherosclerosis plaque rupture in symptomatic carotid artery stenosis. J Vasc Surg 12:755–766

Carroll BA (1991) Carotid sonography. Radiology 178:303–313

Carroll BA, Holder CA (1990) Vertebral artery duplex sonography. J Ultrasound Med 9:S27

Cattin F, Bonneville JF (1995) Echo-Doppler des artères carotides et vertébrales. Aspects pratiques. Masson, Paris

Cave EM, Pugh ND, Wilson RJ (1995) Carotid artery duplex scanning: does plaque echogenicity correlate with patients' symptoms? Eur J Vasc Endovasc Surg 10:77–81

Cesari JB, Blard JM, Kassnasrallah S, Heroum C (1996) Sténoses carotidiennes hypo ou anéchogènes. JEMU 17:309–313

Chang YJ, Lin SK, Ryu SJ, Wai YY (1995) Common carotid artery occlusion: evaluation with duplex sonography. AJNR Am J Neuroradiol 16:1099–1105

Chiras J, Marciano S, Véga-Molina J, Touboul PJ (1985) Spontaneous dissecting aneurysm of the extracranial vertebral artery. Neuroradiology 27:327–333

Comerota AJ, Katz ML, White JV, Grosh JD (1990) The preoperative diagnosis of the ulcerated carotid atheroma. J Vasc Surg 11:505–510

Dauzat M (1991a) L'examen ultrasonographique des axes carotidiens. In: Ultrasonographie vasculaire diagnostique. Théorie et pratique. Vigot, Paris, pp 96–182

Dauzat M (1991b) Les artères subclavières et vertébrales. In: Ultrasonographie vasculaire diagnostique. Théorie et pratique. Vigot, Paris, pp 183–222

De Bray JM, Davinroy M, Gousset D, Maugin D (1980) L'étude par ultrasonographie Doppler des artères vertébrales. Méthodologie et bases d'interprétation. Ultrasons 1:87–92

De Bray JM, Lescalie F, Tachot G, Jeanvoine H (1986) Aspects ultrasonographiques des carotides internes opérées. Artères Veines 5:502–508

De Bray JM, Rozier A, Lescalie F, Merville C (1989) Le duplex peut-il identifier les hyperplasies myo-intimales? Analyse de 33 sténoses sur carotides internes opérées. Artères Veines 8:165–168

De Bray JM, Lhoste P, Dubas F, Emile J (1994) Ultrasonic features of extracranial carotid dissections: 47 cases studied by angiography. J Ultrasound Med 9:659–664

De Bray JM, Baud JM, Gorce P, Pasco A (1996) Le Doppler puissance dans la caractérisation des sténoses de la carotide interne extracrânienne. JEMU 17:175–181

De Bray JM, Penisson-Besnier I, Dubas F, Emile J (1997) Extracranial and intracranial vertebrobasilar dissections: diagnosis and prognosis. J Neurol Neurosurg Psychiatry 63:46–51

Deklunder G, Gautier C, Custoza E (1998) Indication des produits de contraste ultrasonores dans l'exploration des troncs supra-aortiques. JEMU 19:426–430

Erickson SJ, Middleton WD, Mewissen MW (1989) Color Doppler evaluation of arterial stenoses and occlusions involving the neck and thoracic inlet. Radiographics 9:389–406

ESCT (European Carotid Surgery Trialists Collaborative Group) (1991) MRC European Carotid Surgery Trial: interim results for symptomatic patients with severe (70%–99%) or with mild (0%–29%) carotid stenosis. Lancet 337:1235–1243

Feeley TM, Leen EJ, Golgan MP, More DJ (1991) Histologic characteristics of carotid artery plaques. J Vasc Surg 13:719–724

Fraught WE, Mattos MA, Van Bemmelen PS (1994) Colorflow duplex scanning of carotid arteries: new velocity criteria based on receiver operator characteristic analysis for threshold stenosis used in the symptomatic and asymptomatic carotid trials. J Vasc Surg 19:818–828

Frumkin LR, Baloh RW (1990) Wallenberg's syndrome following neck manipulation. Neurology 40:611–615

Furst G, Sitzer M, Meents H, Schlief R (1996) Echo-enhanced color Doppler-assisted duplex imaging of the carotid system. Result of two phase-III studies using Levovist (SHU 508A). Angiology 7:15–21

Geroulakos G, Ramaswami G, Nicolaides A, Labropoulos N (1993) Characterization of symptomatic and asymptomatic carotid plaques using high-resolution real-time ultrasonography. Br J Surg 80:1274–1277

Gibbons GH, Dzau VJ (1994) The emerging concept of vascular remodeling. N Engl J Med 330:1431–1438

Goes E, Janssens W, Maillet B (1990) Tissue characterization of atheromatous plaques: correlation between ultrasound image and histological findings. J Clin Ultrasound 18:611–617

Gortler M, Niethammer R, Widder B (1994) Differentiating subtotal artery stenoses from occlusions by colour-coded duplex sonography. J Neurol 5:301–305

Gray-Weale AC, Graham JC, Burnett JR (1988) Carotid artery atheroma. Comparison of preoperative B-mode ultrasound appearance with carotid endarterectomy specimen pathology. J Cardiovasc Surg 26:676–681

Greselle JF, Zenteno M, Kien P, Castel JP (1987) Dissection spontanée du système vertébro-basilaire. J Neuroradiol 84:115–123

Griewing B, Morgenstern C, Driesner F, Kallwellis G (1996) Cerebrovascular disease assessed by color-flow and power Doppler ultrasonography. Comparison with digital subtraction angiography in internal carotid artery stenosis. Stroke 27:95–100

Hart RG (1988) Vertebral artery dissection. Neurology 38:987–989

Hauser W, Mokri B, Sundt T (1984) Spontaneous cervical cephalic arterial dissection and its angiographic residuum. AJNR Am J Neuroradiol 5:27–34

Hennerici M, Klemm C, Rautenberg W (1988) The subclavian steal phenomenon: a common vascular disorder with rare neurologic deficits. Neurology 38:669–673

Hennerici M, Neuerburg-Heusler D (1998) Extracranial cerebral arteries. In: Vascular diagnosis with ultrasound. Thieme, Stuttgart

Hoskins PR (1996) Accuracy of maximum velocity estimates made using Doppler ultrasound systems. Br J Radiol 69:172–177

Howard G, Baker WH, Chambless LE (1996) An approach for the use of Doppler ultrasound as a screening tool for hemodynamically significant stenosis (despite heterogeneity of Doppler performance). Stroke 27:1951–1957

Iannuzzi A, Wilcosky T, Mercuri M (1995) Ultrasonographic correlates of carotid atherosclerosis in transient ischemic attacks and stroke. Stroke 26:614–619

Jargiello T, Pietura R, Rakowski P, Szczerbo-Trojanowska M (1998) Power-Doppler imaging in the evaluation of extracranial vertebral artery compression in patients with vertebro-basilar insufficiency. Eur J Ultrasound 8:149–156

Johnson JM, Kennelly MM, Decesare D, Morgan S (1985) Natural history of asymptomatic carotid plaque. Arch Surg 120:1010–1012

Kalman PG, Johnston KW, Auech P (1985) In vitro comparison of alternative methods for quantifying the severity of Doppler spectral broadening for the diagnosis of carotid arterial occlusive disease Ultrasound Med Biol 11:435–440

Kessler C, Griewing B (1996) Ultrasound assessment of carotid plaque structure. JEMU 17:357–360

Kirsch JD, Wagner LR, James EM, Charboneau JW (1994) Carotid artery occlusion: positive predictive value of duplex sonography compared with arteriography. J Vasc Surg 4:642–649

Klag MJ, Whelton PK, Seidler AJ (1989) Decline in US stroke mortality. Demographic trends and antihypertensive treatment. Stroke 20:14–21

Koga M, Kimura K, Yasaka M, Otsubo R (1999) Three-dimensional power Doppler imaging of vertebrobasilar circulation in adults. AJNR Am J Neuroradiol 20:943–944

Langlois YE, Greene FM, Roederer GO (1984) Computer-based pattern recognition of carotid artery Doppler signals for disease classification: prospective validation. Ultrasound Med Biol 10:581–595

Langsfeld M, Gray-Weale AC, Lusby RJ (1989) The role of plaque morphology and diameter reduction in the development of new symptoms in asymptomatic carotid arteries. J Vasc Surg 9:548–557

Lee DH, Gao FQ, Rakin RN (1996) Common carotid artery occlusion: evaluation with duplex sonography. AJNR Am J Neuroradiol 16:1009–1015

Lee VS, Hertzberg BS, Kliewer MA, Carroll BA (1999) Assessment of stenosis: implications of variability of Doppler measurements in normal-appearing carotid arteries. Radiology 212:493–498

Lee VS, Hertzberg BS, Workman MJ, Smith TP (2000) Variability of Doppler US measurements along the common carotid artery: effects on estimates of internal carotid arterial stenosis in patients with angiographically proved disease. Radiology 214:387–392

Leonberg SC, Elliott FA (1981) Prevention of recurrent stroke. Stroke 12:731–735

Leys D (1996) Réflexions méthodologiques sur les études réalisées et propositions. JEMU 17:300–301

Li R, Cai J, Teggeler C (1996) Reproducibility of extra-cranial atherosclerotic lesions assessed by B-mode ultrasound: The Atherosclerotic Risk in Communities Study. Ultrasound Med Biol 22:791–799

Li YK, Zhang YK, Lu CM, Zhong SZ (1999) Changes and implications of blood flow velocity of the vertebral artery during rotation and extension of the head. J Manipulative Physiol Ther 22:91–95

Lusby RJ, Ferrel LD, Ehrenfeld WK, Stoney RJ (1982) Carotid plaque hemorrhage: its role in reproduction of cerebral ischaemia. Arch Surg 117:1479–1488

Maiuri F, Gallichio B, Cinalli G (1990) Diagnosis of carotid artery occlusion by duplex scanning. Neurol Res 12:75–77

Manelfe C, Clarisse J, Fredy D (1974) Dysplasie fibromusculaire des artères encéphaliques. A propos de 70 cas. J Neuradiol 1:149–231

Marcade JP (1996) Les aspects macroscopiques de la plaque carotidienne. JEMU 17:383–389

Marosi L, Ehringer H, Pollak C, Minar E (1986) Early postoperative changes after desobliteration of the carotid artery. Subsequent diagnostic control using a high-resolution ultrasonic real-time duplex scanner. J Mal Vasc 11:43–51

Mattos MA, Hodgson KJ, Ramsey DE (1992) Identifying total carotid occlusion with colour flow Doppler scanning. Eur J Vasc Surg 6:204–210

Matula C, Trattnig S, Tschabitscher M, Day JD (1997) The course of prevertebral segment of the vertebral artery: anatomy and clinical significance. Surg Neurol 48:125–131

Mellière D, Becquemin JP, Kassab M, Etienne G (1990) Histoire naturelle et corrigée des artérites radiques oblitérantes. A propos de 14 observations. J Mal Vasc 15:73–81

Middleton WD, Foley WD, Lawson TL (1988a) Flow reversal in the normal carotid bifurcation: color Doppler flow imaging analysis. Radiology 167:207–210

Middleton WD, Foley WD, Lawson TL (1988b) Color flow Doppler imaging of carotid artery abnormalities. AJR Am J Roentgenol 150:419–425

Mokri B, Sundt TM, Houser OW (1979) Spontaneous internal carotid dissection, hemicrania and Horner's syndrome. Acta Neurol 36:677–680

Mokri B, Houser OW, Sandok BA, Piepgras DG (1988) Spontaneous dissections of the vertebral arteries. Neurology 38:880–885

Moneta GL, Edwards JM, Chitwood RW (1993) Correlation of North American Symptomatic Carotid Endarterectomy Trial (NASCET) angiographic definition of 70%–99% internal carotid artery stenosis with duplex scanning. J Vasc Surg 17:152–159

Moneta GL, Edwards JM, Papanicolaou G (1995) Screening for asymptomatic internal carotid artery stenosis: Duplex criteria for discriminating 60%–99% stenosis. J Vasc Surg 21:989–994

Nakamura K, Saku Y, Torigoe R, Ibayashi S (1998) Sonographic detection of haemodynamic changes in a case of vertebro-basilar insufficiency. Neuroradiology 40:164–166

NASCET (North American Symptomatic Carotid Endarterectomy Trial Collaborators) (1991) Beneficial effect of carotid endarterectomy in symptomatic patients with high-grade carotid stenosis. N Engl J Med 325:445–453

Nicolaides AN (1996) The value of computer analysis of ultrasonic plaque echolucency in identifying high-risk carotid bifurcation lesions. JEMU 17:404

Nolsoe CP, Engel U, Karstrup S, Torp-Pedersen S (1990) The aortic wall: an in vitro study of the double line pattern in high-resolution US. Radiology 175:387–390

O'Donnell TF, Erodes L, Maceky WC (1985) Correlation of B-mode ultrasound imaging and arteriography with pathologic findings of carotid endarterectomy. Arch Surg 12:443–449

O'Dwyer JA, Moscow N, Trevor R, Ehrenfeld WK (1980) Spontaneous dissection of the carotid artery. Radiology 137:379–385

O'Leary DH, Holen J, Ricot J (1987) Carotid bifurcation disease: prediction of ulceration with B-mode ultrasound. Radiology 162:523–525

Paivansalo M, Sinituoto TMJ, Tikkakoski TA (1996) Duplex ultrasound of the external artery. Acta Radiol 37:41–43

Paivansalo M, Heikkila O, Tikkakoski T, Leinonen S (1998) Duplex ultrasound in the subclavian steal syndrome. Acta Radiol 39:183–188

Persson AV, Berghorn G, Nanda R, Gupta S (1996) Computerized analysis of carotid plaque density. JEMU 17:402–403

Petro GR, Witver GA, Cacayorin ED, Hodge CJ (1987) Spontaneous dissection of the carotid artery: correlation of arteriography. CT and pathology. AJR Am J Roentgenol 148:393–398

Pfadenhauer K, Müller H (1995) Color-coded duplex ultrasound of the vertebral artery: normal findings and pathologic findings in obstruction of the vertebral artery and remaining cerebral arteries. Ultraschall Med 16:228–233

Picano E, Landini L, Lattanzi F, Salvadori M (1988) Time domain echo pattern evaluations from normal and atherosclerotic arterial walls: a study in vitro. Circulation 3:654–659

Pignoli P, Tremoli E, Poli A, Oreste P (1986) Intimal plus medial thickness of the arterial wall: a direct measurement with ultrasound imaging. Circulation 6:1399–1406

Poli A, Tremoli E, Colombo A (1988) Ultrasonographic measurement of the common carotid arterial wall thickness in hypercholesterolemic patients. Atherosclerosis 70:253–261

Prendes JL, McKinney WM, Buonanno FS, Jones AM (1980) Anatomic variations of carotid bifurcation affecting Doppler scan interpretation. J Clin Ultrasound 8:147–150

Provenzale JM (1995) Dissection of the internal carotid artery and vertebral arteries: Imaging features. AJR Am J Roentgenol 165:1099–1104

Ratiff DA, Gallagher PJ, Hames TK (1985) Characterization of carotid artery disease: comparison of duplex scanning with histology. Ultrasound Med Biol 11:835–840

Reilly MI, Lusby RJ, Hughes L (1993) Carotid plaque histology using real-time ultrasonography. Am J Surg 146:188–193

Reilly MI (1996) Heterogeneous lesions of the carotid bifurcation: detection and clinical significance. JEMU 17:314–321

Ries S, Steinke W, Devuyst G, Artemis N (1998) Power Doppler imaging and color Doppler flow imaging for the evaluation of normal and pathological vertebral arteries. J Neuroimaging 8:71–74

Ringelstein EB (1995) Scepticism toward carotid ultrasonography. A virtue, an attitude or fanaticism? Stroke 26:1743–1746

Robinson ML, Sacks D, Perlmuter GS, Marinelli DL (1988) Diagnostic criteria for carotid duplex sonography. AJR Am J Roentgenol 151:1045–1049

Rohr-Le Floch J, Frey E, Hillion C, Gauthier G (1988) Endartériectomie carotidienne: evaluation ultrasonique à long terme. Rev Neurol 144:332–337

Ross R, Glomset JA (1976) The pathogenesis of atherosclerosis. N Engl J Med 295:369–377

Rubin JM, Bude RO, Carsion PL, Bree RL (1994) Power Doppler US: a potentially useful alternative to mean-frequency base color Doppler US. Radiology 190:853–856

Saloner D, Reilly LM, Anderson CM, Diaz M (1996) Evaluation of disease of carotid bifurcation using magnetic resonance imaging. JEMU 17:348–356

Schwartz K, Becher H, Schimpfky C, Vorwerk D (1994) Doppler enhancement with SHU 508A in multiple vascular regions. Radiology 193:195–201

Sellier N, Chiras J, Benhamou M, Bories J (1983) Dissections spontanées de la carotide interne. Aspects cliniques, radiologiques et évolutifs. A propos de 46 cas. J Neuroradiol 10:243–259

Sidhu PS, Allan PL (1997) Ultrasound assessment of internal carotid artery stenosis. Clin Radiol 52:654–658

Sillesen H (1995) Carotid artery plaque composition. Relation to clinical presentation and ultrasound B-mode imaging. Eur J Endovasc Surg 10:23–30

Sitzer M, Furst G, Fischer H (1993) Between-method correlation in quantifying internal carotid artery stenosis. Stroke 24:1513–1518

Sitzer M, Muller W, Siebler M, Hort W (1995) Plaque ulceration and lumen thrombus are the main source of cerebral microemboli in high-grade internal carotid artery stenosis. Stroke 26:1231–1233

Sitzer M, Fuerst G, Aulich A, Steinmetz H (1996a) Contrast-enhanced characterization of plaque surface morphology in high-grade internal carotid stenoses. JEMU 17:397–400

Sitzer M, Wolfram M, Jorg R (1996b) Color-flow Doppler-assisted duplex imaging fails to detect ulceration in high-grade internal carotid artery stenosis. J Vasc Surg 24:461–465

Sliwka U, Rautenberg W, Schwartz A, Hennerici M (1992) Multimodal ultrasound imaging of the vertebral circulation compared with intra-arterial angiography. J Neurol 239:S38

Steinke W, Kloetzsch C, Hennerici M (1990) Carotid artery disease assessed by color Doppler flow imaging: correlation with standard Doppler sonography and angiography. Am J Roentgenol 154:1061–1068

Steinke W, Meairs S, Ries S, Hennerici M (1996) Sonographic assessment of carotid artery stenosis. Comparison of power Doppler imaging and color Doppler flow imaging. Stroke 27:91–94

Sterpetti AV, Schultz RD, Feldhaus RJ (1988) Ultrasonographic features of carotid plaque and the risk of subsequent neurologic deficits. Surgery 104:652–660

Sutton-Tyrrell K, Wolfson SK, Thompson T, Kelsoey SF (1992) Measurement variability in Duplex scan assessment of carotid atherosclerosis. Stroke 23:215–220

Touboul PJ, Bousser MG, LaPlane D, Castaigne P (1986) Duplex scanning of normal vertebral arteries. Stroke 17:921–923

Touboul PJ, Mas JL, Bousser MG, Laplane D (1988) Duplex scanning in extracranial vertebral artery dissection. Stroke 19:116–121

Trattnig S, Hübsch P, Schuster H, Pötzleitner D (1990) Color-coded Doppler imaging of normal vertebral arteries. Stroke 21:1222–1225

Van Damme H, Martin D, Stassen MP, Limet R (1990) Dissections spontanées de la carotide interne. J Mal Vasc 15:14–22

Visona A, Lusiani L, Castellani V (1986) The echo-Doppler (duplex) system for the detection of vertebral artery occlusive disease: comparison with angiography. J Ultrasound Med 5:247–250

Walker DW, Acker JD, Cole CA (1982) Subclavian steal syndrome detected with duplex pulsed Doppler sonography. AJNR Am J Neuroradiol 3:615–618

Widder B, Paulat K, Hackspacher J (1990) Morphological characterization of carotid artery stenosis by ultrasound duplex scanning. Ultrasound Med Biol 16:349–354

Winter R, Biedert S, Staudacher T, Betz H (1987) Vertebral artery Doppler sonography. Eur Arch Psychiatry Neurol Sci 237:21–28

Wolverson MK, Bashiti HM, Peterson GJ (1983) Ultrasonic tissue characterization of atheromatous plaques using a high resolution real-time scanner. Ultrasound Med Biol 6:669–709

Zierler RE, Phillips DJ, Beach KW (1987) Non-invasive assessment of normal carotid bifurcation hemodynamics with color flow ultrasound imaging. Ultrasound Med Biol 13:471–476

Zukowski AJ, Nicolaides AN, Levis RT (1984) The correlation between carotid plaque ulceration and cerebral infarction seen on CT scan. J Vasc Surg 1:782–787

Zwiebel WJ (1990) Duplex examination of the carotid arteries. Semin Ultrasound CT MR 11:97–135

Zwiebel WJ (2000a) Normal carotid arteries and carotid examination technique. In: Introduction to vascular ultrasonography, 4th edn. Saunders, Philadelphia, pp 113–124

Zwiebel WJ (2000b) Ultrasound assessment of carotid plaque. In: Introduction to vascular ultrasonography, 4th edn. Saunders, Philadelphia, pp 125–135

Zwiebel WJ (2000c) Doppler evaluation of carotid stenosis. In: Introduction to vascular ultrasonography, 4th edn. Saunders, Philadelphia, pp 137–154

Zwiebel WJ (2000d) Ultrasound vertebral examination. In : Introduction to vascular ultrasonography, 4th edn. Saunders, Philadelphia, pp 167–176

Zwiebel WJ, Crummy AB (1981) Sources of error in Doppler diagnosis of carotid occlusive disease. Am J Roentgenol 137:1–2

7 Internal Jugular Vein

Jean Noël Bruneton, Pierre-Yves Marcy, Gilles Poissonnet

CONTENTS

J.N. Bruneton, MD
Service de Radiologie, Hôpital de l'Archet, 151, route de St.-Antoine Ginestière, B.P. 3079, 06202 Nice Cedex 3, France
P.Y. Marcy, MD
Service de Radiodiagnostic, Centre Antoine-Lacassagne, 33 avenue de Valombrose, 06189 Nice Cedex 2, France
G. Poissonnet, MD
Département d'ORL, Centre Antoine-Lacassagne, 33 avenue de Valombrose, 06189 Nice Cedex 2, France

The vascular systems of the lower limbs and the inferior vena cava were the first to benefit from sonographic examination, owing to the frequency of thrombotic disease in these anatomic sites. Over the past decade, however, the development of procedures requiring central venous access (reanimation, cardiology) and safer techniques for venous drug infusion in oncology have prompted numerous studies on the venous system of the upper extremities and the cervical region. Today, the risk of venous thrombosis related to placement of a foreign object – the catheter – in the venous lumen can be predicted both directly and indirectly by sonography (Longley et al. 1993; Patel et al. 1999). The ease of sonographic examination of the internal jugular vein (IJV) logically led to the use of US guidance to reduce the rate of procedural failures and complications related to percutaneous puncture, essentially for the placement of central venous catheters (Bonnet et al. 1989; Gordon et al. 1998; Trerotola et al. 1997).

Sonographic examination of the IJV must be complemented by exploration of the axillary and subclavian veins to accurately assess the quality of venous return from the upper body.

7.1 The Normal Internal Jugular Vein

7.1.1 Anatomy

7.1.1.1 Cervical Veins

The cervical veins can be divided into superficial and deep systems, based on their positions relative to the deep cervical fascia. The superficial veins drain primarily into the external jugular vein. The largest vein in the cervical region, the IJV collects blood from the major part of the neck. Anastomoses with the external jugular vein (EJV) are established either directly or, more commonly, indirectly by collateral veins that drain into one system or the other. The IJV receives the retromandibular vein (which may also drain partly into the EJV), the facial vein, the superficial temporal vein, and the thyroid veins. The EJV receives, directly or indirectly, the occipital vein and the anterior jugular vein. The IJV terminates posterior to the internal aspect of the clavicle, at the root of the neck, where it joins the subclavian vein to form the brachiocephalic trunk.

Although the superior bulb of the IJV cannot be assessed sonographically, the major portion of the vein is readily examined by US, including the inferior bulb that lies in a retroclavicular position. The IJV is related primarily to the common carotid artery (CCA); this relationship must be accurately determined prior to IJV puncture.

7.1.1.2
Diameter

Macchi and Catini (1994) found a mean IJV diameter of 13.8 mm at the ostial level; this diameter was significantly larger in male than in female subjects ($p<0.01$), and the difference tended to increase with age.

The IJVs are often asymmetrical, as revealed by sonographic studies. Lobato et al. (1999) found that in one third of adults the cross-sectional area of the right IJV is more than 50% larger than that of the left IJV, during breath-holding as well as during a Valsalva maneuver or a Trendelenburg tilt.

According to Stickle and McFarlane (1997), the diameter of the IJV is inversely correlated with that of the EJV. In their study, an EJV diameter +7 mm was always associated with an IJV diameter under 15 mm; an EJV diameter of less than 7 mm was consistently correlated with an IJV diameter of at least 20 mm.

Two clinical maneuvers can be used to increase IJV diameter:

- The Valsalva maneuver (Armstrong et al. 1994)
- Trendelenburg tilt: In the study by Mallory et al. (1990), this maneuver increased the cross-sectional area of the IJV lumen from 1.18 to 1.62 cm^2. Knowledge of IJV diameter is useful to optimize catheter placement (Armstrong et al. 1994; Mallory et al. 1990).

7.1.1.3
IJV Valves

Located 0.5–2 cm above the junction of the IJV and the subclavian vein (Imai et al. 1994), the IJV valves play an important role in preventing retrograde blood flow. Patra et al. (1988) emphasized the role of the omohyoid muscle: Contraction of this muscle significantly modifies the surface of the IJV, resulting in modifications in hemodynamics that are especially marked during yawning.

Complete valve closure occurs once per cardiac cycle, during diastole, when atrial contraction transmits pressure backwards into the superior vena cava. Partial valve closure may occur during mid-systole, probably as the result of IJV compression by carotid pulsations.

In their study of 240 jugular veins in 60 men and 60 women, Macchi and Catini (1994) detected a single valvular apparatus in 86% of patients (two cusps were noted in 75%, one cusp in 15%, and three cusps in 10%). No valvular apparatus was found in the remaining 14% of patients (essentially men). In that study, 95% of the valves were considered incompetent. Lepori et al. (1999) detected IJV valves by US in nearly 87% of patients.

7.1.1.4
Relationships with the Common Carotid Artery

Numerous US studies have investigated the relationships of the IJV and the CCA in real-time and as a function of posture, as this anatomic relationship has a direct impact on catheter placement techniques.

Caridi et al. (1998) visualized the right IJV in the typical position, lateral to the CCA, in 71% of individuals; the right IJV was located medially, anterior to the CCA in 16%, and it was positioned more than 1 cm lateral to the artery in 4% of cases; IJV thrombosis was noted in 9%.

Troianos et al. (1996) investigated the anatomic variability of the IJV at the apex of the angle formed by the division of the sternocleidomastoid muscle. The IJV was found to overlie the CCA in 54% of patients; this vascular relationship was more frequent in patients over 60 years of age than in younger subjects. This anatomic situation explains the elevated risk of carotid artery puncture if the cannulating needle traverses the IJV.

Other authors have investigated the benefits of US guidance for IJV cannulation. The IJV lies medial to the CCA in 5.5%–6% of individuals (Gordon et al. 1998; Silberzweig and Mitty 1998); this may explain failures with the anatomic landmark-guided cannulation technique. According to Lin et al. (1998b), 26% of individuals have IJV anatomic variations capable of preventing successful cannulation with the external landmark-guided technique.

Anatomic relationships are modified when patients are examined in a 15° Trendelenburg tilt combined with head rotation of 40° and 80°. SULEK et al. (1996) demonstrated a significant increase in the percent overlap of the CCA and the IJV at 40° and 80° head rotation. Head rotation should thus be kept less than 40° during needle insertion into the IJV to avoid inadvertent puncture of the CCA.

The relationships between the IJV and the CCA vary considerably in children, and sonographic localization of these vessels is essential to minimize the risk of vascular injury.

Between the division of the sternocleidomastoid muscle, the IJV was anterior to the CCA in 56%, anterolateral in 4%, and lateral in 40% for MALLINSON et al. (1999). In contrast, at the level of the cricoid cartilage, the IJV was anterior to the CCA in 24%, anterolateral in 12%, and lateral in 64%.

7.1.2 Sonography

7.1.2.1 Examination Techniques

Sonographic examination of the superficial portion of the IJV must be completed by analysis of the retroclavicular area in order to follow this vein to its termination. A probe of at least 7.5 MHz generally suffices for gray-scale imaging, associated with a 6-MHz transducer for color-Doppler (CD) studies. A number of situations require use of lower frequency probes: short neck, obesity, post-therapy cervical modifications (surgery, radiotherapy). The other venous structures of the neck, and especially the EJV, the termination of the IJV, and the subclavian veins, must also be examined sonographically. Visualization of all portions of the subclavian veins is not always easy, even with a subclavian approach.

Proper vascular examination should include bilateral evaluation of the IJV, the brachiocephalic trunks, and the subclavian and axillary veins. Asymmetry in the Doppler spectra may have significant diagnostic implications in case of central thrombosis.

The three steps in sonographic examination include real-time morphological analysis with gray-scale imaging, CD or power-Doppler (PD) sonography, and Doppler waveform analysis.

- Gray scale imaging is performed during normal respiration and then during a Valsalva maneuver. The Trendelenburg position offers no particular advantage. Visualization of an endoluminal abnormality or a cervical mass closely related to the IJV necessitates both axial and longitudinal scanning during a Valsalva maneuver. Real-time dynamic study can be performed during venous compression (Figs. 7.1, 7.2).
- CD and PD permit rapid localization of the vessels, differentiation of arteries from veins, and identification of any lesions. In case of thrombosis, CD readily demonstrates the presence of collateral veins.
- Doppler waveform analysis provides no complementary information in cases of obvious IJV thrombosis. However, when the IJVs appear morphologically normal, waveform analysis can be performed whenever central venous thrombosis is suspected (LONGLEY et al. 1993).

a 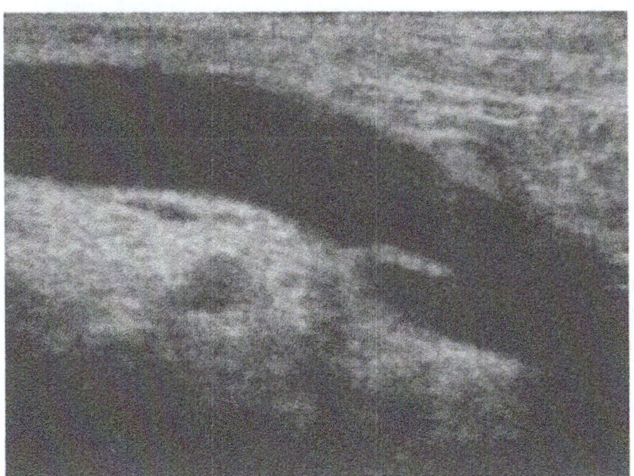

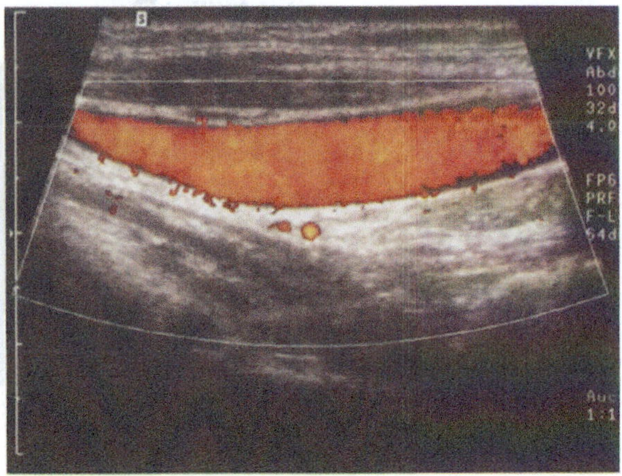 b

Fig. 7.1a,b. Normal internal jugular vein (IJV). **a** IJV valve (sagittal scan); **b** power Doppler (PD) study

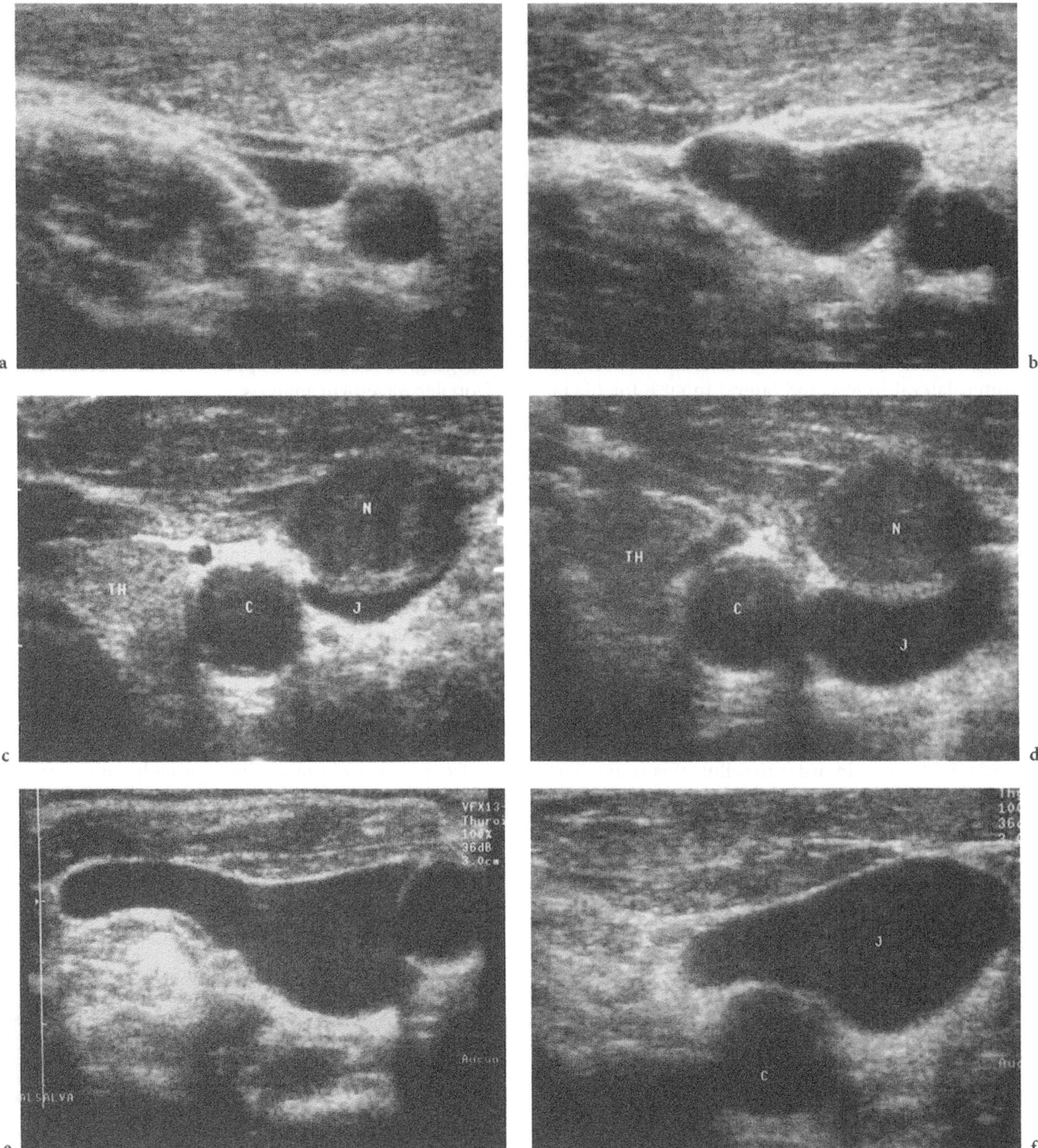

Fig. 7.2a–f. Benefits of the Valsalva maneuver. **a** Pre-Valsalva study. **b** Same patient as in **a**, during a Valsalva maneuver: dilatation of the IJV lateral to the common carotid artery (*CCA*). **c** Enlarged lymph node (*N*) anterior to the IJV (*J*); note the extensive imprint of the nodal lesion on the anterior aspect of the IJV, from which it is separated by a clear echogenic image (*TH* thyroid; *C* CCA). **d** Same patient as in **c**; the Valsalva maneuver produced satisfactory distension of the IJV (*J*). **e** Spectacular dilatation of the IJV lateral to the CCA during a Valsalva maneuver. **f** The IJV (*J*) is positioned anterior to the CCA (*C*) following a Valsalva maneuver

7.1.2.2 Sonographic Features of the IJV

In contrast to arteries, veins have a thin, highly echoic wall without layers. The lumen is typically echogenic, although mobile intraluminal echoes may be visible, especially in zones of turbulence. The Valsalva maneuver causes distension of the IJV but the extent of dilatation of each side is variable. This same phenomenon has been observed for the subclavian vein. The terminal portion of the IJV is usually larger than the proximal portion in the upper cervical region (Figs. 7.3–7.5).

CD and PD often visualize turbulent flow opposite the inferior bulb, but this finding has no pathological significance. Analysis of the upper portion of the jugular vein usually reveals a laminar flow pattern.

Lepori et al. (1999) found valves in nearly 87% of patients, generally on the right side because US of the left IJV is often more difficult. This contrasts with the 93% noted in anatomic evaluations of cadavers. This difference can be explained by the fact that valves are frequently located in the distal portion of the IJV, and examination of the retroclavicular region can be difficult in patients with a short neck. This also explains why, in contrast to autopsy data that highlight the frequency of bicuspid valves, bicuspid valves were demonstrated by US in only 38.2% of living patients. Sonography demonstrates bilateral valves in 60% of patients; the majority of unilateral valves are right-sided (Figs. 7.6–7.9).

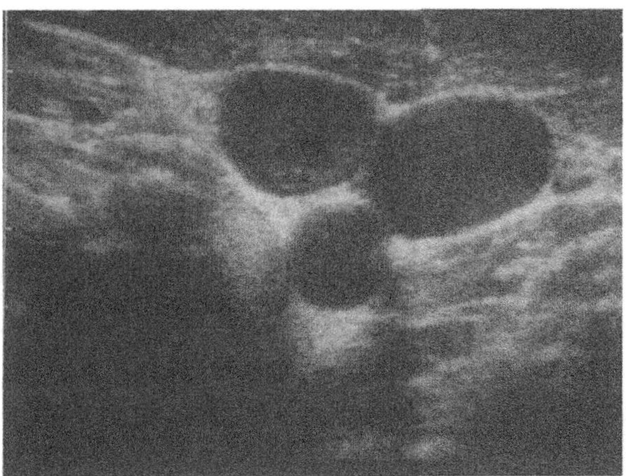

a

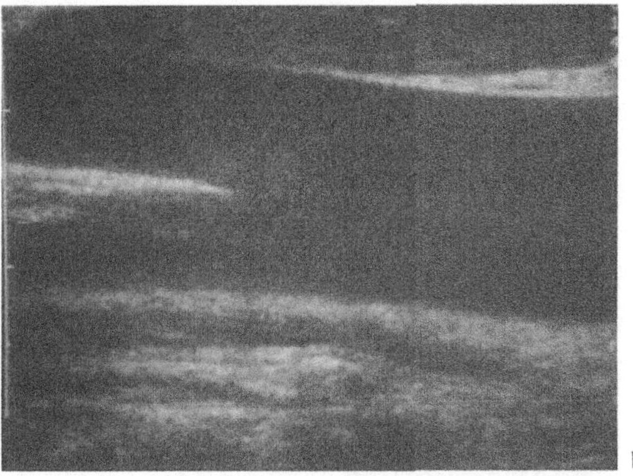

b

Fig. 7.3a,b. Congenital anomaly of the left IJV, which is duplicated over nearly its entire length. **a** Presence of two IJVs anterior to the CCA (axial scan). **b** Duplication of the upper portion of the IJV; the two structures unite distally (sagittal scan)

7.1.2.3 Doppler Sonography

Doppler US of the IJV demonstrated symmetrical, biphasic blood flow in 57% of 148 patients, continuous flow in 29%, and monophasic flow in 13% in the study of Pucheu et al. (1994). These authors considered blood flow velocity normal when it is less than 1 m/s and varies with both respiration and the heart rate. Muller et al. (1990) found an average right-plus-left jugular vein flow of 740±209 ml/min. Flow was 8.7% lower in female than in male subjects, but normalization of flow to 100 g brain tissue failed to reveal any significant sex difference. These authors also failed to note any decrease in IJV flow with age.

Normal Doppler waveforms are characterized by two physiological variations (Patel et al. 1999):

- Cardiac pulsatility, due to the retrograde pressure waves of right atrial contraction, is synchronized to the pulse rate and frequently results in a biphasic signal.

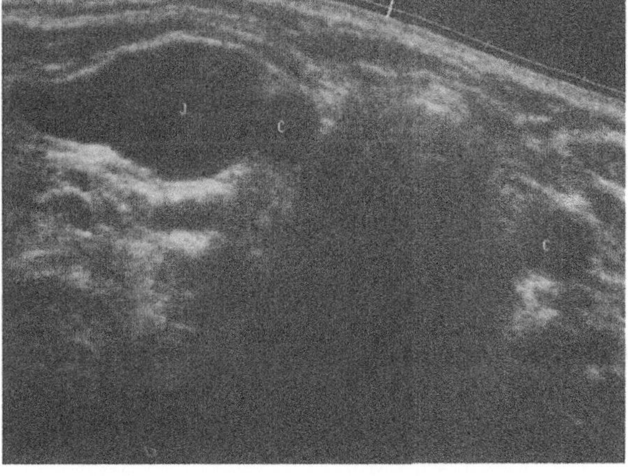

Fig. 7.4. SieScape study of the cervical region after total thyroidectomy: large right IJV (*J*) contrasting with absence of visualization of the left IJV, which was hypoplastic but not thrombosed. *C* CCA

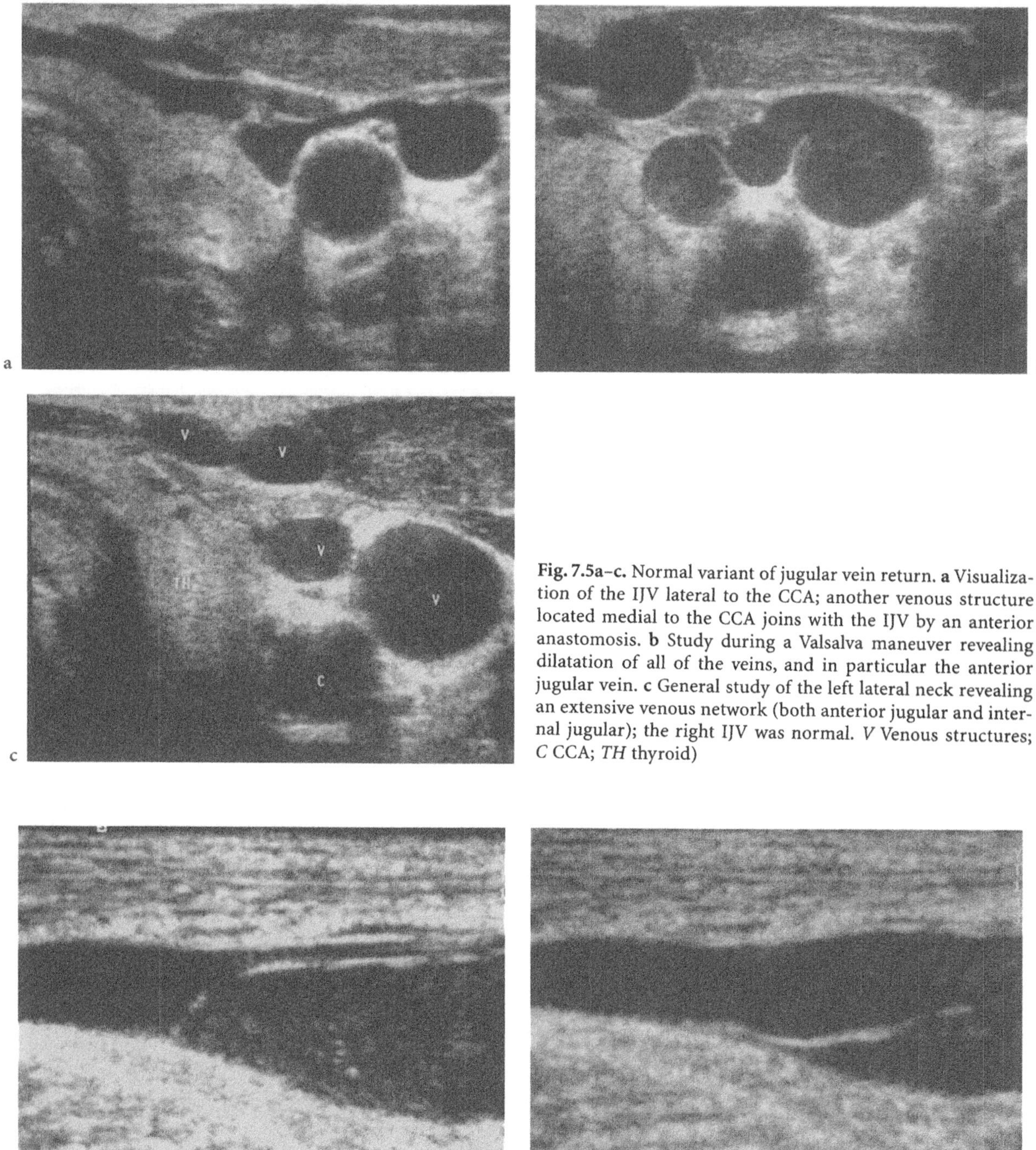

Fig. 7.5a–c. Normal variant of jugular vein return. **a** Visualization of the IJV lateral to the CCA; another venous structure located medial to the CCA joins with the IJV by an anterior anastomosis. **b** Study during a Valsalva maneuver revealing dilatation of all of the veins, and in particular the anterior jugular vein. **c** General study of the left lateral neck revealing an extensive venous network (both anterior jugular and internal jugular); the right IJV was normal. *V* Venous structures; *C* CCA; *TH* thyroid)

Fig. 7.6a,b. Study of the IJV valves at successive times (**a** and **b**)

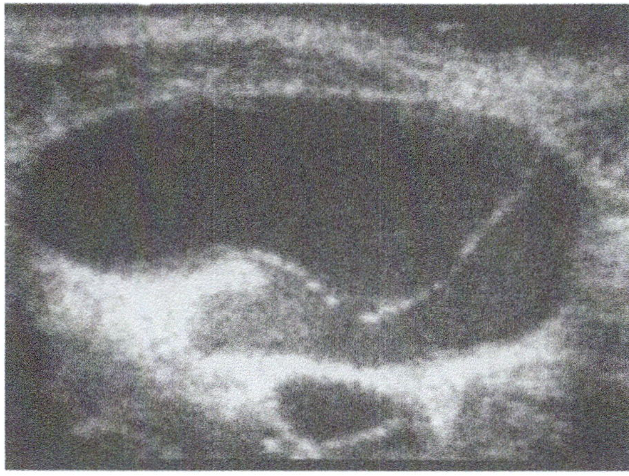

a

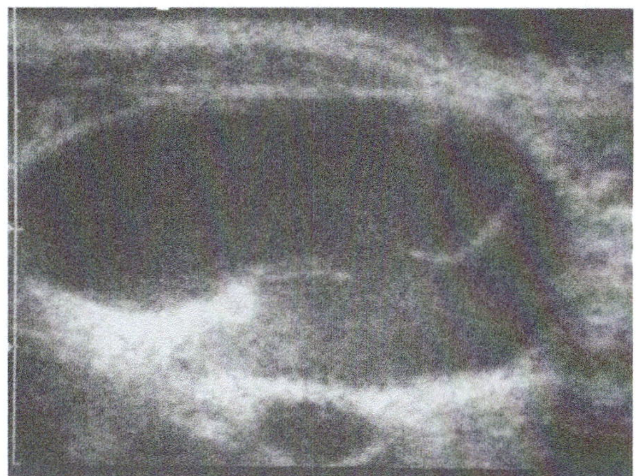

b

Fig. 7.7a,b. Left IJV valve at two different times (**a** and **b**) (axial scan)

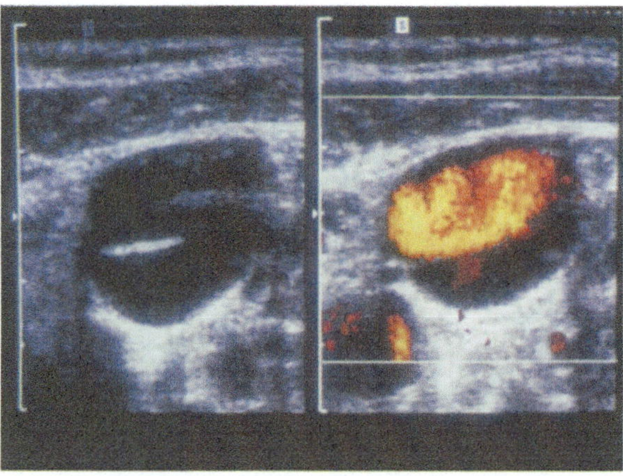

Fig. 7.8. US and PD study of the lower portion of the left IJV: echogenic image of the valves within the vessel; absence of signals below the valve at PD merely reflects physiological modifications in blood flow

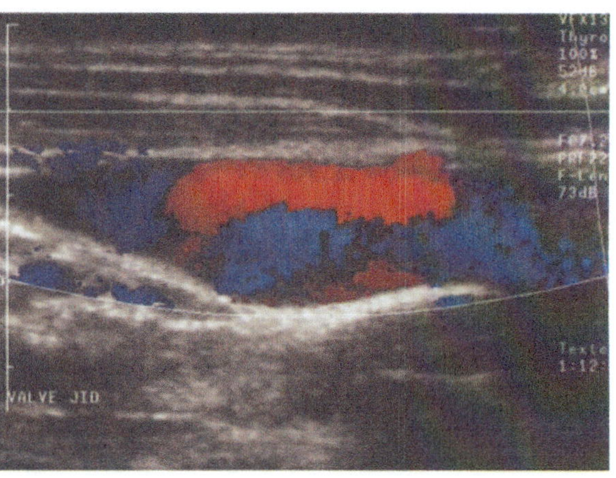

Fig. 7.9. Right IJV valve studied by CD: the numerous artifacts induced by the valve have no pathological significance

- Superimposed variations related to the respiratory cycle, with an increase on inspiration and a decrease on expiration.
  These modifications are easy to detect and identify, if necessary by comparing the cardiac pulsatility and the radial artery pulse and by requesting the patient to modify his or her respiratory rate (Figs. 7.10–7.13). Awareness of these physiological variations is a simple means of indirectly detecting anomalies in venous return in the mediastinum.

A 45-min Trendelenburg tilt reduces the flow velocity in the CCA and the IJV (Hu et al. 1999). Measurement 1 min after mild tilting (10°) revealed a decrease in IJV flow velocity and an increase in the IJV cross-sectional area, but both factors returned to baseline 10 min after tilting (Terai et al. 1995).

7.1.2.4
Other Venous Axes

As mentioned previously, examination of the IJV alone is insufficient in patients with thrombotic disease, and systematic analysis of the axillary and subclavian veins appears to be obligatory. The axillary vein is easily examined in the axilla using an intercostal or subclavicular approach. This vein is readily identified, in particular thanks to CD, because it lies adjacent to the axillary and subclavian arteries. The subclavian vein is difficult to visualize owing to the presence of bony structures, but real-time scanning

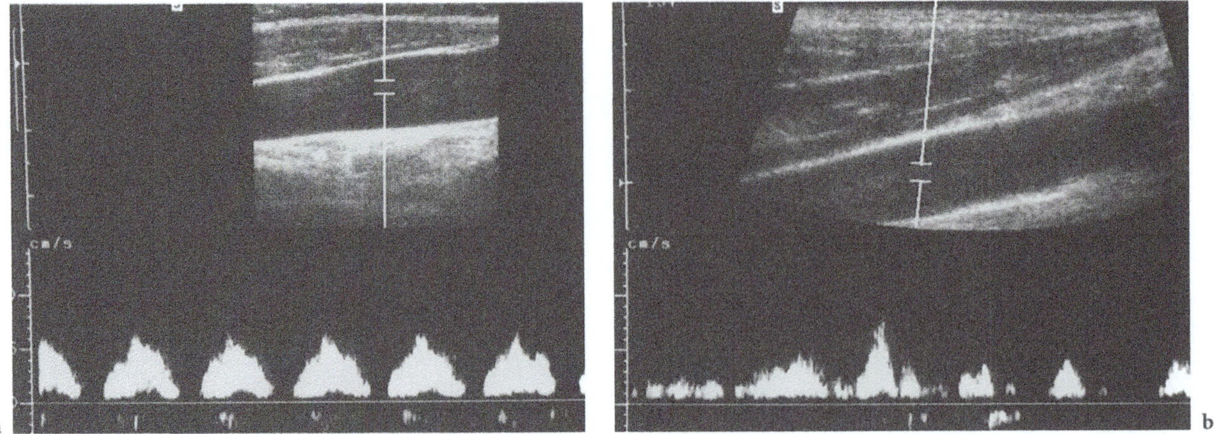

Fig. 7.10a,b. Doppler study of the IJV. **a** Study during breath-holding revealing cardiac pulsatility. **b** Study during normal respiration revealing the variations superimposed by the respiratory cycle

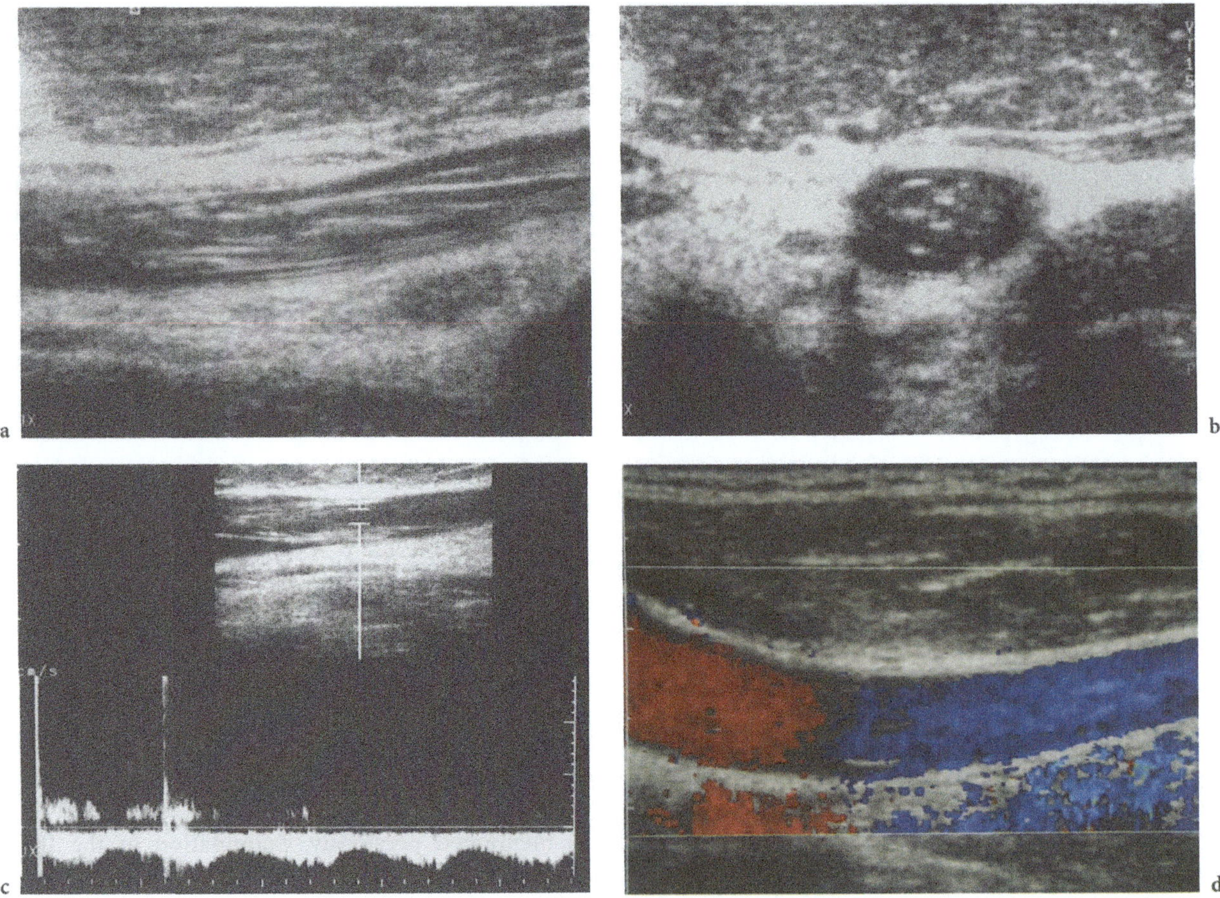

Fig. 7.11a–d. Spontaneous reflux in the left IJV. **a** Echogenic images of flow without any visible obstacle (sagittal scan). **b** Identical nonpathological echogenic endovenous images (axial scan). **c** Doppler study of reflux into the IJV. **d** Less extensive reflux in another patient: CD visualizes the normal return flow and the spontaneous reflux

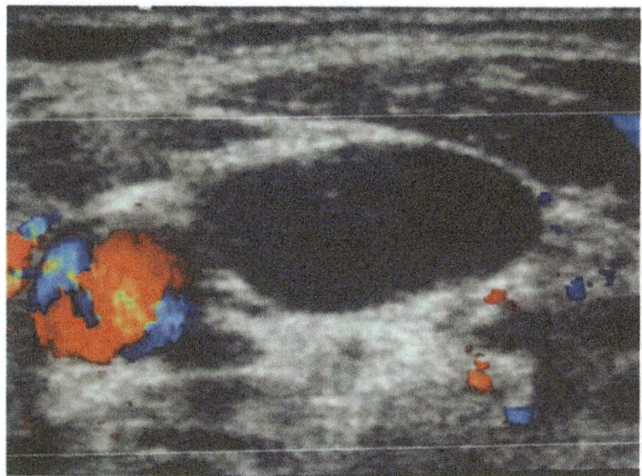
a

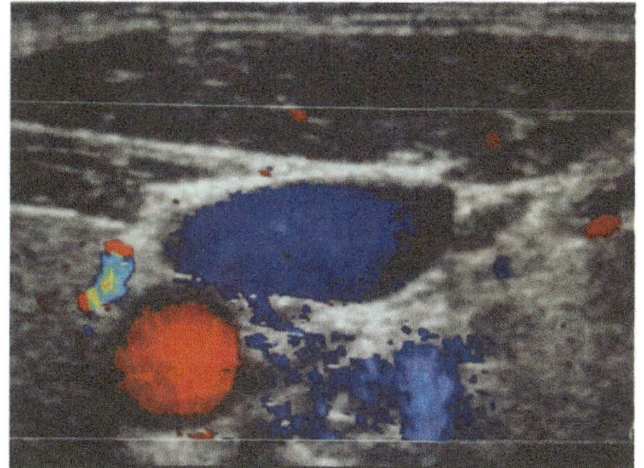
b

Fig. 7.12a,b. Pseudosign of left IJV thrombosis at CD. **a** Absence of visualization of signal in the left IJV. **b** Visualization of flow during a Valsalva maneuver ruled out a diagnosis of thrombosis

generally permits satisfactory evaluation of the entire course of this vessel, which is adjacent to the artery.

KROGER et al. (1998a) emphasized the need for thorough CD examination of the IJV and subclavian veins whenever upper limb venous thrombosis is suspected. In their series of 213 patients, they found solitary subclavian thrombosis in 43.7%; IJV thrombosis was isolated in 26.3% but was combined with thrombosis of the subclavian vein in 30%.

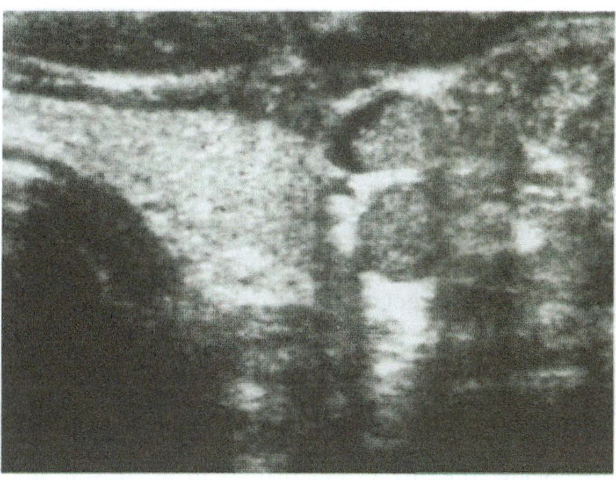

Fig. 7.13. Echogenic appearance of the lumen of the CCA and the IJV after injection of a contrast medium

7.2 Venous Thrombosis

7.2.1 IJV Thrombosis

IJV and subclavian vein thrombosis are increasingly encountered as common, and sometimes asymptomatic, complications of central venous catheter placement (BONNET et al. 1989; KARNIK et al. 1993). Deep venous thrombosis of the upper body is responsible for approximately 10% of all cases of pulmonary embolism.

7.2.1.1 Frequency and Etiology

Compared with the lower extremities, the upper part of the body, and in particular the IJV, is relatively less affected by thrombosis. KROGER et al. (1998b) reviewed 334 cases of upper limb venous thrombosis diagnosed over a 4-year period at a university hospital treating over 40,000 patients annually. In their series, isolated jugular vein thrombosis was noted in only 17% of cases, and combined thromboses (IJV and subclavian veins) in just 19%; 28.7% of cases were related to a central venous catheter or venous port system, and 54.5% of the patients had been treated for cancer.

Other investigators have reported comparable frequencies. In the series of MARIE et al. (1998) upper limb thrombosis represented only 2% of all cases of deep venous limb thrombosis, and IJV involvement (isolated or combined) occurred in 24.5% of these cases. These authors identified as causative factors malignancies (32.7% of cases) and venous catheters (22.4%). BALBARINI et al. (1998) confirmed the low frequency of IJV thrombosis among all cases of deep venous thrombosis.

The principal etiologies of IJV thrombosis include deep neck infections, mastoiditis, Lemierre syndrome, central venous catheterization (TOVI et al. 1993), malignancy, and a hypercoagulable condition. While some causes of IJV thrombosis such as ovarian hyperstimulation syndrome (Moutos et al. 1997) are rare, asymptomatic thrombosis appears commonplace during placement of central venous catheters. Karnik et al. (1993) systematically removed catheters under US guidance or performed duplex US after catheter removal; they found thrombosis in 69.5% of patients but were unable to correlate thrombus formation with any particular factor (basic disease, duration of cannulation, type of catheter, or mode of heparinization).

Lemierre syndrome is a rare cause of thrombophlebitis today. This septic disease of the IJV, isolated or associated with involvement of the cervical and mediastinal veins, is a complication of bacterial pharyngitis resulting in metastatic intrapulmonary abscesses. The pathogen at cause is an anaerobic germ, usually *Fusobacterium necrophorum* (Sinave et al. 1989). Lemierre syndrome had a mortality of 90% prior to the introduction of antibiotics. Screaton et al. (1999) described anaerobic pulmonary sepsis with IJV thrombosis (isolated or combined) or, less often, with isolated thrombosis of the mediastinal veins. (In such cases Doppler analysis of the IJV can provide indirect diagnostic data.)

7.2.1.2 Sonographic Features

Gray-scale imaging is performed in an initial step to assess venous morphology (vein diameter, shape and dimensions of the thrombus, presence of collateral veins); dynamic scanning is then performed to determine the response to direct compression and respiratory maneuvers (Weissleder et al. 1987). In cases of complete thrombosis, US features include an echogenic intraluminal mass, loss of respiratory variability and vessel pulsations, absence of venous response to respiratory maneuvers (especially the Valsalva maneuver), and loss of compressibility of the thrombosed vein (Albertyn and Alcock 1987; Gaitini et al. 1988). The separation between the mass and the venous lumen is clear. With long-standing occlusions, care must be taken not to mistake a large, distended collateral vein for an intact IJV. In case of partial thrombosis, examination may reveal the persistence of flow as an anechoic image associated with a parietal clot. Recent clots may not have the characteristic echogenic pattern of thrombus that permits identification without difficulty. CD is helpful to avoid overlooking a recent thrombus; gray-scale imaging can also suggest the diagnosis when no valve beating is detected, when the vein is noncompressible, or in the absence of venous response to a Valsalva maneuver (Figs. 7.14–7.16).

7.2.1.3 Color Doppler and Doppler Studies

The introduction of CD has improved the credibility of Doppler studies for diagnosis of thrombosis, particularly in the cervical region. Complete workup of the IJVs and the subclavian and axillary veins is usually performed before proposing anticoagulant therapy, thus sparing patients invasive examinations.

In case of complete venous occlusion, Doppler studies reveal the absence of flow. Partial, focal venous occlusion is characterized by increased flow velocity and turbulence at the site of stenosis. Partial occlu-

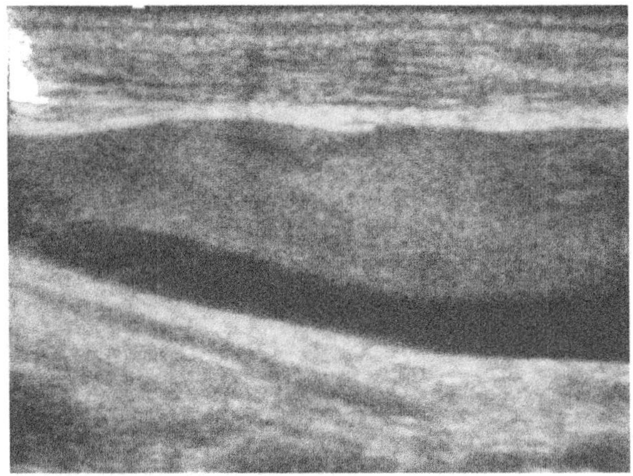

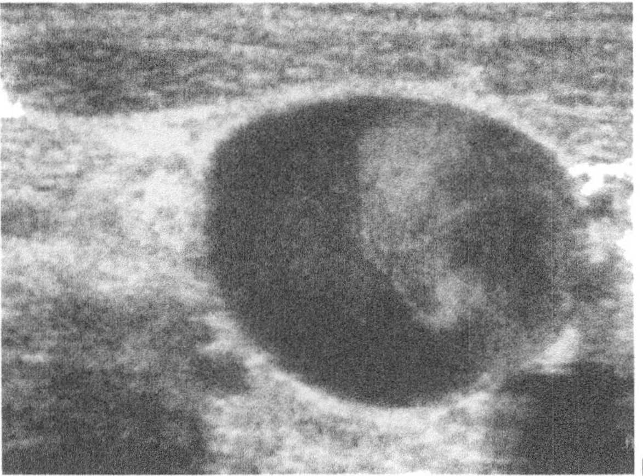

Fig. 7.14a,b. Partial, recent thrombosis of the right IJV. **a** Floating thrombus with a channel less than 1 cm in diameter posteriorly (sagittal scan). **b** Study during a Valsalva maneuver showing the thrombus floating within the lumen of the IJV (transverse scan)

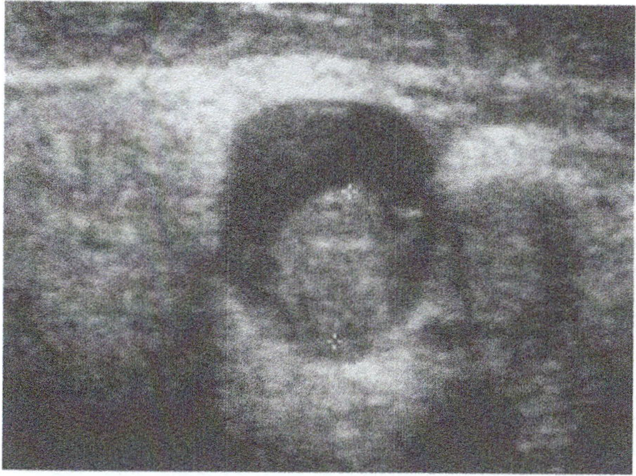

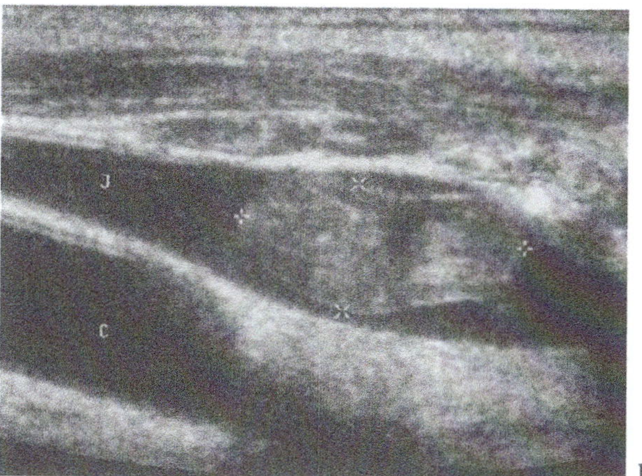

Fig. 7.15a,b. Long-standing focal thrombosis of the IJV. **a** Small (1.5/1.7 cm between the *crosses*) and highly echoic thrombus; this incomplete thrombosis was a sequela of Lemierre syndrome (*C* CCA; *J* IJV) (sagittal scan). **b** Partial echogenic thrombus within the left IJV (axial scan)

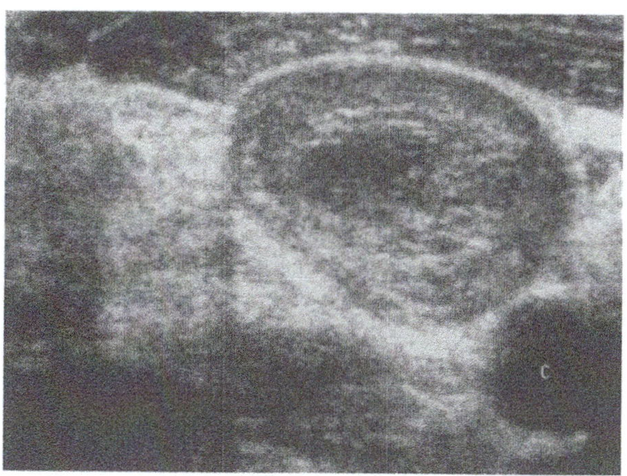

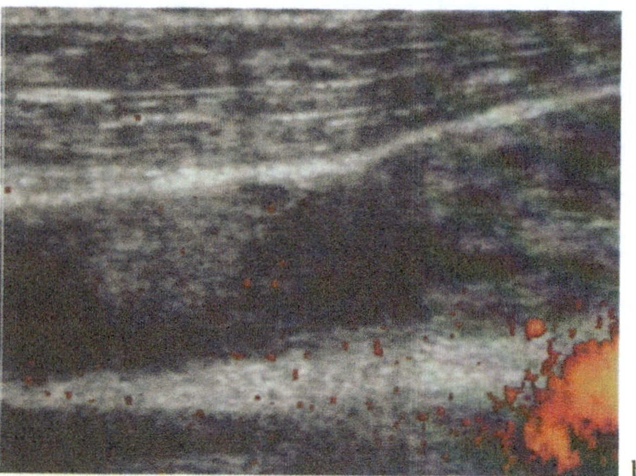

Fig. 7.16a,b. Complete occlusion of the IJV. **a** Complete thrombosis of the right IJV (*C* CCA; axial scan). **b** CD confirmed the absence of vascularity within the IJV (sagittal scan)

sion of a long venous segment creates abnormal Doppler waveforms upstream of the occluded segment and absence of the normal physiological variations associated with respiration.

Kroger and Rudofsky (1998) investigated the echogenicity of an aging venous thrombus with CD. The vascularity visible in 50% of cases corresponded to arterial signals from vessels that develop during organization of the thrombus and are visible for a short time (11th to the 25th day). Vascularity of the thrombus was not associated with any particularly visible arteries in the tissues surrounding the vein.

Following complete US examination of the IJV, there are few if any diagnostic difficulties; both false-positive and false-negative findings are infrequent. False-negative errors may occur during the staging of venous involvement when US is difficult (patients with a short neck, obese individuals, elderly patients with severe cervical arthrosis, etc., for whom sonographic examination of the lower neck is unsatisfactory). In such cases, it may be difficult to confirm the existence of subclavian thrombosis if dilated collateral veins are present (however, the typical proximity of the subclavian vein and artery should help to avoid this pitfall).

In patients with thrombotic disease affecting the IJV, US obviates the need for venography and allows immediate initiation of anticoagulant therapy (Fig. 7.17).

7.2.1.4
Evaluation of Response to Treatment

Sonography allows accurate assessment of the response of cervicothoracic venous thrombosis to

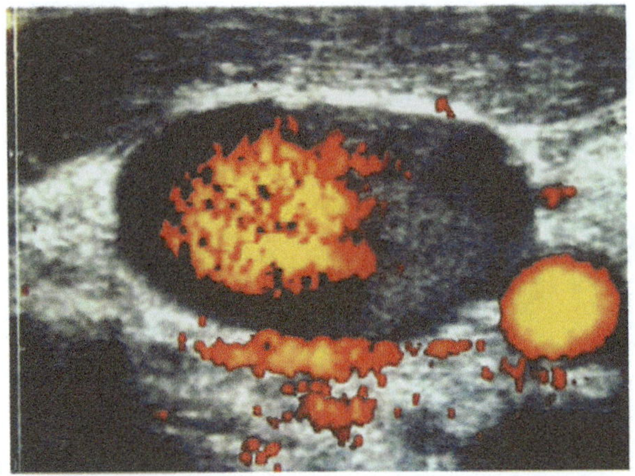

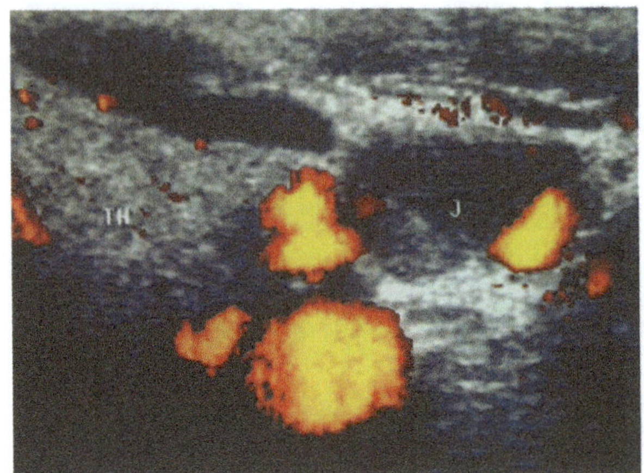

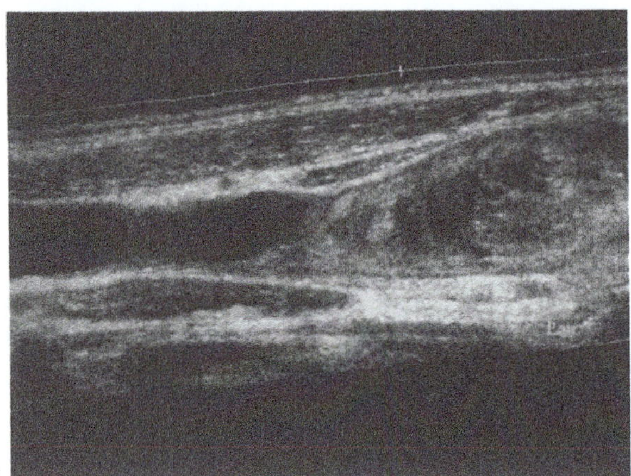

Fig. 7.17a–c. Recent sonographic techniques for the diagnosis of IJV thrombosis. a PD revealed the functional nature of the external portion of the IJV, which is partially occluded (axial scan). b Complete thrombosis of the left IJV (*J*); visualization of perithyroidal and subcutaneous peripheral venous dilatations (*TH* thyroid) (axial scan). c Siescape demonstrates complete occlusion of the inferior part of the left IJV (sagittal scan)

anticoagulant therapy (Patel et al. 1999). Venography is reserved for inconclusive cases that are often related to patient morphology. Near-complete resolution of the intraluminal clot may be seen on serial sonograms in response to anticoagulant therapy, and possible sequelae can be evaluated (Wing and Scheible 1983).

7.2.2 Sonography and IJV Cannulation

7.2.2.1 *Comparative Studies in the Literature*

Table 7.1 lists data from six series that analyzed the difficulties encountered during IJV puncture for placement of a catheter with and without sonographic localization. US improved the safety of the procedure at all stages by limiting the number of failures and incidents (puncture of the CCA, hematoma).

Generally speaking, placement of a venous catheter by IJV cannulation has several potential complications: pneumothorax, hemothorax, neck hematoma, mediastinal hematoma, vascular injury, and catheter migration.

7.2.2.2 *US-guided IJV Access Approaches*

Silberzweig and Mitty (1998) pointed out the danger of a high IJV puncture site owing to the possibility of secondary catheter obstruction by angulation as the catheter exits the IJV. Catheter kinking may occur during head rotation, contraction of the sternocleidomastoid muscle, or neck flexion.

The IJV should be accessed lower, around 2 cm above the clavicle, because the base of the neck remains relatively stable during head rotation, and kinking is thus exceptional. The puncture site should be selected between the sternal and clavicular insertions of the sternocleidomastoid muscle (Bazaral and Harlan 1981).

The patient is examined while supine, with the head turned opposite the side of catheter insertion. The ultrasound probe is placed axially with respect to the long axis of the IJV; percutaneous puncture of the IJV is performed using the Seldinger technique. Constant US visualization of the needle tip prevents accidental transfixion of the vein and ensures that the needle remains within the vein during the entire procedure. SILBERZWEIG and MITTY (1998) insert an 0.018-inch guidewire through a 21-gauge needle and guide it into the right atrium under fluoroscopic control. The needle is removed and a dilator sheath is placed; a larger-diameter guidewire (0.035-inch) is then inserted before the catheter is placed definitively. Tunneled catheters are inserted through a subcutaneous tunnel created over the middle third of the clavicle.

The US-assisted technique of SILBERZWEIG and MITTY (1998) requires two operators, one to insert the needle and the other, sitting opposite, to hold the US probe. In the single-operator cannulation technique described by GRAY et al. (1998), the transducer is held in the nondominant hand and the needle in the dominant hand, using an inclination that limits the distance between the cutaneous incision and the entry into the IJV to less than 2 cm.

7.2.2.3
Results of US-guided IJV Cannulation

In their series of nearly 900 cases of sonographically guided IJV cannulation procedures, GORDON et al. (1998) cited a low complication rate (2.3%), and 87% of procedures were achieved with a single pass. FUNAKI et al. (1997) and TREROTOLA et al. (1997) confirmed the excellent technical success rate (100%) achieved with US guidance of chest-port and hemodialysis catheter placement.

LOBATO et al. (1998) suggested use of a Trendelenburg tilt to facilitate IJV cannulation, because the increased intravascular pressure created by the maneuver renders the IJV less collapsible. When a Trendelenburg position is not feasible, positive inspiratory hold and hepatic compression may prove helpful to obtain venous dilatation.

Direct US guidance improves the safety of IJV cannulation, allowing even an inexperienced operator to successfully insert cannulae rapidly, as demonstrated in a prospective comparison of experienced (more than 25 previous central vein cannulae inserted) and inexperienced (fewer than three) operators (GEDDES et al. 1998) (Fig. 7.18).

7.2.2.4
IJV and Subclavian Approaches

MACDONALD et al. (2000) recommend the internal jugular route rather than the subclavian approach for placement of tunneled central venous catheters. Although both routes had similar technical success rates (100% for the IJV versus 97% for the subclavian vein), fewer procedure-related complications occurred with the IJV route, in particular pneumothorax (p=0.023), symptomatic venous thrombosis (p=0.015), and premature catheter removal due to sepsis (p=0.043) (Fig. 7.19).

Table 7.1. Difficulties reported during IJV cannulation for catheter placement with and without US guidance

	Without US guidance	With US guidance
Mean duration of IJV cannulation (in seconds)	51.4[e]	43.7[c]; 44.5[b] 9.8[b]; 15.8[c], 15.2[e]
Number of passes	2.58[c]	1.39[c]
Failure after first pass (%)	45.2[a]; 48[e]; 65.1[c]; 72[b]; 74[d]	4[e]; 16.4[a]; 19.2[c]; 22[b]; 57[d]
Complete failure (%)	11.9[b]; 14[c]; 23[f]; 24[d]	0[b,d,f]; 1[c]
Puncture of the common carotid artery(%)	2.4[a]; 8.3[b]; 12[e]; 13.6[d]; 25[f]	0[e,f]; 1.7[b]; 2.4[a]; 13.6[d]
Hematoma (%)	3.3[b]; 7.8[a]; 10[e]	0[a]; 0.2[b]; 2[e]
Nerve irritation (%)	1.7[b]; 6[e]	0.4[b]; 4[e]

[a]BOCK et al. (1999) 84 cases
[b]DENYS et al. (1993) 302 cases
[c]LIN et al. (1998a) 190 cases
[d]SLAMA et al. (1997) 69 cases
[e]TEICHGRABER et al. (1997) 100 cases
[f]VERGHESE et al. (1999) 95 children

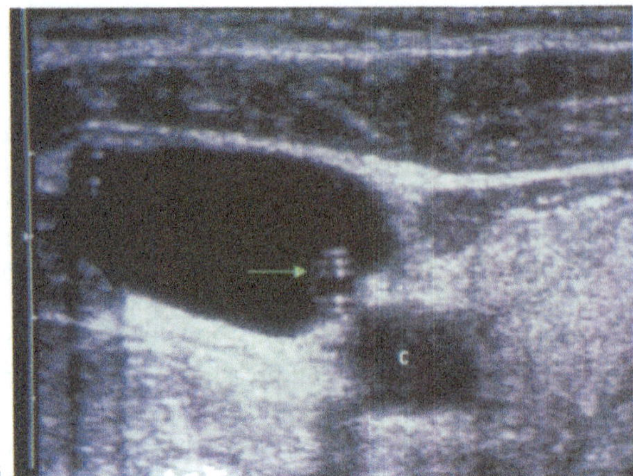
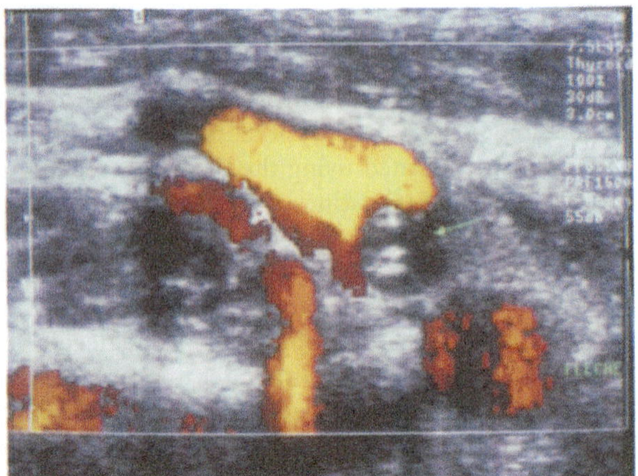

Fig. 7.18a,b. Catheter in the right IJV. **a** The four small echoic images correspond to the wall of the endovascular catheter (*arrow*) (*C* CCA, transverse scan). **b** PD study showing the catheter within the IJV (*arrow*)

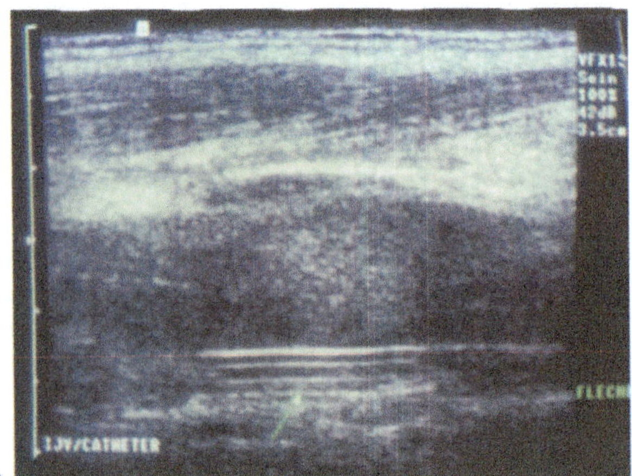

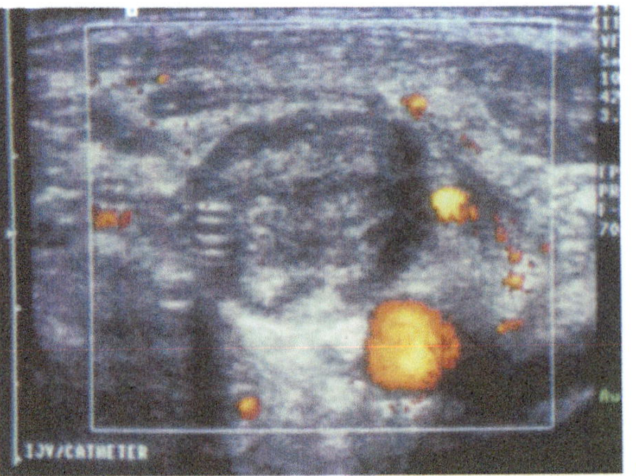

Fig. 7.19a,b. Catheter-related IJV thrombosis **a** Catheter within the IJV, which is completely thrombosed (sagittal scan) **b** PD study confirmed the sonographic findings (catheter visible as four small echogenic images in the external portion of the IJV lumen) (transverse scan)

7.2.2.5
Sonographic Follow-up

Sonographic evaluation of proposed insertion sites prior to IJV catheter placement may reveal significant endoluminal findings. Forauer and Glockner (2000) noted sonographic abnormalities in 35% of their patients (total occlusion in 22.8%, nonocclusive thrombus in 14.1%), 75% of whom required a change in access approach.

7.2.2.6
Indications

In addition to placement of temporary hemodialysis catheters and central venous access catheters, radiologically placed subcutaneous infusion chest ports are being increasingly used for delivery of chemotherapy. This type of venous access is well-tolerated, as Funaki et al. (1997) reported symptomatic catheter-related deep vein thrombosis in just 1% of patients (mean cannulation duration 5 months), and only 5% of catheters had to be removed prematurely. US-guided localization is also indicated for placement of transjugular intrahepatic portosystemic shunts (TIPS) (Roizental et al. 1995). Patel et al. (1999) systematically perform Doppler examination of the cervical veins before insertion of a central venous catheter. Patients with a short neck, obese patients, those with goiter, patients who have undergone cervical surgery, and patients with tracheostomies unquestionably benefit from the increased safety achieved with US guidance of IJV cannulation (Silberzweig and Mitty 1998).

7.2.3 Distal Venous Disease

When mediastinal venous thrombosis impedes blood flow from the IJV to the atrium, and even if the IJV appears morphologically normal, pulsed Doppler can suggest the presence of venous thrombosis involving the brachiocephalic trunks or the superior vena cava. Doppler analysis of the IJVs and the subclavian veins even permits localization of the level of occlusion.

PATEL et al. (1999) demonstrated that reduction or loss of cardiac pulsatility and respiratory phasicity at pulsed Doppler examination predicts central venous thrombus. However, pulsations transmitted from the CCA may be mistaken for normal venous cardiac pulsatility.

The probable site of occlusion can be predicted from the location of abnormal Doppler signals (PATEL et al. 1999). A thrombus in the right innominate vein is associated with normal signals in the left IJV and left subclavian vein but with abnormal signals in the right IJV and the right subclavian vein. Thrombus in the superior vena cava is indicated by abnormal signals in both IJVs and both subclavian veins (Fig. 7.20).

Reduced or absent cardiac pulsatility had a sensitivity of 100% and a specificity of 100% for the prediction of occlusion; in contrast, the sensitivity of diminished or absent respiratory phasicity was only 75% (PATEL et al. 1999). This indirect method thus has a practical value, because direct US examination of the mediastinal veins is often difficult or impossible (KNUDSON et al. 1990). While this approach is operator dependent, the method is currently considered more accurate than earlier techniques such as continuous-wave Doppler imaging and venous occlusion plethysmography (BONNET et al. 1989).

ROSE et al. (1998) underscored the importance of systematic Doppler flow analysis of the axillary veins and IJVs prior to placement of central venous access catheters in order to detect central vein occlusive disease that was responsible for failure of catheterization in 25% of their patients. A normal polyphasic atrial waveform virtually excludes more central venous occlusion or stenosis greater than 80%, thereby ensuring an adequate route for central venous catheterization.

STEIN et al. (1997) consider clinical estimates of right atrial pressure from the jugular venous pulse accurate when right atrial pressure is normal. In contrast, owing to the increased distance between the IJV and the mid-right atrium, elevated right atrial pressure cannot be detected by analysis of the jugular venous pulse in patients with congestive heart failure.

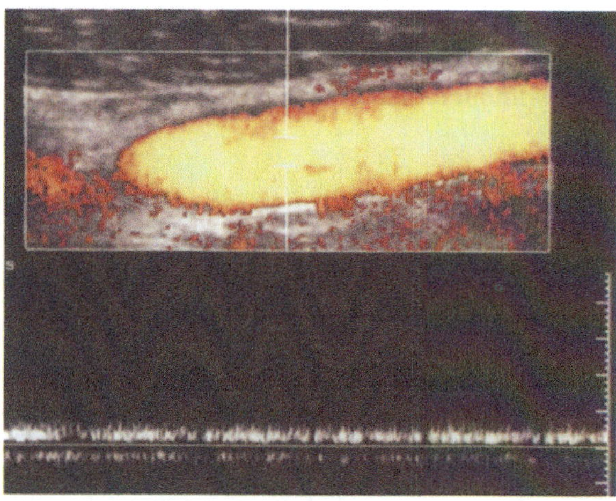

Fig. 7.20. Doppler study of the IJV: Loss of cardiac pulsatility was related to a mediastinal thrombosis

SAKAKIBARA (1978) reported a marked decrease in the IJV inflow velocity in cardiac tamponade. An inspiratory increase in the inflow velocity was observed in mild tamponade but not in severe disease. In constrictive pericarditis, he observed a reverse flow in the jugular vein coexistent with rapidly decelerating inflow in diastole.

7.2.4 Venous Examination after Neck Dissection

QURAISHI et al. (1997) performed Doppler sonography of the IJVs after functional (unilateral or bilateral) neck dissection (FND). Evidence of postoperative IJV thrombosis was seen on early sonograms (postoperative days 1 and 7) in 24.7% of the veins, but the rate then dropped to only 5.8% after 3 months. These findings reflect the relatively high frequency of asymptomatic IJV thrombosis following FND and nearly constant spontaneous recanalization; IJV thrombosis thus need not be sought systematically immediately after neck dissection.

BROWN et al. (1998) reported IJV thrombosis in 14% of patients managed by a free flap; they attributed this complication to the pedicled myocutaneous flap and left-sided jugular vein dissection, rather than to preoperative radiotherapy.

Other investigators have provided complementary data: ZOHAR et al. (1995) reported long-term preservation of IJV patency in 87% of patients after unilateral or bilateral FND. DOCHERTY et al. (1993) noted an increased risk of IJV thrombosis after a combination of radiotherapy and bilateral FND; only 18% of the patients in their study were ultrasonically normal bilaterally after this therapeutic combination. In contrast, the risk of IJV thrombosis is low after FND alone, without radiation therapy (LAKE et al. 1994).

7.3 Other IJV Pathologies

7.3.1 Valve Incompetence

IJV valve incompetence has been documented for many years using pulsed Doppler and M-mode techniques (BROWNLOW and MCKINNEY 1985). It has also been reported as an incidental finding during CT, although much less frequently than with US. YOUSSEFZADEH et al. (1998), for example, reported a CT frequency of only 0.012%.

IJV incompetence was investigated by RATANAKORN et al. (1999) using air-contrast US venography (ACUV), consisting of intravenous brachial injection of agitated air and saline. Sonographic examination of the right IJV by both B-mode monitoring and color flow imaging (CFI) permitted visualization of reflux in half of their patients. ACUV has potential as a noninvasive method to assess IJV valve competency in several pathologies:

- Respirator brain syndrome, which is seen in patients who have been on positive end-expiratory pressure ventilators for a long period; the elevated central pressure, especially in case of chronic tricuspid regurgitation, hinders blood return from the brain, thus triggering headaches.
- Cough headaches (KNAPPERTZ 1996), due to a sudden increase in chest pressure during coughing.
- RUDIKOFF et al. (1980) demonstrated the role of the IJV and thoracic vein valves in cardiopulmonary resuscitation.
- LEPORI et al. (1999) underscored the fact that the presence of IJV valves necessitates precaution during catheter placement, regardless of whether puncture is performed by an antegrade or retrograde (TIPS) route.

7.3.2 Cervical Mass and the IJV

A laterocervical tumor syndrome may affect the venous system, and in particular the IJV; the most common causes are cervical adenopathies. BRUNETON et al. (1990) demonstrated that metastatic nodes have a higher propensity for invasion than lymphomatous nodes. In a series of 78 cases of IJV thrombosis due to cervical adenopathies, 75 were due to nodal metastases of head and neck cancers; only three were related to lymphoma. IJV compression without thrombosis was observed in 65 cases (35 nodal metastases, 30 lymphomatous nodes) (Fig. 7.21).

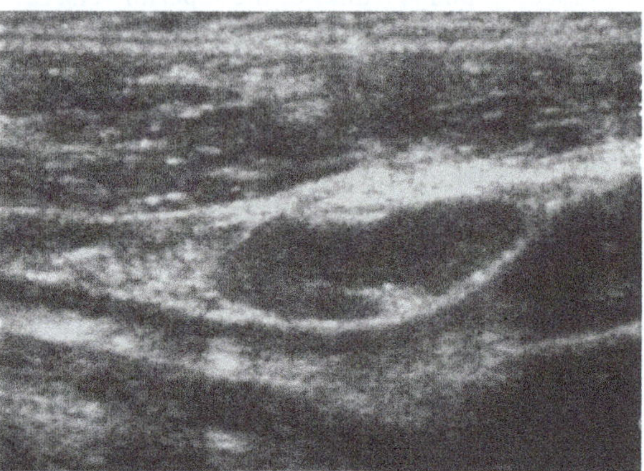
a

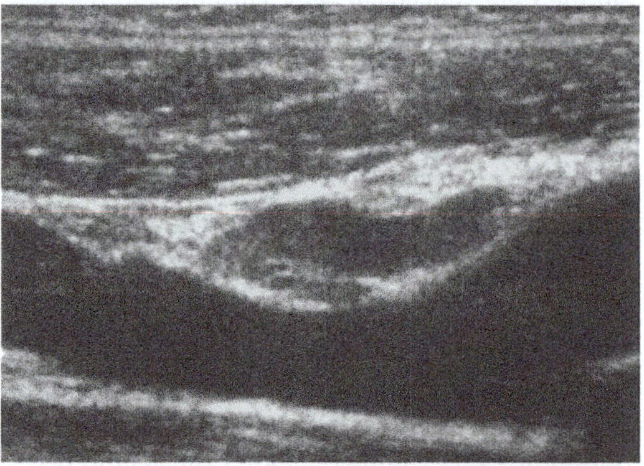
b

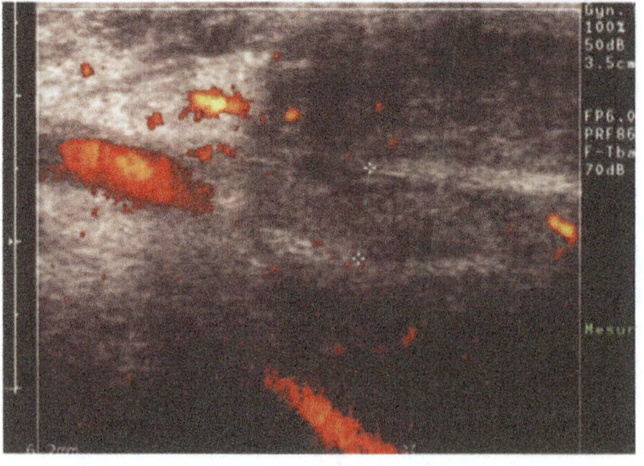

c

Fig. 7.21a,b. Valsalva study of the impact of an adenopathy on the IJV. **a** Interface between the enlarged node and the IJV. **b** No nodal invasion of the IJV wall was detected during examination using the Valsalva maneuver. **c** Anaplastic carcinoma of the thyroid gland involving the IJV

Examination of the cervical lymph nodes should include dynamic scanning with analysis of the IJVs during a Valsalva maneuver. Detection of nodal involvement that appears to extend into the mediastinum requires Doppler examination of the IJV, because loss of cardiac pulsatility and respiratory phasicity may suggest mediastinal vein thrombosis.

7.3.3 Other IJV Pathologies

Other IJV pathologies have been reported:

- Arteriovenous fistula: Porcu et al. (1998) found 20 reports of an abnormal communication between the external carotid artery and the IJV in adults in a review of the literature up until 1996. Fistulas between the CCA and the IJV are often diagnosed rapidly after puncture (Chen et al. 1995). However, Arning (1998) described a long-standing case secondary to insertion of a central venous catheter; prolonged anticoagulation therapy had prevented spontaneous closure of the vascular injury. CD revealed an increased IJV diameter and extremely rapid systolic inflow of arterial blood into the venous lumen.
- Phlebectasia: this benign phenomenon is not uncommon in children (Chao et al. 1999) and usually does not require treatment. CD demonstrates the vascular flow and zones of turbulence. Sonography permits measurement of the IJV diameter, which can increase from a mean of 0.79 cm to 1.58 cm during a Valsalva maneuver. Uzun et al. (1999) reported a case of unilateral IJV phlebectasia in a 56-year-old man that manifested as neck swelling during speech. Sonography allowed recognition of this rare anomaly and ruled out a laryngocele.
- Aneurysm: venous aneurysms of the neck are infrequent lesions without any particular topographic features that are readily detected by US. The sonographic image is rarely circular, as both external jugular vein aneurysms described by Verbeeck et al. (1997) had a saccular appearance.
- Hemangioma: these very rare lesions may manifest as cervical mass. Sarteschi et al. (1999) reported a case of EJV hemangioma in an adult. Gray-scale imaging of the 2-cm-diameter palpable mass showed a well-defined hypoechoic nodule with endoluminal involvement of the EJV but no invasion of surrounding structures; these findings suggested a partial internal thrombus, as the sonographic appearance resembled an intravascular thrombus adherent to the venous wall. Exertion of pressure by the transducer revealed that the vessel was collapsible, whereas the nodule was firm. CD corrected the diagnosis by revealing a network of microvessels, with arterial flow within the nodule (Fig. 7.22).

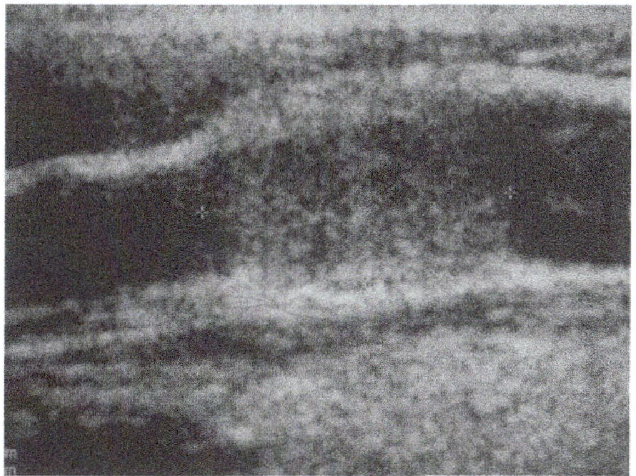

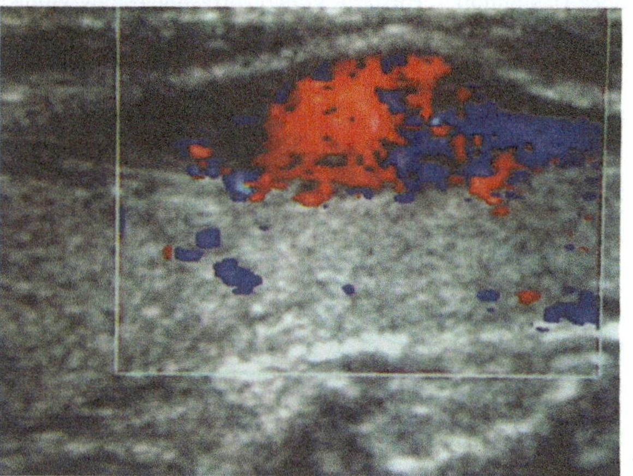

Fig. 7.22a,b. Hemangioma of the EJV (courtesy Sarteschi et al. 1999). **a** Echogenic image within the venous lumen (1.4–0/7 cm) (sagittal scan). **b** CD revealed the hypervascularity of the lesion

References

Albertyn LE, Alcock MK (1987) Diagnosis of internal jugular vein thrombosis. Radiology 162:505–508

Armstrong PJ, Sutherland R, Scott DH (1994) The effect of position and different manoeuvres on internal jugular vein diameter size. Acta Anaesthesiol Scand 38:229–231

Arning C (1998) Arteriovenous fistula of the jugular vein: detection and follow-up with color-coded duplex ultrasound. Vasa 27:183–186

Balbarini A, Rugolotto M, Buttitta F, Mariotti R, Strata G, Mariani M (1998) Deep venous thrombosis: epidemiologic, diagnostic and therapeutic aspects. Cardiologia 43:605–615

Bazaral M, Harlan S (1981) Ultrasonographic anatomy of the internal jugular vein relevant to percutaneous cannulation. Crit Care Med 4:307–310

Bock U, Mollhoff T, Forster R (1999) Ultrasonography-guided versus anatomically oriented puncture of the internal jugular vein for central venous catheterization. Ultraschall Med 20:98–103

Bonnet F, Loriferne JF, Texier JP, Texier M, Salvat A, Vasile N (1989) Evaluation of Doppler examination for diagnosis of catheter-related deep vein thrombosis. Intensive Care Med 15:238–240

Brown DH, Mulholland S, Yoo JH, et al (1998) Internal jugular vein thrombosis following modified neck dissection: implications for head and neck flap reconstruction. Head Neck 20:169–174

Brownlow RL Jr, McKinney WM (1985) Ultrasonic evaluation of jugular venous valve competence. J Ultrasound Med 4:169–172

Bruneton JN, Balu-Maestro C, Merran D, et al (1990) Rapports veineux des adénopathies cervicales. Revue d'une série de 300 cas. J Radiol 71:57–60

Caridi JG, Hawkins IF Jr, Wiechmann BN, Pevarski DJ, Tonkin JC (1998) Sonographic guidance when using the right internal jugular vein for central vein access. AJR Am J Roentgenol 171:1259–1263

Chao HC, Wong KS, Lin SJ, Kong MS, Lin TY (1999) Ultrasonographic diagnosis and color flow Doppler sonography of internal jugular venous ectasia in children. J Ultrasound Med 18:411–416

Chen YW, Yip PK, Hwang BS, Jeng JS, Lin WH (1995) Color Doppler sonographic study of an iatrogenic fistula between the common carotid artery and internal jugular vein. J Ultrasound Med 14:777–780

Denys BG, Uretsky BF, Reddy PS (1993) Ultrasound-assisted cannulation of the internal jugular vein. A prospective comparison to the external landmark-guided technique. Circulation 87:1557–1562

Docherty JG, Carter R, Sheldon CD, et al (1993) Relative effect of surgery and radiotherapy on the internal jugular vein following functional neck dissection. Head Neck 15:553–556

Forauer AR, Glockner JF (2000) Importance of US findings in access planning during jugular vein hemodialysis catheter placements. J Vasc Interv Radiol 11:233–238

Funaki B, Szymski GX, Hackworth CA, et al (1997) Radiologic placement of subcutaneous infusion chest ports for long-term central venous access. AJR Am J Roentgenol 169:1431–1434

Gaitini D, Kaftori JK, Pery M, Engel A (1988) High-resolution real-time ultrasonography. Diagnosis and follow-up of jugular and subclavian vein thrombosis. J Ultrasound Med 7:621–627

Geddes CC, Walbaum D, Fox JG, Mactier RA (1998) Insertion of internal jugular temporary hemodialysis cannulae by direct ultrasound guidance. A prospective comparison of experienced and inexperienced operators. Clin Nephrol 50:320–325

Gordon AC, Saliken JC, Johns D, Owen R, Gray RR (1998) US-guided puncture of the internal jugular vein: complications and anatomic considerations. J Vasc Interv Radiol 9:333–338

Gray RR, Saliken JC, So CB, Sadler CB (1998) Sonographic guidance for central venous access. AJR Am J Roentgenol 171:894

Hu Z, Zhao G, Xiao Z, Chen X, Zhong C, Yang J (1999) Different responses of cerebral vessels to 30 head-down tilt in humans. Aviat Space Environ Med 70:674–680

Imai M, Hanaoka Y, Kemmotsu O (1994) Valve injury: a new complication of internal jugular vein cannulation. Anesth Analg 78:1041–1046

Karnik R, Valentin A, Winkler WB, Donath P, Slany J (1993) Duplex sonographic detection of internal jugular venous thrombosis after removal of central venous catheters. Clin Cardiol 16:26–29

Knappertz VA (1996) Cough headache and the competency of jugular venous valves. Neurology 45:1497

Knudson GJ, Wiedmeyer DA, Erickson SJ, et al (1990) Color Doppler sonographic imaging in the assessment of upper-extremity deep venous thrombosis. AJR Am J Roentgenol 154:399–403

Kroger K, Rudofsky G (1998) Duplex sonography of vascularization of venous thrombosis. Int Angiol 17:103–107

Kroger K, Gocke C, Schelo C, Hinrichs A, Rudofsky G (1998a) Association of subclavian and jugular vein thrombosis: color doppler sonographic evaluation. Angiology 49:189–191

Kroger K, Schelo C, Gocke C, Rudofsky G (1998b) Colour Doppler sonographic diagnosis of upper limb venous thromboses. Clin Sci (Colch) 9:567–661

Lake GM III, Dinardo LJ, Demeo JH (1994) Performance of the internal jugular vein after functional neck dissection. Head Neck Surg 111:201–204

Lepori D, Capasso P, Fournier P, Genton CY, Schnyder P (1999) High-resolution ultrasound evaluation of internal jugular venous valves. Eur Radiol 9:1222–1226

Lin BS, Huang TP, Tang GJ, Tarng DC, Kong CW (1998a) Ultrasound-guided cannulation of the internal jugular vein for dialysis vascular access in uremic patients. Nephron 78:423–428

Lin BS, Kong CW, Tarng DC, Huang TP, Tang GJ (1998b) Anatomical variation of the internal jugular vein and its impact on temporary haemodialysis vascular access: an ultrasonographic survey in uraemic patients. Nephrol Dial Transplant 13:134–138

Lobato EB, Florete DG jr, Paige GB, Morey TE (1998) Cross-sectional area and intravascular pressure of the right internal jugular vein during anesthesia: effects of Trendelenburg position, positive intrathoracic pressure, and hepatic compression. J Clin Anesth 10:1–5

Lobato EB, Sulek CA, Moody RL, Morey TE (1999) Cross-sectional area of the right and left internal jugular veins. J Cardiothorac Vasc Anesth 13:136–138

Longley DG, Finlay DE, Letourneau JG (1993) Sonography of the upper extremity and jugular veins. AJR 160:957–962
Macchi C, Catini C (1994) The valves of the internal jugular veins: a statistical investigation in 120 living subjects using ultrasonic tomography. Ital J Anat Embryol 99:123–127
Macdonald S, Wyatt AJ, McNally D, Edwards RD, Moss JG (2000) Comparison of technical success and outcome of tunneled catheters inserted via the jugular and subclavian approaches. J Vasc Intern Radiol 11:225–231
Mallinson C, Bennett J, Hodgson P, Petros AJ (1999) Position of the internal jugular vein in children. A study of the anatomy using ultrasonography. Paediatr Anaesth 9:111–114
Mallory DL, Shawker T, Evans RG, et al (1990) Effects of clinical maneuvers on sonographically determined internal jugular vein size during venous cannulation. Crit Care Med 18:1269–1273
Marie I, Levesque H, Cailleux V, et al (1998) Deep venous thrombosis of the upper limbs. A propos of 49 cases. Rev Med Interne 19:399–308
Moutos DM, Miller MM, Mahadevan MM (1997) Bilateral internal jugular venous thrombosis complicating severe ovarian hyperstimulation syndrome after prophylactic albumin administration. Fertil Steril 68:174–176
Muller HR, Hinn G, Buser MW (1990) Internal jugular venous flow measurement by means of a duplex scanner. J Ultrasound Med 9:261–265
Patel MC, Berman LH, Moss HA, McPherson SJ (1999) Subclavian and internal jugular veins at Doppler US: abnormal cardiac pulsatility and respiratory phasicity as a predictor of complete central occlusion. Radiology 211:579–583
Patra P, Gunness TK, Robert R, et al (1988) Physiologic variations of the internal jugular vein surface, role of the omohyoid muscle, a preliminary echographic study. Surg Radiol Anat 10:107–112
Porcu A, Dessanti A, Scanu AM, Feo CF, Dettori G (1998) Congenital carotid-jugular fistula in an elderly patient. Minerva Chir 53:853–855
Pucheu A, Evans J, Thomas D, Scheuble C, Pucheu M (1994) Doppler ultrasonography of normal neck veins. J Clin Ultrasound 22:367–373
Quraishi HA, Wax MK, Granke K, Rodman SM (1997) Internal jugular vein thrombosis after functional and selective neck dissection. Arch Otolaryngol Head Neck Surg 123:969–973
Ratanakorn D, Tesh PE, Tegeler CH (1999) A new dynamic method for detection of internal jugular valve incompetence using air contrast ultrasonography. J Neuroimaging 9:10–14
Roizental M, Kane RA, Takahashi J, et al (1995) Portal vein: US-guided localization prior to transjugular intrahepetic portosystemic shunt placement. Radiology 196:868–870
Rose SC, Kinney TB, Bundens WP, Valji K, Roberts AC (1998) Importance of Doppler analysis of transmitted atrial waveforms prior to placement of central venous access catheters. J Vasc Interv Radiol 9:927–934
Rudikoff MT, Maughan WL, Effron M, Freund P, Weisfeld ML (1980) Mechanisms of blood flow during cardiopulmonary resuscitation. Circulation 61:345–352
Sakakibara H (1978) Application of the ultrasonic technique for the pathophysiological analysis of pericardial disease. Jpn Circ J 42:139–148
Sarteschi LM, Bonanomi G, Mosca F, Ferrari M (1999) External jugular vein hemangioma occurring as a lateral neck mass. J Ultrasound Med 18:719–721
Screaton NJ, Ravenel JG, Lehner PJ, Heitzman ER, Flower CD (1999) Lemierre syndrome: forgotten but not extinct. Report of four cases. Radiology 213:369–374
Silberzweig JE, Mitty HA (1998) Central venous access: low internal jugular vein approach using imaging guidance. AJR Am J Roentgenol 170:1617–1620
Sinave CP, Hardy GJ, Fardy PW (1989) The Lemierre syndrome: suppurative thrombophlebitis of the internal jugular vein secondary to oropharyngeal infection. Medicine 68:85–94
Slama M, Novara A, Safavian A, Ossart M, Safar M, Fagon JY (1997) Improvement of internal jugular vein cannulation using an ultrasound-guided technique. Intensive Care Med 23:916–919
Stein JH, Neumann A, Marcus RH (1997) Comparison of estimates of right atrial pressure by physical examination and echocardiography in patients with congestive heart failure and reasons for discrepancies. Am J Cardiol 80:1615–1618
Stickle BR, McFarlane H (1997) Prediction of a small internal jugular vein by external jugular vein diameter. Anesthesia 52:220–222
Sulek CA, Gravenstein N, Blackshear RH, Weiss L (1996) Head rotation during internal jugular vein cannulation and the risk of carotid artery puncture. Anesth Analg 82:125–128
Teichgraber UKM, Benter T, Gebel M, Manns MP (1997) A sonographically guided technique for central venous access. AJR Am J Roentgenol 169:731–733
Terai C, Anada H, Matsushima S, Shimizu S, Okada Y (1995) Effects of mild Trendelenburg on central hemodynamics and internal jugular vein velocity, cross-sectional area, and flow. Am J Emerg Med 13:255–258
Tovi F, Fliss DM, Novak AM (1993) Septic internal jugular vein thrombosis. J Otolaryngol 22:415–420
Trerotola SO, Johnson MS, Harris VJ et al (1997) Outcome of tunneled hemodialysis catheters placed via the right internal jugular vein by interventional radiologists. Radiology 203:489–495
Troianos CA, Kuwik RJ, Pasqual JR, Lim AJ, Odasso DP (1996) Internal jugular vein and carotid artery anatomic relation as determined by ultrasonography. Anesthesiology 85:43–48
Uzun C, Taskinalp O, Koten M, Adali MR, Karasalihoglu AR, Pekindil G (1999) Phlebectasia of left anterior jugular vein. J Laryngol Otol 113:858–860
Verbeeck N, Hammer F, Gofette P, Mathurin P (1997) Saccular aneurysm of the external jugular vein, an unusual cause of neck swelling. J Belge Radiol 80:63–64
Verghese ST, McGill WA, Patel RI, Sell JF, Midgley FM, Ruttimann UE (1999) Ultrasound-guided internal jugular venous cannulation in infants: a prospective comparison with the traditional palpation method. Anesthesiology 91:71–77
Weissleder R, Elizondo G, Stark DD (1987) Sonographic diagnosis of subclavian and internal jugular vein thrombosis. J Ultrasound Med 10:577–587
Wing V, Scheible W (1983) Sonography of jugular vein thrombosis. AJR Am J Roentgenol 140:333–336
Youssefzadeh S, Liskutin J, Dorffner R, Bankier A, Hubsch P (1998) Venous contract fluid level in computed tomography. Clin Radiol J 53:528–531
Zohar Y, Strauss M, Sabo R, Sadov R, Sabo G, Lehman J (1995) Internal jugular vein patency after functional neck dissection: venous duplex imaging. Ann Otol Rhinol Laryngol 104:5

8 Miscellaneous

Jean Noël Bruneton, François Tranquart, PPhilippe Brunner, Michel-Yves Mourou

CONTENTS

J.N. Bruneton, MD
Service de Radiologie, Hôpital de l'Archet, 151, route de St.-Antoine Ginestière, B.P. 3079, 06202 Nice Cedex 3, France
F. Tranquart, MD
Médecine Nucléaire et Ultrasons, INSERM U 316, CHU Bretonneau, 37044 Tours Cedex, France
P. Brunner, MD
Service de Radiologie, Centre Hospitalier Princesse Grace, Avenue Pasteur, 98000 Monaco, Monaco
M.Y. Mourou, MD
Service de Radiologie, Centre Hospitalier Princesse Grace, Avenue Pasteur, MC-98000 Monaco, Monaco

8.1 Congenital Cervical Anomalies

8.1.1 Thyroglossal Duct Cyst

Cystic lesions of the neck have a number of etiologies: hemorrhagic thyroid cyst, thyroglossal duct cyst, branchial cleft cyst, cystic hygroma, parotid abscess, cystic degeneration of a malignant cervical lesion, sebaceous cyst, cold abscess (El-Silimy and Corney 1993). Thyroglossal duct cysts are the most common developmental cyst in the neck (70%) (Allard 1982).

8.1.1.1 General Features

Thyroglossal duct cysts are generally discovered in infancy, and 83.3% are diagnosed before the age of 30 years (al-Dousary 1997). In the embryo, the thyroglossal duct extends from the thyroid to the foramen cecum of the tongue; a thyroglossal duct cyst may thus develop at any level between the base of the tongue and the suprasternal region (WEISMAN 1996).

Histologically, these cysts contain a squamous and ciliated pseudostratified epithelium; thyroid follicles are often present in the cyst wall. Lesion growth is considered a response to recurrent local infections or inflammatory processes (ALLARD 1982).

Although thyroglossal duct cysts are classically considered to occur exclusively along the midline, 37% in the study by AHUJA et al. (1999) were located elsewhere. Thyroglossal duct cysts have also been described in a submandibular location (O'HANLON et al. 1994; WADSWORTH and SIEGEL 1994). According to ALLARD (1982), 1%–2% of thyroglossal duct cysts occur at the base of the tongue, 25% in the suprahyoid region, 60% between the hyoid bone and the thyroid cartilage, and 13%–14% in a suprasternal location.

Clinically, the cervical mass is often not tender; anterior neck swelling was noted in 79% of cases by AL-DOUSARY (1997). Recurrence is more common after mere excision (40%) than after a Sistrunk procedure (7%) (AL-DOUSARY 1997). Only 1% of all thyroglossal duct cysts are complicated by a carcinoma (usually a papillary carcinoma; MARTINS et al. 1999). RANIERI et al. (1996) found only ten cases of carcinoma arising in a thyroglossal duct cyst reported in the English-language literature; associated lymphadenopathy may suggest this classic but rare pathology.

8.1.1.2
Sonography

A combination of physical examination and sonography nearly always permits diagnosis of thyroglossal duct cysts, despite the great variability of their US features. In particular, modifications in their sonographic appearance are not always correlated with the presence or absence of inflammation or infection (Wadsworth and Siegel 1994). The spectrum of sonographic features includes (Fig. 8.1):

- Anechoic lesions with no perceptible wall (42% of the cases in the series of WADSWORTH and SIEGEL 1994). According to HAUSEGGER et al. (1990), thyroglossal duct cysts and branchial cysts have a characteristic anechoic appearance in 68.2% of cases. However, in the adult, AHUJA et al. (1999) found that "typical" anechoic cysts represented only 28% of cases; this may be due to the greater frequency of inflammatory episodes associated with increased age.
- Hypoechoic lesions (homogeneous or heterogeneous) have also been described, predominantly hypoechoic lesions with multiple small anechoic spaces, or cystic lesions with multiple dense internal echoes and thick walls (at least 5 mm) (WADSWORTH and SIEGEL 1994); homogeneously hypoechoic lesions with internal debris accounted for 18% of the cases in the study of AHUJA et al. (1999).
There have been no reports to date of a thyroglossal duct cyst hyperechoic to the adjacent soft tissues.

Sonography may also reveal posterior enhancement (88% of cases for AHUJA et al. 1999) or a thin cyst wall (50% of cases for AHUJA et al. 1999); in some cases there is no sonographically visible fistula or hemorrhagic lesion (WADSWORTH and SIEGEL 1994).

When the cyst is associated with an adenoma, the mass appears solid, more or less homogeneous, and generally hypoechoic to the adjacent structures (Figs. 8.2 and 8.3). Carcinoma in a thyroglossal duct cyst (essentially papillary type) may image as a cystic nodule containing a solid area that corresponds to the malignant thyroid tissue (MARTINS et al. 1999). US examination of the lateral neck may reveal adenopathies.

Overall, clinical findings and the strictly cystic sonographic appearance nearly always permit diagnosis before surgery. Depending on the size of the lesion, it may or may not be palpable; five of the 24 patients examined by BAATENBURG DE JONG et al. (1993c) were asymptomatic, and the cyst was a sonographic discovery.

Differential diagnosis is usually not a problem, even when the sonographic appearance is not completely cystic. Dermoid cysts also occur in the midline, but they are hyperechoic to the adjacent soft tissues. Branchial cleft cysts develop in the lateral neck rather than along the midline, although differential diagnosis from a lateral thyroglossal duct cyst is not possible. Hydatid cysts of the neck are encountered only in geographical regions where this pathology is endemic (EROGLU et al. 1999). Diagnosis of an ectopic thyroid may require scintigraphy (AL-DOUSARY 1997).

8.1.1.3
Other Imaging Modalities

Scintigraphy is unnecessary when clinical examination and sonography suggest the diagnosis; furthermore, US can visualize the entire thyroid gland. On CT scans, thyroglossal duct cysts image as a thin-walled, fluid-density mass; cyst wall thickening and hypervascularization may be observed in case of

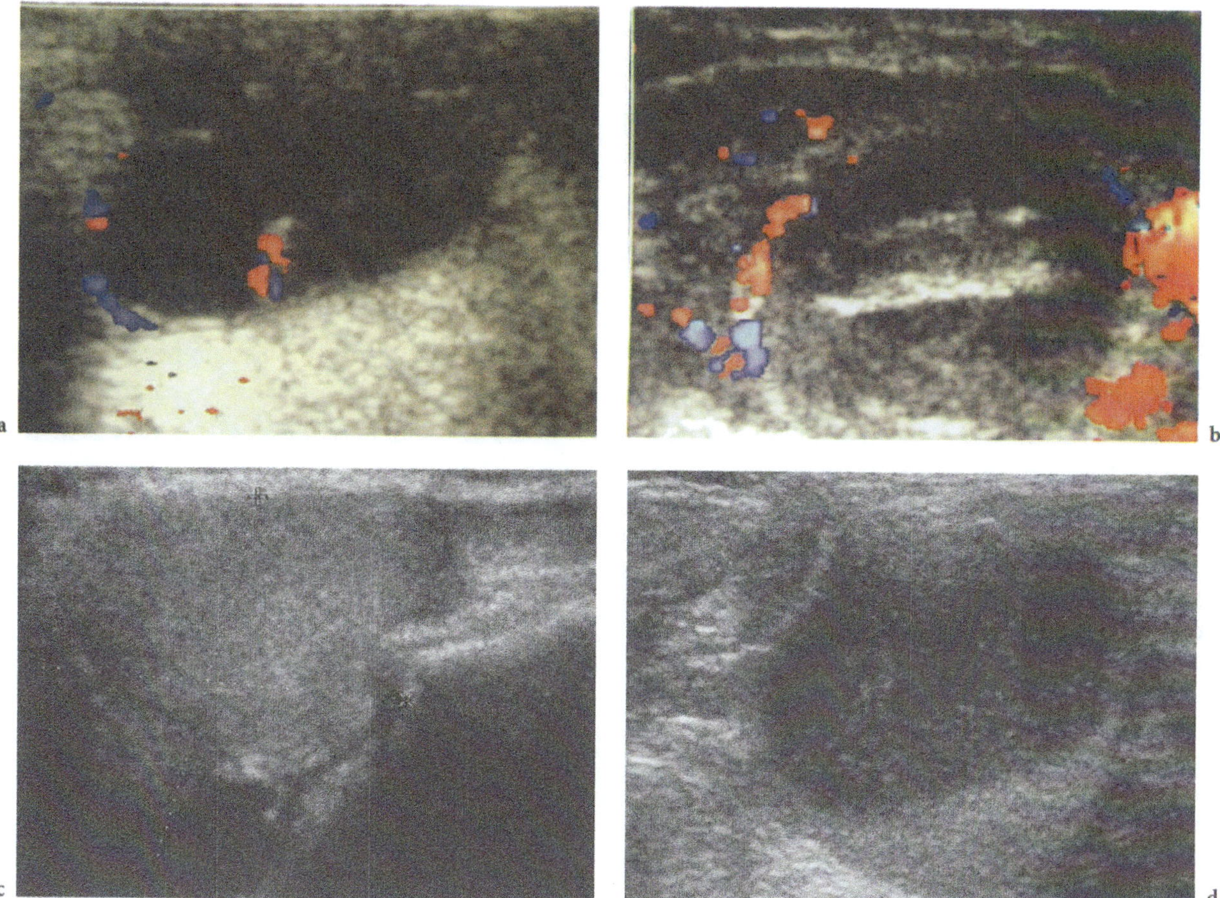

Fig. 8.1a–d. Thyroglossal duct cyst. **a** Septate cyst with parietal vascularity. Owing to this anomaly, a diagnosis of cystic lymphangioma was proposed; a reorganized thyroglossal duct cyst was found at surgery. **b** Thyroglossal duct cyst with internal echoes (recurrent infections). **c** Inhomogeneous appearance of a thyroglossal duct cyst (2.9/2.8 cm between the *two crosses*): solid homogeneous mass anterior to a fluid-like zone (sagittal scan). **d** Fluid-like mass with internal echoes related to previous bleeding episodes

inflammation. On MRI, thyroglossal duct cysts have a low signal intensity on T_1-weighted images and a high signal intensity on T_2-weighted sequences (Miller et al. 1992; Sigal 1999).

8.1.2 Branchial Cleft Cysts

8.1.2.1 General Features

The most common cystic masses of the lateral neck, branchial cleft cysts are detected essentially in young subjects; first and second branchial cleft cysts predominate. Branchial developmental anomalies are divided into three types: sinuses, fistulae, and cysts. Cysts are the result of failed obliteration of the bran-

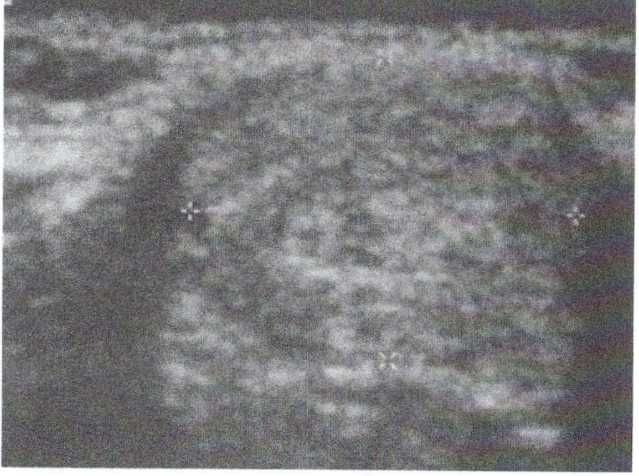

Fig. 8.2. Adenoma of the thyroglossal duct. Solid midline mass (0.9/1.1 cm between the *crosses*) located at a distance from the thyroid; no associated laterocervical adenopathy. The diagnosis was not made until surgery

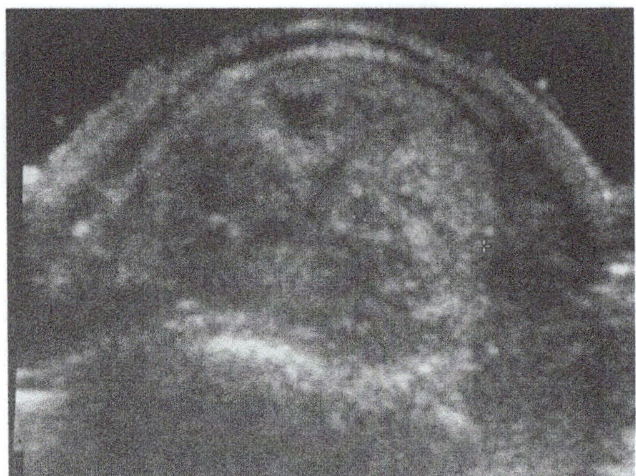

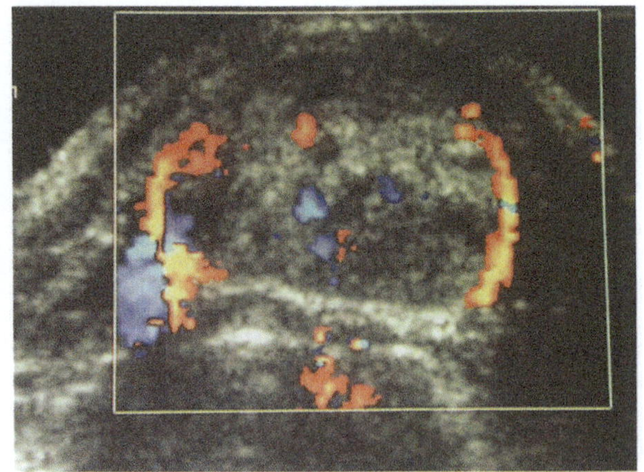

Fig. 8.3a, b. Adenoma of the thyroglossal duct. **a** Solid midline mass (2 cm between the *two crosses*) at a distance from t he thyroid, without any satellite nodes (axial scan). **b** Color Doppler analysis revealing the peripheral and central vascularity of the lesion; surgery confirmed the preoperative diagnosis of adenoma of the thyroglossal duct

chial clefts, and according to Agaton-Bonilla and Gay-Escoda (1996), they represent 80.8% of all branchial arch anomalies.

First branchial cleft anomalies account for approximately 8% of all branchiogenic anomalies (Mukherji et al. 1993). They manifest as a cystic lesion at the inferior pole of the parotid and are usually discovered in a middle-aged subject. The differential diagnosis is a parotid pathology.

Second branchial cleft lesions are the most common, representing 80%–90% of cases. Sometimes subclinical, these lesions are often sonographic discoveries today. In contrast, earlier clinical studies cited a much lower frequency, e.g., only 64% of cases for Bailey (1923). Second branchial arch cysts occur between the angle of the mandible and the supraclavicular region. Four categories have been defined as a function of location: superficial cysts anterior to the sternocleidomastoid muscle, cysts lying below the middle cervical fascia and anterior to the great vessels (the most common variety), branchial extensions towards the pharynx, and cysts between the great vessels and the lateral pharyngeal wall.

Third and fourth branchial cleft anomalies are rare (only 30 cases were reported in the literature in 1999). A piriform sinus fistula or a lateral neck mass reflects a recurrent inflammatory process. Owing to the infrequency of third and fourth cleft lesions, other diagnoses are usually suggested: cystic hygroma, laryngocele, adenopathy, epidermoid cyst, salivary gland lesion (Yang et al. 1999).

Malignant transformation or association with a carcinoma is exceptional (Kukwa et al. 1995) and postoperative recurrence is uncommon (the overall recurrence rate after 2 years of follow-up was only 4.9% in the study of Agaton-Bonilla and Gay-Escoda 1996).

The wide spectrum of clinical pictures ranges from a simple, painless mass (such as cysts) to recurrent infections (as is common when a cutaneous fistula is present).

8.1.2.2
Sonography

The occasionally nonpalpable lesions can reach 4 cm in greatest dimension; generally cystic, their fluid-like appearance is highly suggestive of the diagnosis Baatenburg de Jong et al. 1993b). Branchial cleft cysts occasionally image as a pseudosolid mass owing to their mucoid or cholesterol contents; in other cases, the lesion displays uniform low echogenicity (Reynolds and Wolinski 1993). A fistula, when present, is usually not visible by US. Hemorrhagic complications may create internal echoes; if infection has occurred, fluid levels are visible and the poorly delimited lesion may extend towards the muscles or the thyroid gland (Barberet et al. 1999). US-guided fine-needle aspiration (FNA) is indicated whenever the diagnosis remains in doubt, and in 86% of cases it provides the diagnosis (Engzell and Zajicek 1970). (Fig. 8.4).

Differential diagnoses include a cervical bronchogenic cyst (Brown and Tschen 2000), ectopic cervical thymic cyst (Terzakis et al. 2000), laryngocele, laryngeal mucocele (Swartz et al. 1990), and especially cystic degeneration of a nodal metastasis of thyroid cancer, in which case the lesion may be solitary (Ahuja et al. 1998b). Detection of a cystic mass in the

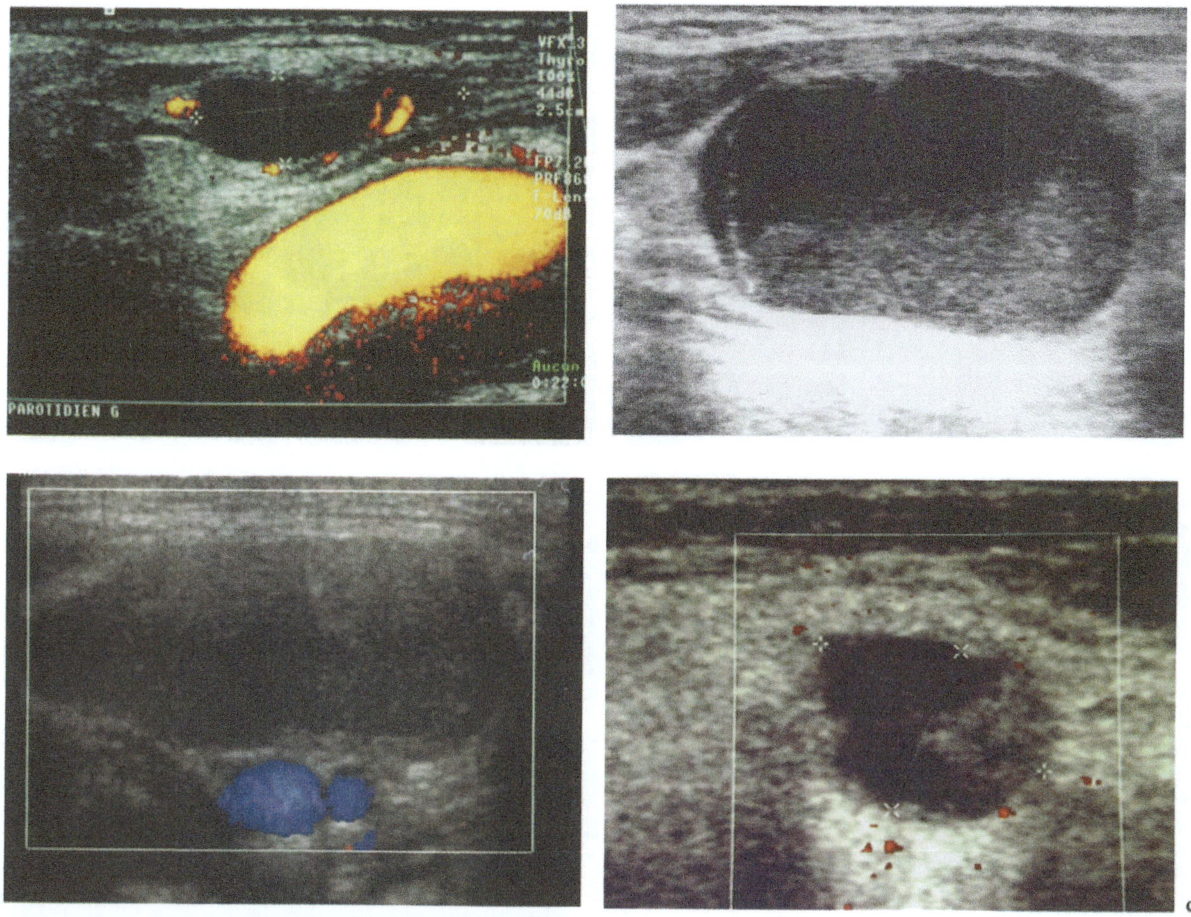

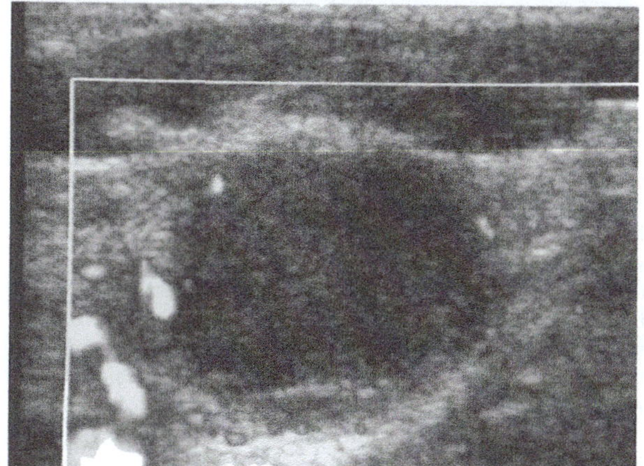

Fig. 8.4a–e. Branchial cleft cysts. **a** This small anechoic branchial cyst (1.7/1 cm between the *crosses*) was avascular at power Doppler analysis. **b** Cystic mass in the lateral neck containing distal echoes (history of hemorrhage), without any other anomaly. **c** Well-defined, discretely heterogeneous hypoechoic lesion in a prevascular, laterocervical position. **d** Infraparotid branchial cyst (1.1/0.7 cm between the *crosses*); power Doppler revealed the absence of vascularity; a preoperative diagnosis of adenitis was made owing to a history of numerous inflammatory episodes; a first branchial arch cyst was discovered at surgery. **e** Small hypoechoic branchial cyst (recurrent infections) with discrete parietal vascularity

lateral neck should always prompt a search for possible association with a thyroid nodule; the difficulties of detecting nodules smaller than 5 mm should be kept in mind. However, there are no sonographic features permitting differentiation of a cystic nodal metastasis of thyroid cancer (sometimes not visible sonographically) from a complicated branchial cyst; such cases require US-guided FNA for definitive diagnosis.

8.1.2.3 Other Imaging Modalities

A barium swallow study performed during a quiescent period may provide definitive diagnostic information for third and fourth branchial arch anomalies (Park et al. 2000; Yang et al. 1999). CT usually reveals a thin-walled, fluid-density mass. Sonographic find-

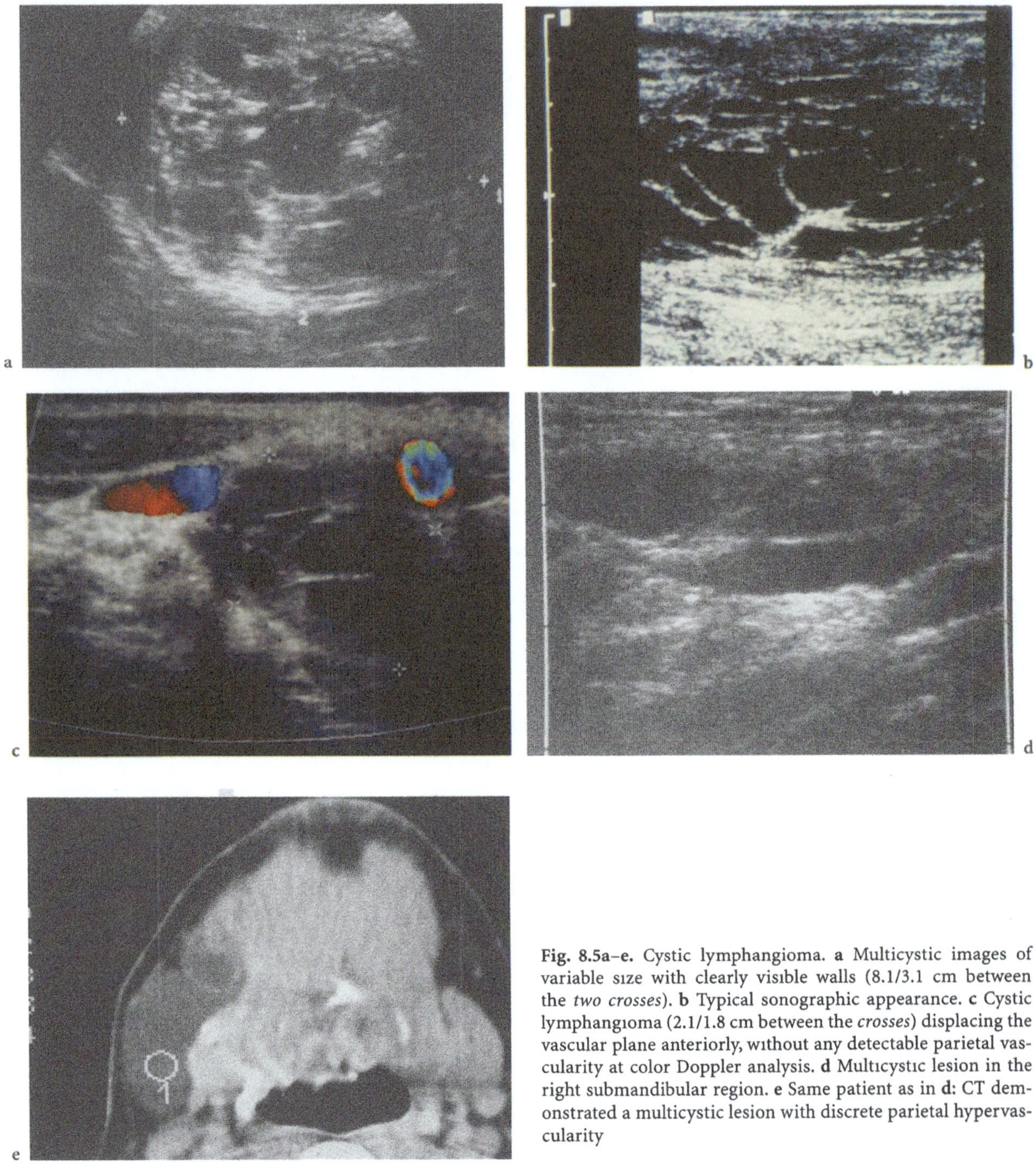

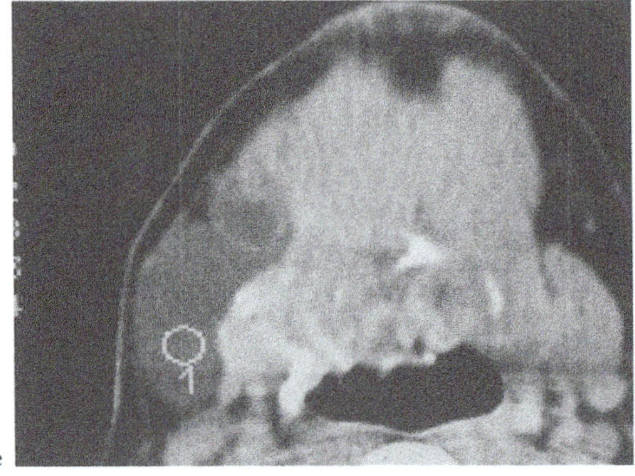

Fig. 8.5a–e. Cystic lymphangioma. **a** Multicystic images of variable size with clearly visible walls (8.1/3.1 cm between the *two crosses*). **b** Typical sonographic appearance. **c** Cystic lymphangioma (2.1/1.8 cm between the *crosses*) displacing the vascular plane anteriorly, without any detectable parietal vascularity at color Doppler analysis. **d** Multicystic lesion in the right submandibular region. **e** Same patient as in **d**: CT demonstrated a multicystic lesion with discrete parietal hypervascularity

ings may include uniform low echogenicity and rim enhancement after intravenous injection of contrast medium, reflecting old or recent inflammatory phenomena (Reynolds and Wolinski 1993). In patients with a fourth branchial arch anomaly, a Valsalva maneuver forces air into the soft tissues (Barberet et al. 1999). MRI can depict the sinus tract; rim enhancement reflecting inflammation may be seen after intravenous gadolinium injection (Mukherji et al. 1993).

8.1.3 Other Congenital Anomalies

8.1.3.1 Cystic Lymphangioma

Discovered essentially during infancy (90% of cases are detected before the age of 2 years), cystic lymphangioma is the result of anomalous sequestration of primitive lymph sacs in one or more of the five branchial clefts that give rise to the lymphatic system. Histologically, lesions are classified as cystic hygroma or cavernous or capillary lymphangioma.

Two forms have been described: a localized form in the lateral neck and a diffuse form involving the tongue, the floor of the mouth, and the parotid region that can produce severe clinical symptoms.

The risk of malignant transformation is low. Imaging-guided percutaneous sclerotherapy using doxycycline has been proposed for unresectable lymphangiomas (MOLITCH et al. 1995).

Sonography typically demonstrates a multicystic mass containing thin septa posterior to the sternocleidomastoid muscle. Color Doppler US may reveal flow signals within the septa (BRUNETON and GEOFFRAY 1995) (Fig. 8.5).

CT and MRI give comparable results. With MRI, a low-intensity signal is noted on T_1-weighted images (except in case of hemorrhage) while a high signal intensity is seen on T_2-weighted sequences; enhancement of the septa is noted after contrast administration with both CT and MRI (SIGAL 1999).

The differential diagnosis is nodal metastases.

8.1.3.2 Epidermoid Cyst

This rare cystic lesion is often diagnosed after the age of 20 or 30 years, when clinical symptoms develop. There is no sex predilection or risk of malignant transformation; complete excision is curative. Submental locations predominate (LOHAUS et al. 1999).

Histopathologically, three types of cyst have been defined (dermoid, epidermoid, and teratoid), but the term dermoid cyst is usually used for all three categories (TURETSCHEK et al. 1995).

Sonographically (Fig. 8.6), the lesion appears homogeneously hyperechoic owing to its contents (cholesterol crystals, keratin). Areas of calcifications

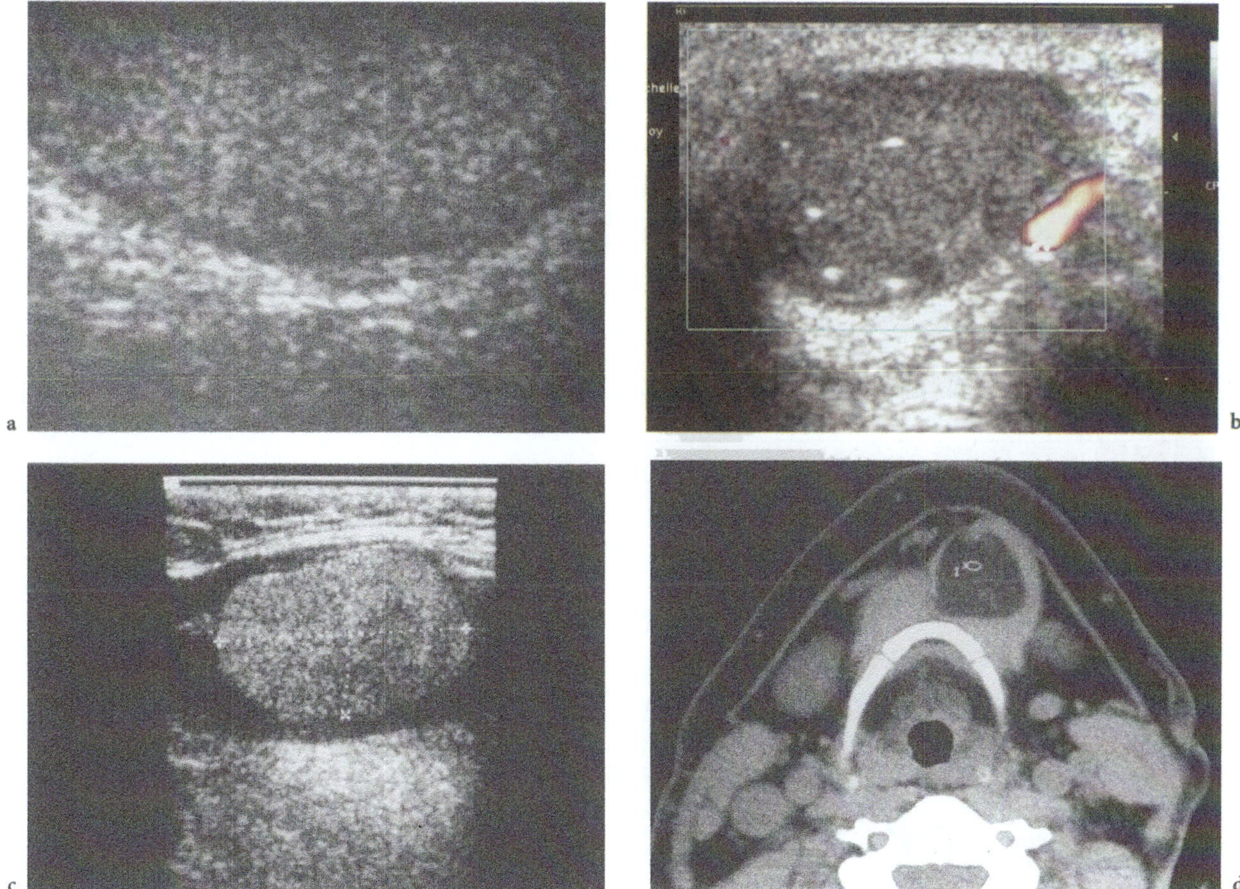

Fig. 8.6a–d. Epidermoid cyst. **a** Well-delimited, homogeneous lesion (2 cm in greatest dimension). **b** Hypoechoic US lesion with small internal echoes but no intranodular vascularity. **c** Homogeneously echogenic solitary cervical mass along the midline. **d** Same patient as in **c**: CT revealed the typical low density of this type of lesion (dermoid cyst)

are possible. The most remarkable feature, however, is the presence of multiple spherical formations corresponding to keratin (LOHAUS et al. 1999). According to YASUMOTO et al. (1991) these lesions show little or no posterior enhancement; for these authors, epidermoid cysts are sonographically indistinguishable from lipoma. Differential diagnoses include a thyroglossal duct cyst, branchial cleft cyst, cystic hygroma, or a ranula.

CT can differentiate an epidermoid cyst from a lipoma because fatty lesions have a lower density. MRI reveals an intermediate intensity signal on T_1-weighted images and a high T_2-weighted signal intensity.

8.1.3.4 Hemangioma

These vascular remnants known as hemangiomas are classified as cavernous, capillary, or mixed. The sonographic appearance of cervical lesions is reportedly similar to that of hemangiomas in other localizations (KANG et al. 1997). US reveals a well-defined, hypoechoic mass, often with a heterogeneous echotexture and cystic spaces (YANG et al. 1997a). Phleboliths occur occasionally and image as hyperechoic punctate structures.

Color Doppler analysis of lesion vascularity has given inconsistent results in the literature, although YANG et al. (1997a) reported color Doppler demonstration of flow in 12 of 13 lesions. When CD fails to depict hypervascularity, use of a contrast medium may permit visualization of vascular elements within an apparently solid lesion, thus allowing differential diagnosis, in particular from a cystic lymphangioma (CHOU et al. 1999) (Fig. 8.7).

Voluminous hemangiomas have been treated by US-guided interstitial Nd:YAG laser (WERNER et al. 1998).

a 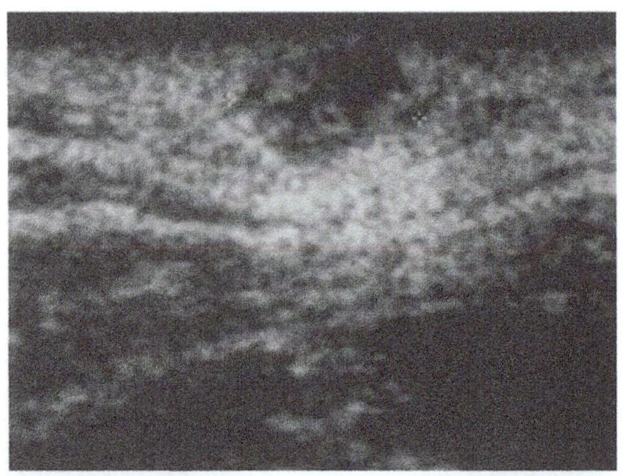

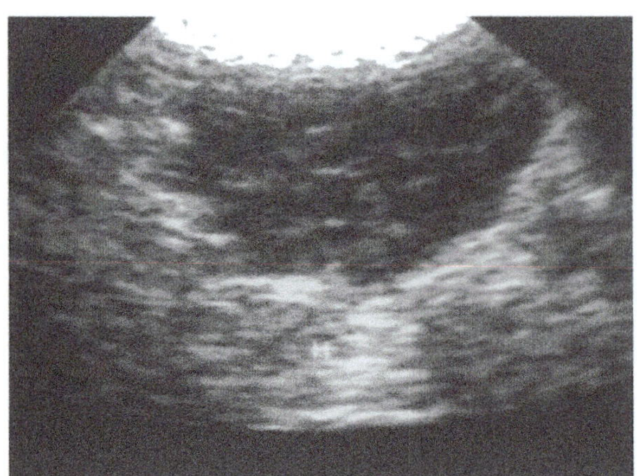 b

c 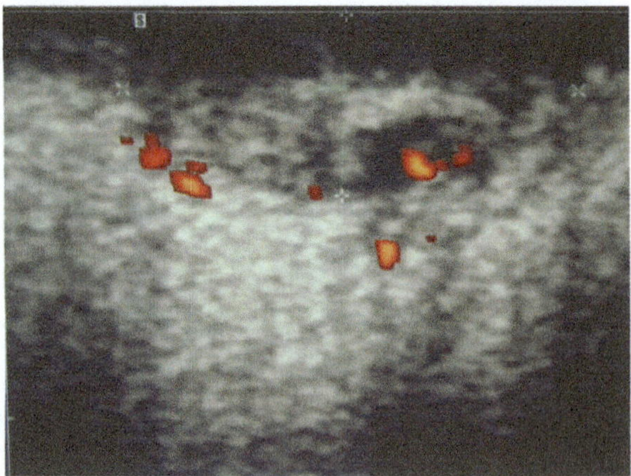

Fig. 8.7a–c. Hemangioma. **a** Small subcutaneous cervical hemangioma (0.5 cm between the *two crosses*). **b** Well-delimited mass in the right lower neck with numerous homogeneous internal echoes. **c** Inhomogeneous lesion (1.1/0.4 cm between the *crosses*) containing zones hyperechoic and hypoechoic compared with the surrounding tissue; the discrete vascularity was not significant at color Doppler

8.2 Inflammation and Infection

8.2.1 Post-radiation Features

The acute and chronic secondary effects of irradiation have been described in detail (MALKINSON and KEANE 1981). In patients with head and neck cancer treated by radiotherapy, subsequent thickening of the cutaneous and subcutaneous tissues is less of a problem than the acute mucosal reaction that peaks during the fourth week of irradiation (MISZCZYK and PRZEOREK 1999). Furthermore, while post-radiation skin reactions are constant, they are also of lesser severity than infrequent radiation-induced complications such as CNS reactions (myelopathy, cranial nerve palsy) that can be evaluated by MRI, bone involvement (osteonecrosis) that is best assessed by CT, laryngopharynx involvement with stenosis amenable to examination by CT, and arteriopathy, which is an indication for US (BECKER et al. 1997).

Most studies on radiation-induced skin changes have dealt with breast cancer patients (WARSZAWSKI et al. 1998). Sonography with a 20- or 30-MHz probe reveals an increase in dermal thickness that is greater in the early phase (less than 3 months after the end of radiotherapy) than in the late phase, dedifferentiation of the limit between the corium and the subcutaneous space, and a reduction in echogenicity compared with the non-irradiated skin (Fig. 8.8).

Osteonecrosis of the mandible is best investigated with CT and especially with MRI (EPSTEIN 1997; LARHEIM et al. 1999). However, US can visualize the lesions, involvement of the adjacent soft tissues, and even the trajectory of a fistula.

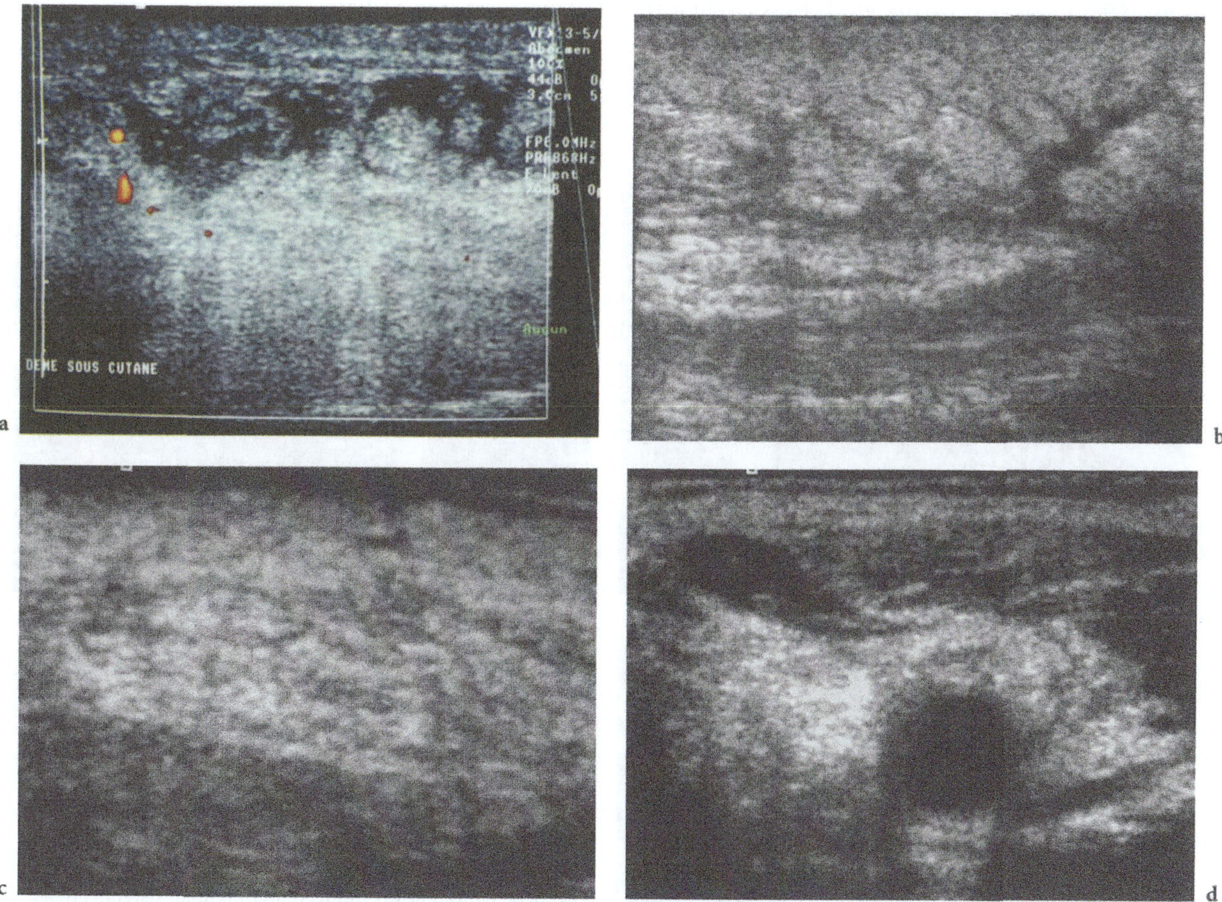

Fig. 8.8a–d. Post-radiation appearance of the subcutaneous space. **a** Severe subcutaneous edema without any notable hypervascularity. **b** Subcutaneous edema with lymphatic ectasia. **c** Long-standing post-radiation appearance, with dedifferentiation of the subcutaneous space. **d** Subcutaneous reorganization after radical neck dissection and radiotherapy

8.2.2
Abscess and Postoperative Inflammation

8.2.2.1
General Features

Deep neck infections have numerous etiologies: bone lesions with prevertebral spread (Talmi et al. 2000), recurrent infection of a branchial cleft cyst or another congenital anomaly (Nusbaum et al. 1999; Park et al. 2000), acute phlegmonous oropharyngitis, acute tonsillitis, peritonsillar space infections (the main cause in children; Ojiri et al. 1998; Ungkanont et al. 1995), perforation of the esophagus, chronic otitis, lymphoma, trauma, a foreign body that is not always identified by imaging – in particular, objects of wood or plastic (Coales et al. 1999).

Head and neck cancers rarely cause deep neck infections (Lee et al. 1996). In contrast, an odontogenic origin should be sought systematically (Peleg et al. 1998; Constantinidis et al. 1998). When the diagnostic workup is negative, a nodal etiology is generally suspected, in particular for lesions in the lateral neck (Jovic et al. 1999).

Sakaguchi et al. (1997) classed the localizations of these lesions in decreasing order of frequency: peritonsillar space, parapharyngeal space, submandibular space, retropharyngeal space, superficial space, anterior visceral space, vascular visceral space.

Contiguous spread of a deep neck infection to the IJV may cause thrombophlebitis that generally responds to treatment (El Sayed and al-Dousary 1996; Lin et al. 1999). Cervical abscesses may be complicated by a mediastinal extension.

The most common causative organisms are streptococci and staphylococci (Gidley et al. 1997); however, only 56.2% of cultures were positive in the study by El Sayed and al-Dousary (1996).

8.2.2.2
Sonography

As cervical infections are seen essentially during childhood, most descriptions of their sonographic features concern pediatric populations (Quraishi et al. 1997) (Figs. 8.9–8.11).

The abscess manifests as a hypoechoic or occasionally anechoic structure with thin septa, sur-

a 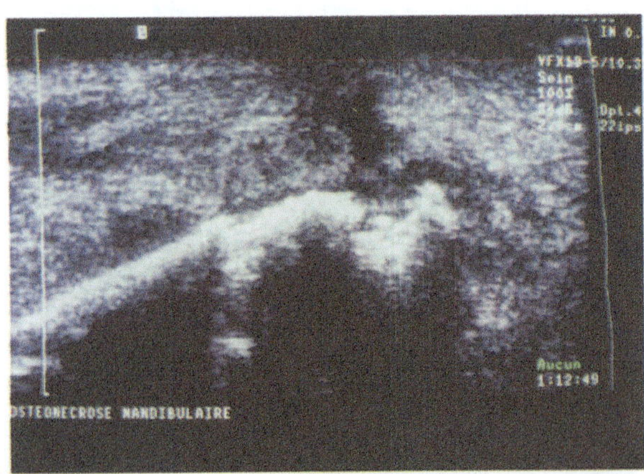

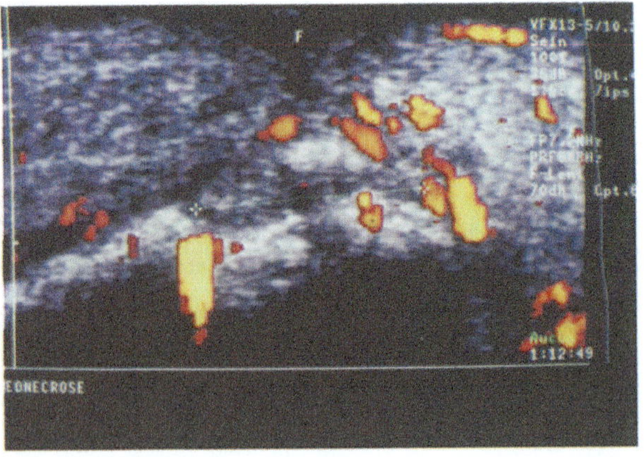 b

c 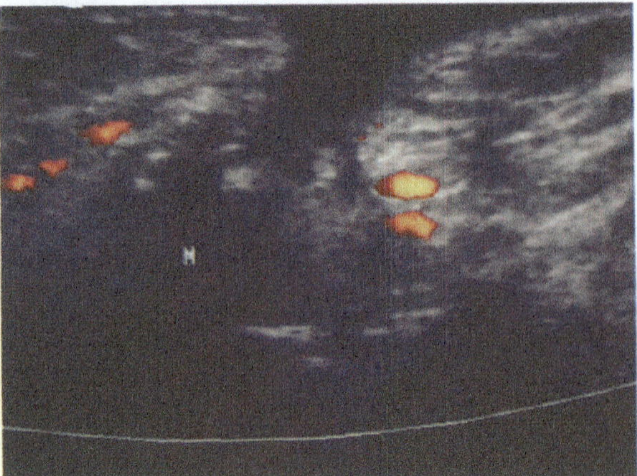

Fig. 8.9a–c. Radiation-induced mandibular osteonecrosis. **a** Mandibular bone defect; the loss of soft tissue substance opposite the defect corresponds to a cutaneous fistula. **b** Same patient as in **a**: power Doppler revealed the perimandibular hypervascularity (*F* cutaneous orifice of the fistula). **c** Mandibular osteonecrosis with a 1-cm-diameter fistula and moderate peripheral hypervascularity (*M* mandible)

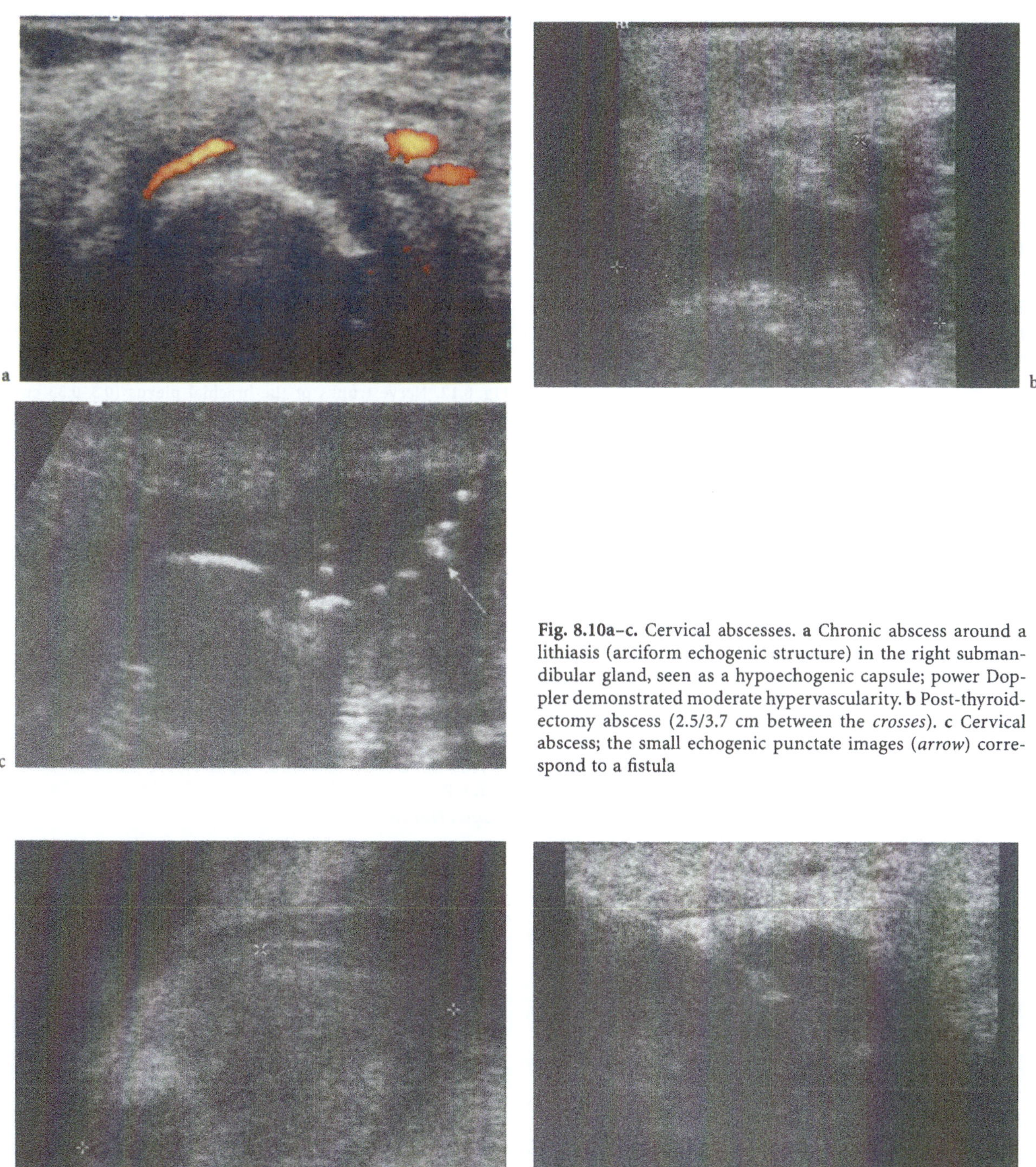

Fig. 8.10a–c. Cervical abscesses. **a** Chronic abscess around a lithiasis (arciform echogenic structure) in the right submandibular gland, seen as a hypoechogenic capsule; power Doppler demonstrated moderate hypervascularity. **b** Post-thyroidectomy abscess (2.5/3.7 cm between the *crosses*). **c** Cervical abscess; the small echogenic punctate images (*arrow*) correspond to a fistula

Fig. 8.11a, b. Submental abscess. **a** Inhomogeneous hypoechoic mass (3.3/2.2 cm between the *crosses*). **b** Drainage of the abscess by percutaneous incision (the catheter is visible as an oblique linear structure within the abscess)

rounded by a more echoic zone of variable thickness. CD reveals more or less extensive hypervascularity that depends on the age of the abscess. Demonstration of an echo-free mass affirms the diagnosis of an abscess, permits subsequent FNA, and rules out uncomplicated cellulitis (PELEG et al. 1998). US guidance of catheter placement for drainage and surveillance constitutes an alternative to open surgery (OCHI et al. 1996; TORANZO et al. 1999).

US is insufficient for analysis of the deep cervical region and cannot demonstrate mediastinal extension. In contrast, involvement of the IJV is readily visualized sonographically.

8.2.2.3
Other Imaging Modalities

As CT has no topographical limitations (in contrast to US), it is the most commonly used technique, even in children (ELIASHAR et al. 1999). CT is particularly useful for lesions in a posterior localization (osseous etiology), even though it is not always easy to distinguish a retropharyngeal space abscess from retropharyngeal cellulitis (BOUCHER et al. 1999). CT demonstration of mediastinal extension of a deep neck abscess usually permits percutaneous CT-guided drainage (POE et al. 1996). MRI is more accurate than CT for examination of the parapharyngeal space (SIEVERS et al. 2000).

8.3
Neurogenic Tumors

8.3.1
Sonography of the Peripheral Nerves

8.3.1.1
Brachial Plexus

Transverse US scans through the supraclavicular region (C-6) demonstrate the nerves of the brachial plexus, between the anterior and middle scalene muscles (YANG et al. 1998). The nerve trunks image as three discrete, rounded, hypoechoic structures that split inferolaterally into anterior and posterior divisions at the outer border of the first rib (Fig. 8.12).

An intact nerve is seen as a hypoechoic tubular structure; fine linear internal echoes are seen inconsistently. Color Doppler (CD) does not reveal any vascularity.

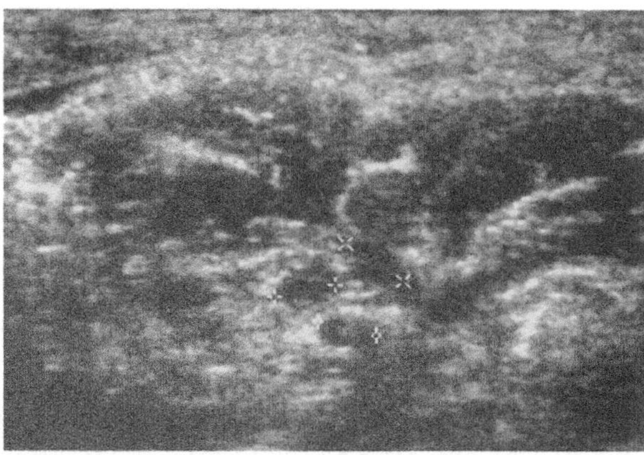

Fig. 8.12. Nerve trunks of the brachial plexus (0.3–0.35 cm between the *crosses*) between the scalene muscles

The major clinical application of sonographic data is regional brachial plexus anesthesia; US guidance increases the efficacy of the catheter-based procedure and reduces the risk of complications (TING and SIVAGNANARATNAM 1989; YANG et al. 1998).

An intraforaminal lesion created by traction injury of the brachial plexus can be visualized sonographically as a thick, irregularly shaped structure with internal echoes simulating nerve continuity (HAYAMIZU et al. 1995).

8.3.1.2
Vagus Nerve

Located between the IJV and the common carotid artery (SOLBIATI et al. 1985; WIEL MARIN et al. 1998) (Fig. 8.13), this tubular structure with a low echogenicity center and a hyperechoic wall (interface with

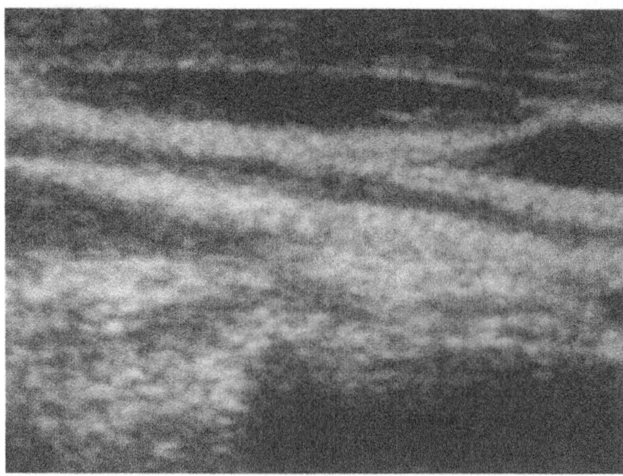

Fig. 8.13. The vagus nerve is visible posterior to the IJV as a low echogenicity structure with hyperechoic walls (sagittal scan)

the peripheral fat) was visible sonographically in 97% of cases for KNAPPERTZ et al. (1998).

8.3.1.3 Paraspinal Sonography

Paraspinal US is not accurate for evaluation of the nerve roots. In particular, its specificity is much too low for satisfactory analysis of the facets of the cervical vertebrae (NAZARIAN et al. 1998).

8.3.2 Glomus Tumors

The term "glomus tumor" is synonymous with non-chromaffin paraganglioma and glomus jugulare tumor.

8.3.2.1 General Features

This usually benign, slow-growing hypervascular tumor arises from the neuroendocrine cells of the extra-adrenal paraganglia. It occurs between the base of the skull and the cross of the aorta. The most common sites, in decreasing order of frequency, are the carotid bifurcation, the vagal glomus, the tympanic glomus, and the jugular glomus; mediastinal localizations are very rare (BLANCO PEREZ et al. 2000; GHILARDI et al. 1991; JANSEN et al. 1997).

Carotid chemodectomas are exceedingly rare, representing only 0.036% of all cervical tumors (KRUPSKI et al. 1982). However, WESTERBAND et al. (1998) reported sonographic discovery of a carotid chemodectoma in 28% of their cases.

Despite their low propensity for malignant transformation (fewer than 10% of cases; ARSLAN et al. 2000; WIN and LEWIN 1995), glomus tumors tend to invade the adjacent nerve, vascular, and osseous structures. Multiple lesions occur in fewer than 5% of cases, either simultaneously or successively. A familial character is observed in 10% of cases (MYSSIOREK and PALESTRO 1998), and is associated with increased risks of multiple lesions (30%) and malignancy.

Clinically, these tumors are usually asymptomatic. In 97% of cases, a non-tender mass prompts the patient to consult a physician (PADBERG et al. 1983); diagnosis is usually made around the age of 40 years. There is no sex predilection.

8.3.2.2 Sonography

The first-line imaging modality for glomus tumors, US demonstrates a homogeneous or discretely inhomogeneous polycyclic mass in the carotid bifurcation, which is splayed (GOODING 1979; MAKARAINEN et al. 1986; TRATTNIG et al. 1991). The diameter of these well-limited lesions ranges from 1 to 6 cm. Echogenicity is variable, but the tumor is often hypoechoic and never cystic. The internal carotid artery is displaced posteriorly while the external carotid artery is displaced anteromedially (Fig. 8.14). US examination of the cervical region must be completed by a search for contralateral involvement.

a 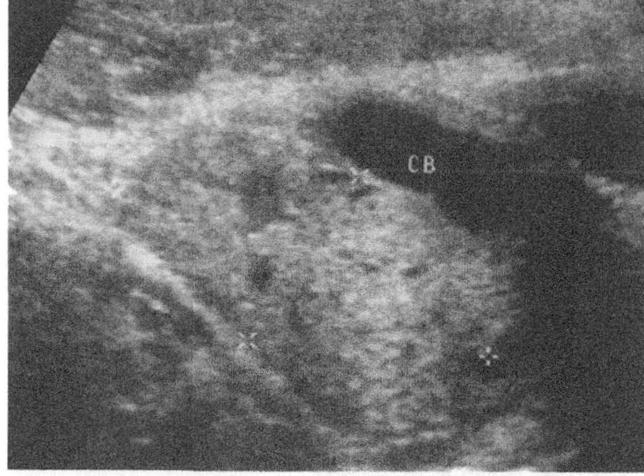

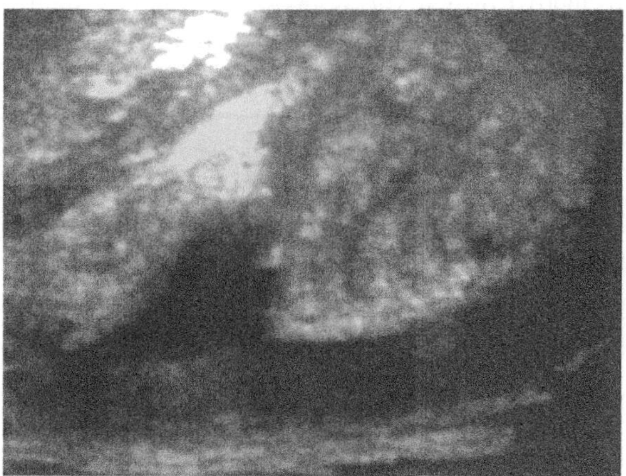 b

Fig. 8.14a, b. Chemodectoma. **a** Echogenic mass displacing the carotid bifurcation (*CB*) anteriorly; the small echogenic zones correspond to vascular structures (3.4/1.7 cm between the *crosses*). **b** Echogenic tissue is visible at the level of the carotid bifurcation (sagittal scan)

Lesions at the level of the vagus nerve have a similar sonographic appearance and generally displace the common carotid artery and the IJV anteriorly (Raby 1987).

Sonography is complemented by Doppler analysis, which nearly always demonstrates flow with a low resistive index (Barry et al. 1993; Derchi et al. 1992; Jansen et al. 1997).

CD reveals abundant flow signals and an intense tumoral blush with capillary images comparable to those observed on angiography (Arslan et al. 2000; Schreiber et al. 1996; Zidi et al. 2000). Infrequently, problems occur for differential diagnosis from an adenopathy, an aneurysm of the common carotid artery, a salivary gland tumor, a branchial cleft cyst, or another neurogenic tumor (Muhm et al. 2000). A hypervascular mass at the level of the carotid bifurcation is highly suggestive of a chemodectoma (Fig. 8.15).

8.3.2.3
Other Imaging Modalities

CT shows a well-defined, round or oval mass that enhances concomitantly with the carotid arteries after iodine injection; analysis of lesion size and its relationship with the vascular axes is satisfactory. Multiple lesions can be demonstrated, along with any extension towards the base of the skull; complete CT examination from the base of the skull down to the upper portion of the thorax is thus mandatory.

On MRI, glomus tumors are iso- or hyperintense to muscle on T_1-weighted images and hyperintense on T_2-weighted sequences; intense enhancement is observed after gadolinium administration (Zidi et al. 2000). Coronal MRI scans are helpful to visualize the upper and lower limits of the lesion. Oblique sagittal scans along the axis of the carotid bifurcation accurately demonstrate the relationship between the lesion and the bifurcation.

Owing to the efficacy of noninvasive imaging techniques, the only current indication for arteriography is assessment of a voluminous tumor prior to embolization.

Technetium-99m-sestamibi scintigraphy reportedly reveals intense early and transient contrast uptake (Piga et al. 1999), and somatostatin receptor scintigraphy has been used to diagnose postoperative recurrence (Schumacher et al. 1996).

8.3.3
Other Neurogenic Tumors

8.3.3.1
Schwannoma

This benign, neurogenic tumor arises from the Schwann cells of the neurilemma. Typically solitary, spherical or oval lesions with an indolent course, they are characterized by their eccentric development along the course of the nerve. This growth pattern permits surgical excision without sacrifice of the nerve, as to opposed to neurofibroma of the cervical vagus nerve (Gilmer-Hill and Kline 2000). Cervical localizations represent only 2.5% of all schwannomas (Andratschke et al. 2000; Torossian et al. 1999); a female predilection has been observed.

The lesion remains asymptomatic for a long period. Schwannomas involving the vagus nerve manifest as a lateral neck mass, on rare occasion associated with neurological symptoms. Postoperative recurrence is rare (Torossian et al. 1999).

a 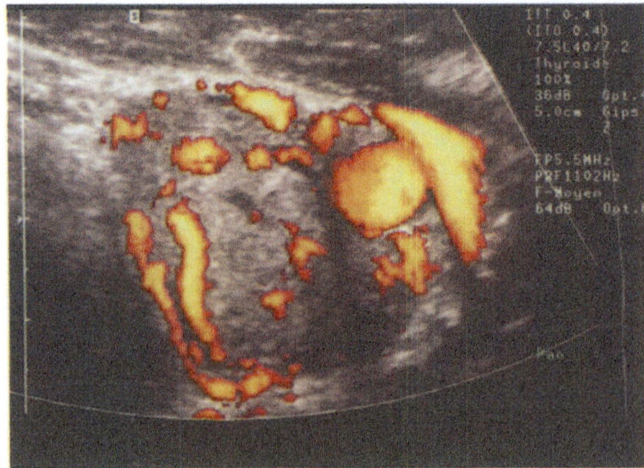

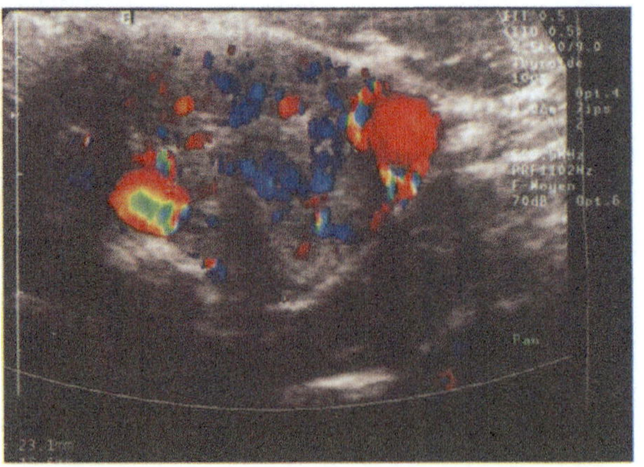 b

Fig. 8.15a, b. Power Doppler and color Doppler analysis of chemodectomas. **a** Hypervascular chemodectoma. **b** Splaying of the external and internal carotid arteries by a hypervascular chemodectoma (2.3/1.6 cm between the *crosses*)

Regardless of the localization (cervical nerves, vagus nerve, cervical sympathetic chain), sonography consistently reveals a well-delimited, hypoechoic nodule with posterior enhancement (NGUYEN et al. 2000; HOOD et al. 2000; TOROSSIAN et al. 1999; WIEL MARIN et al. 1998). One particular variety of schwannoma has a cystic appearance (MIYAWAKI et al. 1999), but when microcysts are present, they are usually too small to be seen sonographically (Fig. 8.16).

HOOD et al. (2000) and TOROSSIAN et al. (1999) emphasized the value of CT and MRI for preoperative diagnosis. Aside from differential diagnosis (principally from a chemodectoma, which is hypervascular on CD), the main problem, regardless of the technique, is accurate localization of the apparently solitary nodular lesion, except when the normal nerve is visualized without interruption of its continuity, as is sometimes possible for the vagus nerve (DE PRA et al. 1995; WIEL MARIN et al. 1998). In other cases, imaging-guided FNA can be performed, but results are rarely conclusive; in the series of YU et al. (1999), FNA provided the preoperative diagnosis in only one of eight cases.

8.3.3.2 Neurofibroma

Neurofibroma develops in the endoneurium as the result of concentric growth in and around the nerve; this complicates surgery because excision always requires sacrificing the nerve. Malignant transformation is possible in neurofibromatosis type I (TOROSSIAN et al. 1999).

Plexiform neurofibromas are characterized by diffuse involvement of the nerve; US demonstrates a hyperechoic mass with coarse internal echoes and lobulated contours (DE PRA et al. 1995).

Non-plexiform neurofibromas and neurofibromas in patients with von Recklinghausen's disease image as solitary or multiple solid nodules that may contain cystic spaces (BRUNETON and GEOFFRAY 1995).

8.3.3.3 Malignant Schwannoma

This extremely rare tumor has no specific features, although signs of necrosis and satellite nodes are

a
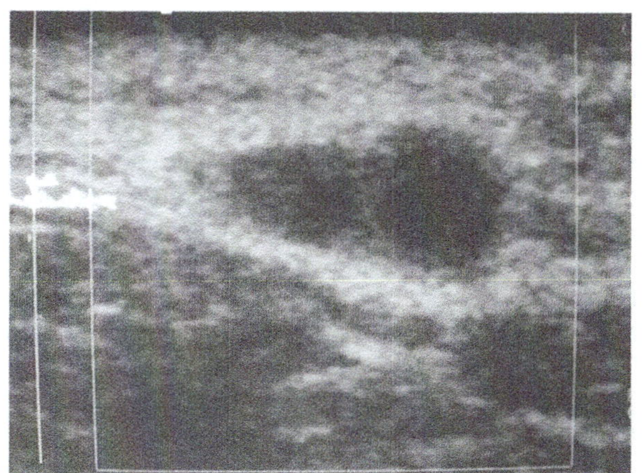

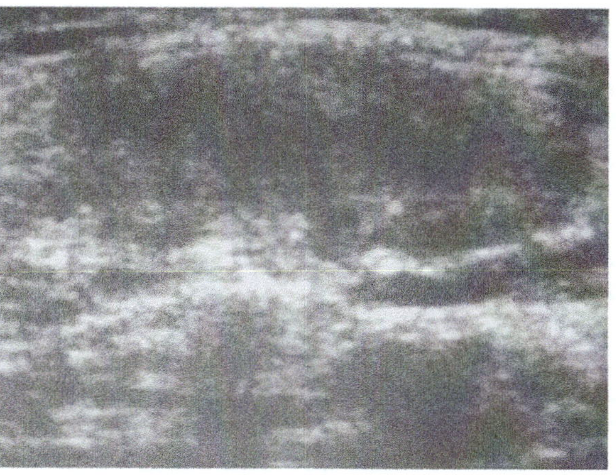
b

c
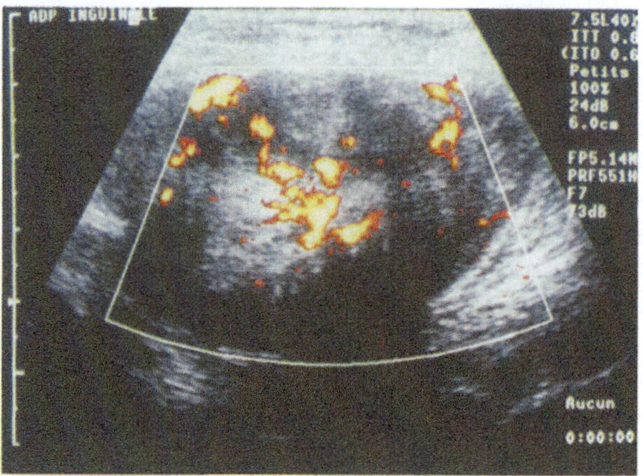

Fig. 8.16a–c. Cervical schwannoma. **a** Spinal schwannoma presenting as a nearly echo-free mass with posterior enhancement and septa. **b** The discrete inhomogeneity of this hypoechoic lesion was probably related to the presence of microcysts undetected by examination with a 12-MHz probe. **c** Power Doppler study of a lesion with a hypervascular hyperechogenic center suggesting an inflammatory node; the final diagnosis was a schwannoma

sometimes noted (Barrios et al. 1999; Colreavy et al. 2000).

On imaging studies, this ill-defined invasive tumor appears hypoechoic to the adjacent structures; adenopathies may be present. The diagnosis cannot be suggested sonographically, and the lesion is usually incorrectly diagnosed as an adenopathy or, less often, a sarcoma.

8.4 Oropharynx and Esophagus

8.4.1 Tongue

A component of the upper level of the floor of the mouth, the tongue lies above the line formed by the mylohyoid muscles. Lateral to the tongue lies the sublingual region.

This organ comprises 17 muscles, eight of which are paired. The largest muscle is the transversally flattened triangular genioglossus muscle, which lies superior to the geniohyoid muscle. The geniohyoid muscle lies immediately above the line formed by the mylohyoid muscles. The genioglossus muscle, as well as the other paired muscles, is separated from the muscle on the contralateral side by the median fibrous lingual septum superiorly and by a thin layer of connective tissue inferiorly.

8.4.1.1 Sonographic Techniques

US examination of the tongue allows assessment of both anatomy and function (speech, swallowing). Numerous techniques have been described.

Using a submental approach, a high-frequency probe permits examination of the floor of the mouth and the deep part of the tongue; however, a low-frequency probe is needed for complete exploration including the superficial portion of the tongue (Maniere-Ezvan et al. 1993).

Intraoral examination can be performed with a high-frequency transducer (endoscopic or intraoperative US probe) (Nagasawa 1999; Yoshida et al. 1987).

Dynamic studies require specific techniques:

- Speech can be investigated by analyzing tongue contours (Akgul et al. 1999); this method requires complete lingual rest, however, and often proves difficult in practice.
- Dynamic studies are generally performed in a sagittal plane using a submental approach and a probe of appropriate frequency (often a low-frequency transducer) (Neuschaefer-Rube et al. 1997).
- The base of the tongue can be imaged using a computer-controlled, bi-directional US system (Kwok et al. 1994).
- M-mode imaging can be used for all dynamic studies, in particular for evaluation of swallowing (Miller and Watkin 1997; Peng et al. 2000).
- Artifacts due to movement of the submental area during function can be reduced using the cushion scanning technique (Peng et al. 2000).
- 3-D tongue surface shapes can be reconstructed by black-and-white 3-D surface reconstruction (Lundberg and Stone 1999) or power Doppler US (Keberle et al. 2000).

8.4.1.2 Morphological Analysis

Standard gray-scale imaging using a submental approach requires a compromise between the high-quality proximal analysis achieved with a high-frequency probe and the need to examine the entire tongue, which mandates use of a lower frequency transducer in adults.

High-frequency analysis of the floor of the mouth reveals, from the surface downwards into the tongue, the plane formed by the two digastric muscles (anterior belly), the plane formed by the mylohyoid muscles that separate the lingual and sublingual regions from the suprahyoid region, the geniohyoid muscles, and the inferior portion of the genioglossus muscles. The midline can also be identified.

Use of a low-frequency probe permits analysis of the entire tongue, from the apex to the posterior portion of the base, but cannot differentiate the lateral muscles (inferior longitudinal, hyoglossus, styloglossus, palatoglossus). Transverse scans permit correct analysis of the midline over its entire height, while sagittal scans show the arciform muscle fibers of the genioglossus muscle (Bruneton et al. 1986; Neuhold et al. 1986). Examination of the normal tongue with a very high frequency intraoral probe reveals three zones: the mucosal epithelium (mean thickness 2.1 mm), the lamina propria, and the tongue muscle (Nagasawa 1999).

CD analysis provides no particularly contributory information. The lingual artery and adjacent venous structures can be visualized, but these anatomic elements have no real interest for management of lingual disease or pathologies affecting the floor of the mouth (Fig. 8.17).

8.4.1.3 Dynamic Study

Tongue movement during swallowing can be accurately evaluated by sonography using a submental approach.

PENG et al. (2000) describe five physiologic phases of swallowing: I (shovel phase); IIa (early transport phase); IIb (late transport phase); IIIa (early final phase); IIIb (late final phase). The average duration of swallowing was 2.43 s (phase IIa was the shortest); the mean speed was 10.34±4.92 mm/s. HIRAI et al. (1991) described age-related changes in tongue motor behavior; in particular, the rhythm of tongue movements is slower in elderly individuals than in younger subjects.

KAWASHIMA et al. (1999) consider reconstructed ultrasound M-mode waveforms just as effective for measurement of tongue movement during swallowing as sequential X-ray TV imaging.

CHI-FISHMAN et al. (1998) underscored the difference between discrete swallowing (single swallows) and continuous drinking, seen as differences in timing and patterns of tongue-palate contact. Continuous drinking is characterized by a shorter duration of tongue movement and overlapping of gestures during sequential swallowing. According to FANUCCI et al. (1992), the average physiologic fluid bolus is 7 ml.

Sonographic study of tongue motion during speech was described in the 1980s by SHAWKER and SONIES (1985); US biofeedback therapy has been proposed for correction of persistent articulatory speech defects (the patient compares the position of his or her tongue with the correct position pre-recorded on a videotape). Tongue movements can also be assessed during mastication (IMAI et al. 1995).

8.4.1.4 Carcinoma of the Tongue

Carcinoma of the tongue manifests as a mass of decreased echogenicity relative to the adjacent normal muscles; fluid or debris in an ulcerated area may image as zones of higher echogenicity.

Tumor margins can be difficult to determine using a submental approach; intraoral examination more accurately visualizes the limits between the neoplastic and healthy tissue (Figs. 8.18–8.23).

Sonography (submental or intraoral) permits accurate determination of the depth of tumor invasion; intraoral US data in particular are well correlated with histological measurements (SHINTANI et al. 1997).

In addition to volumetric information and determination of the depth of invasion, US can demonstrate tumor extension to the floor of the mouth or the tonsillar region (IKEZOE et al. 1991; NAGASAWA 1999). PAVELKA et al. (1986) emphasized the effectiveness of US for demonstrating spread across the midline, a parameter that indicates the feasibility of hemiglossectomy.

The accuracy of sonographic demonstration of the depth of invasion following intraoral and submental examination can be used to predict the post-therapy prognosis (BYERS et al. 1998). NAGASAWA (1999) found that 75% of patients with a mean tumor depth greater than 8 mm had nodal metastases; their 5-year survival was only 45.7%. In contrast, only 29.5% of patients with a depth of invasion less than 8 mm had nodal metastases, and their 5-year survival was 87.5%.

Sonography is more accurate than clinical examination for pretherapy staging of tumors of the mobile tongue (FRUEHWALD et al. 1987; IKEZOE et al. 1991). Intraoral sonography, in particular, is highly accurate for the workup of T1 and T2 tumors.

The main limitations of sonography concern morphological analysis of T1 tumors, unless a very high frequency intraoral probe is available (CALICETI et al. 1992; NARAYANA et al. 1996); inability to differentiate residual disease from post-radiation fibrosis; and, for large lesions especially, difficulty of staging large lesions satisfactorily. CT or MRI should be preferred in these situations (CRECCO et al. 1994; NITSCHE et al. 1991). Parapharyngeal and retropharyngeal tumor spread is best demonstrated by CT and MRI (BONGERS et al. 1990; BRUNETON et al. 1986; FRUEHWALD 1988).

YOSHIDA et al. (1999) used sonographic monitoring during brachytherapy of lingual cancers to position the needles using a submandibular approach.

As mentioned previously, postoperative differentiation of fibrosis from a possible recurrence is impossible on the basis of morphological data, even with CD (Fig. 8.24). US allows repeat evaluation of any dynamic alterations following complete surgical resection.

Sonographic examination of the tongue should always be completed by exploration of the submandibular and laterocervical nodes (BRUNETON et al. 1986).

8.4.2 Floor of the Mouth

As US consistently visualizes the mylohyoid muscles, the floor of the mouth can be distinguished from the

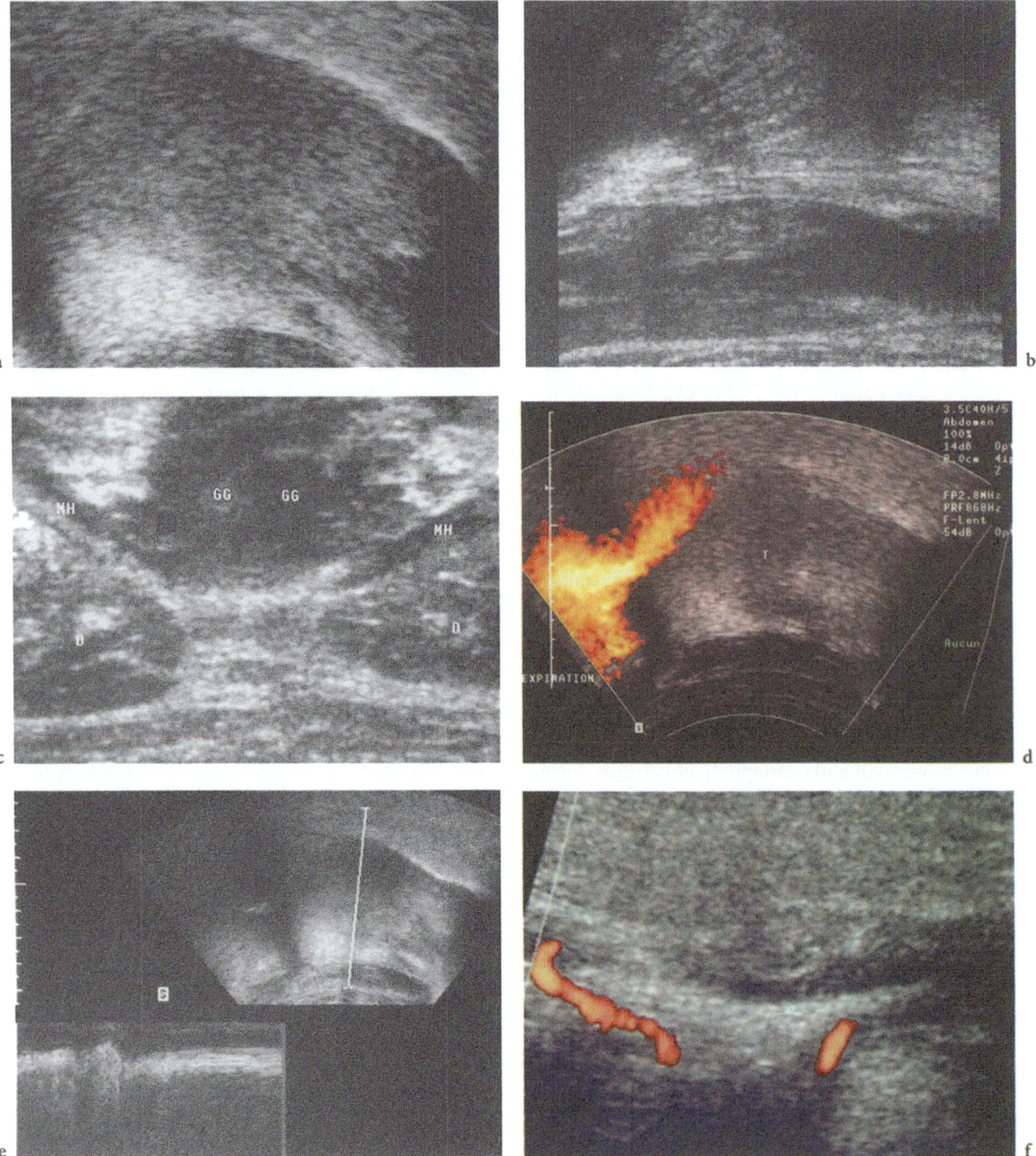

Fig. 8.17a–f. Normal US appearance of the tongue and the floor of the mouth. **a** Normal US appearance of the tongue (3.4-MHz transducer, sagittal scan). **b** Sagittal scan of the inferior portion of the tongue (striated appearance of the genioglossus muscle, linear appearance of the geniohyoid muscle immediately beneath the skin) (8-MHz transducer). **c** Upwardly concave, arciform appearance of the mylohyoid muscles (*MH*); the anterior bellies of the digastric muscles are visible underneath (*D*); above, the mylohyoid muscles are in contact with the two geniohyoid muscles (*GG*) (axial scan). **d** Power color Doppler during an expiratory phase permits satisfactory molding of the base of the tongue (*T*) (sagittal scan). **e** M-mode imaging. **f** Arterial vascularity of the lateral tongue (sagittal scan)

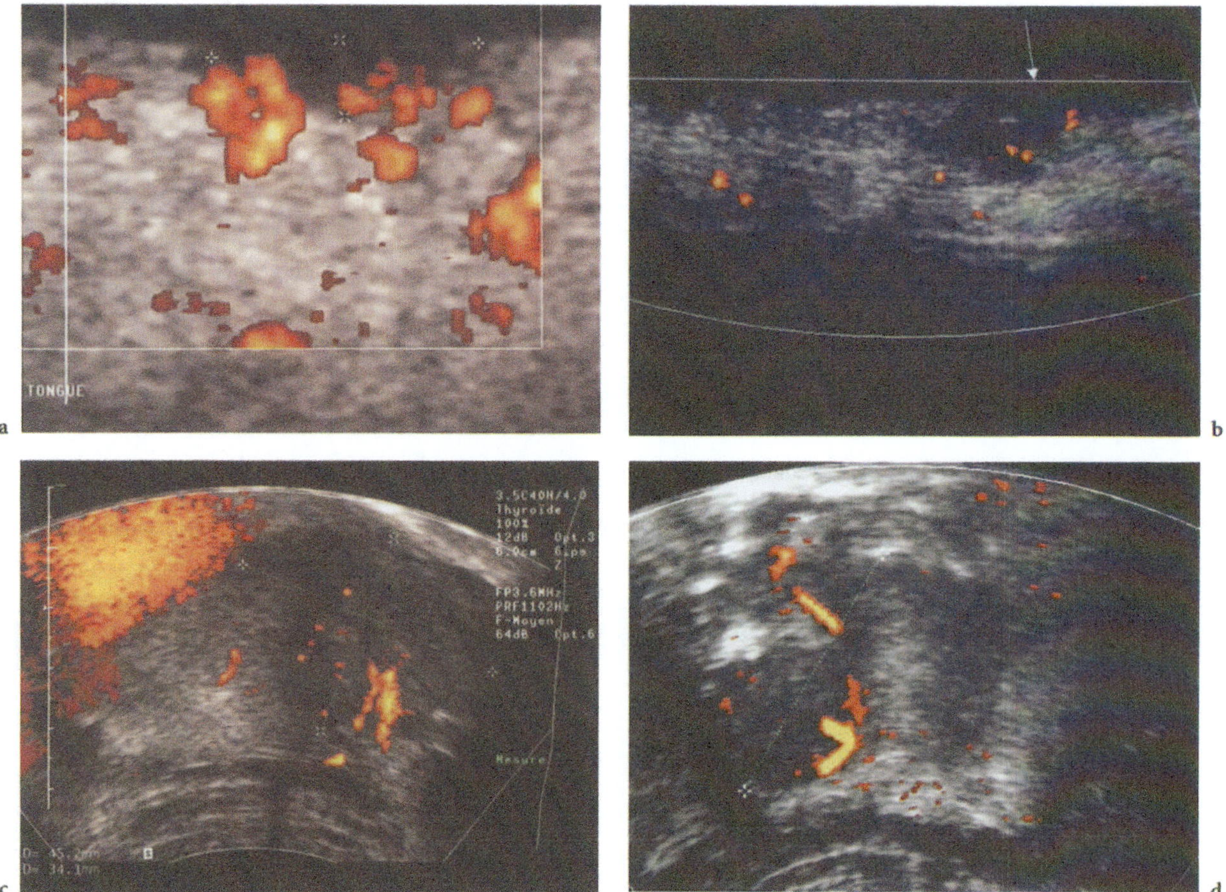

Fig. 8.18a–d. Power Doppler analysis of carcinoma of the tongue. **a** Small T1 tumor (0.6/0.2 cm between the *crosses*); both intra- and peritumoral hypervascularity are visible (intraoral probe). **b** Intraoral examination of this small lingual tumor (*arrow*) revealed nonspecific peripheral and tumoral hypervascularity. **c** Carcinoma of the right side of the tongue (4.5/3.4 cm between the *crosses*): tumor vascularity (sagittal scan). **d** Same patient as in **c**: the lingual tumor (3.6 cm between the *two crosses*) visible as a vertical echogenic mass has not crossed the midline; no signs of spread towards the floor of the mouth (axial scan)

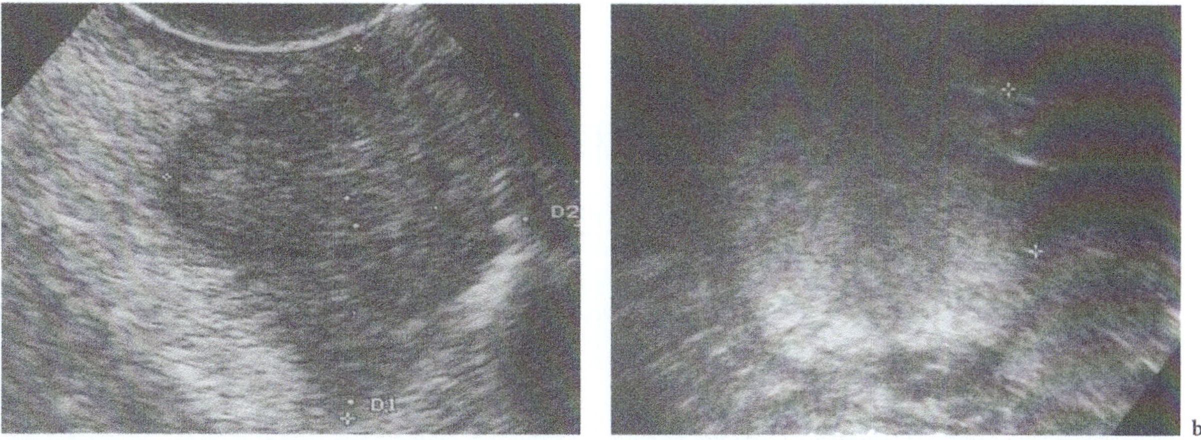

Fig. 8.19a, b. Comparison of intraoral and submental sonography. **a** Intraoral US demonstrated a lingual carcinoma spreading towards the left tonsillar pillar (2.1/2.3 cm between the *crosses*). **b** Same patient as in **a**: submental sonography visualized the tumor (2.4 cm between the *two crosses*); the images are less precise but confirm the absence of spread towards the midline

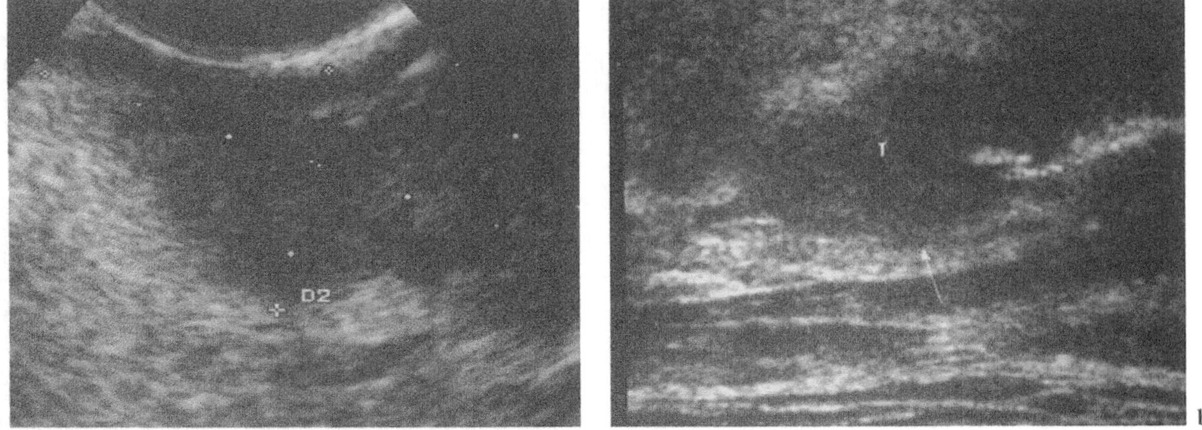

Fig. 8.20a, b. Comparison of intraoral and submental sonography. a Intraoral US revealed a carcinoma of the side of the tongue extending towards the floor of the mouth (3.2/1.3 cm between the *crosses*). b Lateral sagittal scanning using a submental approach permits visualization of tumor invasion (*T*) of the floor of the mouth following infiltration of the mylohyoid muscles (*arrow*)

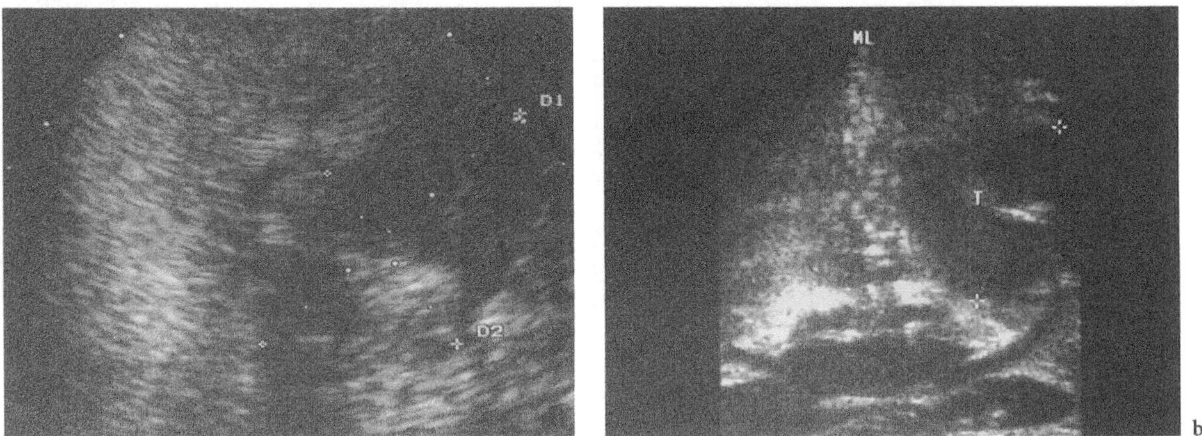

Fig. 8.21a, b. Comparison of intraoral and submental sonography. a Intraoral sonography revealed an ill-defined tumor with necrosis (echogenic area within the hypoechoic mass) extending to the midline (3.1/1.9 cm between the *crosses*). b Submental examination revealing a tumor with an echogenic zone of central necrosis that does not reach the midline on this axial scan (*ML* midline; *T* tumor; 2 cm between the *two crosses*)

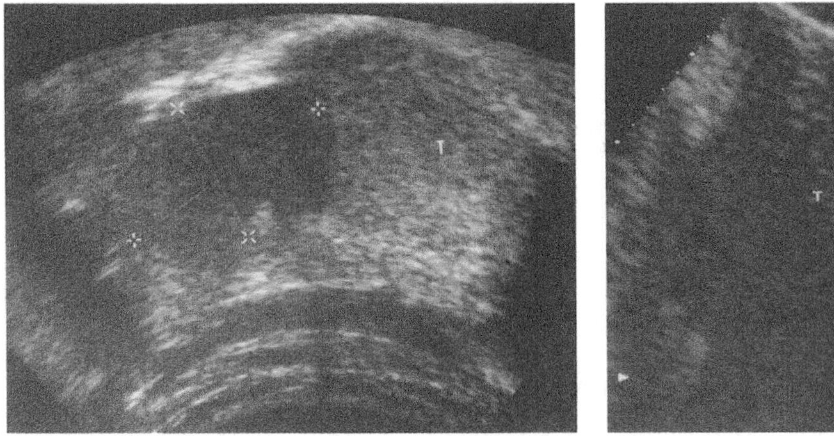

Fig. 8.22. Cancer of the base of the tongue (3.5/2.3 cm between the *crosses*): hypoechoic mass without spread towards the tonsil (sagittal scan, 4 MHz)

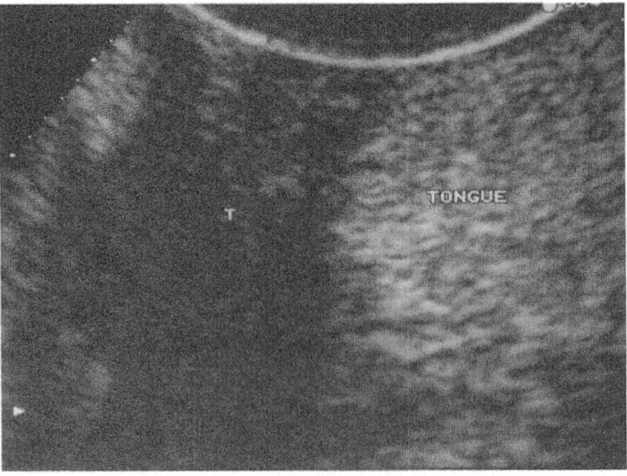

Fig. 8.23. Intraoral sonography of a tumor (*T*) of the posterior part of the tongue

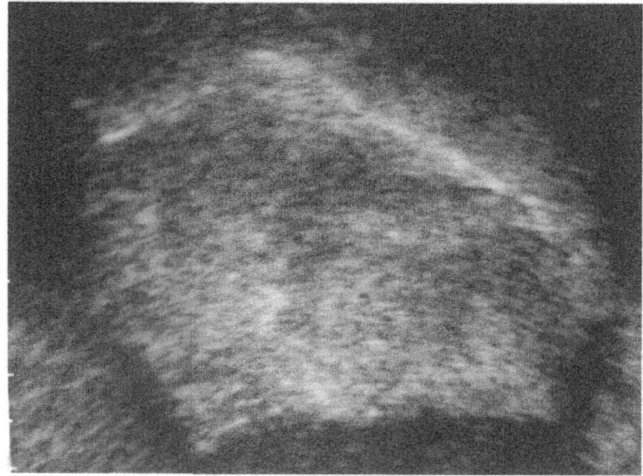

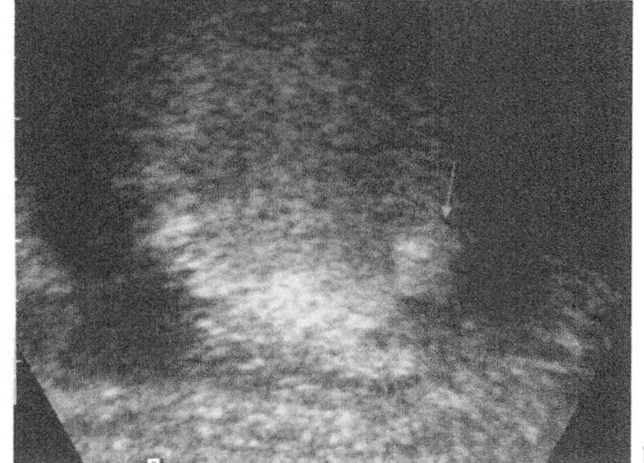

Fig. 8.24a,b. Post-therapy US appearance of the oral cavity. **a** Sequelae of left hemiglossectomy (axial scan, submental approach). **b** Small postoperative area of low echogenicity between the tongue and the floor of the mouth; no clinical signs of tumor recurrence

suprajacent lingual and sublingual regions on sonograms (Fig. 8.25). Sonography is satisfactory for analysis of tumors of the floor of the mouth (volume, extension between the inferior and superior levels or between the sublingual and lingual regions, involvement of the mandible). According to HEPPT and ISSING (1993), US is a sensitive technique for detection of mandibular invasion, and in particular can distinguish cortical and cancellous bone involvement.

For patients who have been treated by radiotherapy, US is better than clinical examination to evaluate regression in tumor size. Here again, however, US has limitations for the differentiation of fibrosis from early disease recurrence; it is not until a tumor has reached a sufficient size that US can confirm recurrence. US-guided FNA is indicated whenever a diagnostic doubt persists.

8.4.3 Tonsil

8.4.3.1 Examination Technique and Normal Appearance

Sonographic examination by a submandibular approach is facilitated by several anatomic landmarks (tongue, air in the oropharynx, submandibular gland). When possible (during preoperative workup under anesthesia), intraoral scanning can be performed with a high-frequency probe; in this case, examination is aided by the position of the external carotid artery, the palatopharyngeal muscle, and the air in the oropharynx (BUCKLEY et al. 1994).

Sonographically, the normal tonsil images as a small, oval structure with low echogenicity and is thus often difficult to visualize (Fig. 8.26).

8.4.3.2 Inflammatory Disease

Acute tonsillitis can be investigated using a submandibular or intraoral approach; such studies are especially interesting owing to the proximity of the carotid artery (8.6 mm to the left and 8.25 mm to the right, according to KUTLUHAN et al. 1998). If no fluid collection is visualized, systematic aspiration biopsy of the tonsil in search of an abscess appears unnecessary.

BUCKLEY et al. (1994) reported successful intraoral US differentiation of peritonsillar cellulitis, which has a homogeneous or a striated appearance, from peritonsillar abscess, which manifests as a heterogeneous or cystic mass containing anechoic spaces. Although transcutaneous submandibular examination is not sensitive enough to detect small anechoic spaces, intraoral US examination can obviate the need for blind FNA of the tonsillar fossa prior to surgical drainage. In the study of STEINHART et al. (1996), intraoral US performed under local anesthesia had a sensitivity of 84%.

8.4.3.3 Carcinoma of the Tonsil

Sonography has an accuracy of 92%–96% for the staging of tonsillar cancer (HELMER et al. 1990; KUPPERS et al. 1991) and is particularly helpful in dem-

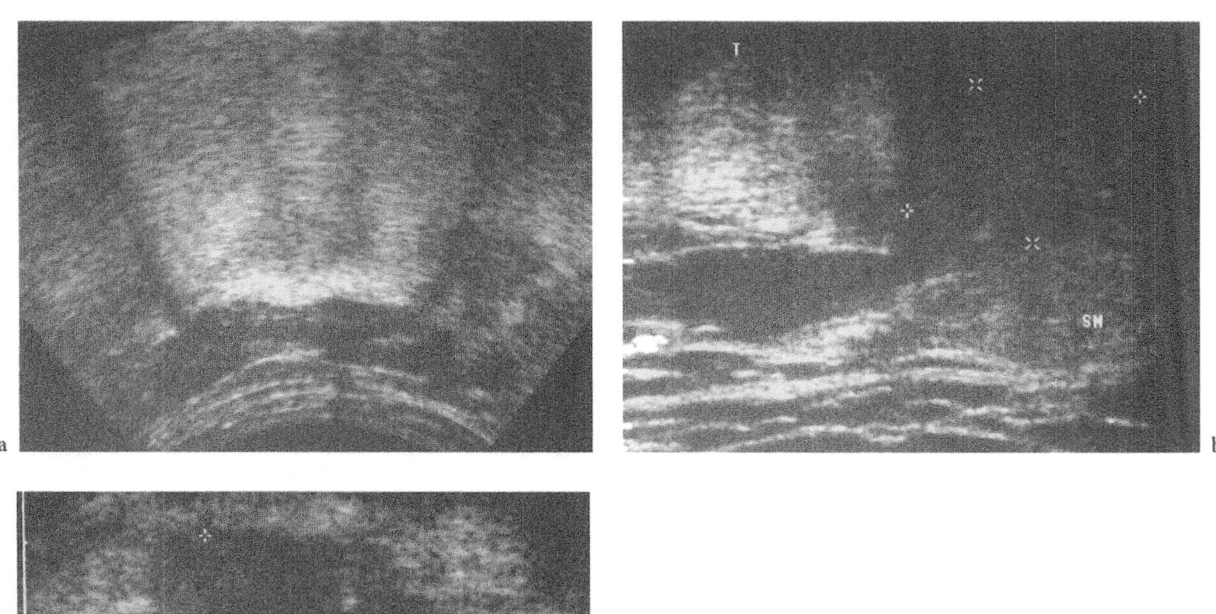

c

Fig. 8.25a–c. Carcinoma of the floor of the mouth. **a** Small (13 mm) hypoechoic lesion on the left side of the floor of the mouth, without any signs of spread to adjacent structures. **b** Carcinoma of the floor of the mouth (1.7/1.5 cm between the *crosses*) extending towards the tongue (*SM* submandibular gland; *T* tongue). **c** Mixed pattern of a large carcinoma of the floor of the mouth (3 cm in greatest dimension)

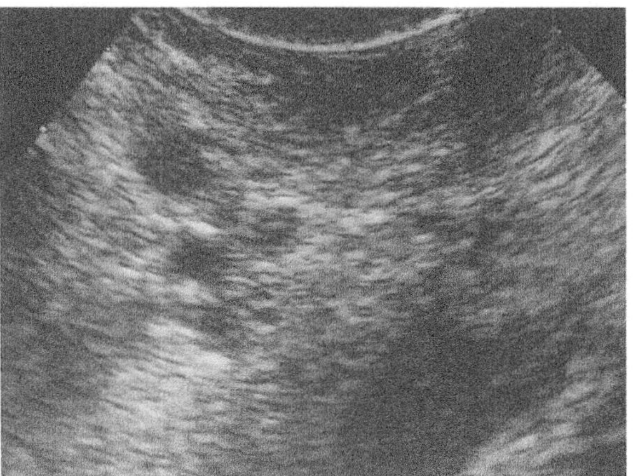

Fig. 8.26. Intraoral sonogram of a normal tonsil

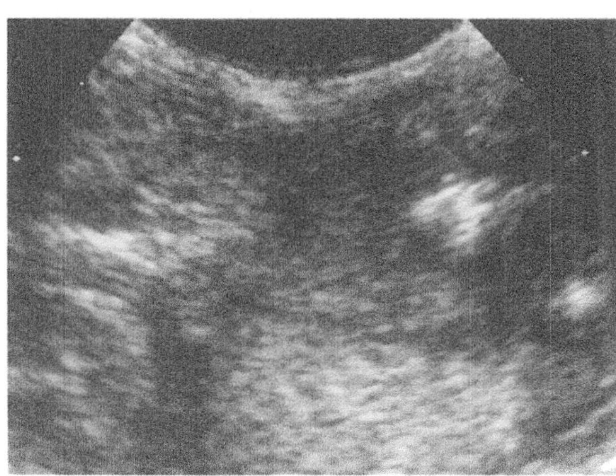

Fig. 8.27. Intraoral sonogram of a partially necrotic tonsillar cancer (central echogenic zone)

onstrating spread to the base of the tongue (METTLER et al. 1979). Mandibular involvement is also demonstrated well by US (HEPPT and ISSING 1993; MILLESI et al. 1990 (Figs. 8.27 and 8.28). Patients who do not undergo surgery may benefit from US surveillance of lesion diameter in response to radiotherapy (HASHIMOTO et al. 1995).

8.4.4 Pharynx

8.4.4.1 Endosonography

Posterior or lateral pharyngeal tumors can be correctly evaluated by US under general anesthesia; tumor relationships with the internal carotid artery are particularly well demonstrated by US (STEINHART et al. 1996). Retropharyngeal adenopathies can also be visualized, but the possibilities for US examination of the nasopharynx and the piriform sinuses are limited. Endosonography of the deepest portions of the pharynx is difficult with standard probes; examination can be facilitated by placing a fingertip US probe on the tip of a support (STEINHART et al. 1996).

Invasion of the mandible by oropharyngeal tumors is difficult to demonstrate sonographically because the medial surface of the mandibular ramus is not accessible to transcutaneous sonography; endosonography is preferable in such cases (HEPPT and ISSING 1993) (Figs. 8.29, 8.30).

In practice, laryngeal endosonography is highly operator dependent. MRI is increasingly preferred for examination of the base of the tongue and the oropharynx whenever tumor invasion is suspected (MAROLDI et al. 1999).

8.4.4.2 Neopharynx after Total Laryngectomy

After total laryngectomy, the neopharynx images sonographically as an oval or round structure (LEE et al. 2000). The wall contains five sonographically distinguishable layers, from inside out: an internal hyperechoic layer (superficial mucosa), a hypoechoic internal layer (deep mucosa), a hyperechoic layer (submucosa), a hypoechoic layer (muscle), and a hyperechoic layer (adventitia) (Fig. 8.31).

8.4.5 Cervical Esophagus

Sonographically, the cervical esophagus is visible between C-5 and T-5 as a tubular structure. The esophageal wall can easily be evaluated posterior to the thyroid, on the left side (Fig. 8.32). Dynamic imaging while the patient swallows water may facilitate identification of a lesion. DOLDI et al. (1997) reported US detection of malignant esophageal tumors larger than 5 mm; the lesion is usually hypoechoic to the adjacent structures and deforms the esophageal wall (Fig. 8.33). Anterior extension of an esophageal cancer or posterior spread of a thyroid cancer to the esophagus is not always seen sonographically.

Transcutaneous cervical sonography is performed primarily to search for lymph node metastases in patients with esophageal cancer; metastatic nodes are especially frequent with supracarinal esoph-

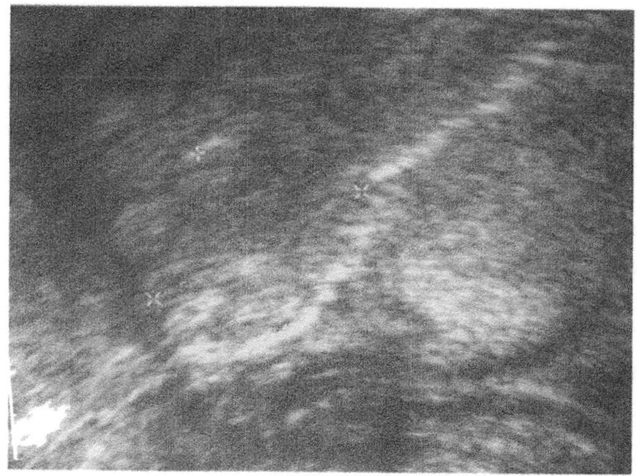

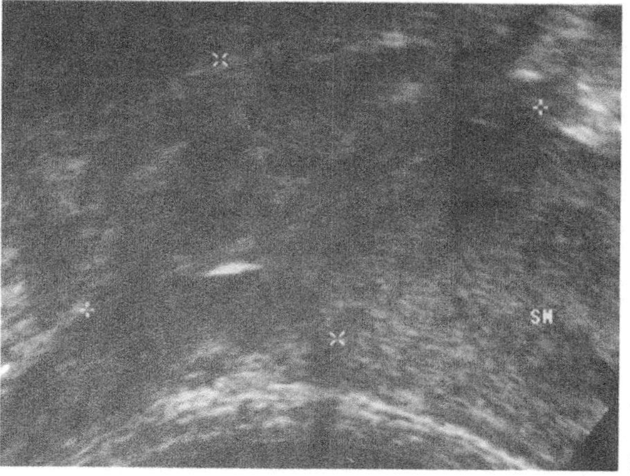

Fig. 8.28a,b. Tonsillar carcinoma visualized using a submental approach. **a** Harmonic imaging: round inhomogeneous lesion (2.7/2.3 mm between the *crosses*). **b** Tonsillar tumor (5.5/3.3 cm between the *crosses*) invading the submandibular space (*SM*)

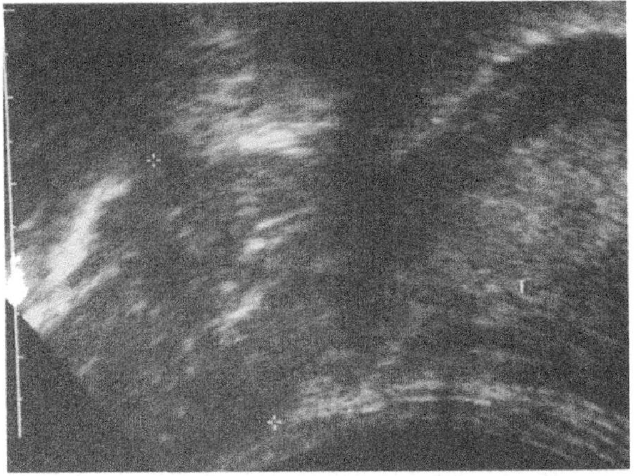

Fig. 8.29. Oropharyngeal carcinoma (3.3 cm between the *two crosses*) (*T* tongue)

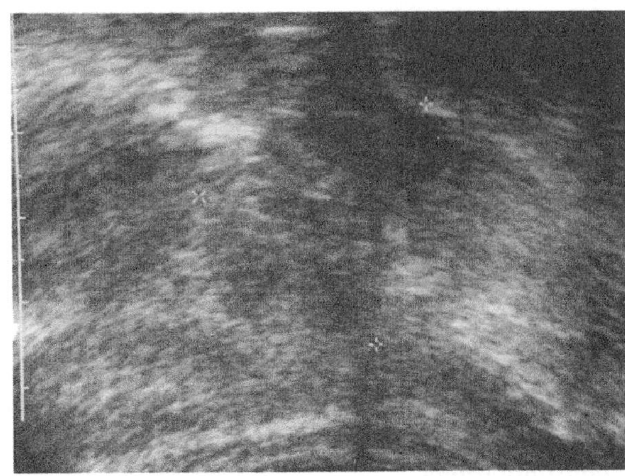

Fig. 8.30. Bulky oropharyngeal carcinoma: tumor size (5.5/3 cm between the *crosses*) prevented complete staging by US

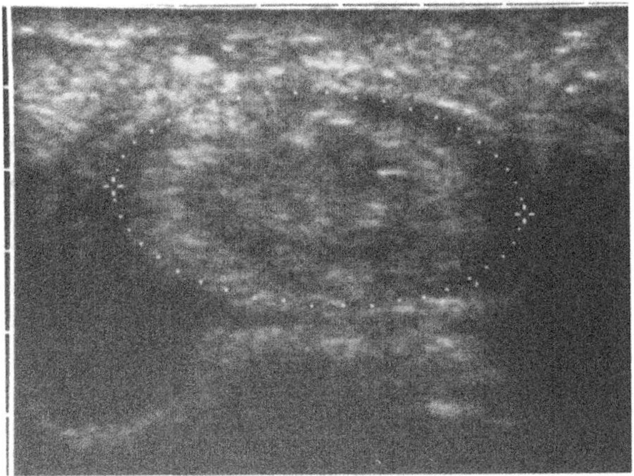

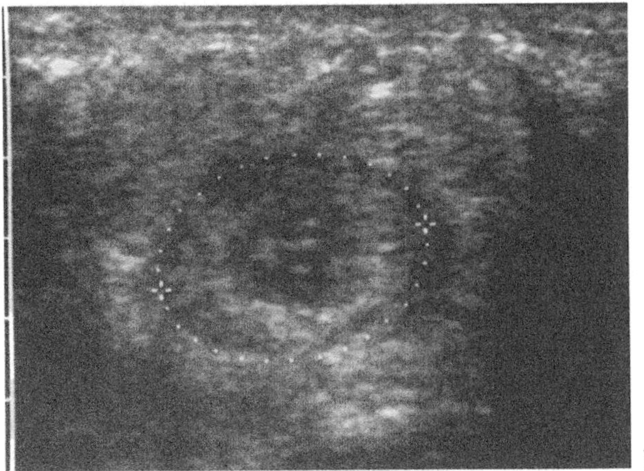

Fig. 8.31a, b. Neopharynx. a Axial scan (1.4/1.6 cm between the *two crosses*). b Sagittal scan permitting analysis of the anterior wall (3 mm between the *two crosses*)

ageal tumors (Doldi et al. 1998). US has a sensitivity of 68%–78.9% for the diagnosis of cervical nodal metastases in esophageal carcinoma; specificity varies between 94% and 97% (Bonvalot et al. 1996; Natsugoe et al. 1999; Tachimori et al. 1994).

Sonography can also occasionally visualize an esophageal pathology (diverticulum, postoperative modifications) manifesting clinically as a cervical mass (Ohshima et al. 2000) (Fig. 8.34).

8.5 Soft Tissue Sarcomas

The rare malignancies known as soft tissue sarcomas correspond to various histologies (Figs. 8.35–8.39): leiomyosarcoma, fibrosarcoma, malignant fibrous histiocytoma (Weber et al. 1992), synovial sarcoma, alveolar soft-part sarcoma (Castillo et al. 1992). These tumors are more common in children than in adults; this is particularly true for rhabdomyosarcomas (Fernandez Perez et al. 1999; Yang et al. 1997b).

Sonographically, cervical sarcomas typically image as hypoechoic or heterogeneous masses with poorly defined margins reflecting their invasive nature. Vascularization is variable, but any hypervascularity is readily detectable by CD. Akata et al. (1999) described a case of multicentric leiomyosarcomatosis with multiple well-delimited, hypoechoic nodular structures throughout the thyroid, the salivary glands, and the muscles.

Sonography is helpful for superficial tumor staging because it can evaluate any vascular (and especially

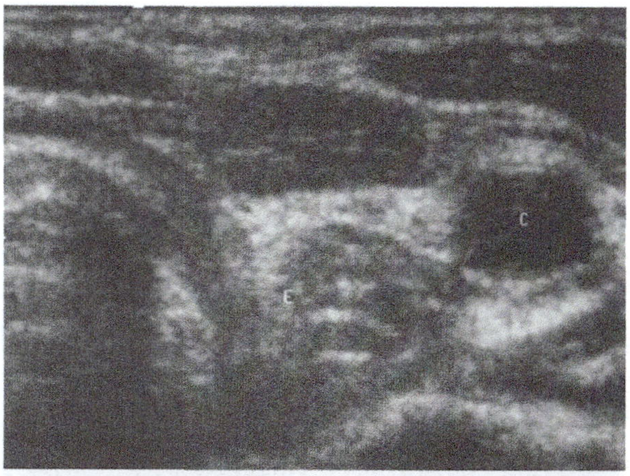

Fig. 8.32a–c. Normal esophagus. **a** US appearance after total thyroidectomy (*E* esophagus; *C* common carotid artery) (axial scan). **b** Sagittal scan. **c** US appearance of the esophagus after total laryngectomy (sagittal scan; 0.6 cm between the *two crosses*)

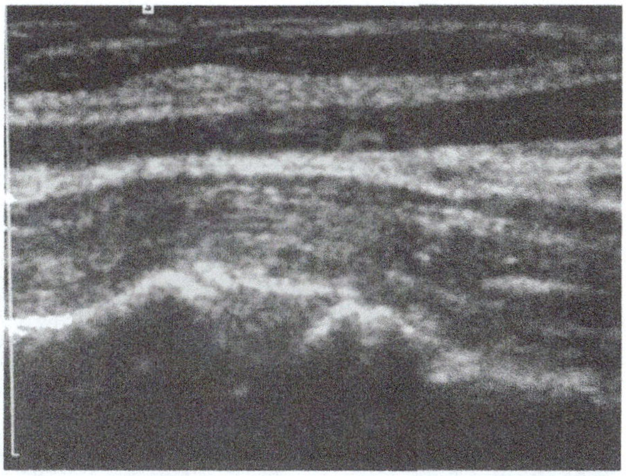

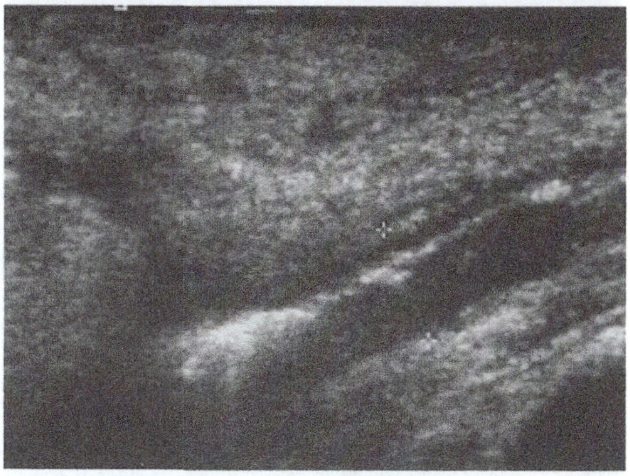

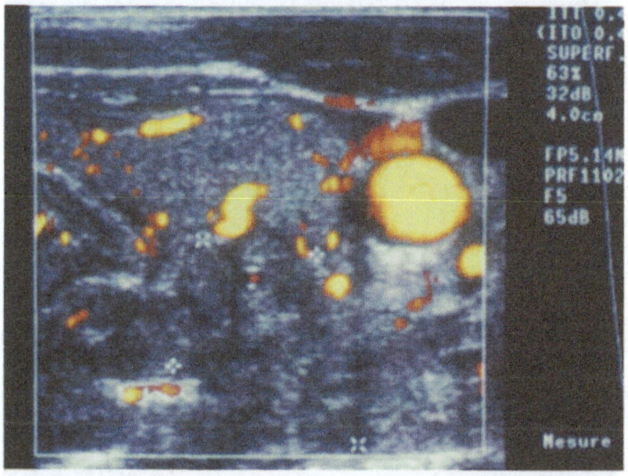

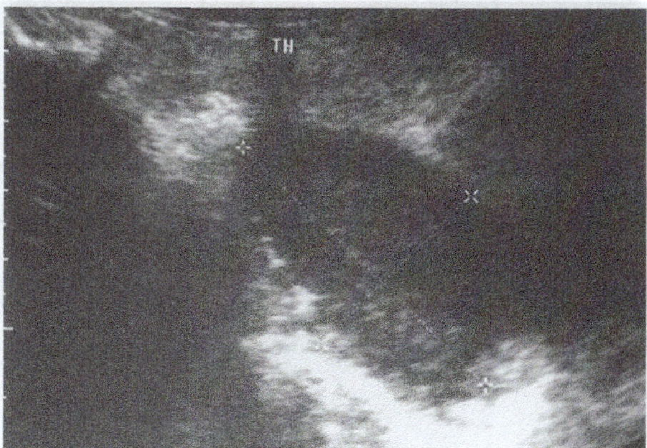

Fig. 8.33a–c. Cancer of the esophagus. **a** Inhomogeneous retrothyroid tumoral syndrome (2/1.4 cm between the *crosses*); the absence of a sharp interface between the esophageal tumor and the thyroid and the presence of vessels traversing both structures permitted detection of tumor invasion of the thyroid (axial scan, power Doppler). **b** Cancer of the cervicothoracic esophagus; examination with a 7-MHz probe was insufficient to determine the depth of invasion of this hypoechoic lesion (4.9/3 cm between the *crosses*). **c** Same patient as in **b**; a lower frequency probe permitted complete examination of the tumor; the limits are better delineated, especially in depth (*TH* thyroid; 5/3.1 cm between the *crosses*)

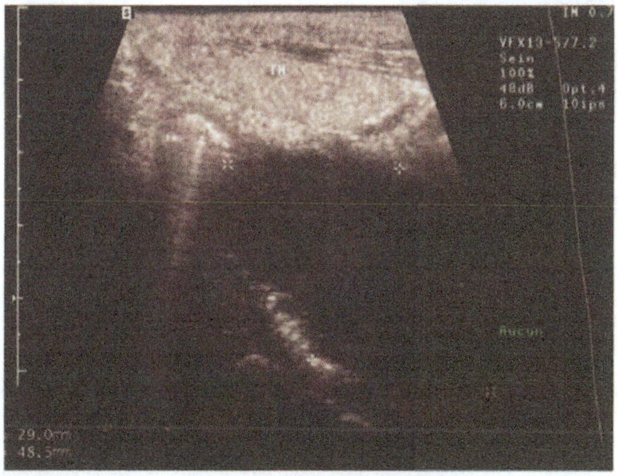

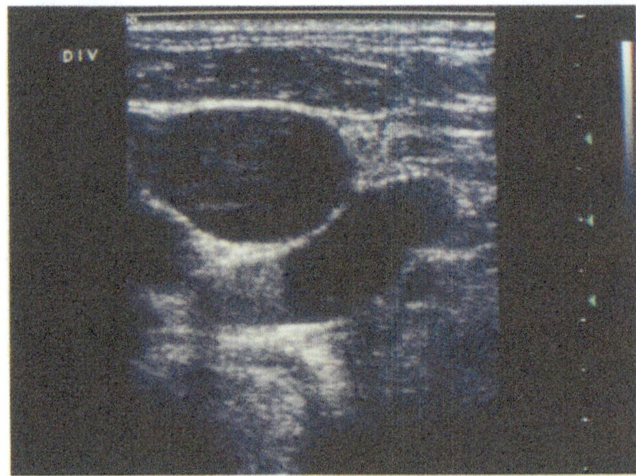

Fig. 8.34. Diverticulum of the cervical esophagus (axial scan)

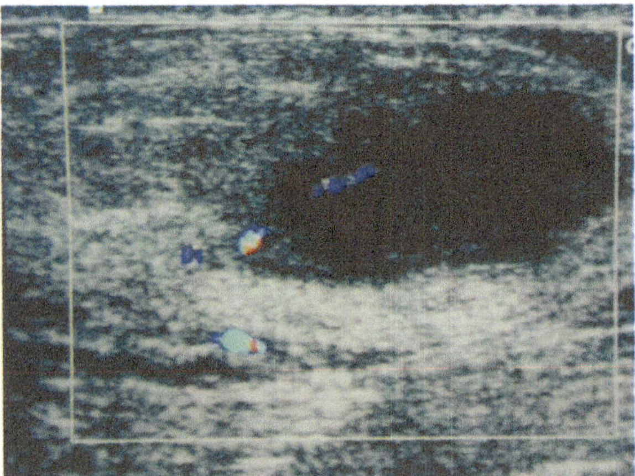

Fig. 8.35. This hypoechoic mass, weakly vascular on color Doppler, corresponded to a plasmocytoma

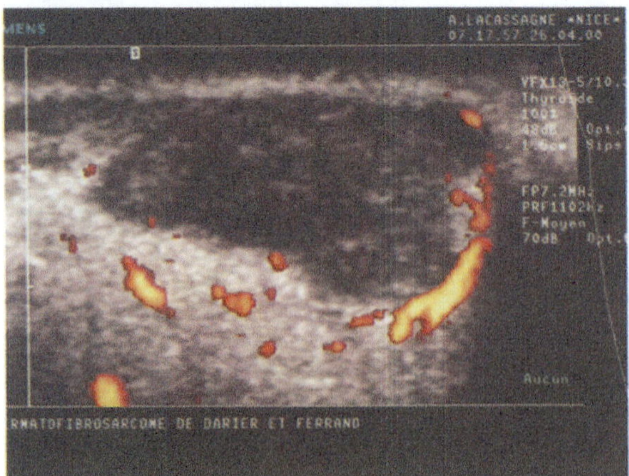

Fig. 8.36. Superficial hypoechogenic mass: second recurrence of a dermatofibrosarcoma

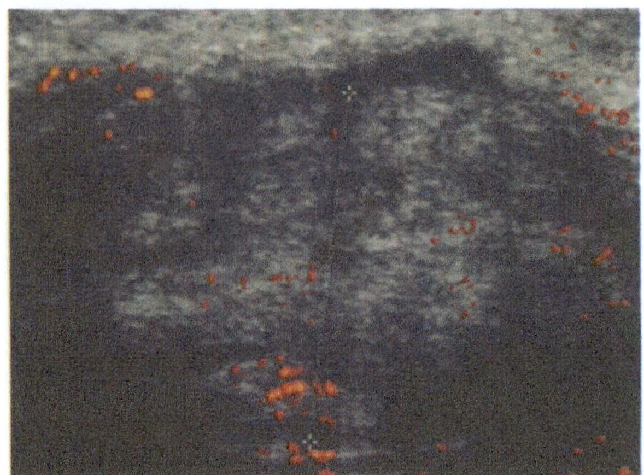

a

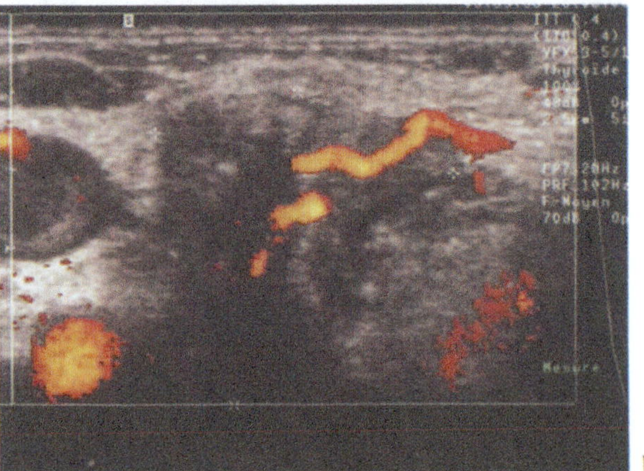

b

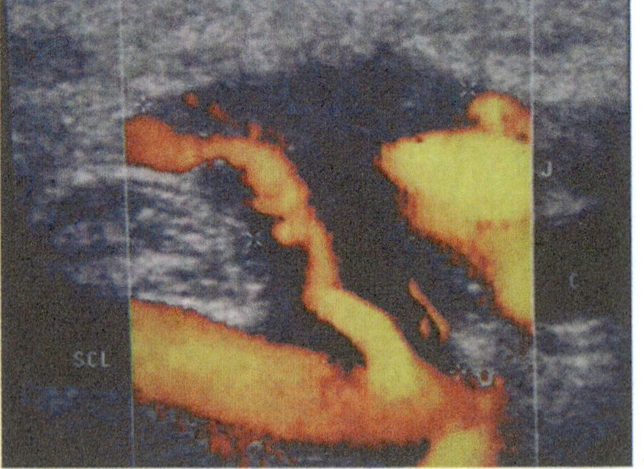

c

Fig. 8.37a–c. Invasive cervical sarcomas. **a** This invasive rhabdomyosarcoma was weakly vascular on power Doppler analysis. **b** Left laterocervical fibrosarcoma (2.1/2 cm between the *crosses*); poorly delimited medially, this lesion is traversed by vascular structures demonstrated by power Doppler. **c** Radiation-induced right cervico-supraclavicular sarcoma (2.6/1.7 cm between the *crosses*) invading the thyrocervical trunk (*SCL* subclavian artery; *C* common carotid artery; *J* internal jugular vein)

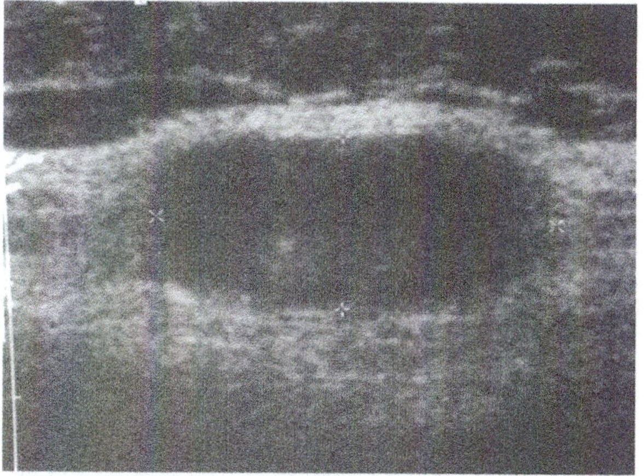

Fig. 8.38. Subcutaneous cervical metastasis of a renal cancer (1.8/0.8 cm between the *crosses*)

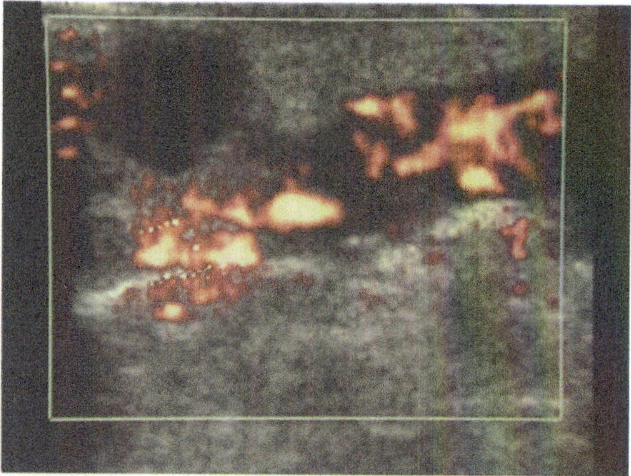

Fig. 8.39. Mandibular sarcoma; spread towards the soft tissues is seen as a hypervascular zone on power Doppler

venous) involvement. For lesions that are not managed surgically, US can readily assess the reduction in tumor size in response to treatment; it can also determine the volume of any residual neoplastic tissue, although the low specificity of sonographic findings in this situation makes US-guided FNA mandatory.

Although sonography is an easy means of following up response to therapy, other imaging modalities are often necessary for pretherapy staging and post-treatment evaluation, in particular MRI (Patel et al. 1999; Varma 1999).

8.6 Nonmalignant Lesions of the Soft Tissues of the Neck

8.6.1 Lipoma

Lipomas, i.e., benign, compressible painless masses, are often diagnosed by clinical examination. CT demonstration of their typical fat density permits pathognomonic diagnosis.

Sonography can readily confirm the clinical diagnostic hypothesis by revealing a well-defined elliptical mass with its longest diameter parallel to the skin surface and multiple echoic lines at a right angle to the US beam. There is no posterior enhancement or flow on color Doppler analysis. Ahuja et al. (1998a) reported that lipomas are hyperechoic to adjacent muscle in 76% of cases, isoechoic in 8%, and hypoechoic in 16%. According to these authors, the three major signs of lipoma are an elliptical mass, hyperechoic pattern, and multiple echogenic lines parallel to the skin surface (Figs. 8.40 and 8.41).

8.6.2 Hematoma

The echotexture of a hematoma depends on its age. Uncomplicated subcutaneous hematomas in an immediately postoperative setting do not require sonography, as they are managed right away by surgery. Postoperative US examination of the cervical region is performed basically to search for a deep hematoma, a task made difficult by the limited availability of acoustic windows. An apparently normal US examination thus does not rule out a diagnosis of hematoma, and CT remains indispensable if the erythrocyte count drops (Fig. 8.42).

When visualized sonographically, hematomas appear globally anechoic and contain numerous small echogenic images. An old hematoma (relatively rare in the cervical region) manifests as an echo-free mass. Post-hematoma sequelae, particularly in the sternocleidomastoid muscle, are hyperechoic (Fig. 8.43).

8.6.3 Laryngocele

A laryngocele is a herniation of the saccule of the laryngeal ventricle. This rare anomaly is frequently associated with a laryngeal tumor or a profession requiring forced expiration through the mouth. Three types have been described: internal laryngocele (confined to the inside of the larynx), external laryngo-

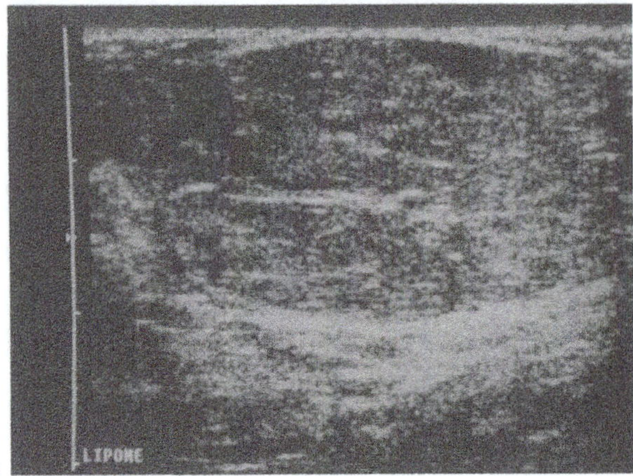

a

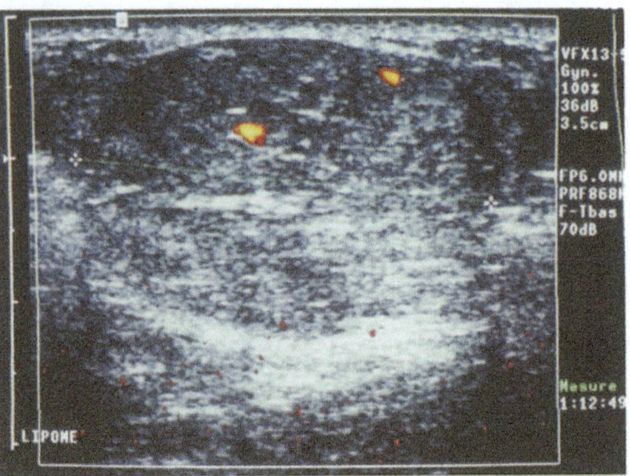

b

Fig. 8.40a, b. Cervical lipoma. **a** Typical sonographic appearance. **b** Power Doppler revealed the presence of two small vessels within the lipoma, which is globally avascular

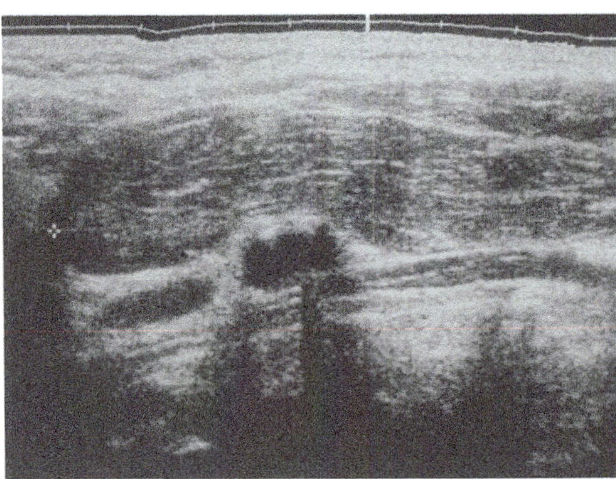

Fig. 8.41. SieScape study of a cervico-supraclavicular lipoma (8.3/1.8 cm between the *crosses*)

cele (extending towards the neck), and mixed type (a combination of both).

Sonographically, the mass is typically fluid-like, but relatively homogeneous echoes may be visible (Fig. 8.44). Internal laryngoceles occur within the thyroid cartilage. While strictly fluid-like lesions may be suggestive of a laryngocele, a mixed laryngocele filled with air is more difficult to diagnose (Baatenburg de Jong et al. 1993a).

8.6.4 Other Pathologies

As sonography is performed as a second-line procedure, immediately after physical examination, it not uncommonly reveals rare lesions such as mediastinal pathologies with a cervical extension or a muscular anomaly such as torticollis (Figs. 8.45 and 8.46). Whenever an associated mediastinal pathology is suspected, CT or MRI is indispensable owing to the topographical limitations of US.

8.7 Trachea

Sonography is rarely used to examine the trachea because the air in this passageway between the larynx and the bronchi hampers US examination. However, the thickness of the tracheal wall can be measured. Shih et al. (1997) reported a mean thickness of 1.54 mm in men and 1.22 mm in women. On sagittal scans, the cartilaginous tracheal rings are seen as highly echoic structures (Fig. 8.47).

Sonography cannot examine the entire trachea; in particular, the posterior wall and the distal portion of the trachea up to the carina are inaccessible to US. Parietal calcifications are indistinguishable from the air in the trachea. However, US may prove helpful to detect an extrinsic lesion compressing the trachea, or, more rarely, an endotracheal lesion in an anterior location (Fig. 8.48).

Deviation or even anteroposterior narrowing of the trachea are fairly common findings during US examination of a voluminous goiter. Tracheal narrowing may also be detected after surgery, especially after tracheotomy. However, sonographic data are generally insufficient to obviate the need for CT.

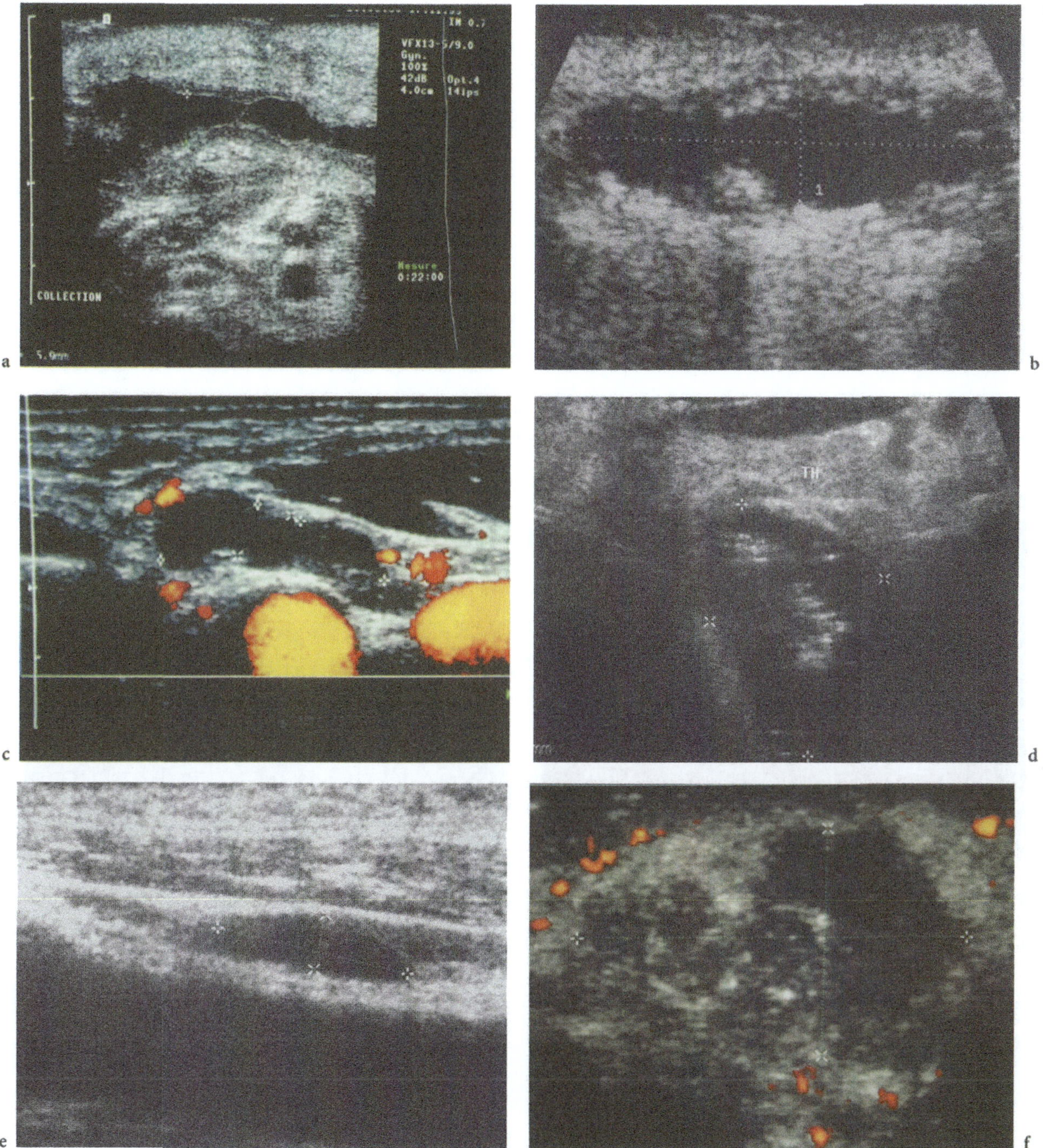

Fig. 8.42a–f. Cervical hematoma. **a** Postoperative hematoma (0.6 cm between the *two crosses*). **b** Post-traumatic jugal hematoma (2.9/0.8 cm between the *crosses*). **c** Small postoperative hematoma (0.5/0.8 cm between the *crosses*) anterior to the common carotid artery and the IJV. **d** Postlaryngectomy hematoma (2.4/1.7 cm between the *crosses*) deep to the thyroid (*TH*); this anechoic mass contains central echogenic elements. **e** Small hematoma (1.2/0.4 cm between the *crosses*) secondary to accidental puncture of the anterior wall of the internal carotid artery during a US-guided FNA procedure. **f** Residual hematoma, 2 cm in diameter (2 months after surgery)

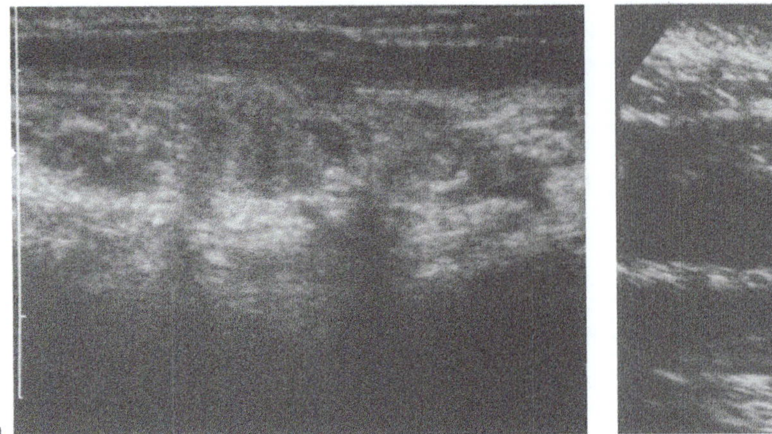

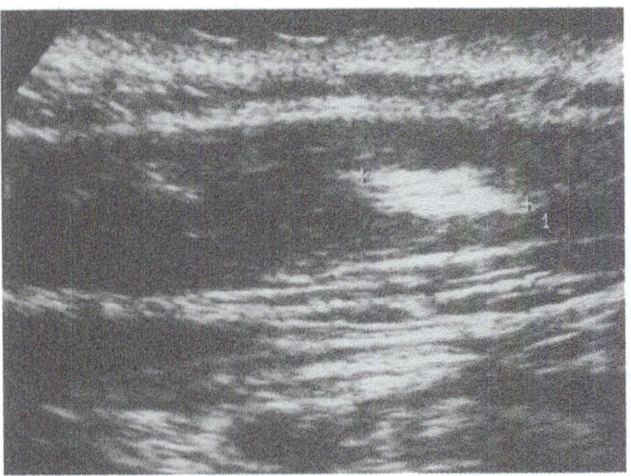

Fig. 8.43a, b. Sequelae of hematoma. **a** Sequela of a hematoma of the sternocleidomastoid muscle. **b** Fibrosis corresponding to an old hematoma of the right sternocleidomastoid muscle (1 cm between the *two crosses*)

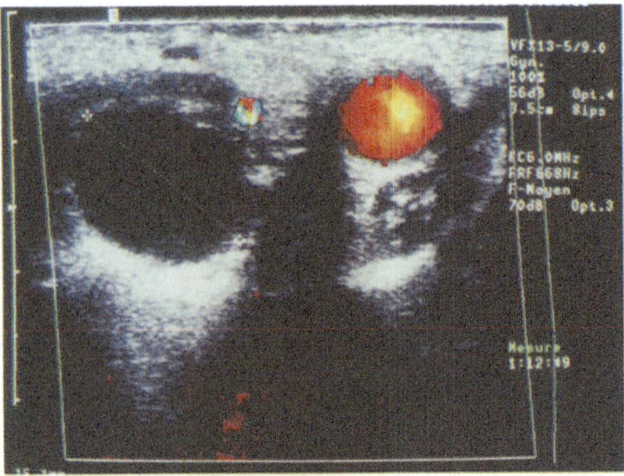

Fig. 8.44. Left-sided laryngocele (1.5 cm between the *two crosses*) medial to the common carotid artery; no demonstrable vascularity

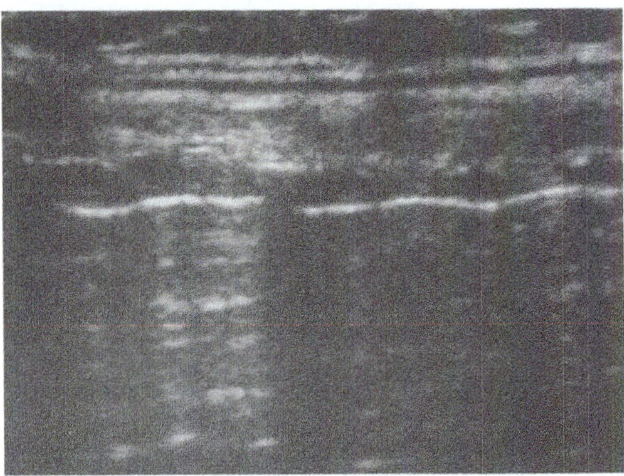

Fig. 8.45. Torticollis with permanent contraction of the left sternocleidomastoid muscle (*C* common carotid artery; *J* internal jugular vein)

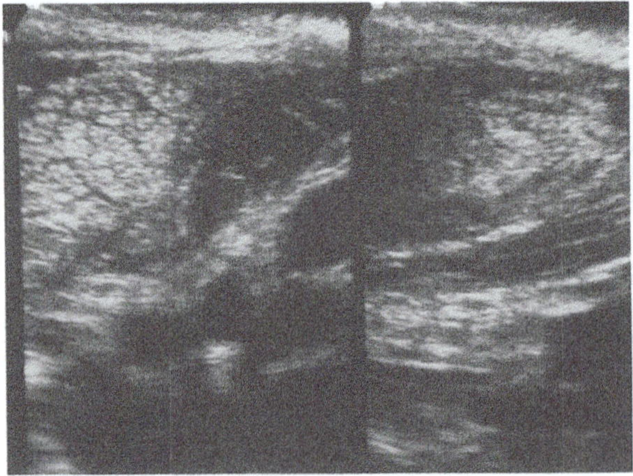

Fig. 8.46. Echogenic appearance of myositis of the sternocleidomastoid muscle (sagittal and axial scans)

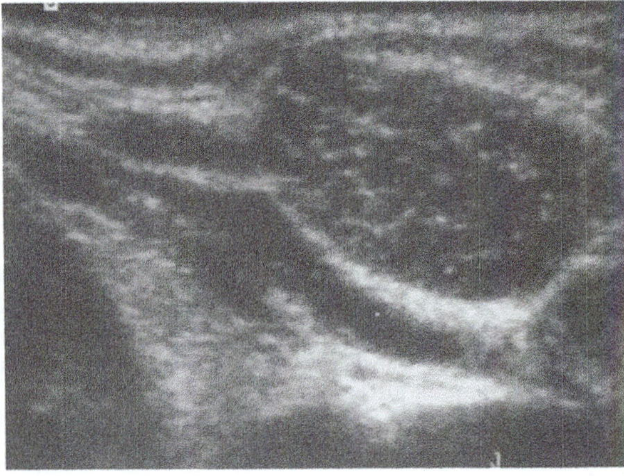

Fig. 8.47. Echogenic appearance of the tracheal rings (sagittal scan)

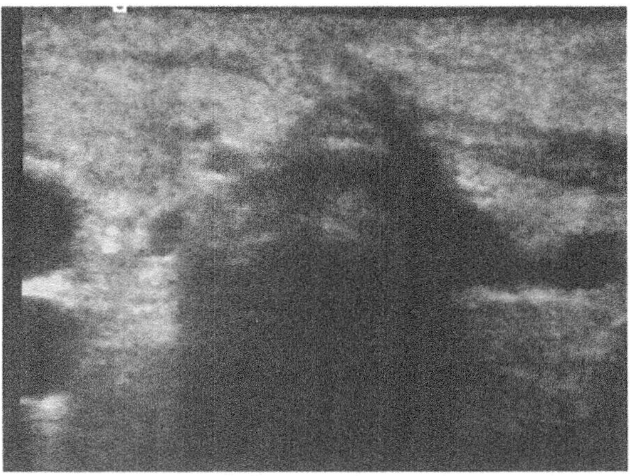

Fig. 8.48. Sequela of tracheotomy (axial transverse scan)

References

Agaton-Bonilla FC, Gay-Escoda C (1996) Diagnosis and treatment of branchial cleft cysts and fistulae. A retrospective study of 183 patients. Int J Oral Maxillofac Surg 25:449–452

Ahuja AT, King AD, Kew J, King W, Metreweli C (1998a) Head and neck lipomas: sonographic appearance. AJNR Am J Neuroradiol 19:505–508

Ahuja A, Ng CF, King W, Metreweli C (1998b) Solitary cystic nodal metastasis from occult papillary carcinoma of the thyroid mimicking a branchial cyst: a potential pitfall. Clin Radiol 53:61–63

Ahuja AT, King AD, King W, Metreweli C (1999) Thyroglossal duct cysts: sonographic appearances in adults. AJNR Am J Neuroradiol 20:579–582

Akata D, Aralasmak A, Ozmen MN, Akhan O, Altundag K, Gullu I (1999) US and CT findings of multicentric leiomyosarcomatosis. Eur Radiol 9:711–714

Akgul YS, Kambhamettu C, Stone M (1999) Automatic extraction and tracking of the tongue contours. IEEE Trans Med Imaging 18:1035–1045

al-Dousary S (1997) Current management of thyroglossal-duct remnant. J Otolaryngol 26:259–265

Allard RHB (1982) The thyroglossal cyst. Head Neck Surg 5:134–136

Andratschke M, Helmberger R, Mees K (2000) Differential diagnosis of parapharyngical mass. Laryngorhinootologie 79:174–179

Arslan H, Unal O, Kutluhan A, Sakarya E (2000) Power Doppler scanning in the diagnosis of carotid body tumors. J Ultrasound Med 19:367–370

Baatenburg de Jong RJ, Rongen RJ, Lameris JS, Knegt P, Verwoerd CDA (1993a) Ultrasound in the diagnosis of laryngoceles. ORL J Otorhinolaryngol Relat Spec 55:290–293

Baatenburg de Jong RJ, Rongen RJ, Lameris JS, Knegt P, Verwoerd CD (1993b) Evaluation of brachiogenic cysts by ultrasound. ORL J Otorhinolaryngol Relat Spec 55: 294–298

Baatenburg de Jong RJ, Rongen RJ, Lameris JS, Knegt P, Verwoerd CD (1993c) Ultrasound characteristics of thyroglossal duct anomalies. ORL J Otorhinolaryngol Relat Spec 55:299–302

Bailey H (1923) Clinical aspects of branchial cysts. Br J Surg 10:565–572

Barberet G, Diakhate I, Conessa C, Moriniere S (1999) TDM et diagnostic des fistules de la quatrième poche branchiale chez l'adulte. J Radiol 80:1676–1678

Barrios JM, Lopez Castanier MY, Razquin J (1999) Malignant schwannoma of the neck An Otorrinolaringol Ibero Am 26:477–486

Barry R, Piennar A, Piennar C, Browning NG, Nel CJ (1993) Duplex Doppler investigation of suspect vascular lesions at the carotid bifurcation. Ann Vasc Surg 7: 140–144

Becker M, Schroth G, Zbaren P, et al (1997) Long-term changes induced by high-dose irradiation of the head and neck region: imaging findings. Radiographics 17:5–26

Blanco Perez P, Gomez Benito M, Santa Cruz S, et al (2000) Vagal chemodectoma with atypical cells. Case report. An Otorrinolaringol Ibero Am 27:5–15

Bongers H, Lenz M, Klier R (1990) T-staging of tongue and mouth floor tumors: comparison of ultrasonography and computerized tomography. Strahlenther Onkol 166: 125–131

Bonvalot S, Bouvard N, Lothaire P, et al (1996) Contributions of cervical ultrasound and ultrasound fine-needle aspiration biopsy to the staging of thoracic oesophageal carcinoma. Eur J Cancer 32A:893–895

Boucher C, Dorion D, Fisch C (1999) Retropharyngeal abscesses: a clinical and radiologic correlation. J Otolaryngol 28:134–137

Brown TJ, Tschen JA (2000) A long-standing dermal nodule on the neck of a young woman. Diagnosis: bronchogenic cyst. Arch Dermatol 136:925–930

Bruneton JN, Geoffray A (1995) In: Solbiati L, Rizzatto G (eds) Ultrasound of superficial structures: high frequencies, Doppler and interventional procedures. Churchill Livingstone, Edinburgh, pp 115–123

Bruneton JN, Roux P, Caramella E, Manzino JJ, Vallicioni J, Demard F (1986) Tongue and tonsil cancer: staging with US. Radiology 158:743–746

Buckley AR, Moss EH, Blokmanis A (1994) Diagnosis of peritonsillar abscess: value of intraoral sonography AJR Am J Roentgenol 162:961–964

Byers RM, El-Naggar AK, Lee YY, et al (1998) Can we detect or predict the presence of occult nodal metastases in patients with squamous carcinoma of the oral tongue? Head Neck 20:138–144

Caliceti U, Sorrenti G, Zironi G, et al (1992) Ultrasound staging research of progressive pathology of the base of the tongue. Acta Otorhinolaryngol Ital 12:345–353

Castillo M, Lee YY, Yamasaki S (1992) Infratemporal alveolar soft part sarcoma: CT, MRI and angiographic findings. Neuroradiology 34:367–369

Chi-Fishman G, Stone M, McCall GN (1998) Lingual action in normal sequential swallowing. J Speech Lang Hear Res 41:771–785

Chou YH, Tiu CM, Chiou HJ, Lai CR, Hsu CC, Yu C (1999) Echo-enhancing sonography of a large-vessel hemangioma of the neck. J Clin Ultrasound 27:465–468

Coales UF, Tandon P, Hinton AF (1999) Limitations of imaging of foreign bodies in parapharyngeal abscess and the importance of surgical exploration. J Laryngol Otol 113: 683–685

Colreavy MP, Lacy PD, Hughes J, et al (2000) Head and neck schwannomas. A 10-year review. J Laryngol Otol 114:119–124

Constantinidis J, Steinhart U, Zenk J, Iro H (1998) Treatment of deep neck infections. Laryngorhinootologie 77:551–556

Crecco M, Vidiri A, Vigili MG, et al (1994) The magnetic resonance estimation of the T parameter in the staging of tumors of the oral cavity and tongue. A correlation with postoperative data and preliminary echotomographic experience. Radiol Med (Torino) 87: 452–459

De Pra L, Derchi LE, Balconi G (1995) Peripheral nerves. In: Solbiati L, Rizzatto G (eds) Ultrasound of superficial structures. High frequencies, Doppler and interventional procedures, Churchill Livingstone, Edinburgh, pp 303–313

Derchi LE, Serafini G, Rabbia C, et al (1992) Carotid body tumors: US evaluation. Radiology 182:457–459

Doldi SB, Lattuada E, Zappa MA, et al (1997) Ultrasonographic imaging of neoplasms of the cervical esophagus. Hepatogastroenterology 44:724–726

Doldi SB, Lattuada E, Zappa MA, et al (1998) Ultrasonographic evaluation of the cervical lymph nodes in preoperative staging of esophageal neoplasms. Abdom Imaging 23:275–277

Eliashar R, Sichel JY, Gomori JM, Saah D, Elidan J (1999) Role of computed tomography scan in the diagnosis and treatment of deep neck infections in children. Laryngoscope 109:844

El Sayed Y, al-Dousary S (1996) Deep-neck space abscesses. J Otolaryngol 25:227–233

el-Silimy O, Corney C (1993) The value of sonography in the management of cystic neck lesions. J Laryngol Otol 107:245–251

Engzell U, Zajicek J (1970) Aspiration biopsy and cytologic findings in 100 cases of congenital cysts. Acta Cytol 14:51–57

Epstein J, Van der Meij E, McKenzie M, Wong F, Lepawsky M, Stevenson-Moore P (1997) Postradiation osteonecrosis of the mandible: a long-term follow-up study. Oral Surg Oral Med Oral Pathol Oral Radiol Endod 83:657–662

Eroglu A, Atabekoglu S, Kocaoglu H (1999) Primary hydatic cyst of the neck. Eur Arch Otorhinolaryngol 256:202–204

Fanucci A, Cerro P, Fanucci E (1992) Sonographic evaluation of physiologic bolus volume in oral swallowing. Am J Physiol Imaging 7:73–76

Fernandez Perez A, Moreno Leon JA, Fernandez-Nogueras Jimenez F, Rubi Uria J (1999) Rhabdomyosarcoma of the neck in adults. Acta Otorhinolaryngol 50:211–214

Fruehwald FX (1988) Clinical examination, CT and US in tongue cancer staging. Eur J Radiol 8:236–241

Fruehwald F, Salomonowitz E, Neuhold A, Pavelka R, Mailath G (1987) Tongue cancer. Sonographic assessment of tumor stage. J Ultrasound Med 6:121–137

Ghilardi G, Bortolani EM, Pizzocari P, Vandone PL, De Monti M (1991) Paraganglioma of the neck. Analysis of 32 operated cases. Minerva Chir 46:1109–1117

Gidley PW, Ghorayeb BY, Stiernberg CM (1997) Contemporary management of deep neck space infections. Otolaryngol Head Neck Surg 116:16–22

Gilmer-Hill HS, Kline DG (2000) Neurogenic tumors of the cervical vague nerve: report of four cases and review of the literature. Neurosurgery 46:1498–1503

Gooding GAW (1979) Gray-scale ultrasound detection of carotid body tumors. Radiology 132:409–410

Hashimoto M, Sato K, Kato H, Hirano H, Tomura N, Watarai J (1995) Oropharyngeal cancer: clinical efficacy of ultrasound. Radiol Med 13:59–61

Hausegger KW, Sukic J, Stering R (1990) Ultrasonography of cervical cysts and their differential diagnosis. Ultraschall Med 11:188–192

Hayamizu K, Naito K, Ito K (1995) Ultrasonography for traction injuries of the brachial plexus. Nippon Igaku Hoshasrn Gakkai Zasshi 55:873–877

Helmer M, Grasl MC, Pavelka R, Steiner E, Gritzmann N (1990) Sonography in malignant tonsillar tumors. Rofo Fortschr Geb Rontgenstr Neuen Bildgeb Verfahr 152: 713–717

Heppt WJ, Issing WJ (1993) Assessment of tumorous mandibular involvement by transcutaneous ultrasound and flexible endosonography. J Craniomaxillofac Surg 21:107–112

Hirai T, Tanaka O, Koshino H, Yajima T (1991) Ultrasound observations of tongue motor behavior. J Prosthet Dent 65:840–844

Hood RJ, Reibel JF, Jensen ME, Levine PA (2000) Schwannoma of the cervical sympathic chain. The Virginia experience. Ann Otol Rhinol Laryngol 109:48–51

Ikezoe J, Nakanishi K, Morimoto S, et al (1991) Sonographic imaging of cancer of the mobile tongue. Acta Radiol 32:6–8

Imai A, Tanaka M, Tatsuta M, Kawazoe T (1995) Ultrasonographic images of tongue movement during mastication. J Osaka Dent Univ 29:61–69

Jansen JL, Baatenburg de Jong RJ, Schipper J, Van der Mey AG, Van Gils AP (1997) Color Doppler imaging of paragangliomas in the neck. J Clin Ultrasound 25:481–485

Jovic R, Vlaski L, Komazec Z, Canji K (1999) Results of treatment of deep neck abscesses and phlegmon. Med Pregl 52:402–408

Kang B, Du J, Huang J (1997) Ultrasonographic diagnosis of hemangiomas of soft tissue. J Tongji Med Univ 17:168–171

Kawashima S, Takahashi Y, Niikuni N, et al (1999) Development of X-ray TV M-mode and reconstructed ultrasound M-mode methods for investigating tongue movement during swallowing in humans. J Oral Sci 41:1–4

Keberle M, Jenett M, Scharfenberger M, Hahn D (2000) 3D Power Doppler ultrasound: new possibilities in the diagnosis and documentation of tumors of the base of the tongue. Laryngorhinootologie 79:197–200

Knappertz VA, Tegeler CH, Hardin SJ, McKinney WM (1998) Vagus nerve imaging with ultrasound: anatomic and in vivo validation. Otolaryngol Head Neck Surg 118:82–85

Krupski WC, Effeney DJ, Ehrenfeld WK, Stoney RJ (1982) Cervical chemodectoma. Am J Surg 144:215–219

Kukwa A, Pietniczka M, Wieclawska M, Sujkowska U, Filipowicz K (1995) Branchial carcinoma in material from a neck cyst. Otolaryngol Pol 49 [Suppl 20]:145–148

Kuppers P, Siegert R, Blessing R (1991) Ultrasonic diagnosis of the tonsillar region. Laryngorhinootologie 70:497–500

Kutluhan A, Sakarya ME, Cankaya H, Akkaya S (1998) Clinical value of preoperative intraoral ultrasonography in tonsillectomy. Auris Nasus Larynx 25:181–185

Kwok W, Wiegand L, Channin DS, Wiegand DA (1994) Development of the bi-directioned ultrasound system for base of tongue imaging. Comput Biol Med 24:295–304

Larheim TA, Westesson PL, Hicks DG, Eriksson L, Brown DA (1999) Osteonecrosis of the temporomandibular joint: correlation of magnetic resonance imaging and histology. J Oral Maxillofac Surg 57:888–898

Lee JH, Sohn JE, Choe DH, Lee BH, Kim K, Chin SY (2000) Sonographic findings of the neopharynx after total laryngectomy: comparison with CT. AJNR Am J Neuroradiol 21: 823–827

Lee WC, Walsh RM, Tse A (1996) Squamous cell carcinoma of the pharynx and larynx presenting as a neck abscess cellulitis. J Laryngol Otol 110:893–895

Lin CH, Chou JC, Lin TL, Lou PJ (1999) Spontaneous resolution of internal jugular vein thrombosis in a Salmonella neck abscess patient. J Laryngol Otol 113:1122–1124

Lohaus M, Hansmann J, Witzel A, Flechtenmacher C, Mende U, Reisser C (1999) Uncommon sonographic findings of an epidermoid cyst in this head and neck. HNO 47: 737–740

Lundberg AJ, Stone M (1999) Three-dimensional tongue surface reconstruction: practical considerations for ultrasound data. J Acoust Soc Am 106:2858–2867

Makarainen H, Paivansalo M, Hyrynkangas K, Leinonen A, Siniluoto T (1986) Sonographic patterns of carotid body tumors JCU 14:373–375

Malkinson FD, Keane JT (1981) Radiobiology of the skin: review of some effects on epidermis and hair. J Invest Dermatol 77:133–138

Maniere-Ezvan A, Duval JM, Darnault P (1993) Ultrasonic assessment of the anatomy and function of the tongue. Surg Radiol Anat 15:55–61

Maroldi R, Battaglia G, Farina D, Maculotti P, Chiesa A (1999) Tumours of the oropharynx and oral cavity: perineural spread and bone invasion. JBR-BTR 82: 94–300

Martins AS, Melo GM, Tincani AJ, Lage HT, Matos PS (1999) Papillary carcinoma in a thyroglossal duct: case report. Sao Paulo Med J 117:248–250

Mettler FA jr, Schultz K, Kelsey CA, Khan K, Sala J, Kligerman M (1979) Gray-scale ultrasonography in the evaluation of neoplastic invasion of the base of the tongue. Radiology 133:781–784

Miller JL, Watkin KL (1997) Lateral pharyngeal wall motion during swallowing using real-time ultrasound. Dysphagia 12:125–132

Miller MB, Rao VM, Barry MT (1992) Cystic masses of the head and neck: pitfalls in CT and MR interpretation. AJR Am J Roentgenol 159:601–607

Millesi W, Prayer L, Helmer M, Gritzmann N (1990) Diagnostic imaging of tumor invasion of the mandible. Int J Oral Maxillofac Surg 19:294–298

Miszczyk L, Przeorek W (1999) Evaluation of severity and clinical course of acute mucosal reaction during postop radiotherapy of laryngeal cancer. Otolaryngol Pol 53: 397–402

Miyawaki T, Nakamura A, Hayashi H, Kurihara K (1999) Macrocystic schwannoma in the seventh cervical nerve. Plast Reconstr Surg 104:789–792

Molitch HI, Unger EC, Witte CL, Vansonnenberg E (1995) Percutaneous sclerotherapy of lymphangiomas. Radiology 194:343–347

Muhm M, Polterauer P, Gstottner W, et al (2000) Glomus caroticum chemodectoma. Review on current diagnosis and therapy. Wien Klin Wochenschr 112:115–120

Mukherji SK, Tart RP, Slattery WH, Stringer SP, Benson MT, Mancuso AA (1993) Evaluation of first branchial anomalies by CT and MR. J Comput Assist Tomogr 17:576–581

Myssiorek D, Palestro CJ (1998) 111 Indium pentetreotide scan detection of familial paragangliomas. Laryngoscope 108:228–231

Nagasawa H (1999) Ultrasonographic diagnosis of tongue cancer using intraoral high-frequency probe. Kokubyo Gakkai Zasshi 66:98–106

Narayana HM, Panda NK, Mann SB, Katariya S, Vasishta RK (1996) Ultrasound versus physical examination in staging carcinoma of the mobile tongue. J Laryngol Otol 110:43–47

Natsugoe S, Yoshinaka H, Shimada M et al (1999) Assessment of cervical lymph node metastasis in esophageal carcinoma using ultrasonography. Ann Surg 229:62–66

Nazarian LN, Zegel HG, Gilbert KR, Edell SL, Bakst BL, Goldberg BB (1998) Paraspinal ultrasonography: lack of accuracy in evaluating patients with cervical or lumbar back pain. J Ultrasound Med 17:117–122

Neuhold A, Fruhwald F, Balogh B, Wicke L (1986) Sonography of the tongue and floor of the mouth. I. Anatomy. Eur J Radiol 6:103–107

Neuschaefer-Rube C, Wein BB, Angerstein W, Klajman S jr, Fischer-Wein G (1997) Sector-related gray-scale analysis of video ultrasound recorded tongue movements in swallowing. HNO 45:556–562

Nguyen CT, Tan J, Blackwell K, Bhuta S, Sercarz JA (2000) Primary melanocytic schwannoma of cervical sympathic chain. Head Neck 22:195–199

Nitsche N, Waitz G, Iro H (1991) Endo-oral sonography in comparison with transcutaneous sonography, computerized tomography and magnetic resonance tomography. HNO 39:247–253

Nusbaum AO, Som PM, Rothschild MA, Shugar JM (1999) Recurrence of a deep neck infection: a clinical indication of an underlying congenital lesion. Arch Otolaryngol Head Neck Surg 125:1379–1382

Ochi K, Ogino S, Fukamizu K, et al (1996) US-guided drainage of deep neck space abscess. Acta Otolaryngol Suppl 522:120–123

O'Hanlon DM, Walsh N, Corry J, Mortimer G, Flynn JR (1994) Aberrant thyroglossal cyst. J Laryngol Otol 108:1105–1107

Ohshima A, Yamashita H, Noguchi S (2000) Endoscopic ultrasonography in the evaluation of thyroid cancer into the esophagus. Surgery 127:478–479

Ojiri H, Tada S, Ujita M, et al (1998) Infrahyoid spread of deep neck abscess: anatomical consideration. Eur Radiol 8:955–959

Padberg FT, Cady B, Persson AV (1983) Carotid body tumor. Am J Surg 145:526–528

Park SW, Han MH, Sung MH, et al (2000) Neck infection associated with pyriform sinus fistula: imaging findings. AJNR Am J Neuroradiol 21:817–822

Patel SC, Silbergleit R, Talati SJ (1999) Sarcomas of the head and neck. Top Magn Reson Imaging 10:362–375

Pavelka R, Streinzer W, Zrunek M, Fruhwald F, Neuhold A, Seidl G (1986) Evaluation of real-time sonography in the pretherapeutic staging of malignant tumors of the tongue and mouth floor. Laryngol Rhinol Otol (Stuttg) 65:632–639

Peleg M, Heyman Z, Akdekian L, Taicher S (1998) The use of ultrasonography as a diagnostic tool for superficial fascial space infections. J Oral Maxillofac Surg 56:1129–1131

Peng CL, Jost-Brinkmann PG, Miethke RR, Lin CT (2000) Ultrasonographic measurement of tongue movement during swallowing J Ultrasound Med 19:15–20

Piga M, Farina GP, Loi GL, et al (1999) Visualisation of a paraganglioma by technetium-99m-sestamibi scintigraphy. J Endrocrinol Invest 22:296–300

Poe LB, Petro GR, Matta I (1996) Percutaneous CT-guided aspiration of deep neck abscesses. AJNR Am J Neuroradiol 17:1359–1363

Quraishi MS, O'Halpin DR, Blayney AW (1997) Ultrasonography in the evaluation of neck abscesses in children. Clin Otolaryngol 22:30–33

Raby N (1987) Ultrasonographic appearances of glomus vagale tumour. Br J Radiol 61:246–249

Ranieri E, D'Andrea MR, Vecchione A (1996) Fine-needle aspiration cytology of squamous cell carcinoma arising in a thyroglossal duct cyst. A case report. Acta Cytol 40:747–750
Reynolds JH, Wolinski AP (1993) Sonographic appearance of branchial cysts. Clin Radiol 48:109–110
Sakaguchi M, Sato S, Ishiyama T, Katsumo S, Taguchi K (1997) Characterization and management of deep neck infections. Int J Oral Maxillo Fac Surg 26:131–134
Schreiber J, Mann W, Ringel K (1996) The role of color duplex ultrasound in diagnosis and differential diagnosis of carotid body tumors. Laryngorhinootologie 75:100–104
Schumacher A, Jonas M, Rummeny E, Schmid SH, Scheld HH, Schober O (1996) Diagnosis of recurrence of a glomus carotid artery tumor by somatostatin receptor scintigraphy. Nuklearmedizin 35:38–41
Shawker TU, Sonies BC (1985) Ultrasound biofeedback for speech training. Instrumentation and preliminary results. Invest Radiol 20:90–93
Shih JY, Lee LN, Wu HD, et al (1997) Sonographic imaging of the trachea. J Ultrasound Med 16:783–790
Shintani S, Nakayama B, Matsuura H, Hasegawa Y (1997) Intraoral ultrasonography is useful to evaluate tumor thickness in tongue carcinoma. Am J Surg 173:345–347
Sievers KW, Greess H, Baum U, Dobritz M, Lenz M (2000) Paranasal sinuses and nasopharynx CT and MRI. Eur J Radiol 33:185–202
Sigal R (1999) Imagerie des masses cervicales. J Radiol 80:1807–1815
Solbiati L, De Pra L, Ierace T, Bellotti E, Derchi LE (1985) High-resolution sonography of the recurrent laryngeal nerve: anatomic and pathologic considerations. AJR Am J Roentgenol 145:989–993
Steinhart H, Mendel M, Schroeder HG (1996) Endosonography of the pharynx. Laryngorhinootologie 75:682–686
Swartz JD, D'Angelo AJ Jr, Harnsberger HR, Zwillenberg S, Marlowe FI (1990) The laryngeal mucocele. Imaging analysis of a rare lesion. Clin Imaging 14:110–115
Tachimori Y, Kato H, Watanabe H, Yamaguchi H (1994) Neck ultrasonography for thoracic esophageal carcinoma. Ann Thorac Surg 57:1180–1183
Talmi YP, Knoller N, Dolev M, et al (2000) Postsurgical prevertebral abscess of the cervical spine. Laryngoscope 110:1137–1141
Terzakis G, Louverdis D, Vlachou S, Anastasopoulos G, Dokianakis G, Tsikou-Papafragou A (2000) Ectopic thymic cyst in the neck. J Laryngol Otol 114:318–320
Ting PL, Sivagnanaratnam V (1989) Ultrasonographic study of the spread of local anaesthesia during axillary brachial plexus bloc. Br J Anaesth 63:326–329
Toranzo JM, Martinez JM, Metlich MA, Hurtado JA (1999) Ultrasonography-guided percutaneous drainage of cervicofacial infections. Dentomaxillofac Radiol 28:257
Torossian JM, Beziat JL, Abou Chebel N, Devouassoux-Shisheboran M, Fischer G (1999) Extracranial cephalic schwannomas: a series of 15 patients. J Craniofac Surg 10:389–394
Trattnig S, Hubsch P, Schwaighofer B, Karnel F, Eilenberger M (1991) Vascular space-occupying lesions of the carotid artery-detection with color-coded Doppler sonography. Comparison with duplex sonography and angiography. Ultraschall Med 12:70–73
Turetschek K, Hospodka H, Steiner E (1995) Case report. Epidermoid cyst of the floor of the mouth: diagnostic imaging by sonography, computed tomography and magnetic resonance imaging. Br J Radiol 68: 205–207
Ungkanont K, Yellon RF, Weissman JL, et al (1995) Head and neck space infections in infants and children. Otolaryngol Head Neck Surg 112:375–382
Varma DG (1999) Optimal radiologic imaging of soft tissue sarcomas. Semin Surg Oncol 17: 2–10
Wadsworth DT, Siegel MJ (1994) Thyroglossal duct cysts: variability of sonographic finding. AJR Am J Roentgenol 163:1475–1477
Warszawski A, Rottinger EM, Vogel R, Warszawski N (1998) 20 MHz ultrasonic imaging for quantitative assessment and documentation of early and late postirradiation skin reactions in breast cancer patients. Radiother Oncol 47:241–247
Weber BP, Kempf HG, Kaiserling E (1992) Malignant fibrous histiocytoma in the area of the head and neck. Laryngorhinootologie 71:43–49
Weisman J (1996) Non-nodal masses of the neck. In: Som PM, Curtin HD (eds) Head and neck imaging, Mosby, Baltimore, pp 794–822
Werner JA, Lippert BM, Gottschlich S et al. (1998) Ultrasound-guided interstitial Nd:YAG laser treatment of voluminous hemangiomas and vascular malformations in 92 patients. Laryngoscope 108:463–470
Westerband A, Hunter GC, Cintora I, et al. (1998) Current trends in the detection and management of carotid body tumors. J Vasc Surg 28:84–92
Wiel Marin A, Zucchetti F, Butti A, et al (1998) Neurinoma of the vagus verve. Description of 2 cases and review of the literature. G Chir 19:31–34
Win T, Lewin JS (1995) Imaging characteristics of carotid body tumors. Am J Otolaryngol 16:325–328
Yang C, Cohen J, Everts E, Smith J, Caro J, Andersen P (1999) Fourth branchial arch sinus: clinical presentation, diagnostic workup, and surgical treatment. Laryngoscope 109:442–446
Yang WT, Ahuja A, Metreweli C (1997a) Sonographic features of head and neck hemangiomas and vascular malformations: review of 23 patients. J Ultrasound Med 16:39–44
Yang WT, Kwan WH, Li CK, Metreweli C (1997b) Imaging of pediatric head and neck rhabdomyosarcomas with emphasis on MRI and a review of the literature. Pediatr Hematol Oncol 14:243–257
Yang WT, Chui PT, Meterweli C (1998) Anatomy of the normal brachial plexus revealed by sonography and the role of sonographic guidance in anesthesia of the branchial plexus. AJR Am J Roentgenol 171:1631–1636
Yasumoto M, Shibuya H, Gomi N, Kasuga T (1991) Ultrasonographic appearance of dermoid and epidermoid cysts in the head and neck. J Clin Ultrasound 19:455–461
Yoshida H, Akizuki H, Michi K (1987) Intraoral ultrasonic scanning as a diagnostic aid. Craniomaxillofac Surg 15:306–311
Yoshida K, Shimizutami K, Tanaka E, et al (1999) Ultrasonographic monitoring of high dose rate interstitial implant using template technique for oral tongue cancer. Radiol Med 17:337–341
Yu GH, Sack MJ, Baloch Z, Gupta PK (1999) Difficulties in the fine-needle aspiration (FNA) diagnosis of schwannoma. Cytopathology 10:186–194
Zidi A, Bonaziz N, Mnif N, et al (2000) Tumeurs du corpuscule carotidien: apport des différentes techniques d'imagerie. A propos de six observations. J Radiol 81:953–957

9 Pediatric Cervical Ultrasonography

Anne Geoffray, Catherine Garel

CONTENTS

A. Geoffray, MD
Hôpital Lenval, Service de Radiodiagnostic, 57 avenue de la Californie, 06200 Nice, France
C. Garel, MD
Service de Radiologie, Hôpital Robert Debré, 75935 Paris Cedex 19, France

9.1 Congenital Anomalies

9.1.1 Thyroglossal Cysts

9.1.1.1 General Features

Thyroglossal cysts are secondary to the persistence of portions of Bochdalek's duct (thyrolingual duct), the embryologic pathway of descent of the thyroid gland. This duct runs from the foramen cecum at the base of the tongue, through the lingual muscles, the mylohyoid muscle, and the anterior cervical triangle, passes around the hyoid bone from the front to the back, then courses anterior to the hyothyroid membrane and terminates at the level of the thyroid isthmus (Diagram 9.1). Defective closure of this duct results in

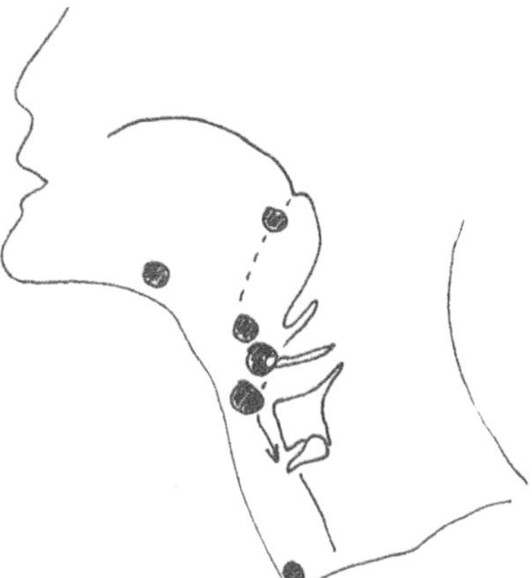

Diagram 9.1. Embryologic pathway of descent of the thyroid gland

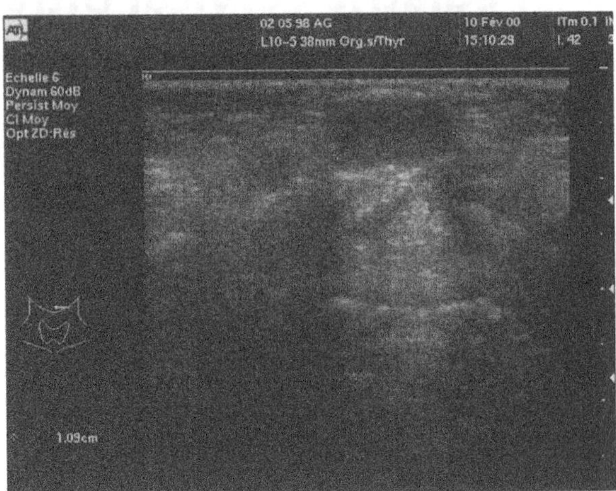

Fig. 9.1. Well-defined hypoechoic nodule in a 2-year-old boy: uncomplicated thyroglossal duct cyst

formation of a cyst that is always midline or near-midline. These cysts may develop at any point between the base of the tongue and the manubrium sternum. Suprahyoid sites predominate, but submental, suprahyoid and, less often, suprasternal or occasionally mediastinal thyroglossal cysts are also encountered. These frequent developmental lesions, representing 70% of all congenital cysts of the neck, are often diagnosed in childhood, although some go undetected until later in life. Thyroglossal cysts are asymptomatic except when superinfected. Diagnosis is made clinically by palpation of a small, well-limited, rounded midline mass in the anterior neck.

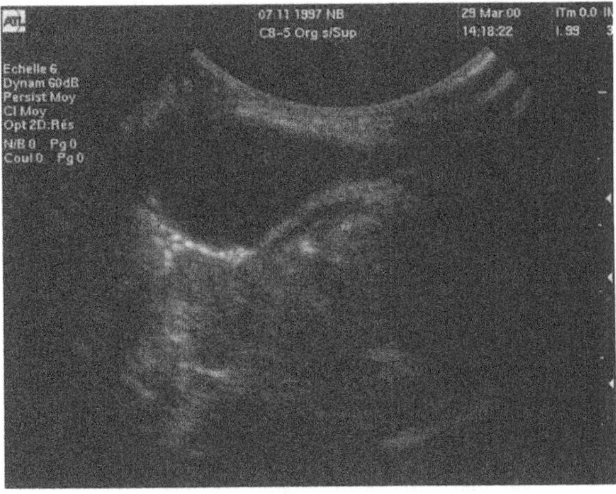

Fig. 9.2. Anechoic near-midline mass: thyroglossal duct cyst

9.1.1.2 Sonographic Features

Ultrasonography typically reveals a cystic midline mass, but sonographic findings are actually variable, as the mass may also be anechoic, homogeneously or heterogeneously hypoechoic containing small anechoic spaces, or even hyperechoic (Figs. 9.1–9.3). There may thus be difficulties may with differential diagnosis from a tumor. The midline or near-midline cervical location of these cysts, between the tongue base and the thyroid, should suggest the diagnosis. No correlation exists between the sonographic features of these cysts and their pathological (infectious or inflammatory) nature (WADSWORTH and SIEGEL 1994). A sinus tract connecting the cyst to the hyoid bone is occasionally demonstrated sonographically (Fig. 9.4). Ultrasonography plays an essential role, not so much for diagnosis of the thyroglossal cyst itself, which is generally suspected clinically, but to docu-

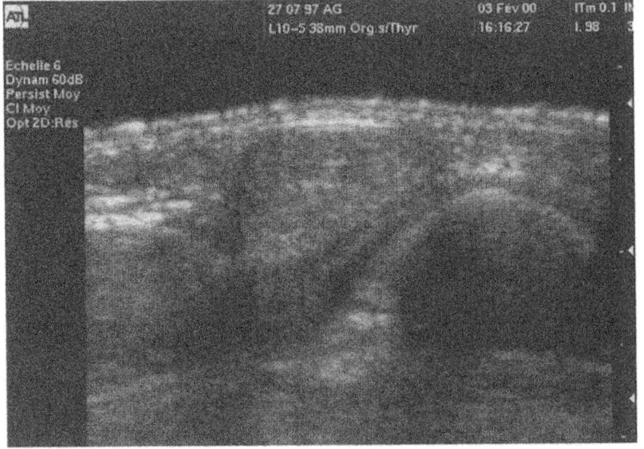

Fig. 9.3. Three-year-old boy with a hyperechoic, right near-midline mass anterior to the hyoid bone: thyroglossal duct cyst

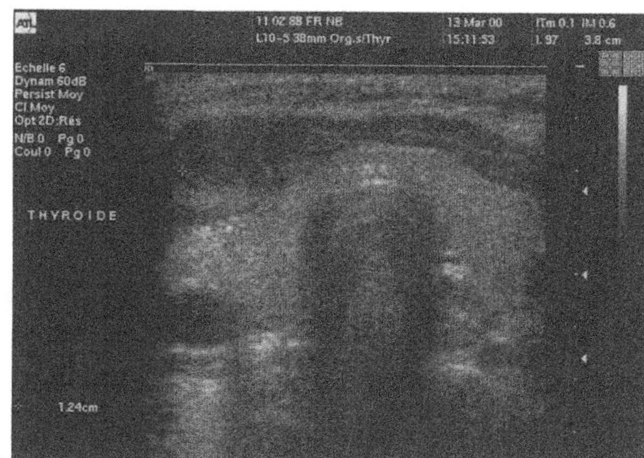

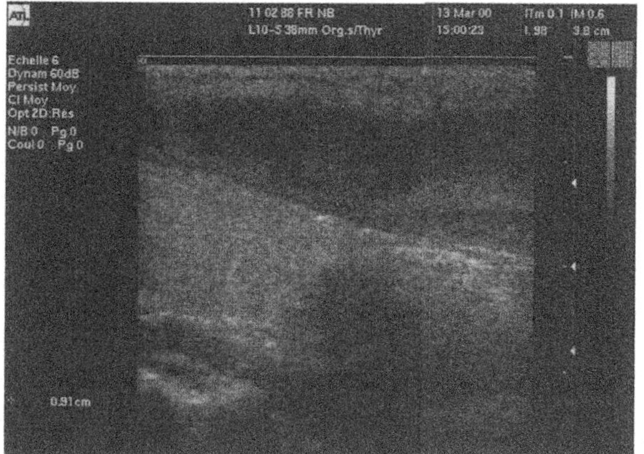

Fig. 9.4a, b. Twelve-year-old girl with a highly inflammatory anterior neck. **a** Well-defined hypoechoic mass anterior to the right thyroid lobe. **b** The tract is visible as a 9-mm-thick hypoechoic band connecting the cyst to the hyoid bone

ment the presence of the thyroid gland. The differential diagnosis, an ectopic thyroid, contraindicates surgical excision. Visualization of a normally located thyroid with normal sonographic features obviates the need for scintigraphy (Lin-Dunham et al. 1995). In contrast, if a normal thyroid is not found in the expected anatomic location, thyroid scintigraphy is indispensable to search for ectopic thyroid tissue. There have been rare reports of intrathyroid thyroglossal cysts presenting as thyroid nodules (McHenry et al. 1993).

Ultrasonography combined with physical examination suffices for the diagnosis of thyroglossal cysts (Brewis et al. 2000). Computed tomography (CT) merely confirms the lesion and provides no additional data.

9.1.1.3 Course

Recurrence is possible following surgical resection, especially in patients with a recent preoperative infection and those with multiple thyroglossal duct tracts (Ducic et al. 1998). Wide excision, using an appropriate technique and removing the anterior two thirds of the hyoid bone, generally leads to cure without recurrence.

Malignant transformation occurs in approximately 1% of cases, resulting in papillary thyroid carcinoma (Heshmati et al. 1997; O'Connell et al. 1998) or, exceptionally, another histological type of cancer (Hama et al. 1997). Most such neoplasms are discovered at histopathological examination of the surgical specimen. The majority have been described in adults, and pediatric cases remain uncommon (Patti et al. 2000; Yoo et al. 1998).

9.1.2 Branchial Cysts, Sinuses and Fistulas

Branchial cysts, sinuses, and fistulas are developmental anomalies arising essentially from remnants of the branchial arches forming the embryonic lateral cervical wall that normally disappear during fetal development. There are initially six pairs of branchial arches (Diagram 9.2):

- *Branchial sinuses* are small cutaneous orifices without any deep communication. Although they cannot be visualized sonographically, this imaging modality is helpful to rule out a subjacent cyst.
- *Branchial fistulas* are connected to both the skin and the pharynx. US rarely demonstrates the fistulous tract (Fig. 9.5), and they are best explored with fistulography.
- *Branchial cysts*, located lateral to the laryngopharynx, without connection to the skin or pharynx, are the most common branchial anomaly and are examined well with US.

9.1.2.1 First Branchial Arch Cysts

First branchial arch cysts are located at the inferior pole of the parotid gland. Often undetected until adulthood, the most frequent diagnosis is a parotid cyst. Sonographic visualization of a well-defined cystic mass suspended from the inferior pole of the parotid

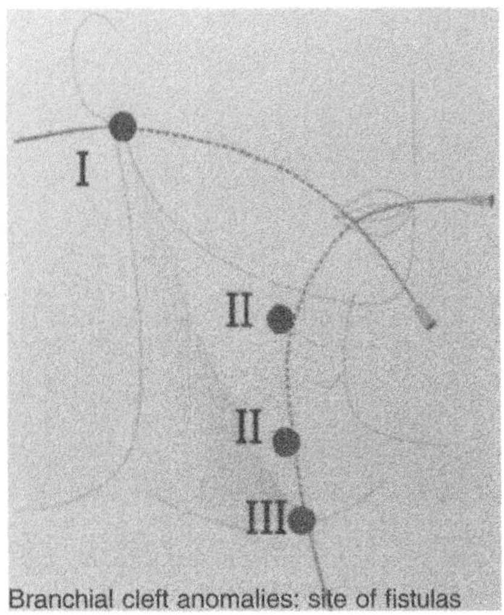

Diagram 9.2. Branchial arches

(Fig. 9.6) is suggestive of a first arch cyst (Baader and Lewis 1994; Nofsinger et al. 1997). The inconstant association with a fistula, the external orifice of which lies in the triangle of Poncet, limited by the external acoustic meatus, the hyoid bone, and the mandible, facilitates diagnosis. An extension towards the external acoustic meatus, which is better demonstrated by CT or MRI, is also suggestive of the diagnosis.

9.1.2.2
Second Branchial Arch Cysts

Second branchial arch cysts occur in the lateral neck, anterior to the sternocleidomastoid muscle, near the angle of the mandible and in the supraclavicular region. The most frequent (70%) of all branchial cleft anomalies (Marsot-Dupuch et al. 1995), these cysts account for 2% of all cervical tumors. Diagnosis is generally made early following detection of a lateral cervical mass. Sonographically, the mass is well-defined and anechoic or only weakly echoic. The highly uniform echogenicity of the mass is rather characteristic (Reynolds and Wolinski 1993). Aspiration cytology may be helpful for diagnosis (Perez et al. 1994); a straw-colored or sometimes purulent aspirate may be obtained if superinfection has occurred (Fig. 9.7). The differential diagnosis is adenitis. An internal extension towards the paratonsillar space or between the internal and external carotid arteries, or a posterior extension occasionally creates problems for differential diagnosis from cystic lymphangioma. Bilateral cysts have been described. Treatment consists in surgical resection.

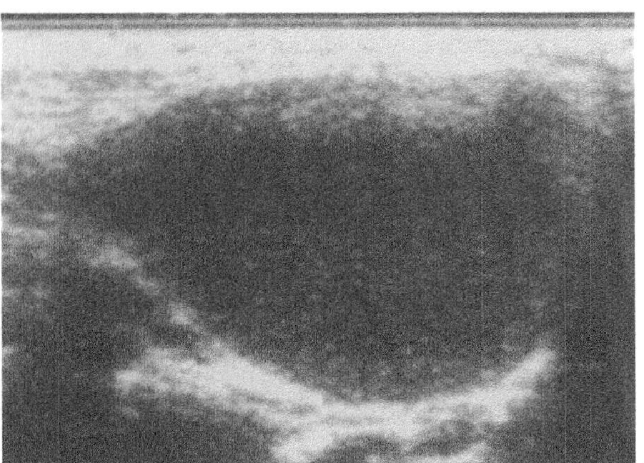
a

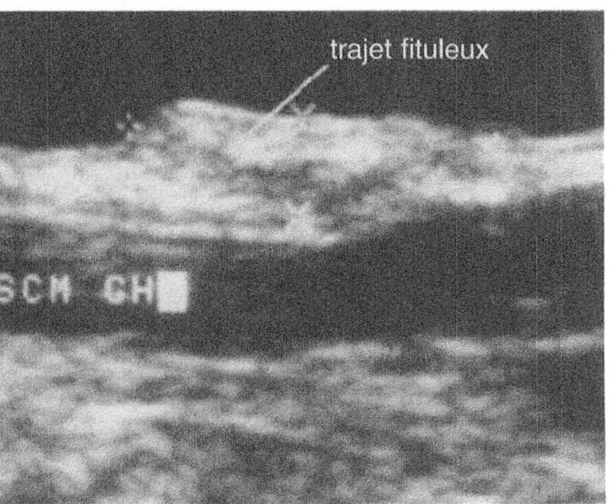

b

Fig. 9.5a, b. Homogeneously hypoechoic mass in the lateral neck. **a** Note the uniform echogenicity. second arch cyst. **b** Demonstration of a subcutaneous fistulous tract. (Courtesy Prof P Devred, Marseilles, France)

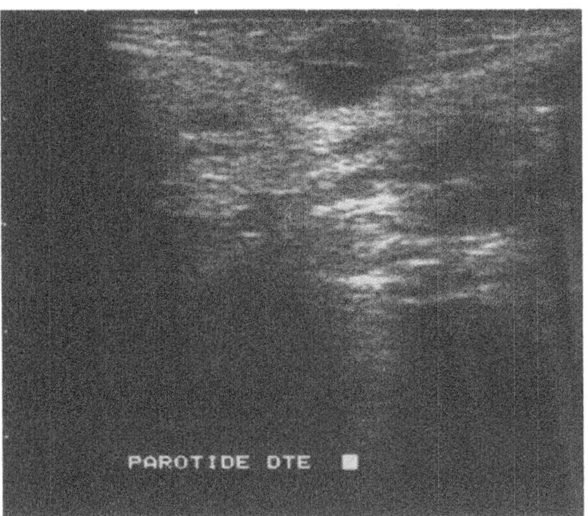

Fig. 9.6. Cystic intraparotid nodule: first arch cyst

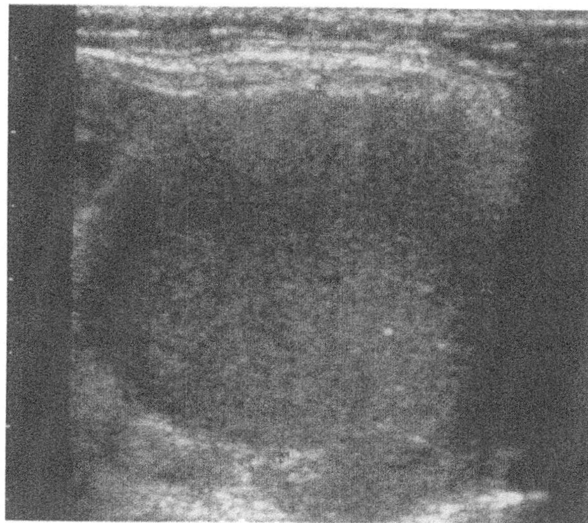

Fig. 9.7. Large hypoechoic mass with uniform echogenicity: superinfected second arch cyst

9.1.2.3
Third Branchial Arch Anomalies

Anomalies of the third arch are rare. Noncommunicating cysts are indistinguishable from second arch cysts. High-lying, prelaryngeal cysts mimic a thyroglossal duct cyst (Fig. 9.8). Surgical demonstration of the fistulous tract communicating with the piriform sinus corrects the diagnosis.

9.1.2.4
Fourth Branchial Arch Anomalies

The most common fourth arch anomalies are piriform sinus fistulas, which are usually left-sided. The fistula runs anteroinferiorly from the apex of the piriform sinus through the constrictor muscle of the pharynx or directly through the laryngeal cartilage. Such congenital anomalies can cause phlegmonous adenitis of the mid portion of the neck that can become quite bulky, causing dyspnea and/or dysphagia, especially in young children. Phlegmonous adenitis tends to recur after treatment until the fistula is correctly diagnosed. Sonographic findings for phlegmonous adenitis are nonspecific: an avascular anechoic or hypoechoic mass corresponding to a necrotic node. A left-sided lesion in the mid portion of the neck should suggest the diagnosis. The presence of air, visible small, punctate, echoic areas within the cervical or thyroid mass, is highly suggestive of the diagnosis (Fig. 9.9). A plain neck film may reveal the presence of air and contribute to the diagnosis. The fistulous orifice can then be sought by laryngoscopy of the base of the left piriform sinus. A barium swallow or CT may also be helpful for diagnosis (Bar-Ziv et al. 1996; Nicollas et al. 1998; Yang et al. 1999). Fourth arch anomalies are often not diagnosed until adulthood (Barberet et al. 1999).

Infection through a piriform sinus fistula may lead to acute suppurative thyroiditis or an anterior neck abscess (Lucaya et al. 1990), imaged as a hypoechoic intrathyroid nodule with inflammatory features (Fig. 9.10).

9.1.3
Laryngeal Cysts

Laryngeal cysts are rare but serious lesions that can cause respiratory distress. They develop in an aryepiglottic fold or a vallecula following occlusion of a

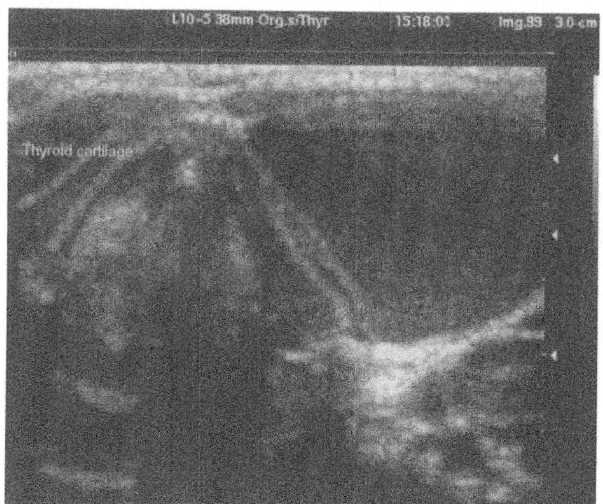

a

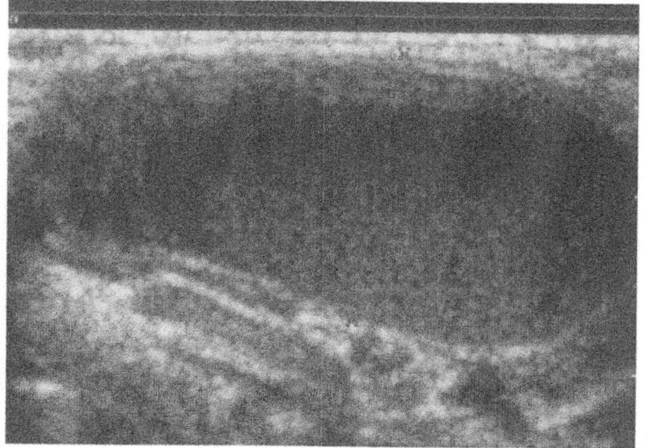

b

Fig. 9.8a, b. Prelaryngeal cystic mass: third arch cyst. **a** Transverse scan, **b** sagittal scan

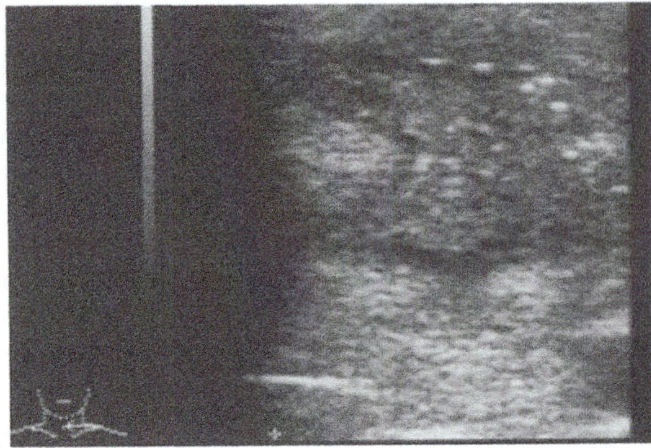

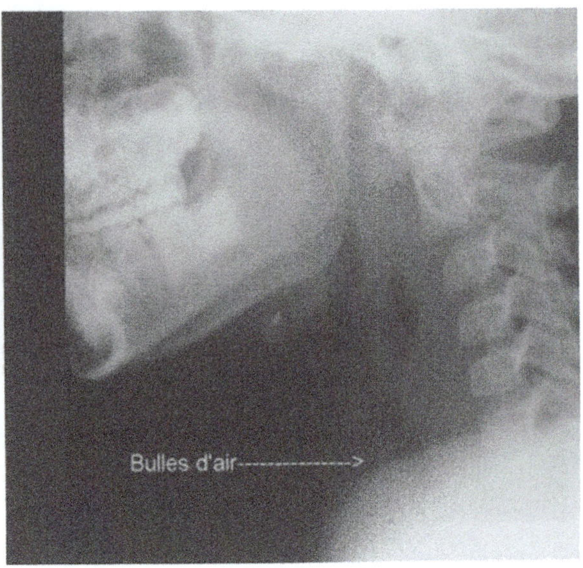

Fig. 9.9 a Echoic lateral neck mass containing hyperechoic punctate spaces corresponding to small air bubbles. fourth arch fistula **b** The air bubbles are clearly visible on the standard profile film of the neck

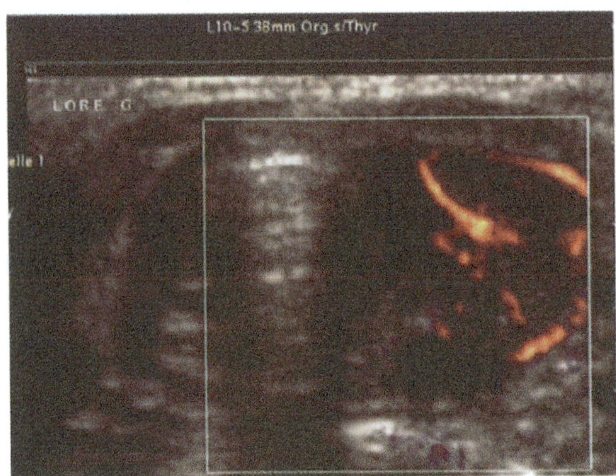

Fig. 9.10. Left lobe of an inflammatory, hypoechoic, and hypervascular (CD) thyroid suppurative thyroiditis secondary to a fourth arch fistula

laryngeal mucous gland or secondary to atresia of the laryngeal saccule orifice (Ward et al. 1995). Ultrasonography can accurately localize the laryngeal mass and confirm its cystic nature. Treatment is surgical, generally by endoscopic excision (Shita et al. 1999). A lateral cervical approach may be required for recurrent cysts (Civantos and Holinger 1992).

9.1.4 Other Cysts

Other cystic cervical lesions include epidermoid cysts and dermoid cysts that arise from inclusion of a portion of ectoderm. Epidermoid cysts have only squamous epithelium (Fig. 9.11), whereas dermoid cysts contain hair, sebaceous and sweat glands, and squamous epithelium (Smirniotopoulos and Chiechi 1995). These neck lesions typically image at CT as a unilocular cystic mass (Fig. 9.12) (Vittore et al. 1998). Differential diagnosis from a thyroglossal duct cyst can be difficult. The existence of calcifications may suggest the diagnosis, which is usually made by histopathological examination.

9.1.5 Thymic Anomalies

The normal thymus lies in the anterior mediastinum, and presence of thymic tissue at any other level reflects an anomaly in embryonic descent. A distinction is made between *aberrant thymus*, as may occur in the lateral neck or suprasternal area, anywhere along the normal pathway of thymic descent, and *ectopic thymus*, lying in any other position (e.g., pharynx, trachea, esophagus, posterior neck, or mediastinum) (Koumanidou et al. 1998). When the aberrant thymus is connected by a bridge to the thymus in the normal mediastinal location, diagnosis is easy. Diagnosis is more difficult when there is no connecting bridge, and surgical resection may be required (Duroux et al. 1993). Ultrasonography reveals a well-defined, homogeneous, weakly echoic mass with the same echotexture as the thymus (Fig. 9.13).

Cervical thymic cysts present as cystic masses with no specific features other than their atypically low infrahyoid position, sometimes with an extension into the upper mediastinum (Riechelmann et al. 1992).

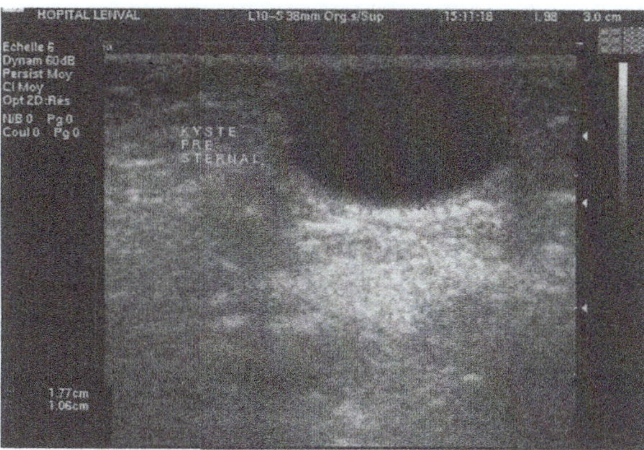

Fig. 9.11. Completely anechoic, fluid-like, high presternal mass: epidermoid cyst

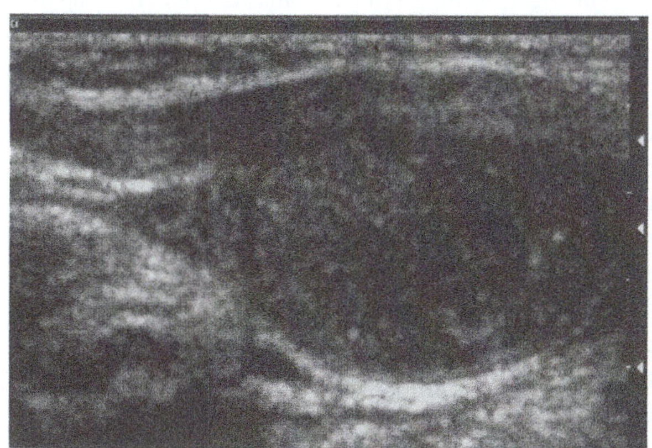

Fig. 9.12. Well-delimited, finely inhomogeneous midline cystic mass containing small, dense, punctate echoes: dermoid cyst

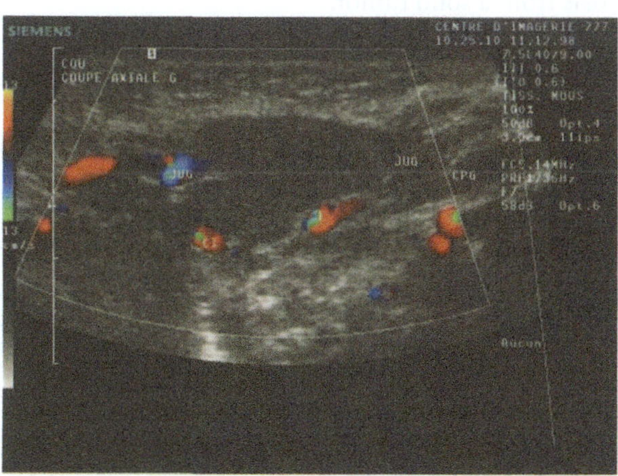

Fig. 9.13. Uniform weakly echoic mass between the large vessels of the neck: aberrant thymus. *CI* Internal carotid artery; *CE* external carotid artery; *CPG* left primary carotid artery; *JUG* internal jugular vein

9.2 Fibromatosis Colli

Hematoma of the sternocleidomastoid muscle (sternocleidomastoid "tumor") is often secondary to birth trauma (0.4% of all births). Diagnosis is clinical. An elongated unilateral mass is present within the muscle and may be associated with torticollis. Sonography demonstrates a mass (Fig. 9.14) of variable echotexture that is often inhomogeneous in the sternocleidomastoid muscle, a mass with fusiform muscle enlargement compared with the healthy side, or muscle enlargement alone (Bedi et al. 1998). The intramuscular location and comparison with the contralateral side (Fig. 9.15) facilitate the diagnosis given the context and the child's age (first 8 weeks of life). Resolution is spontaneous but usually slow; sonographic follow-up is unnecessary. Physical therapy (stretching exercises) is often required to prevent fibrous contracture of the muscle.

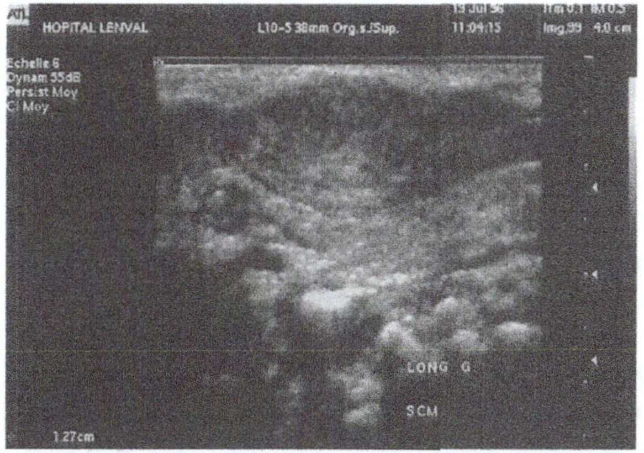

a

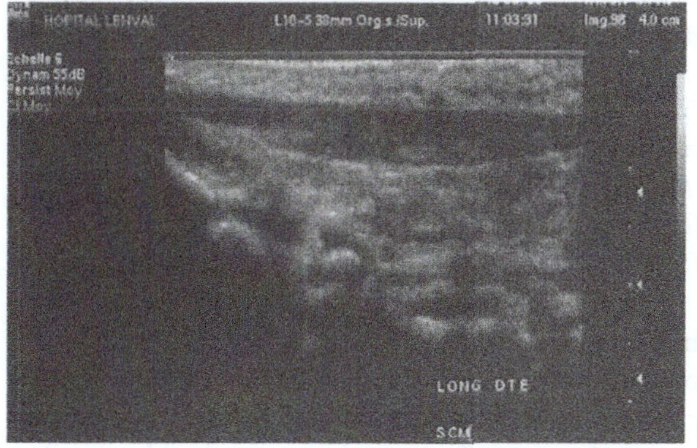

b

Fig. 9.14. Hyperechoic mass in the sternocleidomastoid muscle

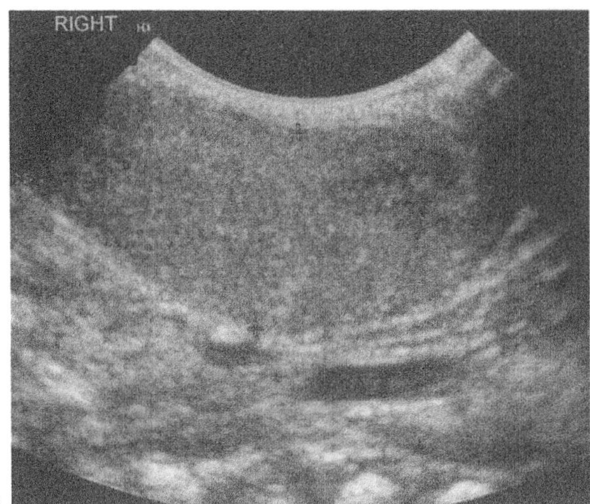

a

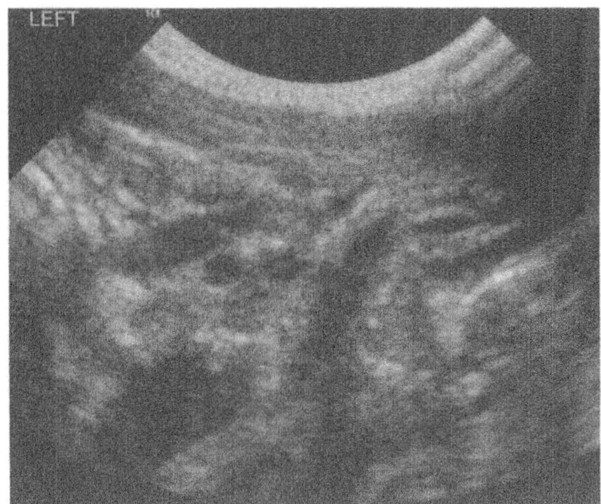

b

Fig. 9.15. Discretely hyperechoic, inhomogeneous fusiform enlargement (*right*) of the sternocleidomastoid muscle compared with the healthy contralateral side: fibromatosis colli

Use of fine-needle aspiration cytology has been suggested for diagnosis (Peireira et al. 1999) because smears reveal mature fibroblasts and fragments of striated muscle fibers. We feel that diagnosis should remain clinical, when necessary complemented by US; additional examinations can be reserved for infrequent cases with an inconclusive diagnosis.

9.3 Nodal Masses

9.3.1 Infections

9.3.1.1 *Bacterial Lymphadenopathy*

Infectious lymphadenopathy is very frequent in the pediatric age-group. Diagnosis is made clinically. US is of no diagnostic value in itself but can be useful for examination of large nodes to search for abscess formation.

Enlarged cervical lymph nodes due to common infections usually occur below the angle of the mandible and in the jugulocarotid region. Sonography typically demonstrates multiple, weakly echoic, elongated nodes (Fig. 9.16). These nodes appear highly vascular on color Doppler and power Doppler (Fig. 9.17). Progression to abscess formation manifests as an area of very low echogenicity within an often large, tender node; in advanced stages the lesion may appear avascular, with a markedly anechoic central fluid-like component (Fig. 9.18). Sonography permits evaluation of response to treatment and assessment of the potential benefits of incision and drainage (Quraishi et al. 1997).

Retropharyngeal abscesses are particular to children, in that they commonly result from a tonsil infection. Ultrasonography may contribute to diagnosis by revealing a weakly echogenic or sometimes anechoic prespinal mass. A lateral film of the neck depicts the anterior displacement of the airway (Fig. 9.19). CT may be necessary to confirm the diagnosis prior to surgical incision. Necrosis or an infectious context are suggestive of an abscess and permit differential diagnosis from a solid tumor.

9.3.1.2 *Infectious Mononucleosis*

Cervical lymphadenopathy is a consistent feature of infectious mononucleosis. The lymph nodes are voluminous and only weakly echoic (Fig. 9.20).

9.3.1.3 *Cat-scratch Disease*

Cervical lymphadenopathy is frequent in cat-scratch disease, a benign, self-limited regional lymphadenitis. The nodes have no specific features except for their often large dimensions and a more marked propensity for abscess formation (Fig. 9.21). The existence of concomitant hepatic or splenic nodules is highly suggestive of the diagnosis.

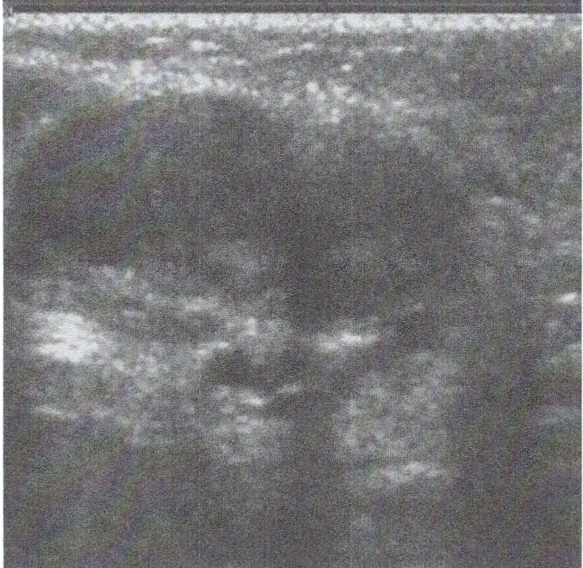

Fig. 9.16. Adenitis

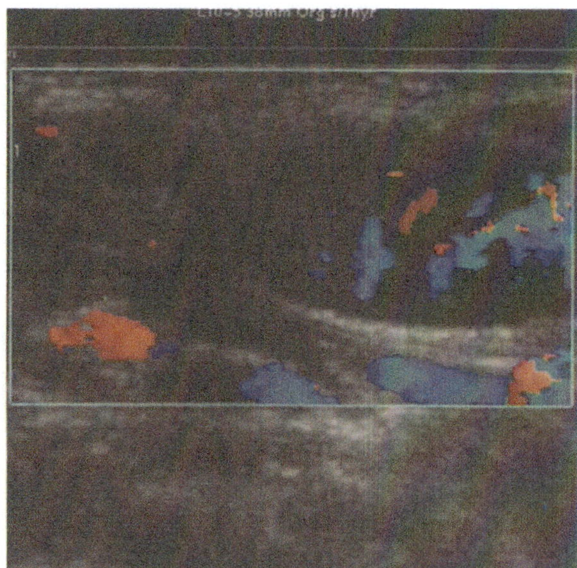

Fig. 9.17. Highly vascular infectious node

a

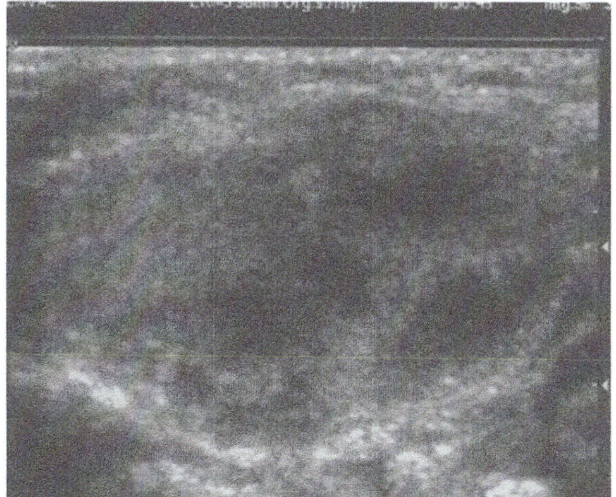

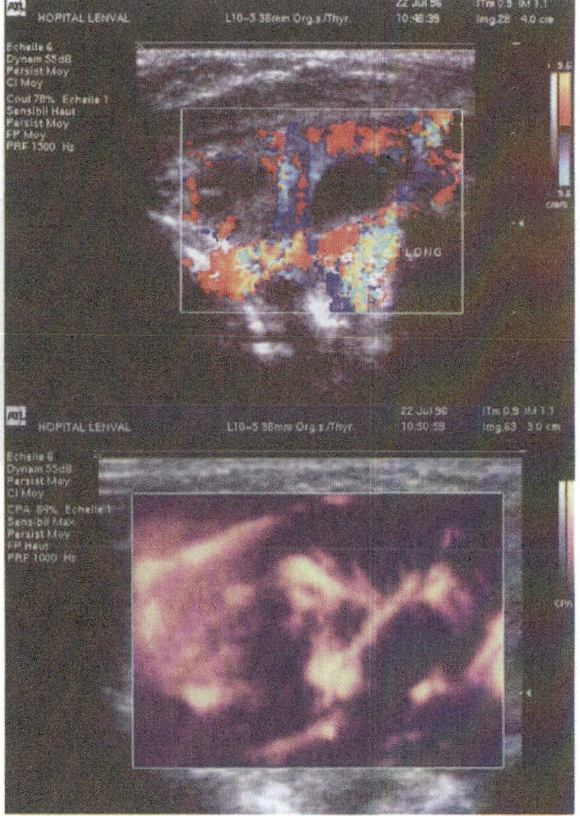

b

Fig. 9.18a, b. Necrotic lymph node. **a** Lymph node containing anechoic areas. **b** The avascular anechoic spaces correspond to areas of necrosis (color Doppler)

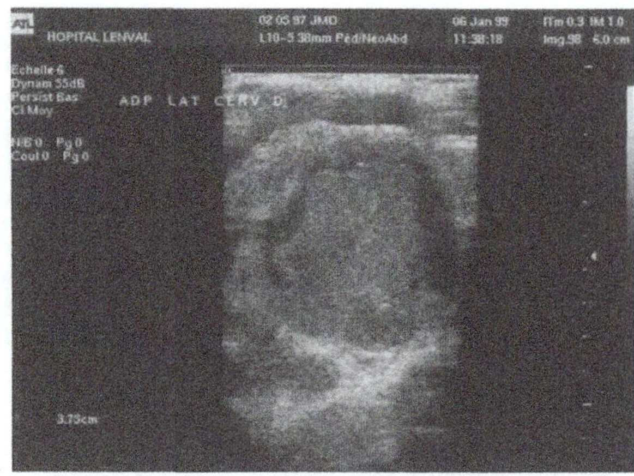

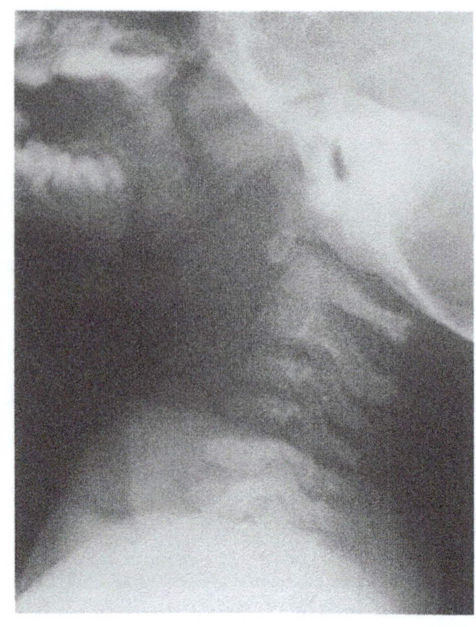

Fig. 9.19a, b. Retropharyngeal abscess. **a** Prespinal cervical mass in a febrile patient: retropharyngeal abscess. **b** Lateral neck film demonstrating extensive thickening of the prespinal soft tissues caused by the retropharyngeal abscess

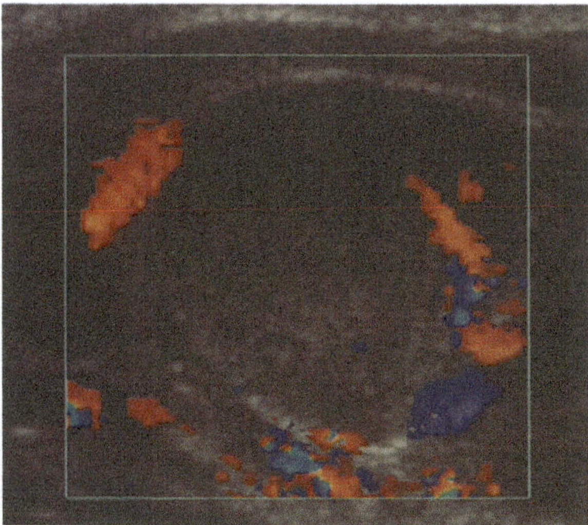

Fig. 9.20. Rounded hypoechoic adenopathy: infectious mononucleosis

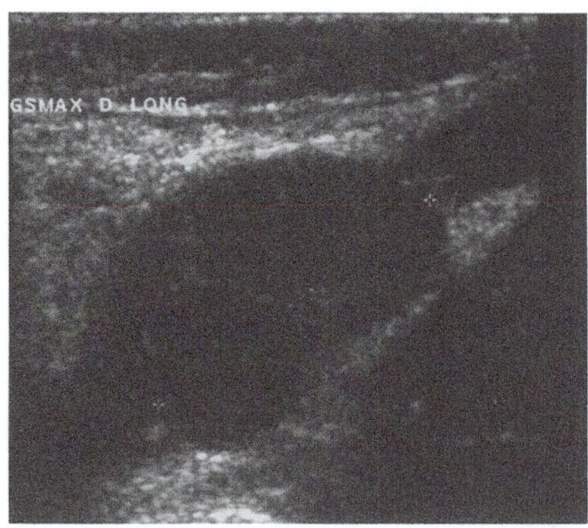

Fig. 9.21. Highly necrotic lymph nodes: cat-scratch disease

9.3.1.4 *Tuberculous and Atypical Mycobacterial Adenitis*

Chronic lymphadenopathy, namely in the posterior cervical triangle (Vazquez et al. 1995), is highly suggestive of the diagnosis, especially if the nodes have a hyperechoic center (Fig. 9.22) or calcifications are present. Sonographic findings may be nonspecific, and bulky nodes may contain areas of necrosis (Fig. 9.23).

9.3.2 Malignancy

9.3.2.1 *Hemopathies*

The cervical adenopathies encountered in hemopathies tend to be larger, more rounded, and more markedly hypoechoic (Fig. 9.24) than infectious nodes. They are also more diffuse, involving in par-

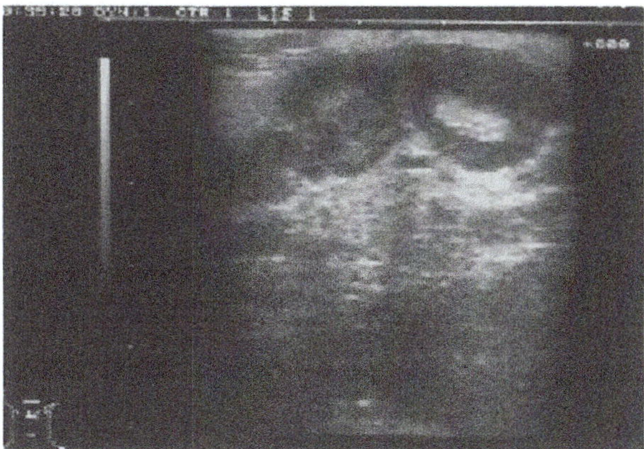

Fig. 9.22. Lymph nodes with an extremely hyperechoic center: atypical mycobacterial infection

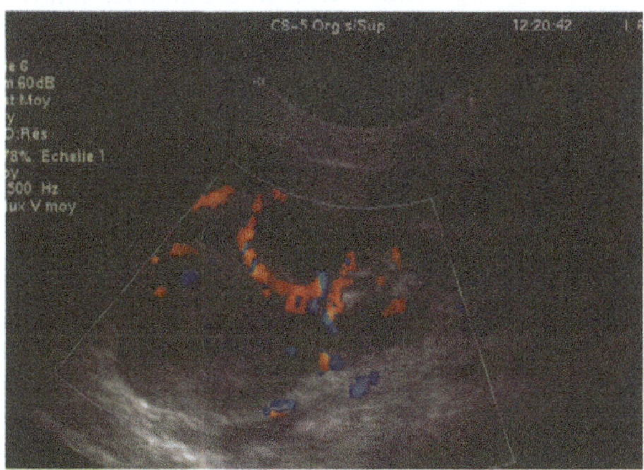

Fig. 9.23. Large lymph node with a necrotic component: tuberculosis

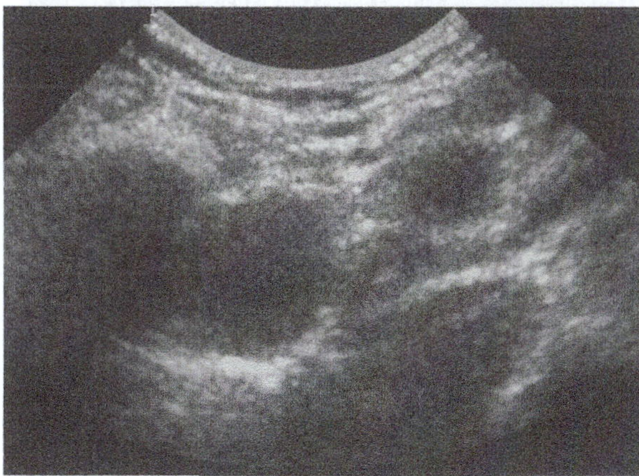

Fig. 9.24. Multiple, hypoechoic lymph nodes extending to the thymic bed: leukemia

ticular the posterior chains and the supraclavicular region (Redondo Granado et al. 1992). The vascular pattern is variable, ranging from poor to rich vascularity, both at the center and at the periphery of the nodes. Owing to the absence of any formal characteristics, the clinical context orients the diagnosis. Aspiration cytology is required for conclusive diagnosis whenever doubt persists.

9.3.2.2
Solid Tumors

The metastases of solid tumors do not have any specific characteristics. Nodal metastases reportedly have a spotted, peripheral, or mixed vascular pattern (Issing et al. 1999; Wu et al. 1998).

9.3.3
Characterization of Lymph Nodes

There are no specific features allowing the classification of lymph nodes and confirmation of their benign or malignant nature. Numerous authors (Steinkamp et al. 1999; Ying et al. 1998) have attempted to define criteria allowing differentiation of benign from malignant nodes. Results are conflicting, and no investigation has dealt solely with children. In fact, the problem is different in pediatric patients from that in adults, owing to the frequency of benign reactive cervical adenopathies of infectious origin in young children, particularly during the winter. In contrast, when doubt persists concerning chronic adenopathies or unexplained nodal enlargement, cytological aspiration biopsy is indicated for diagnosis, as no other feature (nodal size, echogenicity, vascularity) is conclusive.

9.4
Non-nodal Tumoral Pathologies

9.4.1
Vascular Tumors and Malformations

9.4.1.1
Hemangiomas

Hemangiomas are the most frequent tumors in children (Dubois and Garel 1999); 60% occur in the cervicofacial region (Fig. 9.25). These benign tumors appear soon after birth and have a rapid course the

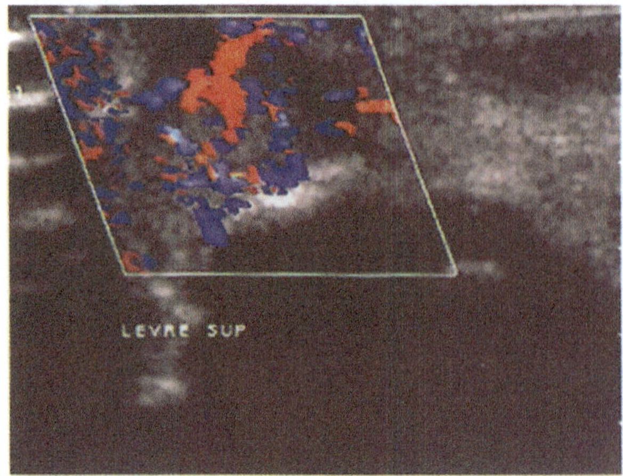

Fig. 9.25. Vascular mass in the upper lip: progressive hemangioma

first months of life, then regress spontaneously. The diagnosis is usually made clinically (Enjolras 1999). Ultrasonography is helpful for deep-seated hemangiomas because it permits differential diagnosis from masses of other origins. Examination is often performed in the acute growth phase. The echotexture of the mass is variable and calcifications are possible. Color Doppler demonstrates the high vessel density (more than 5 vessels per square centimeter; Fig. 9.26). The Doppler shift is over 2 kHz (Dubois et al. 1998); the resistive index is low. During the period of involution, the lesion decreases in size and the number of vessels decreases, but the Doppler shift remains elevated.

Forty percent of all venous malformations involve the cervicofacial region. Present at birth as a soft bluish mass that expands with maneuvers that increase the venous pressure, they are often asymptomatic. Sonography demonstrates a hypoechoic mass (Fig. 9.27) that is nearly always inhomogeneous; iso- and hyperechogenic masses are less common (Trop et al. 1999). The presence of calcifications corresponding to phleboliths is pathognomonic. Doppler studies demonstrate a slow and usually monophasic flow. A biphasic flow suggests a mixed lesion with a capillary component. Sometimes no blood flow is perceptible owing to thrombosis or to very slow velocity.

9.4.1.2 Lymphangiomas

Cystic lymphangiomas are congenital malformations due to a developmental defect in communication of lymphatic sacs with their drainage channels. These generally rare lesions are seen most commonly in infancy, as 80% appear before the age of 2 years (Pia et al. 1999). Cervical localizations predominate (70%–80% of cases), with most lesions arising in the posterior cervical triangle (Dubois et al. 1997). Lymphangiomas are subdivided into macrocystic and microcystic pathological types. *Macrocystic lymphangiomas* consist of large, multiloculated cystic masses containing fluid separated by septa; flow is perceptible only at the level of the septa (Fig. 9.28). *Microcystic lymphangiomas* may appear hyperechoic, owing to the multiple interphases created by the juxtaposed septa (Fig. 9.29); no flow is perceptible. CT or MRI may be helpful in determining the exact limits of extensive lesions prior to treatment. In particular, care must be

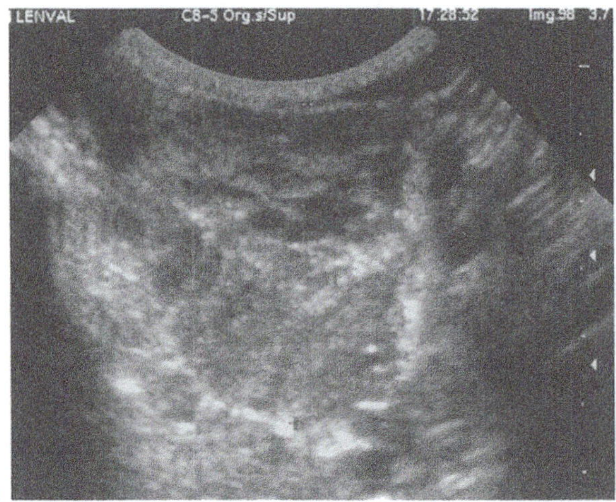

a

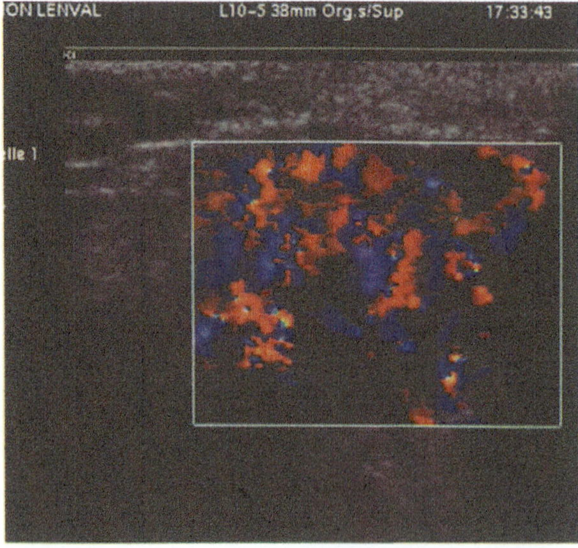

b

Fig. 9.26. Inhomogeneous parotid mass (**a**): this angioma appeared highly vascular on color Doppler (**b**)

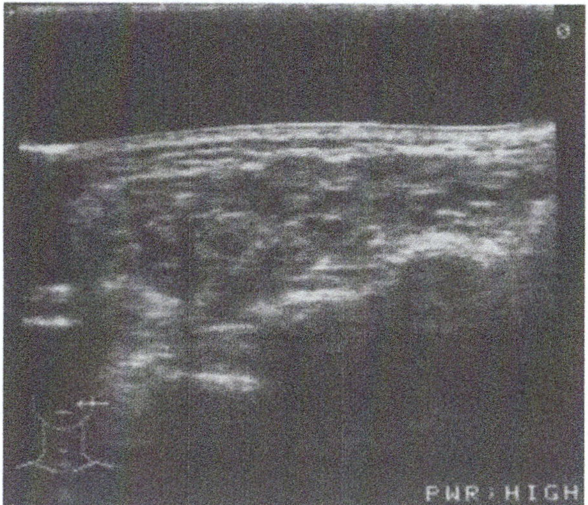

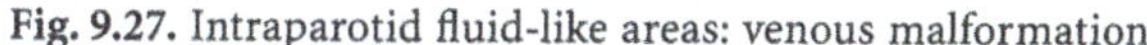

Fig. 9.27. Intraparotid fluid-like areas: venous malformation

taken to find any mediastinal extension. Surgery is the treatment of choice. Increasing use is being made of sclerosing agents such as Ethibloc (BREVIÈRE et al. 1992; DUBOIS et al. 1997; ESTEBAN et al. 1996), OK-432 (GREINWALD et al. 1999), and ethanol. Ultrasonography permits localization of the largest cysts, verification of the needle trajectory, and monitoring of injection (Fig. 9.30). Sonography is also helpful for follow-up and can demonstrate cyst disappearance or recurrence. Lesions commonly increase in size immediately after injection. External leakage of the sclerosing agent is frequent, and such fistulization appears to be related to a favorable response. Several injection sessions are often required. Sclerotherapy gives the best results for lymphangiomas with few relatively large cysts. Treatment of microcystic lymphangiomas is often less satisfactory.

9.4.2 Cervical Neurogenic Tumors

Cervical neurogenic tumors include *ganglioneuromas* and *neuroblastomas*. Cervical localizations of such neoplasms are relatively rare (<5% of all neuroblastomas; ABRAMSON et al. 1993). These tumors arise from the cranial nerves, the cervical sympathetic chain, or the paraganglion cells of the parasympathetic chain (DE HEYN 1990). Sonography is usually nonspecific, revealing a solid hypoechoic or complex mass along a nerve trajectory or in the posterior neck that sometimes contains small calcifications. A complementary imaging modality (CT or

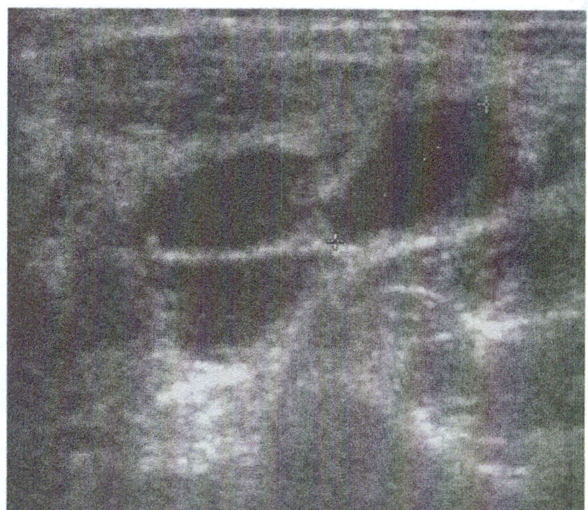

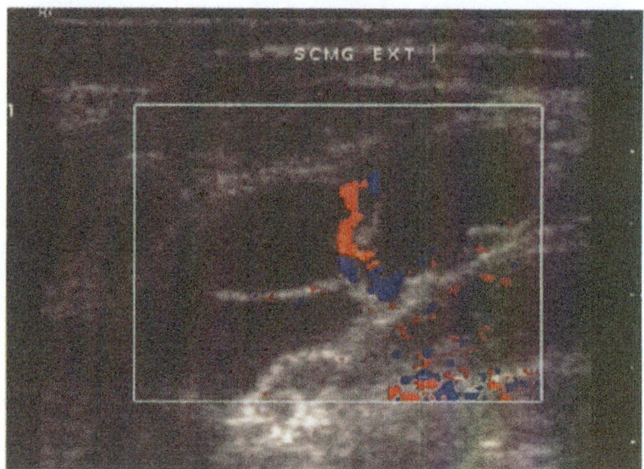

Fig. 9.28a, b. Macrocystic lymphangioma. **a** Cervical mass formed by the juxtaposition of fluid-like zones. **b** Only the septa appear vascularized

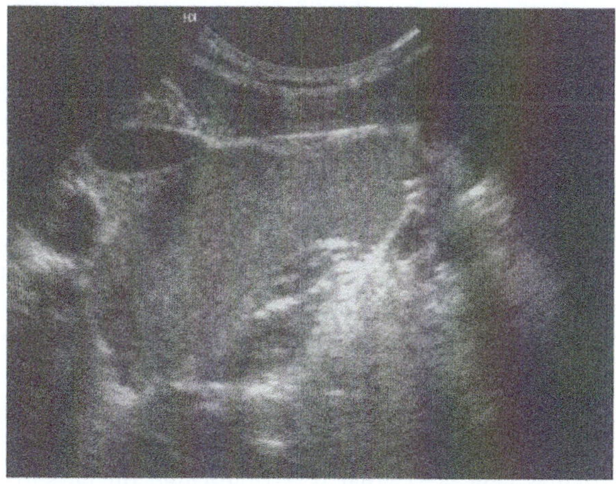

Fig. 9.29. Homogeneous cervical mass composed of fine echoes: microcystic lymphangioma

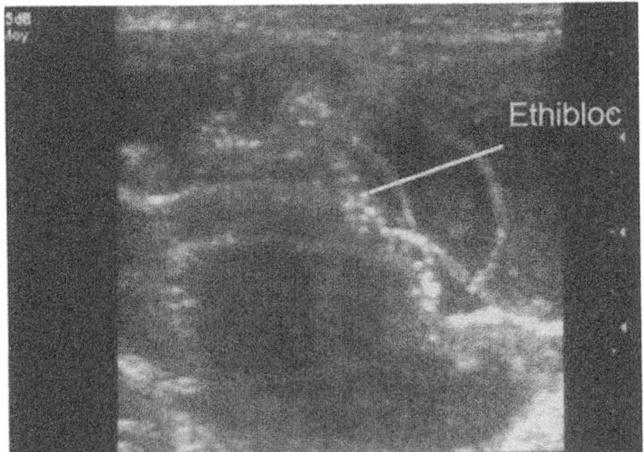

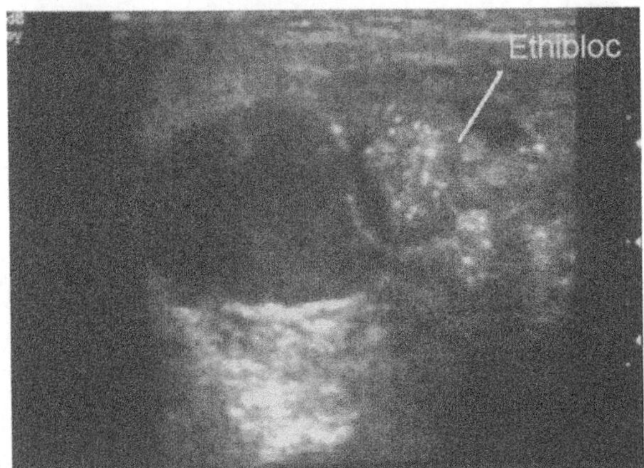

Fig. 9.30. Macrocystic lymphangioma after Ethibloc injection

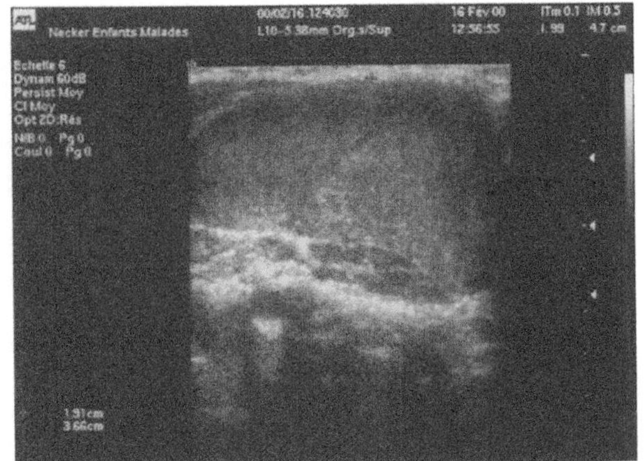

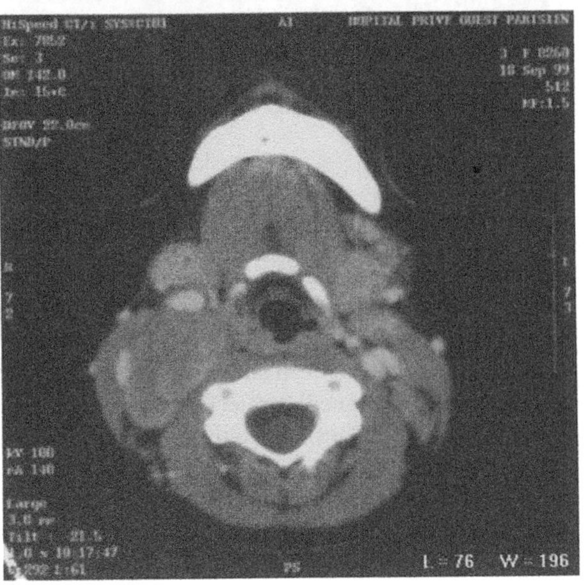

Fig. 9.31a, b. Neuroblastoma. **a** Lateral neck mass: neuroblastoma. **b** On the CT scan, the mass is visible posterior to the jugulocarotid bundle (Courtesy Hôpital des Enfants Malades, Paris, France)

MRI) is indispensable to determine the exact extent of the tumor prior to surgery (Fig. 9.31) and especially to search for an intraspinal extension (dumbbell tumor) (Maggi et al. 1995).

9.4.3 Other Masses

A variety of other tumors are also encountered in the neck. *Lipomas* have variable sonographic features, but are usually hypoechoic (Chikui et al. 1997; Marques Gubern et al. 1990). *Lipoblastomas* are infrequent, rapidly growing benign fatty tumors that may also occur in children. The fatty nature of these tumors is occasionally suggested by sonography, but other techniques are much more contributory. CT demonstrates a negative density while MRI reveals a mass with a high signal intensity on T_1-weighted images (Fig. 9.32) that is extinguished on fat-saturation sequences. These imaging modalities are an indispensable part of the preoperative workup.

Pilomatrixomas are benign tumors derived from a hair follicle and are often mistaken for other tumors (Williams et al. 1991). They image sonographically as well-defined, finely inhomogeneous masses (Fig. 9.33).

Fibromatosis is a rapidly aggressive, sonographically nonspecific mass on sonograms that tends to occur at the base of the tongue (Fig. 9.34) or around the mandible (Fig. 9.35).

Other possible but infrequent cervical tumors include *synovial sarcoma* (Kester 1990), *rhabdomyosarcoma*, and *fibrosarcoma*. These lesions are usually nonspecific at ultrasound examination.

a

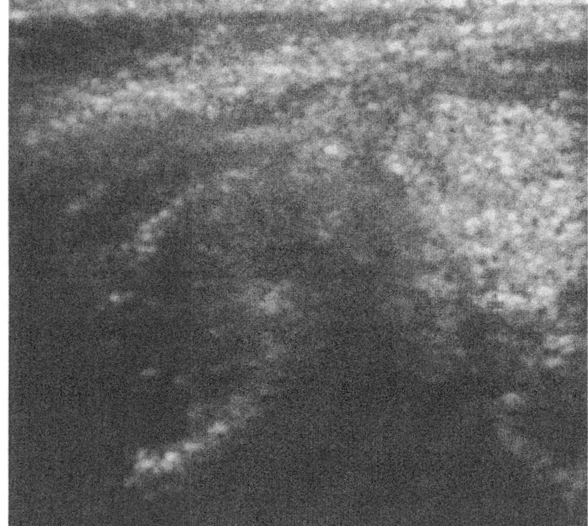

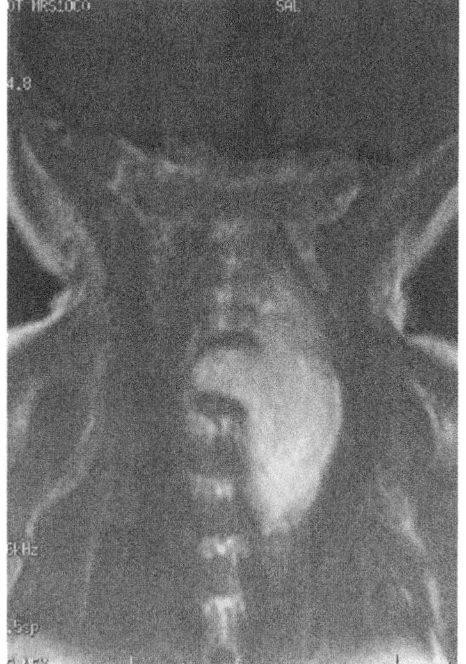

c

b

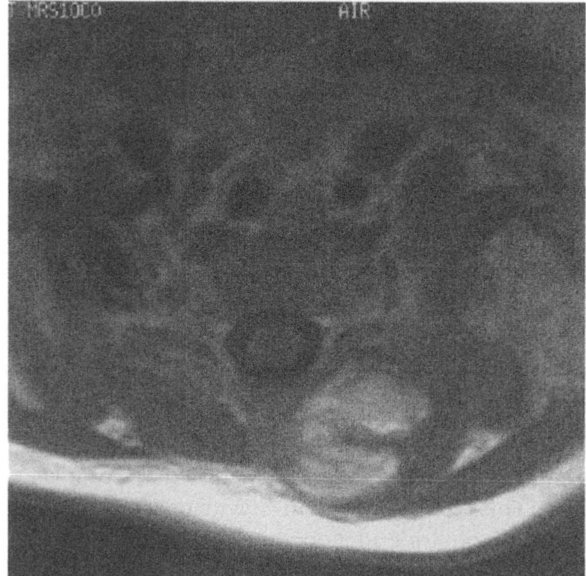

Fig. 9.32a–c. Lipoblastoma in a 1-year-old child. **a** Axial scan of the posterior neck: ill-defined, markedly hyperechoic laterovertebral mass. **b, c** MRI of the same child: axial (**b**) and coronal (**c**) scans revealing a mass with a high signal intensity on T_1-weighted sequences. The extension is better visualized, in particular between the spinal apophyses

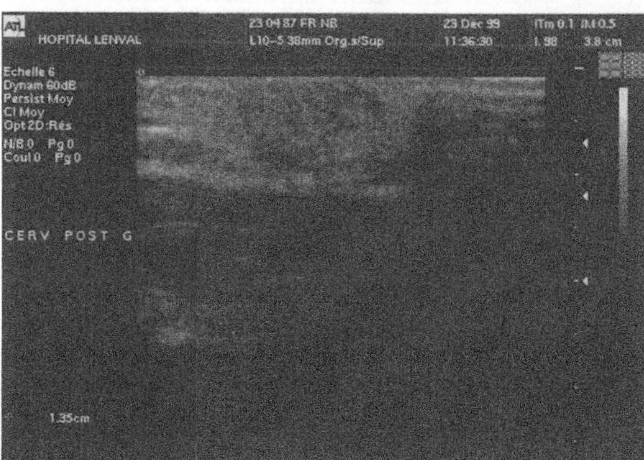

Fig. 9.33. Finely hyperechoic mass with a hypoechoic rim: pilomatrixoma

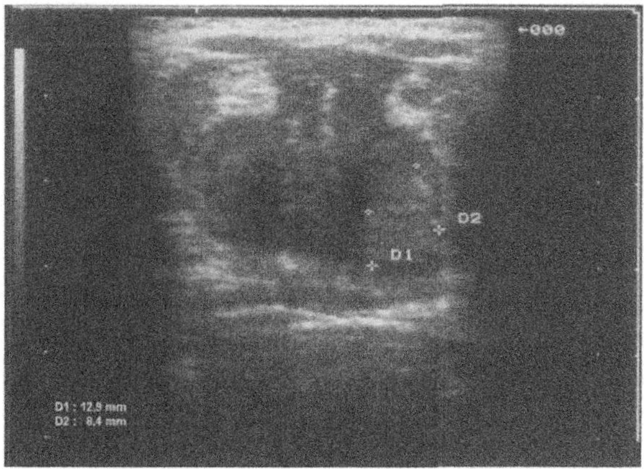

Fig. 9.34. Hyperechoic mass on the right side of the tongue. Scan obtained using an oblique submental approach: lingual fibromatosis

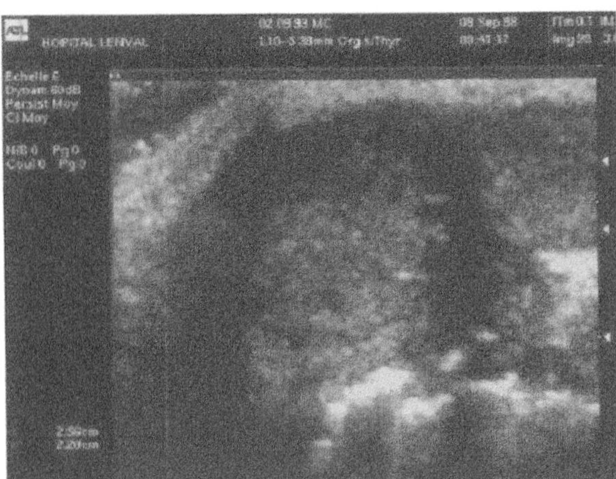
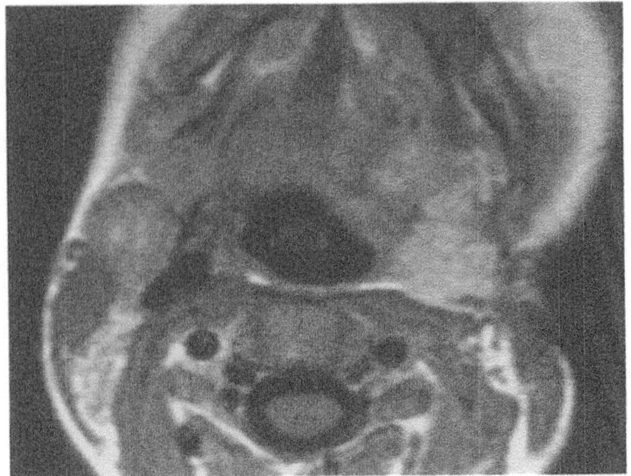

Fig. 9.35a, b. Desmoid fibroma. a Infiltrative mass in the submandibular region associated with adenopathies. b MRI (axial T_2-weighted imaging) revealed a hyperintense mass

9.5 Salivary Glands

9.5.1 Parotid Gland

9.5.1.1 Inflammatory Disease

9.5.1.1.1 Lymphadenitis

Intraparotid lymphadenitis is frequent, and usually associated with cervical lymphadenopathy (Garcia et al. 1998). Sonography demonstrates hypoechoic nodules within the parotid gland (Fig. 9.36). Such nodules have no particular significance. Although intraparotid lymphadenitis also occurs in hemopathies, it is more commonly associated with multiple cervical adenopathies of infectious bacterial origin. As for other enlarged nodes, progression to phlegmonous adenitis is possible (Fig. 9.37), in particular in cat-scratch disease.

9.5.1.1.2 Parotitis

Caused by the mumps virus or by bacteria, *acute parotitis* occurs in a febrile context as tender swelling of the parotid gland. Ultrasonography merely demonstrates a large homogeneous gland (Fig. 9.38) and is of little value.

Chronic parotitis is a bacterial infection manifesting as recurrent painful unilateral or bilateral swelling of the parotid gland, sometimes accompanied by fever. Secondary dilatation of the small salivary gland ducts, probably related to a congenital anomaly of these ducts, favors an ascending infection (Chitre and Premchandra 1997). Sonographic features are characteristic: The echogenic, sometimes enlarged gland contains multiple round hypoechoic areas measuring 2–4 mm in diameter. These hypoechoic areas correspond to the ductal dilatations shown by sialography (Fig. 9.39) and to surrounding lymphocytic infiltration (Encina et al. 1996; Nozaki et al. 1994).

HIV-positive children develop a particular form of chronic parotitis secondary to lymphocytic infiltration. Here, too, sonography reveals multiple small hypoechoic nodules corresponding to lymphoid infiltration. Progression to cyst formation may occur (Fig. 9.40). This type of parotid involvement is seen in children with multiple adenopathies and lymphoid pneumonia (LIP). Parotid mucosa-associated lymphoid

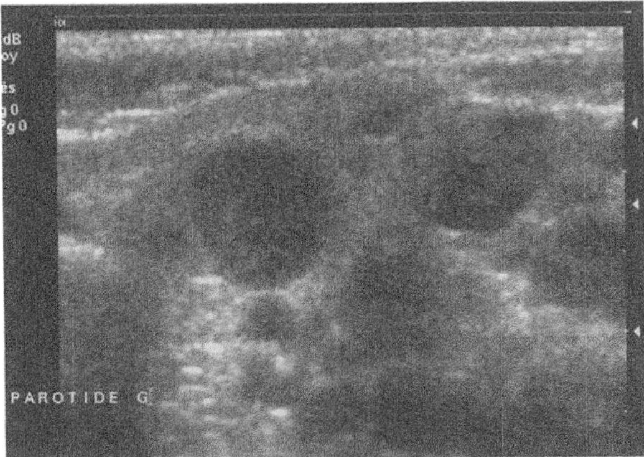

Fig. 9.36. Hypoechoic nodules in an infectious context: enlarged intraparotid nodes

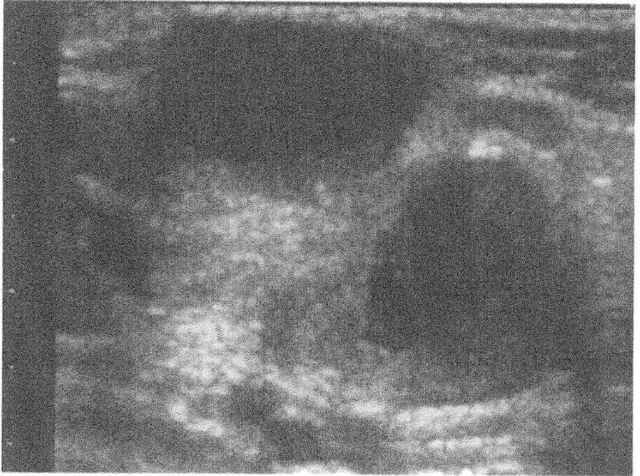

Fig. 9.37. Anechoic nodules: necrotic adenitis

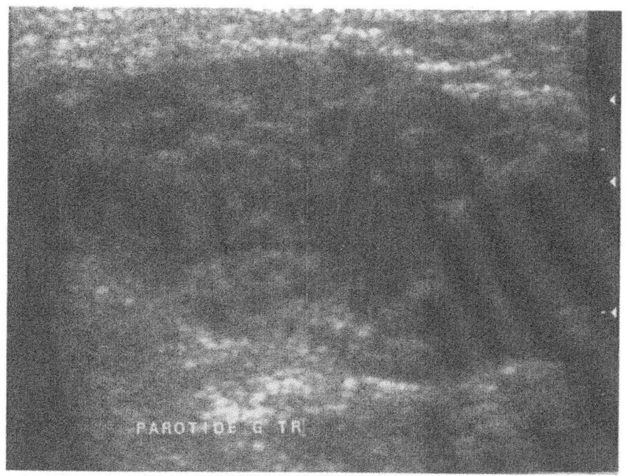

Fig. 9.38. Large, tender parotid with an intraparotid adenopathy: acute parotitis

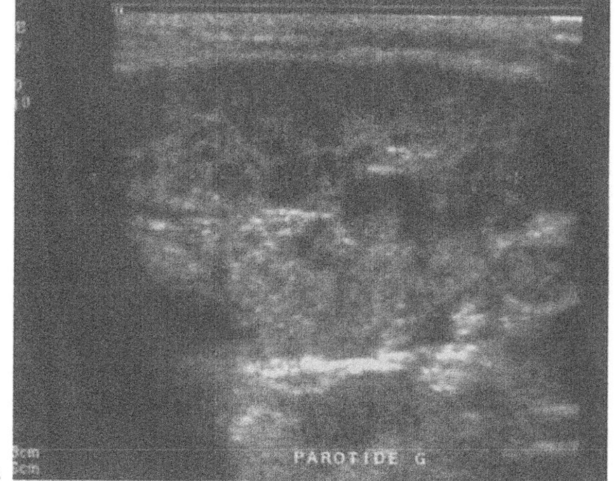

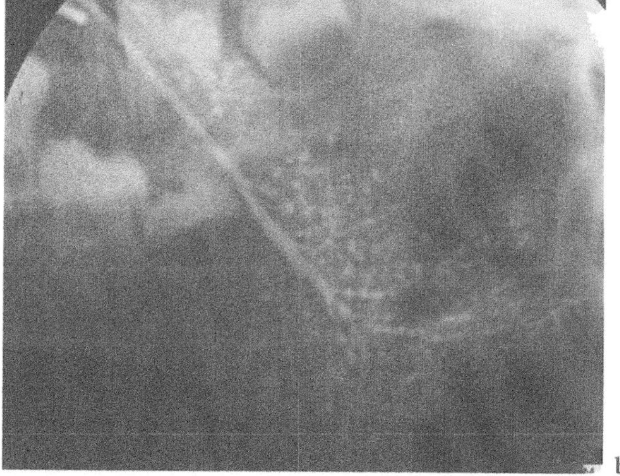

Fig. 9.39a, b. Chronic parotitis. a Multiple small, hypoechoic intraparotid nodules. b Sialography revealed the dilated canaliculi

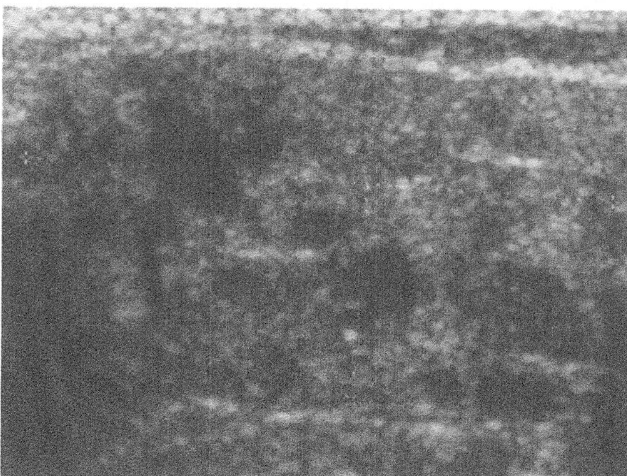

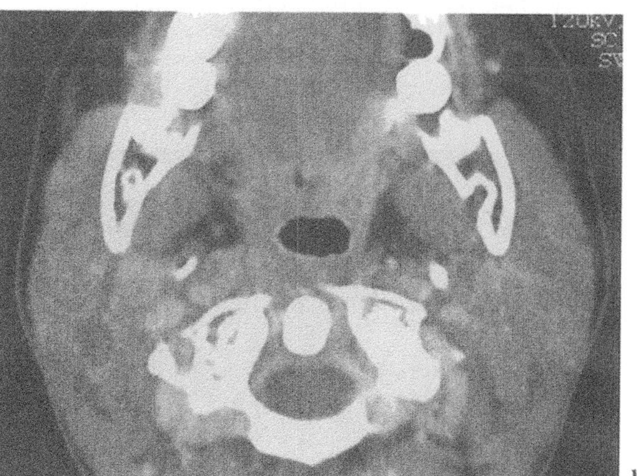

Fig. 9.40a, b. HIV-related parotitis of several years' duration. a Intraparotid microcysts; b CT revealed small intraparotid cysts

tissue (MALT) lymphoma has also been described in HIV-infected children (Corr et al. 1997).

On rare occasions, diffuse infiltration of the parotid is seen in systemic diseases such as sarcoidosis and tuberculosis.

9.5.1.2
Benign Tumors

9.5.1.2.1
Cystic Tumors

A parotid cyst should suggest an anomaly of the first branchial arch (see Sect. 9.1). Cystic hygroma or cystic lymphangioma may also occur within the parotid (Fig. 9.41). Sonography can demonstrate the limits of the lesion, but the deep lobe is best analyzed by CT or MRI. Treatment is generally surgical (Alqahtani et al. 1999), although percutaneous injection of a sclerosing agent is increasingly being used for these difficult-to-manage lesions.

9.5.1.2.2
Angiomas and Vascular Tumors

Vascular tumors account for 60% of all cases of parotid enlargement. The clinical presentation – a soft, bluish mass or presence of an associated angioma cutis – is suggestive of angioma. Sonography demonstrates a more or less homogeneously hypoechoic mass occupying all or part of the enlarged gland.

Color Doppler is helpful for diagnosis. Ultrasonography suffices for the diagnosis of most of these angiomas. Surgery is rarely indicated owing to the localization of the lesions, the surgical risk (namely nerve injury), and especially the frequency of spontaneous regression. Venous malformations are also possible at the level of the parotid gland.

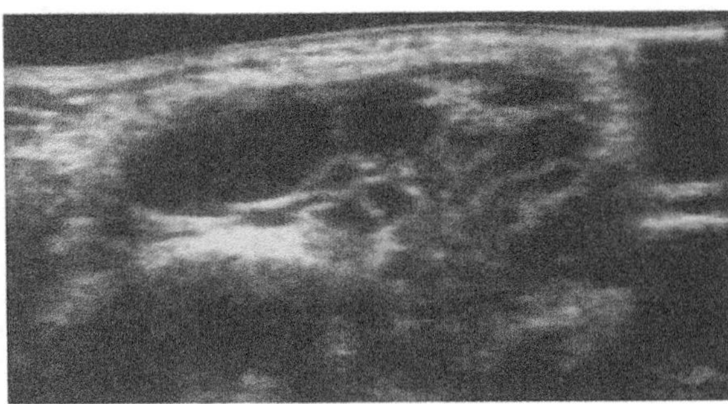

Fig. 9.41. Avascular intraparotid cystic areas: lymphangioma

9.5.1.2.3
Benign Solid Tumors

The infrequent benign parotid tumors include *pleomorphic adenomas* or *mixed tumors* that involve the superficial lobe. These firm, well-limited masses do not cause facial paralysis. Sonographic examination reveals a well-defined, hypoechoic mass (Fig. 9.42).

9.5.1.3
Malignant Tumors

Much more frequent in children than in adults, malignant tumors have a rapid growth pattern and rapidly show fixation to adjacent tissues. *Rhabdomyosarcomas* are characterized by rapid extracapsular spread to the adjacent soft tissues and bony structures. *Lymphomas* and *intraparotid_adenopathies* are encountered in lymphomas with cervical node involvement (Fig. 9.43). As ultrasonography merely confirms the presence of a parotid mass, other imaging modalities (CT or MRI) remain indispensable for diagnosis.

Other malignant tumors, essentially limited to the parotid, include *mucoepidermoid carcinoma* (MEC) (Khadaroo et al. 1998) and *acinar cell carcinoma*. These tumors are usually seen after the age of 10 years. *Adenocarcinoma* and *squamous cell carcinoma* are less common. Sonographic features are generally nonspecific and may suggest a benign intraparotid mass, especially if relatively homogeneous and well-defined (Jones et al. 1997). Such cases require cytologic aspiration biopsy followed by surgery.

9.5.1.4
Lithiasis

The oblique course of Stensen's duct (parotid duct) renders it less susceptible to lithiasis than Wharton's duct (submaxillary duct). Sonographically, stones show up as highly echoic areas associated with posterior reinforcement and ductal dilatation.

9.5.2
Submandibular Glands

As the submandibular glands do not contain lymph nodes, intraglandular adenopathy is not encountered at this level.

Acute inflammation of the submandibular gland is usually secondary to duct obstruction by a stone or, more rarely, to congenital stenosis. Sonography demonstrates an enlarged hypoechoic gland, sometimes

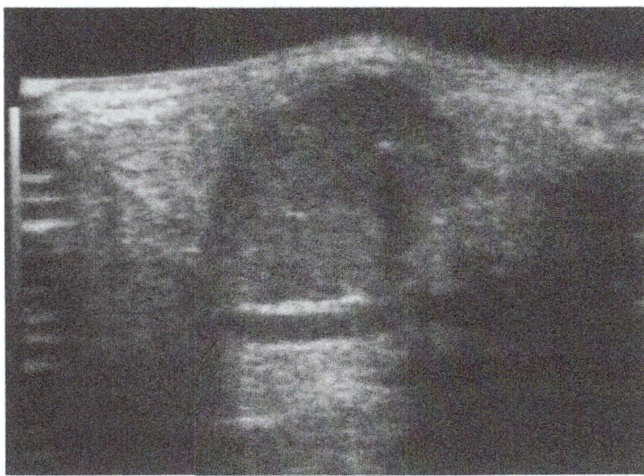

Fig. 9.42. Hypoechoic nodule in the superficial lobe containing a calcification: pleomorphic adenoma

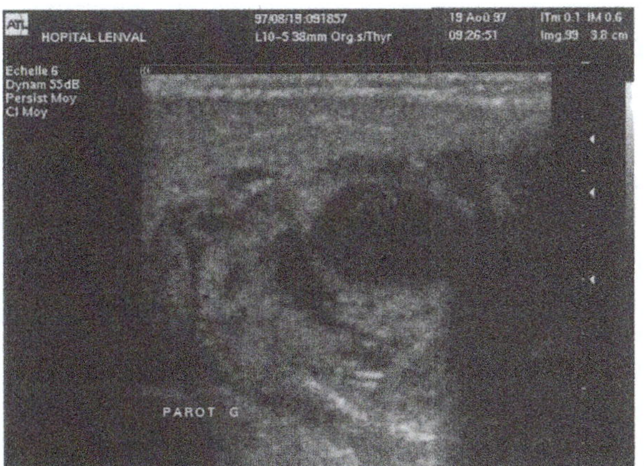

a

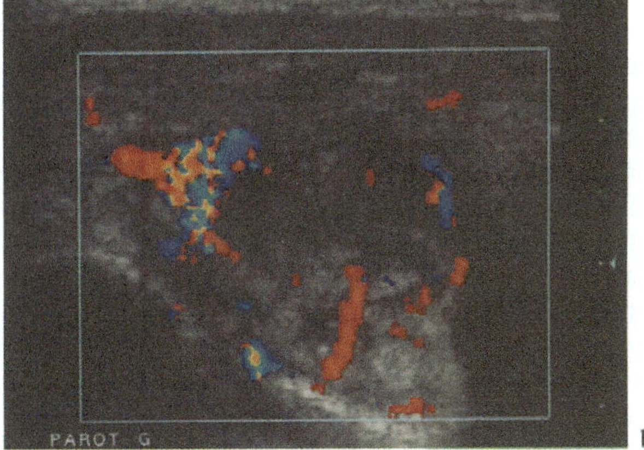

b

Fig. 9.43a, b. Highly hypoechoic intraparotid adenopathies with a peripheral vascular pattern: B-cell lymphoma

with ductal dilatation, and shows the stone in Wharton's duct.

Tumors of the submandibular glands are the same as those affecting the parotid gland (Garcia et al. 1998); angiomas predominate. Less common tumors include pleomorphic adenoma, mucoepidermoid carcinoma, and cystic adenoid carcinoma. US has low specificity (see corresponding chapter on adults).

9.5.3 Submental Gland

Located at the level of the floor of the mouth, anterior to the submaxillary gland, the normal submental gland is difficult to visualize. A cystic dilatation or a ranula corresponding to a mucocele may be encountered at any age. Sonography demonstrates a cystic mass on the floor of the mouth (Fig. 9.44). Treatment is by surgical resection.

9.6 Thyroid Gland

The echotexture of the normal thyroid gland is the same in children as in adults, i.e., homogeneously hyperechoic compared with the adjacent muscles. Nomograms for thyroid size have been established as a function of age, including the antenatal period (Achiron et al. 1998; Chanoine et al. 1991; Ho and Metreweli 1998).

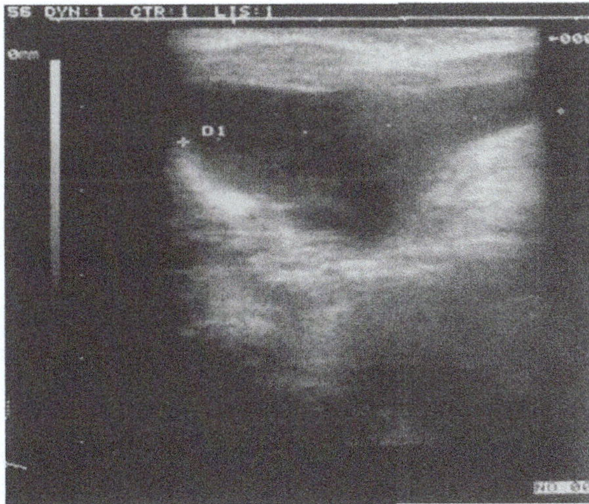

Fig. 9.44. Cystic dilatation of the submental gland

9.6.1
Congenital Anomalies

Mass screening of newborns provides biochemical data that may suggest the diagnosis of congenital hypothyroidism. Suspected congenital hypothyroidism is a therapeutic emergency requiring prompt initiation of replacement therapy. Ultrasonography plays an important role, as it can document the presence of the thyroid; when the thyroid bed is empty, the condition is referred to as athyrosis; when the gland is present, congenital hypothyroidism may be due to dyshormonogenesis.

In term euthyroid neonates, the normal dimensions of the thyroid gland are independent of birth weight (Vade et al. 1997). Attempts should be made to sonographically measure each lobe in all three planes (transverse, anteroposterior, longitudinal). Mean values are: thickness 7±2 mm, width 7.5±2 mm, and long axis 17±5 mm. As the dimensions of the transducer are relatively large compared with the short neck of the child, measurement of the long axis can prove difficult. Certain authors have thus proposed that only width and thickness be measured.

9.6.1.1
Athyrosis

Sonography fails to show a normally located thyroid gland in patients with athyrosis (Fig. 9.45). While the presence of nonthyroid tissue secreting thyrocalcitonin (C cells) can be misleading, the appearance differs from that of a normal thyroid gland. A small tissue density image may be seen in the place of the thyroid; this fairly echogenic and inhomogeneous image is difficult to define and measure and must not be confused with a normal thyroid gland (Fig. 9.46).

In the absence of a normal thyroid in the normal location, sonography is used to search for ectopic thyroid tissue, in particular at the lingual level (Ueda et al. 1992), the most frequent site of ectopias. US is unreliable for demonstration of ectopia. The ectopic thyroid gland may be difficult to define because of its small dimensions or because its echogenicity is similar to that of the surrounding tissues, in particular at the tongue base (Takashima et al. 1995). In cases of athyrosis, ultrasonography is always complemented by scintigraphy to search for functioning thyroid tissue.

9.6.1.2
Hypothyroidism Due to Dyshormonogenesis

In neonates with hypothyroidism due to dyshormonogenesis, sonography shows a thyroid gland in the normal anatomic position. Sonographic features are variable but generally correspond to an enlarged, finely inhomogeneous gland (Fig. 9.47).

9.6.1.3
Transient Hypothyroidism

When hypothyroidism is transient, the thyroid gland is in the normal position and displays normal echogenicity.

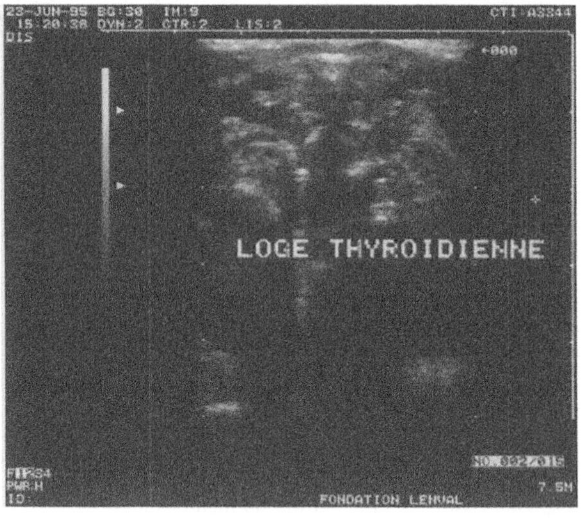

Fig. 9.45. Absence of a visible thyroid at ultrasound examination: athyrosis

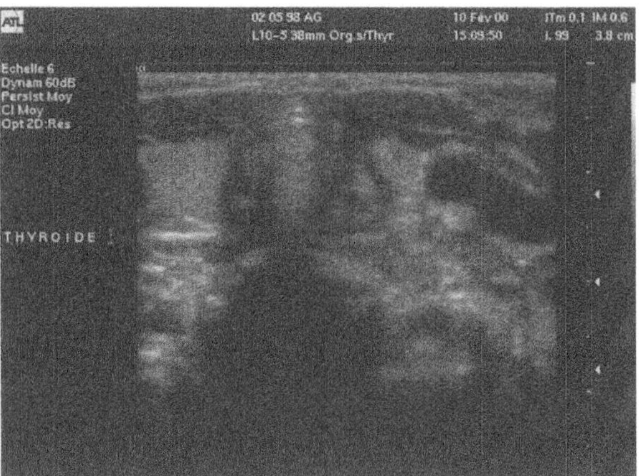

Fig. 9.46. Normal thyroid in a newborn

9.6.2
Hyperthyroidism

Hyperthyroidism is diagnosed on the basis of clinical and biochemical data. US is of little benefit in this pathology. The thyroid is more or less homogeneously enlarged and appears markedly hypervascular on color Doppler studies.

9.6.3
Inflammation (Thyroiditis)

Infectious thyroiditis is rare (Fig. 9.48), and should always prompt a search for a subjacent etiology, in particular a fistula of the fourth branchial arch, which may be the cause of a thyroid abscess.

Autoimmune thyroiditis is the most frequent cause of nonendemic goiter and acquired hypothyroidism in children. Girls are affected much more often than boys (Roth et al. 1997). Goiter is perceptible clinically. Thyroid function tests are normal in 50% of cases, while hypothyroidism and occasionally hyperthyroidism are detected in the remainder. The presence of antithyroid antibodies confirms the diagnosis. At sonography, the echotexture of the enlarged gland may vary from homogeneously hypoechoic (Fig. 9.49) to finely inhomogeneous or multinodular (Fig. 9.50). Hypoechogenicity may be a prognostic factor, because marked hypoechogenicity is indicative of patent or subclinical hypothyroidism.

9.6.4
Benign Tumors

Thyroid cysts are usually solitary, anechoic lesions with posterior reinforcement. Care must be taken to confirm their exclusively fluid-like nature. Any intracystic vegetation is suspicious and should be verified by aspiration cytology or surgical resection (Fig. 9.51) (Yoskovitch et al. 1998). *Colloid cysts* (Fig. 9.52) are particular thyroid lesions that tend to recur after aspiration.

The majority of benign solid thyroid tumors are *adenomas* (Lafferty and Batch 1997). These sonographically solid lesions are usually solitary. Cystic degeneration is possible (Fig. 9.53). Fine-needle aspiration cytology is useful for surgical planning (Lugo-Vicente et al. 1998; Fig. 9.54), as surgical resection is the rule. The incidence of adenoma is increased in children with a history of therapeutic irradiation in infancy (Shore et al. 1993) or accidental exposure to radiation (Nikiforov et al. 1995) and in children

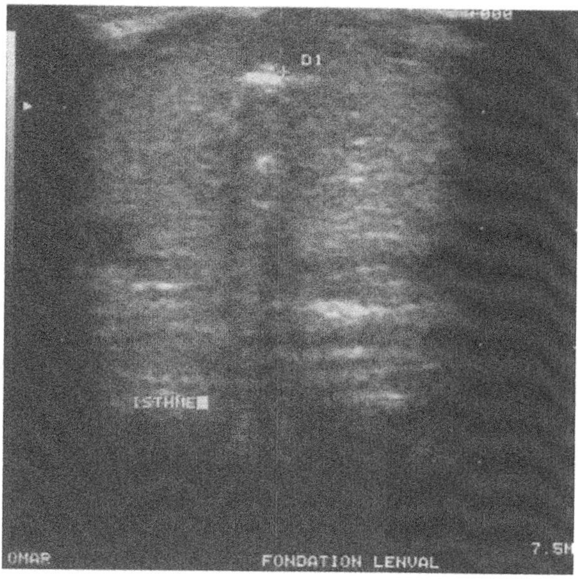

Fig. 9.47. Large neonatal thyroid gland: dyshormonogenesis

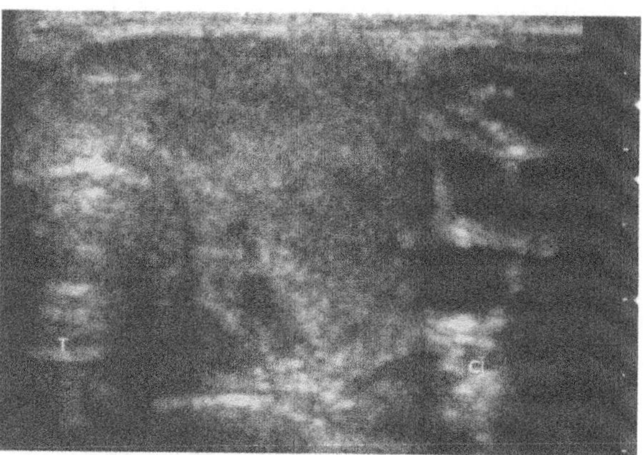

Fig. 9.48. Strongly inhomogeneous left lobe: infectious thyroiditis related to a fourth arch fistula. *T* Trachea; *C* carotid artery

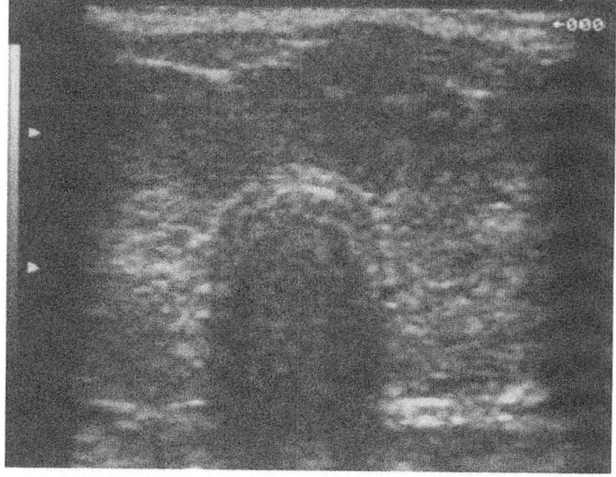

Fig. 9.49. Large hypoechoic thyroid in a 15-year-old girl: Hashimoto's thyroiditis

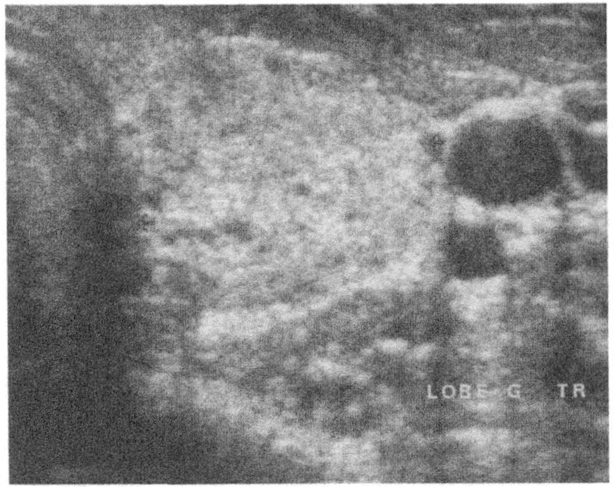

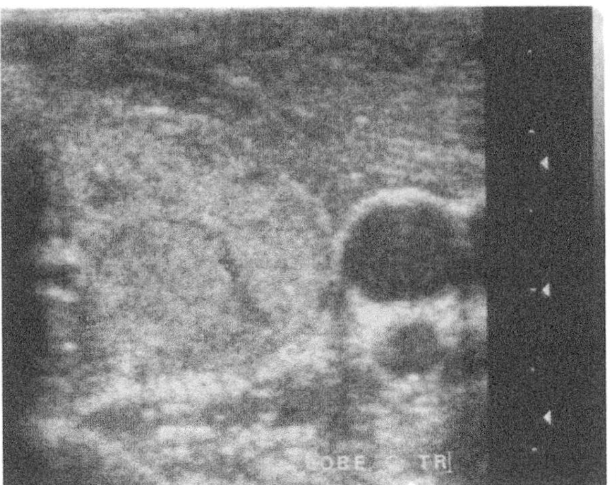

Fig. 9.50a, b. Hashimoto's disease in a 13-year-old boy. **a** Large hyperechoic micronodular thyroid. **b** Appearance of a nodule prompted fine-needle aspiration cytology that diagnosed a vesicular adenoma

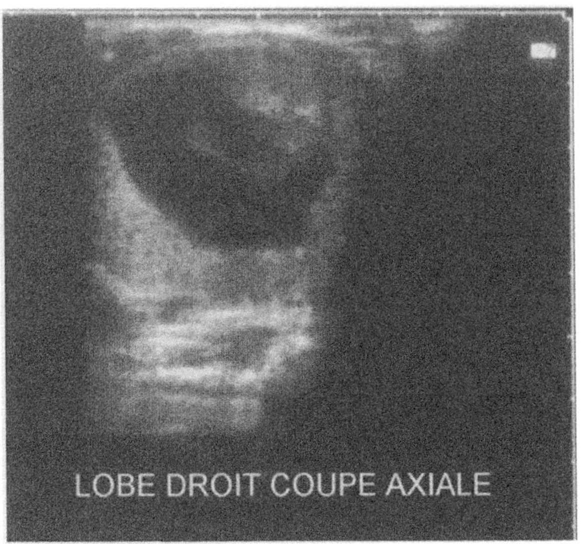

Fig. 9.51. Parietal nodule in a cyst. papillary carcinoma

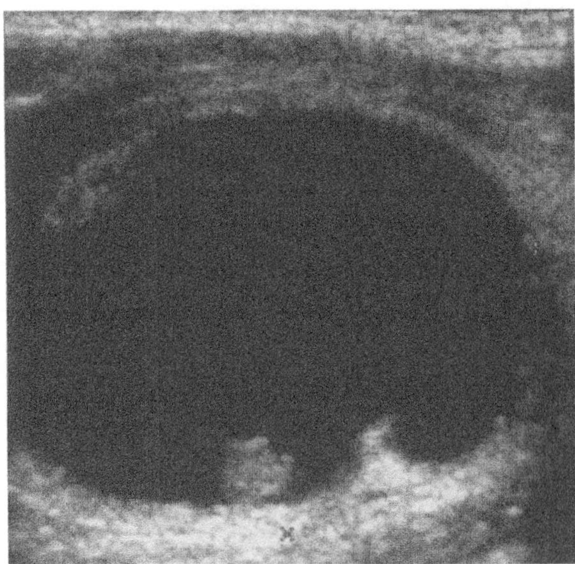

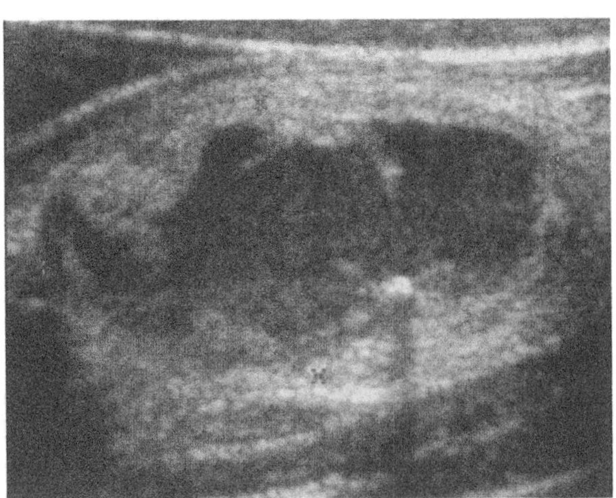

Fig. 9.52a, b. Colloid cyst. **a** Anechoic nodule with focal wall thickening. **b** Two months later. diffuse wall thickening

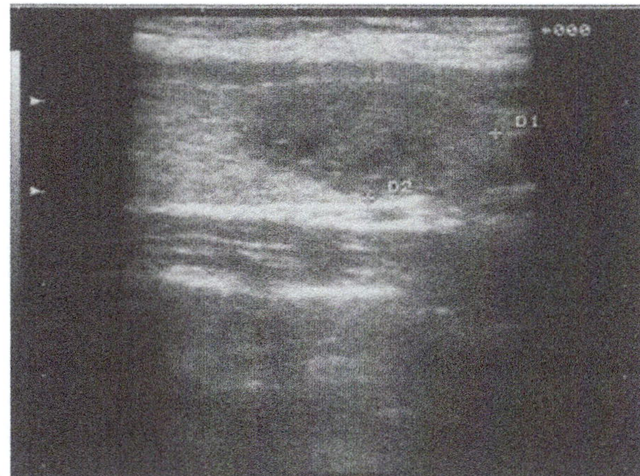

a

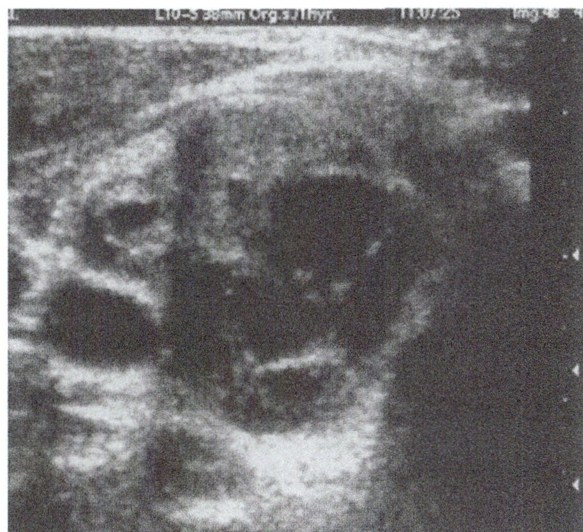
b

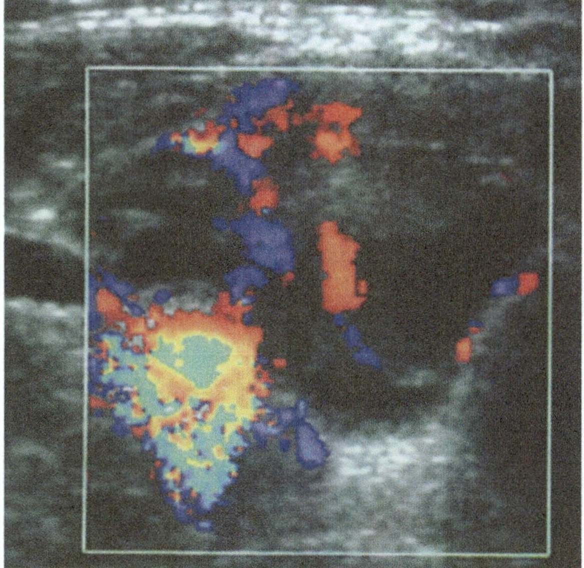
c

Fig. 9.53a–c. Thyroid adenoma. **a** Inhomogeneous nodule containing small cystic areas (aspiration cytology diagnosed an adenoma). **b, c** Two years later, the nodule had increased in size and become cystic; surgery confirmed the diagnosis of adenoma

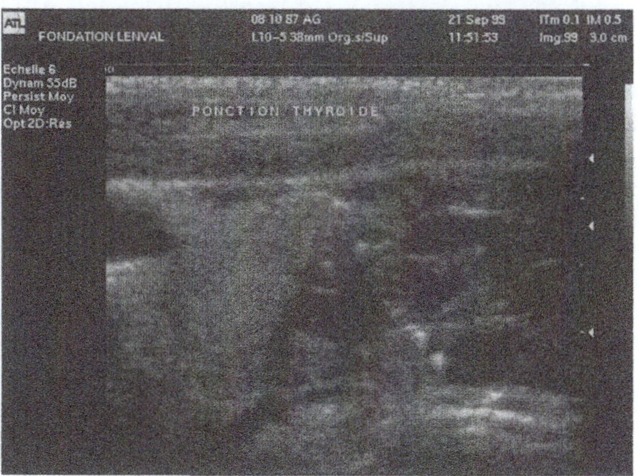

Fig. 9.54. FNA for thyroid adenoma. **a** Inhomogeneous thyroid nodule in a 12-year-old boy. **b** Aspiration cytology was diagnostic for adenoma

who have been treated for congenital hypothyroidism (Alabbasy et al. 1992).

Goiter, corresponding to clinically palpable enlargement of thyroid, may be homogeneous or heterogeneous and multinodular (Fig. 9.55). Iodine-deficient individuals are at particular risk for development of goiter.

9.6.5 Malignant Tumors

Although thyroid carcinoma is uncommon in children (only 1.5% of all pediatric malignancies) (Garcia et al. 1992), the probability of a thyroid nodule being malignant is higher in children than in adults. Papillary carcinomas are much more common than follicular, medullary, and anaplastic histological types.

Sonographic features are nonspecific: a more or less well-defined, hypoechoic single nodule or multiple nodules (Fig. 9.56). More misleading appearances, such as the presence of neoplastic tissue on the walls of a cyst, are also encountered.

9.6.6 Post-therapy Features

Development of a cancer several years after head and neck or total body irradiation is a well-recognized possibility (Crom et al. 1997; Soberman et al. 1991), as is the increased incidence of thyroid nodules and tumors following accidental irradiation (Chernobyl disaster) (Nikiforov et al. 1995). Such children require regular, long-term monitoring by sonography (Fig. 9.57).

Any nodule in a child should be considered suspicious until proven otherwise by aspiration cytology or surgical resection, especially if there is a history of radiotherapy or exposure to ionizing radiation.

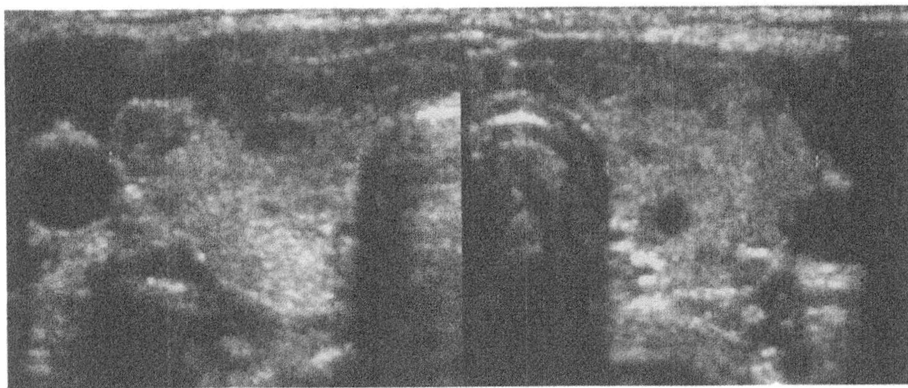

Fig. 9.55. Multinodular goiter

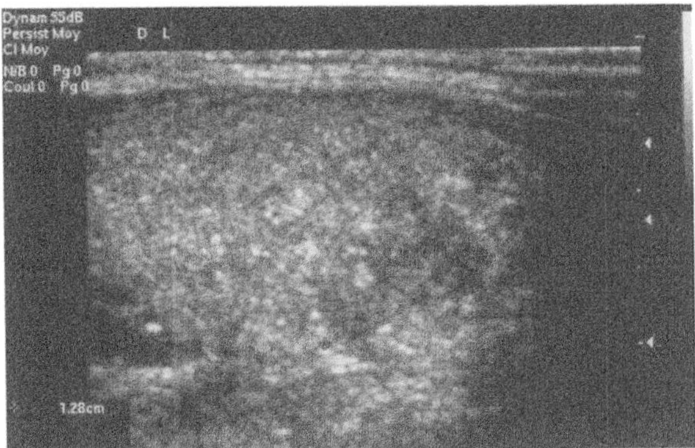

Fig. 9.56. Poorly defined hypoechoic nodule in the right lobe: papillary carcinoma

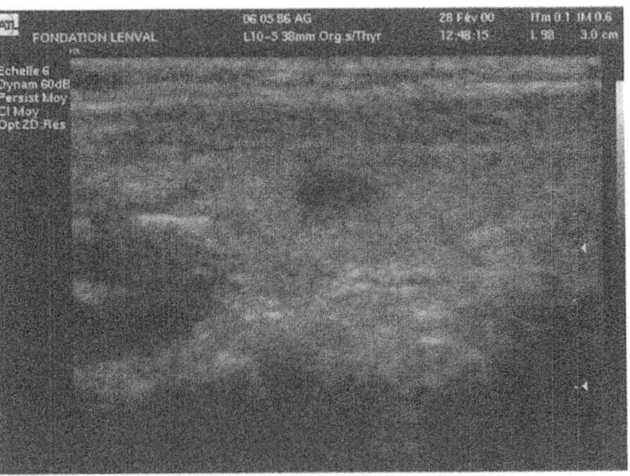

Fig. 9.57. Hypoechoic nodule of recent onset in a 12-year-old girl who had received radiotherapy for cervical Hodgkin's disease; FNA diagnosed a benign cyst

9.7 Larynx

Sonography is particularly suitable for examination of the larynx in children because the absence of ossification of the laryngeal cartilages facilitates visualization of the internal structures. For this same reason, image contrast of the image is poor on MRI and at CT, because the nonossified cartilages are not easily discernable. Ultrasound readily shows the cartilages, and the possibility of real-time observation is an unquestionable advantage for assessment of this mobile organ.

9.7.1 Technique

Sonography of the larynx can be performed at any age, without sedation. Sonography is performed with the child in the supine position and the neck hyperextended. Videotaping or a similar system is indispensable for workup of functional pathologies and in particular of laryngeal paralysis. Observation of movements during phonation may be helpful. Transverse scans are obtained through the three main levels of the larynx.

9.7.2 Sonographic Anatomy (Figs. 9.58–9.60)

The sonographic anatomy of the larynx has been extensively described (GAREL et al. 1991; RAGHAVENDRA et al. 1987; UEDA et al. 1993). The echotexture of the laryngeal cartilages differs depending on their nature: the hyaline cartilages (thyroid, cricoid, and posterior arytenoid cartilages) are hypoechoic, whereas the elastic cartilages (epiglottis and vocal apophysis of the arytenoids) are hyperechoic.

The endolaryngeal (vocal cords) and extralaryngeal muscles are hypoechoic. The false vocal cords (ventricular bands) are hyperechoic. The movements of the vocal cords (abduction and adduction) are well-visualized during inspiration and expiration.

Air, which is hyperechoic, creates posterior shadowing that prevents visualization of the posterior and median structures. Visibility of these structures reflects an abnormal reduction in air flow.

9.7.3 Pathology

Evaluation of the larynx, like that of the tongue, is indispensable during cervical sonography. In general, the pathology is confined to the larynx, and dysphonia and stridor are the major clinical signs. Occasionally, the laryngeal localization is part of a more diffuse cervical pathology.

Infection and inflammatory disease, which are quite common in children, usually do not require US investigation. Sonography is even formally contraindicated in patients with epiglottitis. The technique may be helpful in certain cases of subglottic laryngitis to search for an anomaly within the edematous region (Fig. 9.61), but the majority of cases are diagnosed clinically.

Laryngomalacia, another very frequent laryngeal pathology, is not associated with any specific sonographic features.

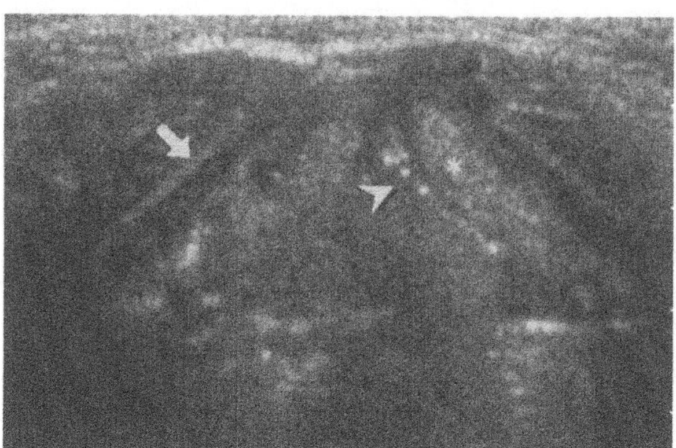

Fig. 9.58. Transverse scan through the supraglottis. *Arrow*: thyroid cartilage; *arrowhead*: supraglottic air; *asterisk*: false vocal cord (ventricular band)

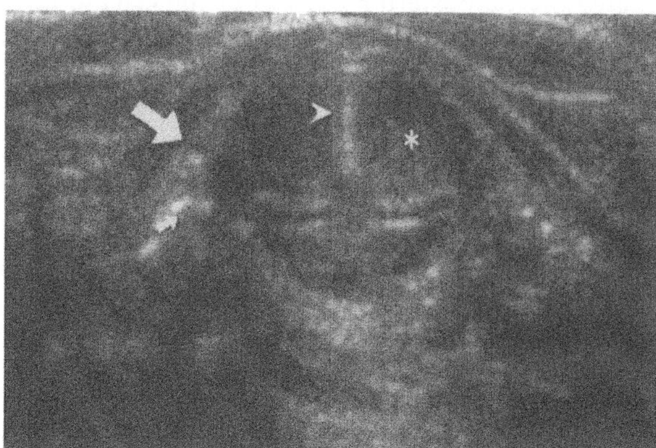

Fig. 9.59. Transverse scan through the glottis. *Large arrow*: thyroid cartilage; *asterisk*: vocal cord; *arrowhead*: glottic air; *small arrow*: arytenoid

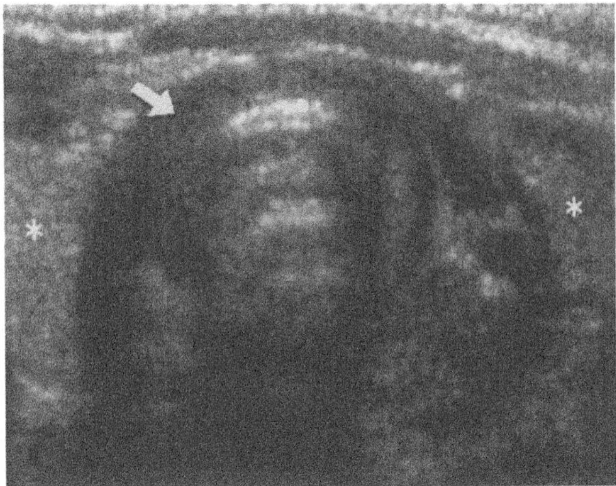

Fig. 9.60. Transverse scan through the subglottis. *Arrow*: cricoid cartilage. The posterior portion of the cricoid ring is not visible due to the posterior shadow created by the subglottic air. *Asterisks*: superior portion of the thyroid lobes

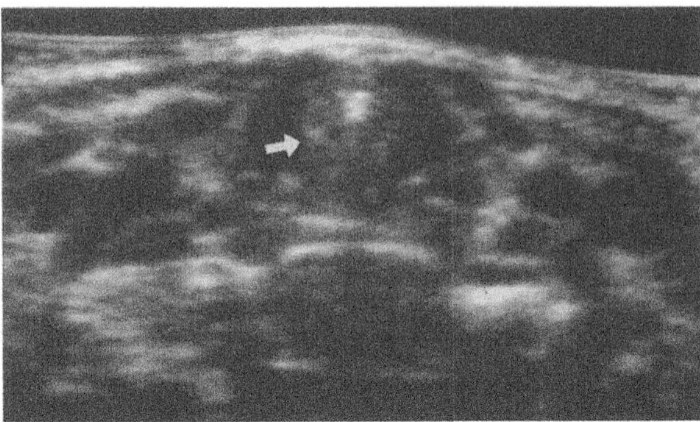

Fig. 9.61. Subglottic angioma revealed by repeated episodes of subglottic laryngitis. Transverse scan through the subglottis. Note the small hyperechoic right-sided posterior mass corresponding to the angioma (*arrow*) within the subglottic edema

Sonography appears particularly indicated for the evaluation of malformations, tumors, and trauma and for laryngeal paralysis (Fig. 9.61).

9.7.3.1 Malformations

All three levels of the larynx may be involved, but usually only the subglottic portion is affected. The cricoid cartilage must be accurately examined to search for hypertrophy of the anterior ring (Fig. 9.62), which displaces the subglottic air posteriorly, for an elliptical cricoid that has lost is typical rounded shape (Fig. 9.63), or for hypertrophy of the entire cartilage, as may exist in severe congenital narrowing or atresia.

A laryngeal diastema, or posterior laryngeal slit, located on the posterior portion of the cricoid in a midline location, is not accessible to sonography and thus cannot be demonstrated by this imaging technique.

At the level of the glottis, a laryngeal web, or congenital diaphragm, connecting the anterior margin of the two vocal cords may be seen sonographically if it is sufficiently thick. Such a finding should always prompt a search for associated subglottic stenosis, which is difficult to diagnose endoscopically.

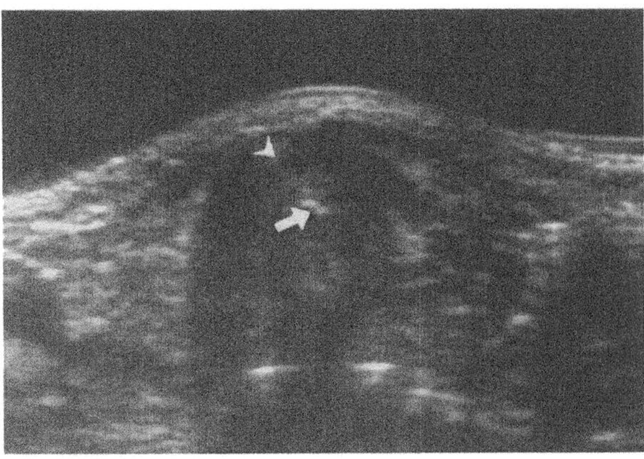

Fig. 9.62. Hypertrophy of the anterior ring of the cricoid cartilage. Transverse scan through the subglottis. Rounded anterior subglottic mass of intermediate echogenicity (*arrowhead*) displacing the subglottic air posteriorly (*arrow*)

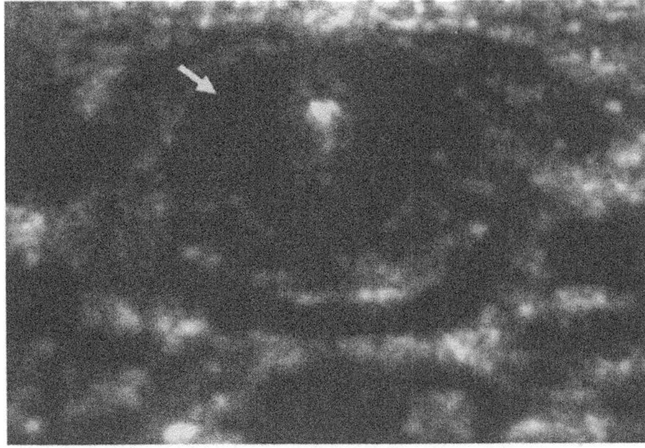

Fig. 9.63. Elliptical cricoid cartilage: stridor and respiratory distress in a 4-month-old child. Transverse scan through the subglottis. The cricoid cartilage has lost its typical rounded shape and appears elliptical (*arrow*)

9.7.3.2 Tumors

Congenital cysts and vascular malformations account for the majority of laryngeal tumors in children.

Angioma is the most frequent benign tumor of the larynx in children and is diagnosed in newborns. The site of predilection is the subglottis; the majority are posterior and left-sided, although midline, horseshoe-shaped, and lateral angiomas also occur. These immature hemangiomas regress spontaneously but may become life threatening during acute phases of progression.

Whereas standard radiographs demonstrate merely indirect signs, sonography permits direct visualization of the angioma. The echotexture is variable, and probably depends on its age, just as for cervical hemangiomas.

Initially hypoechoic and highly vascular, angiomas undergo fatty involution and become hyperechoic. The vascular pattern should theoretically be analyzable by color Doppler. However, because these small dyspneic newborns almost always have very rapid respiration, Doppler studies nearly always contain artifacts and are noncontributory.

The size of the angioma can be evaluated sonographically, which allows surveillance of its course. Sometimes the angioma is visible within an area of subglottic edema (Fig. 9.61).

Glottic and vestibular angiomas are much less common and usually associated with an extralaryngeal component, visible by sonography but not by endoscopy.

Other vascular malformations of the larynx include cystic lymphangiomas, the intralaryngeal location of which is suspected clinically. They may be associated with a cervical lymphangioma and image sonographically as cysts of variable size and location.

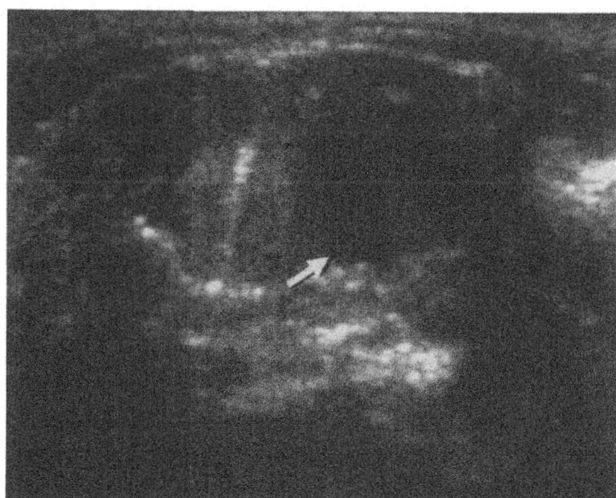

Fig. 9.64. Cyst of the left aryepiglottic fold. Transverse scan through the supraglottis. The anechoic cyst (*arrow*) shows posterior echo reinforcement

Congenital laryngeal cysts, located in a vallecula or an aryepiglottic fold, are readily identified by sonography (Fig. 9.64).

The other tumors of the larynx – neurofibromatosis, amylosis, tumors that develop from the muscles (rhabdomyosarcoma, rhabdomyoma, etc.) – are uncommon in children.

Although sonography cannot make the etiological diagnosis, it can localize the lesion, which may involve one or more levels, and can determine the lesion's relations to the laryngeal structures.

9.7.3.3 Trauma

Sonography is indicated for evaluation of external laryngeal trauma because it can accurately visualize the cartilages. Furthermore, unlike endoscopy, the technique is not hindered by hematoma or edema. A search should always be made for displacement of a cartilaginous structure and possible avulsion.

Ultrasound is rarely contributory for assessment of iatrogenic trauma. It can help to determine the position and mobility of the arytenoids, but it visualizes granulomas poorly and cannot accurately define the extent or severity of stenosis.

9.7.3.4 Functional Disease: Laryngeal Paralysis

Vocal cord mobility can be readily analyzed sonographically, provided the child is not sleeping deeply. In this last situation, the amplitude of motion is too limited and there is a risk of erroneous diagnosis of paralysis.

In cases of unilateral paralysis, the affected vocal cord is not abducted during inspiration; on the contrary, it may be drawn passively towards the healthy side. In such cases the echo created by the air in the glottis appears oblique rather than sagittal (Fig. 9.65), a finding similar to the "twist" effect described at endoscopy.

Sonography cannot differentiate vocal cord paralysis from cricoarytenoid ankylosis.

Most laryngeal pathologies can currently be diagnosed by endoscopy. Sonography has the advantage of being atraumatic and suitable for serial studies. Furthermore, ultrasound is much better adapted to examination of the larynx in children than MRI or CT, allowing evaluation in physiological conditions and real-time observation of this mobile organ.

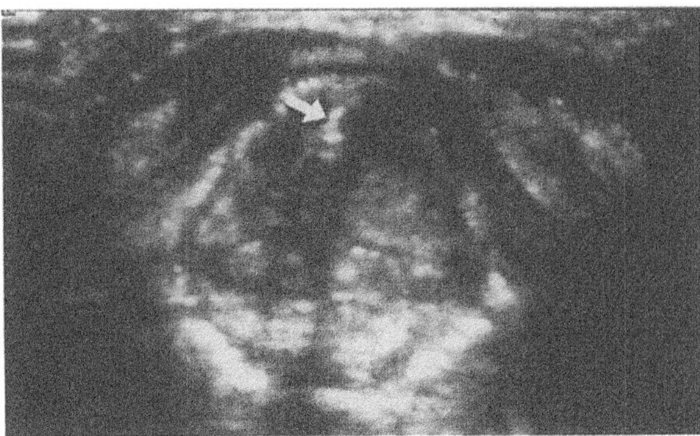

Fig. 9.65. Paralysis of the left vocal cord. Transverse scan through the glottis obtained during inspiration. The right vocal cord is in abduction. The paralyzed left vocal cord is pulled passively to the right side and is in adduction. The echo of the glottic air (*arrow*) is no longer sagittal but oblique

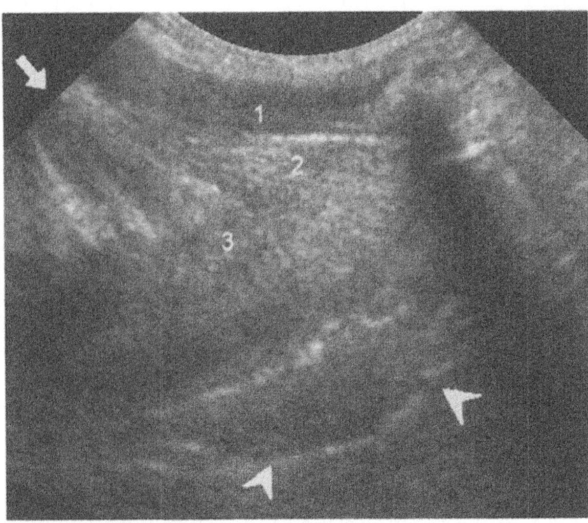

Fig. 9.66. Midline sagittal scan. *Arrow*: hyoid bone; *arrowheads*: dorsum of the tongue. *1* mylohyoid muscle, *2* geniohyoid muscle, *3* genioglossus muscle

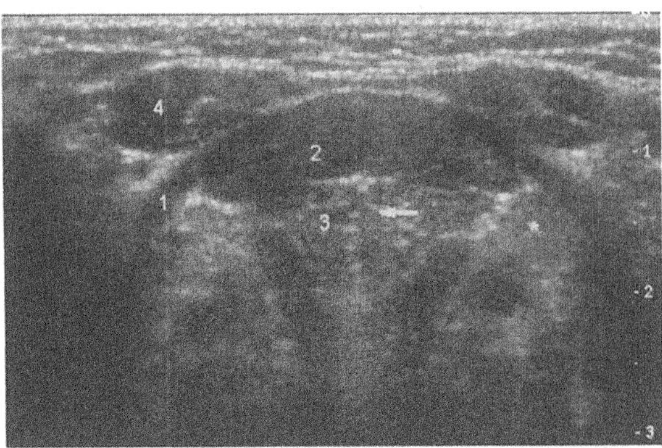

Fig. 9.67. Anterior coronal scan. *1* mylohyoid muscle, *2* geniohyoid muscle, *3* genioglossus muscle, *4* digastric muscle. *Asterisk*: sublingual gland; *arrow*: lingual septum

9.8 Tongue

Relatively few articles have been published on the sonographic anatomy of the tongue (Frühwald et al. 1986; Garel et al. 1994; Neuhold et al. 1986; Shawker et at. 1984; Yasumoto et al. 1993). Sonography is particularly useful in children, owing to the rapidity of examination, the absence of exposure to ionizing radiation, and the accuracy of lingual analysis regardless of the child's age, even in the presence of sucking movements that degrade MR and CT images.

9.8.1 Examination Technique

The child is examined supine with the neck hyperextended. Two types of probes are useful: a high-frequency (7–12 MHz) linear transducer for accurate examination of the most superficial regions and a lower frequency (5–8 MHz) sector probe for analysis of the deeper regions and for sagittal scans in newborns and infants in whom the small dimensions of the neck prevent use of larger probes. Both coronal and sagittal scans are obtained.

9.8.2 Sonographic Anatomy

Owing to the examination position, the image is reversed, and the child's chin is seen at the top of the screen.

On midline sagittal scans (Fig. 9.66), the most important landmark is the hyoid bone, which appears hyperechoic with a marked posterior acoustic shadow.

The mylohyoid and geniohyoid muscles forming the floor of the mouth are readily identified; the genioglossus muscle, located above them, appears more hyperechoic.

The dorsum of the tongue is easily distinguished.

On coronal scans, the appearance depends on the level of the slice.

Anteriorly (Fig. 9.67), the digastric, mylohyoid, and geniohyoid muscles and the hyperechoic sublingual glands can be recognized. At this level, the genioglossus muscle is more or less hypoechoic on either side of the hyperechoic lingual septum. More posteriorly (Fig. 9.68), the mylohyoid and geniohyoid muscles are still visible, and the genioglossus muscle is hyperechoic.

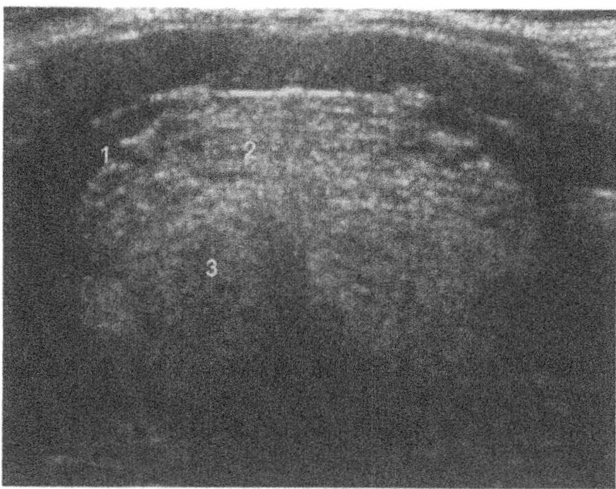

Fig. 9.68. Posterior coronal scan. *1* mylohyoid muscle, *2* geniohyoid muscle, *3* genioglossus muscle

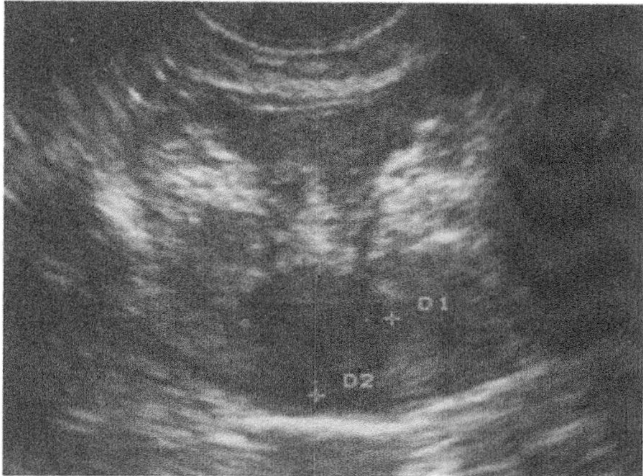

Fig. 9.69. Lingual thyroid in a young boy with dysphagia. Posterior coronal scan. Hypoechoic mass at the base of the tongue (10 mm between the *crosses*). Analysis of the thyroid bed failed to reveal a thyroid in the normal position

9.8.3 Pathology

Regardless of the child's age, the tongue can be affected by a number of pathologies, including malformations, infectious lesions, and tumors. Lingual sonography is an integral part of sonographic examination of the neck. A lingual pathology may be discovered in two different circumstances:

- During clinical examination (the lingual pathology is often the reason for the medical consultation)
- During initial sonographic workup of a cervical pathology that has a potential risk of lingual involvement (the tongue must be systematically examined in such cases)

Discovery of an empty thyroid space should always prompt a search for a lingual thyroid (Fig. 9.69) at the level of the foramen cecum. Inversely, detection of a mass at the base of the tongue should be followed by examination of the thyroid bed.

Workup of a cervical thyroglossal duct cyst must include a search for a possible intralingual prolongation (Fig. 9.70) that requires ablation to avoid recurrence.

Cervical vascular malformations (hemangiomas, venous malformations, and especially cystic lymphangiomas) often include a lingual component. The presence of a lingual component in cystic lymphangioma explains the severity of the disease (Cohen and Thomson 1986; François et al. 1986), because it considerably complicates the surgical procedure. A lingual component must thus be sought systematically (Fig. 9.71). The mylohyoid muscles are an excellent anatomic landmark in such cases.

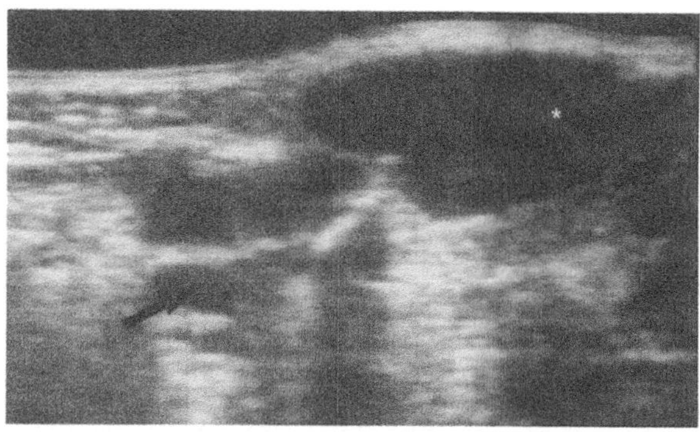

Fig. 9.70. Intralingual component of a thyroglossal duct cyst. Midline sagittal scan. The extralingual component (*star*) of the thyroglossal duct cyst is visible, as is the intralingual cystic component in the genioglossus muscle (*arrow*)

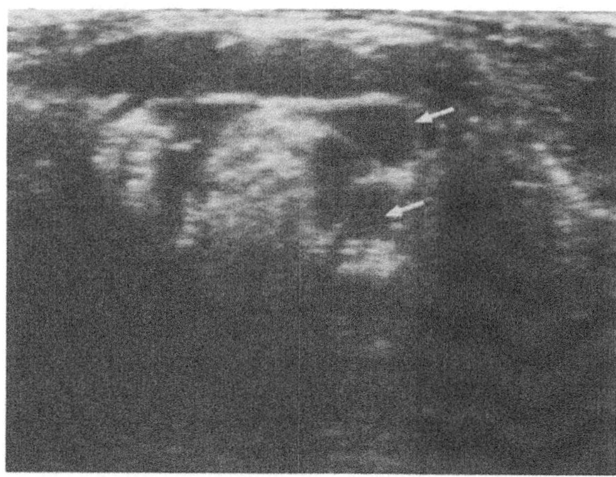

Fig. 9.71. Cystic lymphangioma in a newborn. Anterior coronal scan. The cysts are clearly visible in both sublingual glands (*arrows*) and in the genioglossus muscle

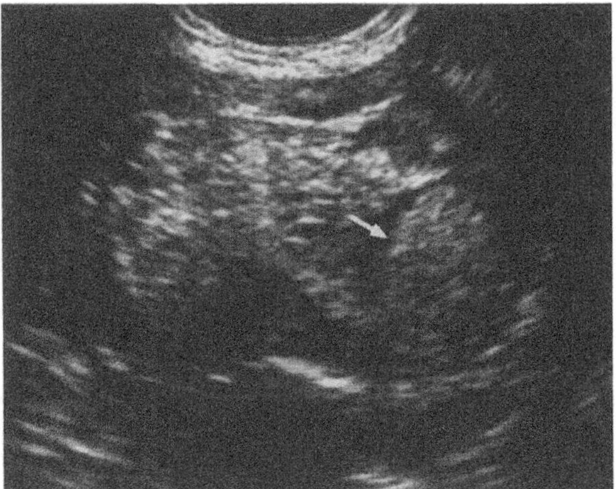

Fig. 9.72. Lingual teratoma in a newborn. Coronal scan. Located on the left side, near the dorsum of the tongue, the mass (*arrow*) appears hyperechoic owing to its essentially fatty content

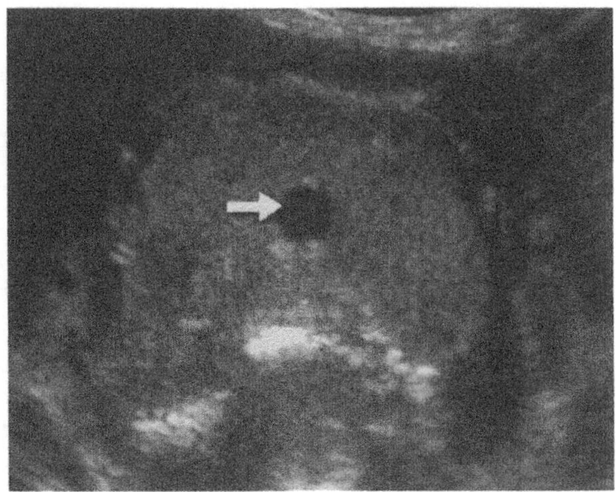

Fig. 9.73. Cyst at the base of the tongue in a newborn who presented with malaise. Posterior coronal scan. An anechoic cyst (*arrow*), measuring several millimeters in diameter, is readily identified at the base of the tongue. The small dimensions of this cyst do not explain the malaise

Certain lesions are confined to the tongue, i.e., a tumoral process involving the genioglossus muscle (fibromatosis, teratoma; Fig. 9.72), a malformation (vascular malformation), or a lesion of infectious origin. In this last case, it is important to differentiate infection of a pre-existent cyst at the base of the tongue (which requires excision) from a de novo abscess (which requires surgical incision and drainage and antibiotic therapy). Small lingual cysts may also be discovered during the workup of newborns with unexplained malaise. The presence of such cysts, suspected clinically, is easily confirmed by sonography (Fig. 9.73).

Pathologies of the tongue and the floor of the mouth are not uncommon and are easily accessible to US examination, which, unlike CT or MRI, is not hampered by sucking movements or swallowing, and can be performed at any age.

References

Abramson SJ, Berdon WE, Ruzal-Shapiro C, Stolar C, Garvin J (1993) Cervical neuroblastoma in eleven infants – a tumor with favorable prognosis. Pediatr Radiol 23:253–257

Achiron R, Rotstein Z, Lipitz S, Karasik, Seidman DS (1998) The development of the foetal thyroid: in utero ultrasonographic measurements. Clin Endocrinol (Oxf) 48:259–264

Alabbasy AJ, Delbridge L, Eckstein R, Cowell C, Silink M (1992) Microfollicular thyroid adenoma and congenital goitrous hypothyroidism. Arch Dis Child 67:1294–1295

Alqahtani A, Nguyen LT, Flageole H, Shaw K, Laberge JM (1999) 25 years' experience with lymphangiomas in children. J Pediatr Surg 34:1164–1168

Baader WM, Lewis JM (1994) First branchial cleft cysts presenting as parotid tumors. Ann Plast Surg 33:72–74

Barberet G, Diakhate I, Conessa C, Moriniere S (1999) CT imaging and fourth branchial pouch fistula in adults. J Radiol 80:1676–1678

Bar-Ziv J, Slasky BS, Sichel JY, Lieberman A, Katz R (1996) Branchial pouch sinus tract from the piriform fossa causing acute suppurative thyroiditis, neck abscess, or both: CT appearance and the use of air as a contrast agent. AJR Am J Roentgenol 167:1569–1572

Bedi DG, John SD, Swischuk LE (1998) Fibromatosis colli of infancy: variability of sonographic appearance. J Clin Ultrasound 26:345–348

Brevière GM, Bonnevalle M, Pruvo JP, et al (1993) Use of Ethibloc in the treatment of cystic and venous angiomas in children. 19 cases. Eur J Pediatr Surg 3:166–170

Brewis C, Mahadevan M, Bailey CM, Drake DP (2000) Investigation and treatment of thyroglossal cysts in children. J R Soc Med 93:18–21

Chanoine JP, Toppet V, Lagasse R, Spehl M, Delange F (1991) Determination of thyroid volume by ultrasound from the neonatal period to late adolescence. Eur J Pediatr 150:395–399

Chikui T, Yonetsu K, Yoshiura K, et al (1997) Imaging findings of lipomas in the orofacial region with CT, US and MRI. Oral Surg Oral Med Oral Pathol Oral Radiol Endod 84:88–495

Chitre VV, Premchandra DJ (1997) Recurrent parotitis. Arch Dis Child 77:359–363

Civantos FJ, Holinger LD (1992) Laryngoceles and saccular cysts in infants and children. Arch Otolaryngol Head Neck Surg 118:296–300

Cohen SR, Thomson JW (1986) Lymphangiomas of the larynx in infant and children: a survey of pediatric lymphagioma. Ann Otol Rhinol Laryngol 127 [Suppl 95]:1–20

Corr P, Vaithilingum M, Thejpal R, Jeena P (1997) Parotid MALT lymphoma in infected children. J Ultrasound Med 16:615–617

Crom DB, Kaste SC, Tubergen DG, Greenwald CA, Sharp GB, Hudson MM (1997) Ultrasonography for thyroid screening after head and neck irradiation in childhood cancer survivors. Med Pediatr Oncol 28:15–21

De Heyn G (1990) Benign cervical tumors of neuroectodermal origin: apropos of 3 clinical cases. Acta Otorhinolaryngol Belg 44:17–20

Dubois J, Garel L (1999) Imaging and therapeutic approach of hemangiomas and vascular malformations in the pediatric age group. Pediatr Radiol 29:879–893

Dubois J, Garel L, Abela A, Laberge L, Yazbeck S (1997) Lymphangiomas in children: percutaneous sclerotherapy with an alcoholic solution of zein. Radiology 204:651–654

Dubois J, Patriquin HB, Garel L, et al (1998) Soft-tissue hemangiomas in infants and children: diagnosis using Doppler sonography. AJR Am J Roentgenol 17:247–252

Ducic Y,Chou S, Drkulec J, Ouellette H, Lamothe A (1998) Recurrent thyroglossal duct cysts: a clinical and pathological analysis. Int J Pediatr Otorhinolaryngol 44:47–50

Duroux S, Guillard JM, Chateil JF, et al (1993) Accessory thymus in cervical ectopy: apropos of a case. Pediatrie 48:301–304

Encina S, Ernst P, Villanueva J, Pizarro E (1996) Ultrasonography: a complement to sialography in recurrent chronic childhood parotitis. Rev Stomatol Chir Maxillofac 97:258–263

Enjolras O (1999) Les angiomes de l'enfant à un tournant dans leur compréhension et dans leur prise en charge. Arch Pediatr 6:1261–1265

Esteban MJ, Gitierrez C, Gomez J, et al (1996) Treatment with Ethibloc of lymphangiomas and venous angiomas. Cir Pediatr 9:158–162

François M, Le Guillou C, Depondt J, Aboucaya JP, Cotencin P, Narcy P (1986) Les lymphangiomes cervico-faciaux chez l'enfant. Ann Otol Laryngol 130:113–117

Frühwald F, Neuhold A, Seidl G, Pavelka R, Meilath G, Zrunek M (1986) Sonography of the tongue and floor of mouth. II. Neoplasms of the tongue. Eur J Radiol 6:108–112

Garcia CJ, Daneman A, McHugh K, Chan H, Daneman D (1992) Sonography in thyroid carcinoma in children. Br J Radiol 65:977–982

Garcia CJ, Flores PA, Arce JD, Chuaqui B, Schwartz DS (1998) Ultrasonography in the study of salivary gland lesions in children. Pediatr Radiol 28:418–425

Garel C, Hassen M, Legrand I, Elmaleh M, Narcy P (1991) Laryngeal ultrasonography in infants and children: pathological findings. Pediatr Radiol 21:164–167

Garel C, Elmaleh M, François M, Narcy P, Hassan M (1994) Ultrasonographic evaluation of the tongue and the floor of the mouth: normal and pathological findings. Pediatr Radiol 24:554–557

Greinwald JH jr, Burke DK, Sato Y, et al (1999) Treatment of lymphangiomas in children: an update of Picibanil (OK-432) sclerotherapy. Otolaryngol Head Neck Surg 21:381–387

Hama Y, Sugenoya A, Kobayashi S, Itoh N, Amano J (1997) Squamous cell carcinoma arising from thyroglossal duct remnants: report of a case and results of immunohistochemical studies. Surg Today 27:1077–1081

Heshmati HM, Fatourechi V, van Heerden JA, Hay ID, Goellner JR (1997) Thyroglossal duct carcinoma: report of 12 cases. Mayo Clin Proc 72:315–319

Ho SS, Metreweli C(1998) Normal foetal thyroid volume. Ultrasound Obstet Gynecol 11:118–122

Issing PR, Kettling T, Kempf HG, Heerman R, Lenarz T (1999) Ultrasound evaluation of characteristics of cervical lymph nodes with special reference to color Doppler ultrasound. A contribution to differentiating reactive from metastatic lymph node involvement in the neck. Laryngorhinootologie 78:556–572

Jones AO, Lam AH, Martin HC (1997) Acinic cell carcinoma of the parotid in children. Australas Radiol 41:44–48

Kester NL (1990) Synovial sarcoma in the neck of an eleven month old girl. Pediatr Radiol 20:487

Khadaroo RG, Walton JM, Ramsay JA, Hicks MJ, Archibald SD (1998) Mucoepidermoid carcinoma of the parotid gland: a rare presentation in a young child. J Pediatr Surg 33:893–395

Koumanidou C, Vakaki M, Theophanopoulou M et al (1998) Aberrant thymus in infants: sonographic evaluation. Pediatr Radiol 28:987–989

Lafferty AR, Batch JA (1997) Thyroid nodules in childhood and adolescence – thirty years of experience. J Pediatr Endocrinol Metab 10:479–486

Lin-Dunham JE, Feinstein KA, Yousefzadeh DK, Ben-Ami T (1995) Sonographic demonstration of a normal thyroid gland excludes ectopic thyroid in patients with thyroglossal duct cyst. AJR Am J Roentgenol 164:1489–1491

Lucaya J, Berdon WE, Enriquez G, Regas J, Carreno JC (1990) Congenital pyriform sinus fistula: a cause of acute left-sided suppurative thyroiditis and neck abscess in children. Pediatr Radiol 21:27–29

Lugo-Vicente H, Ortiz VN, Irizarry H, Camps JI, Pagan V (1998) Pediatric thyroid nodules: management in the era of fine-needle aspiration. J Pediatr Surg 33:1302–1305

Maggi G, Dorato P, Trischitta V, Varone A, Civetta F (1995) Cervical dumbbell ganglioneuroma in an eighteen month old child. A case report. J Neurosurg Sci 39:257–260

Marques Gubern A, Jimenez AI, Martinez Ibanez V, et al (1990) Embryonal fatty tumors. Lipoblastoma-lipoblastomatosis. Cir Pediatr 3:109–112

Marsot-Dupuch K, Levret N, Pharaboz C, Robert Y, el Maleh M, Meriot P, Poncet JL, Chabolle F (1995) Congenital neck masses. Embryonic origin and diagnosis. Report of the CIREOL. J Radiol 76:405–415

McHenry CR, Danish R, Murphy T, Marty JJ (1993) Atypical thyroglossal duct cyst: a rare cause for a solitary cold thyroid nodule in childhood. Am Surg 59:223–228

Neuhold A, Fruhwald F, Balogh B, Wicke L (1986) Sonography of the tongue and floor of mouth. I. Anatomy. Eur J Radiol 6:103–107

Nicollas R, Ducroz V, Garabedian EN, Triglia JM (1998) Fourth branchial pouch anomalies: a study of six cases and review of the literature. Int J Pediatr Otorhinolaryngol 44:5–10

Nikiforov YE, Heffess CS, Korzenko AV, Fagin JA, Gnepp DR (1995) Characteristics of follicular tumors and non-neoplastic thyroid lesions in children and adolescents exposed to radiation as a result of the Chernobyl disaster. Cancer 76:900–909

Nofsinger YC, Tom LW, LaRossa D, Wetmore RF, Handler SD (1997) Periauricular cysts and sinuses. Laryngoscope 107:883–887

Nozaki H, Harasawa A, Hara H, Kohno A, Shigeta A (1994) Ultrasonography features of recurrent parotitis in childhood. Pediatr Radiol 24:98–100

O'Connell M, Grixti M, Harmer C (1998) Thyroglossal duct carcinoma: presentation and management, including eight case reports. Clin Oncol (R Coll Radiol) 10:186–190

Patti G, Ragni G, Calisti A (2000) Papillary thyroid carcinoma in a thyroglossal duct cyst in a child. Med Pediatr Oncol 34:27–29

Pereira S, Tani E, Skoog L (1999) Diagnosis of fibromatosis colli by fine-needle aspiration (FNA)cytology. Cytopathology 10:25–29

Perez JA, Henning E, Valencia V, Schultz C (1994) Cysts of second branchial cleft: review of 32 operated cases. Rev Med Child 122:782–787

Pia F, Aluffi P, Olina M (1999) Cystic lymphangioma in the head and neck region. Acta Otorhinolaryngol Ital 19:87–90

Quraishi MS, O'Halpin DR, Blayney AW (1997) Ultrasonography in the evaluation of neck abscesses in children. Clin Otolaryngol 22:30–33

Raghavendra BN, Horii SC, Reede DL, Rumancik WM, Persky M (1987) Sonographic anatomy of the larynx, with particular reference to the vocal cords. J Ultrasound Med 6:225–230

Redondo Granado MJ, Alvarez Guisasola FJ, Gomez Martin I, Bobillo del Amo H, Blanco Quiros A, Mateos Otero JJ (1992) Diagnostic evaluation of cervical adenopathies in childhood. Ann Esp Pediatr 37:233–237

Reynolds JH, Wolinski AP (1993) Sonographic appearance of branchial cysts. Clin Radiol 48:109–110

Riechelmann H, Wolfensberger M, Coerdt W (1992) Differential diagnosis of children's enlarged necks – cervical thymic cysts. HNO 40:59–63

Roth C, Scortea M, Stubbe P et al (1997) Autoimmune thyroiditis in childhood – epidemiology, clinical and laboratory findings in 61 patients. Exp Clin Endocrinol Diabetes 105 [Suppl 4]:66–69

Shawker TH, Sonies BC, Stones M (1984) Soft tissue anatomy of the tongue and floor of the mouth: an ultrasound demonstration. Brain Lang 21:335–350

Shita L, Rypens F, Hassid S, Vermeylen D, Struyen J (1999) Sonographic demonstration of a congenital laryngeal cyst. J Ultrasound Med 18:665–667

Shore RE, Hildreth N, Dvoretsky P, Pasternack B, Andresen E (1993) Benign thyroid adenomas among persons X-irradiated in infancy for enlarged thymus glands. Radiat Res 134:217–223

Smirniotopoulos JG, Chiechi MV (1995) Teratomas, dermoids and epidermoids of the head and neck. Radiographics 15:1437–1455

Soberman N, Leonidas JC, Cherrick I, Schiff R, Karayalcin G (1991) Sonographic abnormalities of the thyroid gland in long-term survivors of Hodgkin disease. Pediatr Radiol 21:250–253

Steinkamp HJ, Teichgraber UK, Mueffelmann M, Hosten N, Kenzel P, Felix R (1999) Differential diagnosis of lymph node lesions. A semiquantitative approach with power Doppler sonography. Invest Radiol 34:509–515

Takashima S, Nomura N, Tanka H, Yasushi I, Kazunori M, Tokuzo H (1995) Congenital hypothyroidism: assessment with ultrasound. Am J Neuroradiol 16:1117–1123

Trop I, Dubois J, Guibaud L, et al (1999) Soft-tissue venous malformations in pediatric and young adult patients: diagnosis with Doppler US. Radiology 212:841–845

Ueda D, Mitamura R, Suzuki N, Yano K, Okuno A (1992) Sonographic imaging of the thyroid gland in congenital hypothyroidism. Pediatr Radiol 22:102–105

Ueda D, Yano K, Okuno A (1993) Ultrasonic imaging of the tongue, mouth, and vocal cords in normal children: establishment of basic scanning positions. J Clin Ultrasound 21:431–439

Vade A, Gottschalk ME, Yetter EM, Subbaiah P (1997) Sonographic measurements of the neonatal thyroid gland. J Ultrasound Med 16:395–399

Vazquez E, Enriquez G, Castellote A, et al (1995) US, CT, and MR imaging of neck lesions in children. Radiographics 15:105–122

Vittore CP, Goldberg KN, McClatchey KD, Hotaling AJ (1998) Cystic mass at the suprasternal notch of a newborn: congenital suprasternal dermoid cyst. Pediatr Radiol 28:984–986

Wadsworth DT, Siegel MJ (1994) Thyroglossal duct cysts: variability of sonographic findings. AJR Am J Roentgenol 163:1475–1477

Ward RF, Jones J, Arnold JA (1995) Surgical management of congenital saccular cysts of the larynx. Ann Otol Rhinol Laryngol 104:707–710

Williams MD, Pearson MH, Thomas FD (1991) Pilomatrixoma: a rare condition in the differential diagnosis of a parotid swelling. Br J Oral Maxillofacial Surg 29:201–203

Wu CH, Chang YL, Hsu WC, Ko JY, Sheen TS, Hsieh FJ (1998) Usefulness of Doppler spectral analysis and power Doppler sonography in the differentiation of cervical lymphadenopathies. AJR 171:503–509

Yang C, Cohen J, Everts E, Smith J, Caro J, Andersen P (1999) Fourth branchial arch sinus: clinical presentation, diagnostic workup, and surgical treatment. Laryngoscope 109:442–446

Yasumoto M, Nakagawa T, Shibuha H, Suzuki S, Satoh T (1993) Ultrasonography of the sublingual space. J Ultrasound Med 12:723–729

Ying M, Ahuja A, Metreweli C (1998) Diagnostic accuracy of sonographic criteria for evaluation of cervical lymphadenopathy. J Ultrasound Med 17:437–445

Yoo KS, Chengazi VU, O'Mara RE (1998) Thyroglossal duct cyst with papillary carcinoma in an 11-year-old girl. J Pediatr Surg 33:745–746

Yoskovitch A, Laberge JM, Rodd C, Sinsky A, Gaskin D (1998) Cystic thyroid lesions in children. J Pediatr Surg 33:866–870

Subject Index

List of Contributors

Nicolas Amoretti, MD
Service de Radiodiagnostic
Hôpital Pasteur
30, avenue Voie Romaine, BP 69
F-06002 Nice Cedex 1
France

Christopher Arens, MD
HNO-Universitätsklinik
Justus-Liebig-Universität Giessen
Faulgenstraße 10
D-35394 Giessen
Germany

Jean Noël Bruneton, MD
Service de Radiologie
Hôpital de l'Archet
151, route de St.-Antoine Ginestière
B.P. 3079
F-06202 Nice Cedex 3
France

Philippe Brunner, MD
Service de Radiologie
Centre Hospitalier Princesse Grace
Avenue Pasteur
98000 Monaco
Monaco

Bruno Carlotti, MD
Otorhinolaryngologiste
88, boulevard de Cimiez
F-06000 Nice
France

Patrick Chevallier, MD
Service de Radiodiagnostic
Hôpital de l'Archet
151 Chemin de St. Antoine de Ginestière
F-06200 Nice Cedex
France

Olivier Dassonville, MD
Département d'ORL
Centre Antoine-Lacassagne
33 avenue de Valombrose
F-06189 Nice Cedex 2
France

Catherine Garel, MD
Service de Radiologie
Hôpital Robert Debré
75935 Paris Cedex 19
France

Anne Geoffray, MD
Hôpital Lenval
Service de Radiodiagnostic
57 avenue de la Californie
06200 Nice
France

Nathalie Lassau, MD
Département d'Imagerie Médicale
Institut Gustave-Roussy
F-94805 Villejuif Cedex
France

Robin Lecesne, MD
Service de Radiodiagnostic
Hôpital du Haut Lévêque
F-33604 Pessac
France

Laurence Leenhardt, MD
Service Central de Médecine Nucléaire
Hôpital La Pitié-Salpêtrière
83 Boulevard de l'Hôpital
F-75013 Paris
France

Tito Livraghi, MD
Unita Raiologia
Ospedale Civile
Via C. Battisti, 23
I-20059 Vimercate (MI)
Italy

Pierre-Yves Marcy, MD
Service de Radiodiagnostic
Centre Antoine-Lacassagne
33 avenue de Valombrose
F-06189 Nice Cedex 2
France

Denis Matter, MD
Centre d'Imagerie Médicale
85 route de Polygone
F-71000 Strasbourg
France

Francesca Meloni, MD
Unita Raiologia
Ospedale Civile
Via C. Battisti, 23
I-20059 Vimercate (MI)
Italy

Michel-Yves Mourou, MD
Service de Radiologie
Centre Hospitalier Princesse Grace
Avenue Pasteur
MC-98000 Monaco
Monaco

Bernard Padovani, MD
Service de Radiodiagnostic
Hôpital Pasteur
30, avenue Voie Romaine, BP 69
F-06002 Nice Cedex 1
France

Gilles Poissonnet, MD
Département d'ORL
Centre Antoine-Lacassagne
33 avenue de Valombrose
06189 Nice Cedex 2
France

Charles Raffaelli, MD
Service de Radiodiagnostic
Hôpital Pasteur
30, avenue Voie Romaine, BP 69
F-06002 Nice Cedex 1
France

Jean Tramalloni, MD
Cabinet de Radiologie
25 rue du Docteur Paul Bruel
F-95350 Louvres
France

Christine Tran, MD
Service de Radiodiagnostic
Hôpital Pasteur
30, avenue Voie Romaine, BP 69
06002 Nice Cedex 1
France

François Tranquart, MD
Médecine Nucléaire et Ultrasons
INSERM U 316
CHU Bretonneau
37044 Tours Cedex
France

Jocelyne Viateau-Poncin, MD
Clinique d'Aulnay
28-36 avenue du 14 Juillet
F-93604 Aulnay-sous-Bois Cedex
France

Medical Radiology
Diagnostic Imaging and Radiation Oncology

Titles in the series already published

Diagnostic Imaging

Innovations in Diagnostic Imaging
Edited by J. H. Anderson

Radiology of the Upper Urinary Tract
Edited by E. K. Lang

The Thymus - Diagnostic Imaging, Functions, and Pathologic Anatomy
Edited by E. Walter, E. Willich, and W.R. Webb

Interventional Neuroradiology
Edited by A. Valavanis

Radiology of the Pancreas
Edited by A. L. Baert, co-edited by G. Delorme

Radiology of the Lower Urinary Tract
Edited by E. K. Lang

Magnetic Resonance Angiography
Edited by I. P. Arlart, G. M. Bongartz, and G. Marchal

Contrast-Enhanced MRI of the Breast
S. Heywang-Köbrunner and R. Beck

Spiral CT of the Chest
Edited by M. Rémy-Jardin and J. Rémy

Radiological Diagnosis of Breast Diseases
Edited by M. Friedrich and E.A. Sickles

Radiology of the Trauma
Edited by M. Heller and A. Fink

Biliary Tract Radiology
Edited by P. Rossi

Radiological Imaging of Sports Injuries
Edited by C. Masciocchi

Modern Imaging of the Alimentary Tube
Edited by A. R. Margulis

Diagnosis and Therapy of Spinal Tumors
Edited by P. R. Algra, J. Valk, and J. J. Heimans

Interventional Magnetic Resonance Imaging
Edited by J. F. Debatin and G. Adam

Abdominal and Pelvic MRI
Edited by A. Heuck and M. Reiser

Orthopedic Imaging
Techniques and Applications
Edited by A. M. Davies and H. Pettersson

Radiology of the Female Pelvic Organs
Edited by E. K.Lang

Magnetic Resonance of the Heart and Great Vessels
Clinical Applications
Edited by J. Bogaert, A. J. Duerinckx, and F. E. Rademakers

Modern Head and Neck Imaging
Edited by S. K. Mukherji and J. A. Castelijns

Radiological Imaging of Endocrine Diseases
Edited by J. N. Bruneton in collaboration with B. Padovani and M.-Y. Mourou

Trends in Contrast Media
Edited by H. S. Thomsen, R. N. Muller, and R. F. Mattrey

Functional MRI
Edited by C. T. W. Moonen and P. A. Bandettini

Radiology of the Pancreas
2nd Revised Edition
Edited by A. L. Baert
Co-edited by G. Delorme and L. Van Hoe

Emergency Pediatric Radiology
Edited by H. Carty

Spiral CT of the Abdomen
Edited by F. Terrier, M. Grossholz, and C. D. Becker

Liver Malignancies
Diagnostic and Interventional Radiology
Edited by C. Bartolozzi and R. Lencioni

Medical Imaging of the Spleen
Edited by A. M. De Schepper and F. Vanhoenacker

Radiology of Peripheral Vascular Diseases
Edited by E. Zeitler

Diagnostic Nuclear Medicine
Edited by C. Schiepers

Radiology of Blunt Trauma of the Chest
P. Schnyder and M. Wintermark

Portal Hypertension
Diagnostic Imaging-Guided Therapy
Edited by P. Rossi
Co-edited by P. Ricci and L. Broglia

Recent Advances in Diagnostic Neuroradiology
Edited by Ph. Demaerel

Virtual Endoscopy and Related 3D Techniques
Edited by P. Rogalla, J. Terwisscha Van Scheltinga, and B. Hamm

Multislice CT
Edited by M. F. Reiser, M. Takahashi, M. Modic, and R. Bruening

Pediatric Uroradiology
Edited by R. Fotter

Radiology of AIDS
A Practical Approach
Edited by J.W.A.J. Reeders and P.C. Goodman

CT of the Peritoneum
Armando Rossi and Giorgio Rossi

Magnetic Resonance Angiography
2nd Revised Edition
Edited by I. P. Arlart, G. M. Bongratz, and G. Marchal

Pediatric Chest Imaging
Edited by Javier Lucaya and Janet G. Strife

Applications of Sonography in Head and Neck Pathology
Edited by J. N. Bruneton in collaboration with C. Raffaelli and O. Dassonville

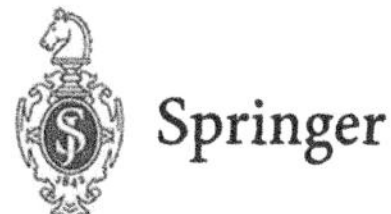

MEDICAL RADIOLOGY
Diagnostic Imaging and Radiation Oncology

Titles in the series already published

RADIATION ONCOLOGY

Lung Cancer
Edited by C.W. Scarantino

Innovations in Radiation Oncology
Edited by H. R. Withers and L. J. Peters

Radiation Therapy of Head and Neck Cancer
Edited by G. E. Laramore

Gastrointestinal Cancer – Radiation Therapy
Edited by R.R. Dobelbower, Jr.

Radiation Exposure and Occupational Risks
Edited by E. Scherer, C. Streffer, and K.-R. Trott

Radiation Therapy of Benign Diseases
A Clinical Guide
S.E. Order and S. S. Donaldson

Interventional Radiation Therapy Techniques – Brachytherapy
Edited by R. Sauer

Radiopathology of Organs and Tissues
Edited by E. Scherer, C. Streffer, and K.-R. Trott

Concomitant Continuous Infusion Chemotherapy and Radiation
Edited by M. Rotman and C. J. Rosenthal

Intraoperative Radiotherapy – Clinical Experiences and Results
Edited by F. A. Calvo, M. Santos, and L.W. Brady

Radiotherapy of Intraocular and Orbital Tumors
Edited by W. E. Alberti and R. H. Sagerman

Interstitial and Intracavitary Thermoradiotherapy
Edited by M. H. Seegenschmiedt and R. Sauer

Non-Disseminated Breast Cancer
Controversial Issues in Management
Edited by G. H. Fletcher and S.H. Levitt

Current Topics in Clinical Radiobiology of Tumors
Edited by H.-P. Beck-Bornholdt

Practical Approaches to Cancer Invasion and Metastases
A Compendium of Radiation Oncologists' Responses to 40 Histories
Edited by A. R. Kagan with the Assistance of R. J. Steckel

Radiation Therapy in Pediatric Oncology
Edited by J. R. Cassady

Radiation Therapy Physics
Edited by A. R. Smith

Late Sequelae in Oncology
Edited by J. Dunst and R. Sauer

Mediastinal Tumors. Update 1995
Edited by D. E. Wood and C. R. Thomas, Jr.

Thermoradiotherapy and Thermochemotherapy
Volume 1:
Biology, Physiology, and Physics
Volume 2:
Clinical Applications
Edited by M.H. Seegenschmiedt, P. Fessenden, and C.C. Vernon

Carcinoma of the Prostate
Innovations in Management
Edited by Z. Petrovich, L. Baert, and L.W. Brady

Radiation Oncology of Gynecological Cancers
Edited by H.W. Vahrson

Carcinoma of the Bladder
Innovations in Management
Edited by Z. Petrovich, L. Baert, and L.W. Brady

Blood Perfusion and Microenvironment of Human Tumors
Implications for Clinical Radiooncology
Edited by M. Molls and P. Vaupel

Radiation Therapy of Benign Diseases
A Clinical Guide
2nd Revised Edition
S. E. Order and S. S. Donaldson

Carcinoma of the Kidney and Testis, and Rare Urologic Malignancies
Innovations in Management
Edited by Z. Petrovich, L. Baert, and L.W. Brady

Progress and Perspectives in the Treatment of Lung Cancer
Edited by P. Van Houtte, J. Klastersky, and P. Rocmans

Combined Modality Therapy of Central Nervous System Tumors
Edited by Z. Petrovich, L. W. Brady, M. L. Apuzzo, and M. Bamberg

Age-Related Macular Degeneration
Current Treatment Concepts
Edited by W. A. Alberti, G. Richard, and R. H. Sagerman

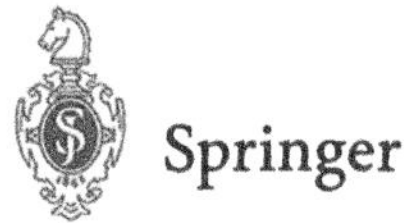

The manufacturer's authorised representative in the EU is Springer Nature Customer Service Centre GmbH, Europaplatz 3, 69115 Heidelberg, Germany. If you have any concerns regarding our products, please contact ProductSafety@springernature.com

Printed and bound by CPI Group (UK) Ltd, Croydon, CR0 4YY

28/04/2026

02098462-0006